The Heart
Physiology, from Cell to Circulation
Third Edition

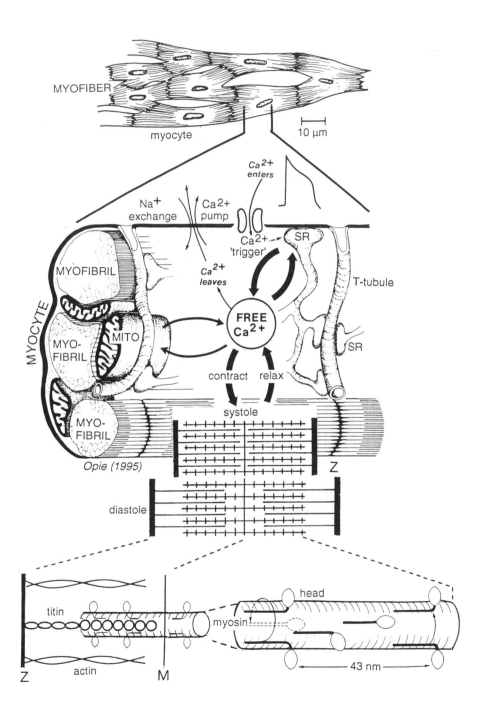

MYOFIBER

myocyte

10 μm

Na⁺ exchange

Ca2+ pump

Ca²⁺ enters

Ca²⁺ leaves

Ca2+ 'trigger'

SR

T-tubule

FREE Ca²⁺

MYOFIBRIL

MITO

MYO-FIBRIL

MYO-FIBRIL

MYOCYTE

Opie (1995)

contract   relax

systole

Z

diastole

SR

titin

myosin

head

actin

Z   M

43 nm

The Heart
Physiology, from Cell to Circulation
Third Edition

Lionel H. Opie, MD, DPhil

Professor of Medicine, University of Cape Town,
South Africa, and Director, Cape Heart Center
and Heart Disease Research Unit of
the Medical Research Council
Visiting Research Fellow (1997), Merton College, and
University Departments of Physiology
and Biochemistry, Oxford, England
Visiting Professor, 1984–1988, Cardiovascular Division,
Stanford University Medical Center,
Stanford, California, U.S.A.

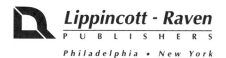

Lippincott - Raven
PUBLISHERS

Philadelphia • New York

Acquisitions Editor: Ruth W. Weinberg
Supervising Editor: Kim Swan
Production Service: Colophon
Indexer: Beta Computer Indexing
Cover Designer: David Levy
Manufacturing Manager: Dennis Teston
Compositor: Lippincott–Raven Electronic Production
Printer: Maple Press

Printed in the United States of America
9 8 7 6 5 4 3 2 1

Library of Congress Cataloging-in-Publication Data
Opie, Lionel H.
    The heart : physiology, from cell to circulation / Lionel H. Opie. — 3rd ed.
        p.   cm.
    Includes bibliographical references and index.
    ISBN 0-7817-1560-1
    1. Heart—Physiology.   2. Heart—Metabolism.   3. Heart cells.
I. Title.
    [DNLM: 1. Heart—physiology.   WG 202 061h 1997]
QP111.4.064   1997
616.1'2—dc21
DNLM/DLC   97–41380
for Library of Congress   CIP

To three outstanding teachers:

Eugene Braunwald
leader among cardiovascular leaders,
and writer among writers

Arnold M. Katz
an inspiring writer,* teacher, and speaker

William Henry Opie
my late father, who taught me that the search for the truth
is the basis of all scientific endeavor

---

*I have read only two books on cardiology virtually from cover to cover, each over one weekend, omitting only one or two chapters. One was Paul Wood's *Diseases of the Heart and Circulation,* read as a clinical medical student in 1954, and the other was Arnold Katz's book *Physiology of the Heart,* when first published in 1977. They both made a profound impression.

Legend to frontispiece: The crux of the contractile process lies in the changing concentrations of Ca^{2+} ions in the myocardial cytosol. Ca^{2+} ions are schematically shown as entering via the calcium channel that opens in response to the wave of depolarization that travels along the sarcolemma. These Ca^{2+} ions trigger the release of more calcium from the sarcoplasmic reticulum (SR) and thereby initiate a contraction–relaxation cycle, which is terminated by the uptake of calcium by the sarcolemmal pump. Calcium stored in the SR will then be liberated by the events associated with the next wave of depolarization. Eventually the small amount of calcium that has entered the cell will leave by a Na^+/Ca^{2+} exchanger. At a molecular level, contraction is driven by the interaction of actin and myosin that is set in motion by the arrival of the calcium ions at the contractile proteins. It is the myosin heads, projecting from the thick myosin bodies, that provide the power stroke that moves the thin actin filaments. Titin is the giant molecule that both supports the myosin molecules by attaching to the Z lines and provides elasticity. (The upper panel is reproduced with permission from Braunwald et al. *Mechanisms of Contraction of the Normal and Failing Heart.* 2nd ed. Boston: Little, Brown, 1976. The other panels are copyright L. H. Opie.)

Contents

Part V. The Circulation

Part VI. Pathophysiology

Foreword by
Eugene Braunwald

Despite the extraordinary advances in cardiology during the twentieth century, cardiovascular disease remains the most common cause of death and serious morbidity in the industrialized world. However, there is substantial cause for optimism; research on cardiovascular diagnosis and therapy has never been more active and productive, and it has brought us to the threshold of great advances in clinical cardiology. Cardiovascular research is based increasingly on advances in basic science. For the past fifty years, physiology, the "queen of the biomedical sciences," provided the principal underpinnings to clinical developments in cardiovascular medicine. More recently, the applications of cellular and molecular biology to cardiovascular medicine have become increasingly evident. This anxiously awaited third edition of Professor Opie's masterful text, *The Heart*, presents an appropriately expanded scientific base for cardiovascular disease.

This marvelous book is a concise, yet comprehensive, presentation of basic cardiovascular science. It presents, in a very readable and eminently understandable fashion, an extraordinary amount of important information critical to our understanding of how the cardiovascular system and its components function and malfunction. Professor Opie has the unique ability to explain in a straightforward manner the key principles of modern cardiovascular science without oversimplifying this complex subject.

While the third edition of this now well-established book builds on the strengths of its predecessors, it has been completely revised and largely rewritten. It is as current as last month's journals. The excellent explanatory diagrams (an Opie trademark) are even better than in previous editions and serve to make even the most complex concepts understandable.

In an era of multi-authored texts, which are often disjointed and present information that is repetitive and sometimes even contradictory, it is refreshing to have a body of information that speaks with a single, authoritative, respected, and accurate voice. *The Heart* is such a book.

This magnificent edition of *The Heart*, clearly the finest yet, will be of immense value and interest to students and teachers of cardiovascular science and to the many scholarly practitioners of cardiovascular medicine and surgery who wish to move beyond practice guidelines and understand the underlying cellular and physiologic bases of cardiovascular disease and its treatment.

Eugene Braunwald, MD
Harvard Medical School
Boston, Massachusetts

Foreword by Arnold M. Katz

The explosive growth of science has made the single-authored cardiology text a rarity. On the one hand, details of molecular biology and signal transduction are becoming critical to the understanding of heart disease pathology; on the other, definitive tests of the clinical relevance of these fundamental concepts are coming from a growing list of clinical trials. However, the interplay between basic science and clinical experience often generates counterintuitive findings. Concepts of disease once viewed as obvious have turned out to be either wrong or, at best, oversimplifications, while the clinical presentation in patients with heart disease commonly obscures the underlying pathophysiological mechanisms. The patient with heart failure, for example, suffers from more than a weakened myocardium, as evidenced by the dismal results of virtually every clinical trial of inotropic therapy and by growing evidence that drugs that weaken the failing heart prolong survival and improve symptoms. Myocardial infarction, we now know, is not primarily a disorder of the heart, but instead is a consequence of blood vessel disease—the heart being the victim of coronary artery occlusion. And clinical trials of drugs intended to prevent sudden cardiac death have demonstrated that modification of abnormal ion channel function can be more proarrhythmic than antiarrhythmic.

There are many reasons why so many of our attempts to apply basic science to clinical cardiology have yielded counterintuitive results. The failure of inotropic drugs to improve outcome in heart failure reflects the fact that the failing heart is deteriorating progressively, and that energy starvation probably plays a role in causing cell death. Limiting myocardial infarct size is generally impossible after coronary artery occlusion unless flow to the ischemic myocardium can be restored. Efforts to prevent lethal arrhythmias by administering drugs that eliminate nonlethal ectopy generally worsen outcome because these drugs depress conduction elsewhere in the heart thereby initating lethal arrhythmias.

These and other errors do not reflect flaws in either clinical observations or basic "facts"; instead, they occur because causal links between basic mechanisms and disease are generally more complex than can be recognized intuitively. This, in turn, reflects the many gaps that remain in our understanding of pathophysiology. Yet it is an oversimplification to assume that the more we know, the better able we will be to manage the cardiac patient. In spite of the dazzling technology now available for diagnosis and treatment of heart disease, real understanding of the mechanisms responsible for heart disease often requires information that is not easily retrieved from the literature. Moreover, to meet the challenges posed by the cardiac patient, we must identify, interpret, integrate, and then apply the appropriate basic science knowledge for each clinical situation. This is best done at the bedside by an informed clinical scientist, rather than in a conference room by a committee.

The ability to integrate basic science and clinical cardiology is facilitated by an authoritative single-authored text that shifts effortlessly and naturally between these two aspects of cardiology. Lionel Opie, who for more than 30 years has made original contributions to our understanding of the mechanisms responsible for clinical heart disease, meets this need. His third edition of *The Heart: Physiology, from Cell to Circulation* demonstrates Professor Opie's broad and expert view of cardiology, his ability to integrate basic science and clinical medicine, and, above all, the lucidity of his writing.

Arnold M. Katz, MD, DMed (Hon.)
Professor of Medicine
The University of Connecticut

Preface

*I must frankly own that, if I had known the labour
which this book has entailed, I should never have
been courageous enough to commence it.*
　　　　　　Mrs. Beaton's Household Management,
　　　　　　London, Ward, Lock & Co., 1820

*Encouraged by the public reception of the former
editions, the author has spared neither labour nor
expense to render this as perfect as his opportunities
and abilities would permit. The progress of
knowledge is so rapid, and the discoveries so
numerous, both at home and abroad, that this may
rather be regarded as a new work than as a re-
publication of an old one. On this account, a short
enumeration of the more important changes may
possibly be expected by the reader.*
　　　　　　William Withering (discoverer of digitalis),
　　　　　　in Botany, Third Edition,
　　　　　　London: Calldel and Davies, 1801

Like Withering, nearly 200 years ago, I am excited by the impossible task of keeping up with the rapid progress of knowledge and discoveries. To bring these changes to students and fellows, seven crucial changes have been made in this third edition:

1. To emphasize that the book leads from cellular biology to the control of the circulation in health and disease, via the new emphasis on vascular biology, the subtitle changes from "Physiology and Metabolism" to "Physiology, from Cell to Circulation."
2. There is a new introductory section on basic cardiovascular physiology, specifically attuned to the needs of medical students and postgraduate research students in biochemistry and molecular biology, who need an easy-to-read working knowledge of cardiovascular physiology; these three chapters may be omitted by those with suitable background such as cardiologists-in-training.

3. New material is added to make the text more practical for students, including a section on the electrocardiogram, increased details on the peripheral circulation, and substantial emphasis on the molecular biology of ion channels, cardiovascular growth, and remodeling.
4. There is a new chapter on blood pressure and peripheral circulation.
5. Questions are given at the end of every chapter, the first set for students and the second for cardiologists-in-training.
6. The new illustrations include a two-color section on the mechanism of contraction. Of the total of 315 illustrations, 54% are new (40%) or substantially modified (14%). Chapters with the most new illustrations are the introductory chapter (89% new); those on channels, pumps, and exchangers (67% new); vascular smooth muscle (69% new); and blood pressure (93% new).
7. References. A concerted attempt has been made to provide the reader with all the major new references for each chapter. The greatest increase in new references (as percentage of the total) is, not surprisingly, in vascular smooth muscle and endothelium (88%), followed by receptors and signal transduction (76%), with ventricular function and load in the third position (67%).

What remains unchanged is the original intent of the book to explain cardiac function to a wide range of potential readers, including fellows in cardiology, research students, and advanced medical students. The line drawings have been carefully created with the aid of Jeanne Walker, to allow a simple visual approach to learning (or teaching) such a complex subject. Hence, it is anticipated that the text will appeal both to teachers and to those taught—those students of cardiology and physiology whose highest standards require a thorough understanding of the physiologic function of this most vital organ.

Because the drawings constitute a diagrammatic text that can stand alone, and because of the new emphasis on the circulation, this book should be seen as a companion and not as competitor to Arnold Katz's book *Physiology of the Heart.* The topic of the present book, physiology from cell to circulation, also makes it a natural smaller companion to Eugene Braunwald's classic *Heart Disease, 3 ed,* Hurst's long-running *The Heart, 8 ed,* and an innovative newcomer, Topol's *Textbook of Cardiovascular Medicine.*

Lionel H. Opie, 1997

Acknowledgments

Among my professional colleagues who generously gave advice and criticism, are the following (and I apologize to those many others inadvertently omitted):

Edward Carmeliet, MD, PhD
Professor
Laboratory of Physiology
Catholic University of Leuven
Leuven, Belgium

Kieran Clarke, PhD
Associate Director
British Heart Foundation
Molecular Cardiology Group
Department of Biochemistry
University of Oxford
Oxford, England

Patrick Commerford, MB ChB, FCP (SA)
Professor of Cardiology
University of Cape Town
Cape Town, South Africa

William F. Ganong, MD
Professor
Department of Physiology
University of California
San Francisco, California, U.S.A.

Gerd Heusch, MD, PhD, FESC
Professor and Director of the
  Department of Pathophysiology

Center for Internal Medicine
University of Essen
Essen, Germany

Gary D. Lopaschuk, PhD
Professor and Director
Cardiovascular Research Group
Heritage Medical Research Centre
University of Alberta
Edmonton, Alberta, Canada

Kathleen G. Morgan, PhD
Director
Boston Biomedical Research
  Institute
Associate Professor of
  Physiology in Medicine
Harvard Medical School
Boston, Massachusetts, U.S.A.

David Paterson, DPhil
University Laboratory of Physiology
Lecturer, University of Oxford
Fellow, Merton College
Oxford, England

Mark G. Perlroth, MD
Professor of Medicine
Stanford University Medical Center
Stanford, California, U.S.A.

J. Caspar Rüegg, MD, PhD
Professor of Physiology
University of Heidelberg
Heidelberg, Germany

Bernard Swynghedauw, MD, PhD
Director
INSERM Unit 127
Paris, France

Jutta Schaper, PhD
Professor
Max-Planck Institute
Bad Nauheim, Germany

Further crucial acknowledgments are due to Jeanne Walker, a wonderful medical illustrator without peer, and to Victor Claasen, better than a computer in remembering and retrieving references. Sylvia Dennis, who joined the team recently, has already added her unique skills.

I was privileged to complete this book in Merton College, Oxford, a most historic, scholarly, and beautiful institution, of which William Harvey was Warden many years ago. I am indebted to Dr. Jessica Rawson, Warden of Merton College, and to Dr. David Paterson and other Fellows of the College, for this most kind invitation.

Last but not least, I cannot overemphasize my gratitude for the love and support given to me by my family. In the words of a Chinese colleague working in Beijing:

> *I believe the results of work is really the truth, it*
> *takes me all my lifetime; sacrifice the happiness*
> *of my family.*

From the Introduction to the First Edition

Richard J. Bing, MD, doyen of cardiac metabolism and physiology, and Professor Emeritus, University of Southern California, turned 87 in October 1997 and is still active in outstanding research. The following is an extract from his Introduction to the first edition of this book:

> Evolution of science, like biological evolution, develops by a zigzag course of trial and error; the errors are soon forgotten though they serve as stepping-stones to new progress. The factors which determine both scientific progress and scientific error are dependent on the ability of the brain to be analytical, curious, critical, observant and imaginative. These are constant factors—qualities of the human brain which have evolved together with other properties of mind and body. There are, on the other hand, variables which determine progress in the natural sciences. Techniques and the spirit of the period, together with the personality of the scientist, make up these variables. Endowed with these constants, and blessed or cursed by these variables, the human mind attempts to discover single stones in the mosaic of the biological system, or if graced with a flash of genius, it can visualize whole parts of nature's mosaic.

> A glance into the early beginnings of cardiac physiology and metabolism is not amiss, because we find that the pioneers wrestled with the same ideas that occupy us today, and that an astonishing amount of scientific truth is contained in early publications. Much of this important work, dating from the 1870s to 1920, was summarized in a remarkable fashion by Tigerstedt in 1923, in a volume on the physiology of the circulation. Tigerstedt himself was an outstanding investigator, to whom we owe the discovery of renin. One section of this remarkable book deals with the "chemical conditions for cardiac action."

> His book contains a wealth of information, for example: the Langendorff perfusion method was first introduced in 1890 by Martin and Applegarth of Johns Hopkins in Baltimore; Langendorff had no knowledge of this work when he described his perfusion method in 1895. Particularly fascinating is the story of the discovery of the role of calcium ions. It is interesting that Ringer was first misled by the use of sodium chloride-enriched tapwater which contained, without his knowledge, not only calcium chloride, but also potassium chloride which antagonized the calcium effect. A year later Ringer discovered that the arrested heart could be made to beat again by the addition of calcium chloride. He concluded in 1883 that calcium is absolutely essential for maintenance of cardiac contraction. Thus Ringer established that calcium increased

the force of contraction and prolonged systole. Yet excess calcium could result in contracture of the heart and could diminish the duration of diastole.

What distinguishes the present volume from the early publication by Tigerstedt are the
continuous advances in physical and biological chemistry, molecular biology, electron
microscopy, electrophysiology and myocardial mechanics. In bringing together these
basic disciplines into a volume that can be assimilated by clinical cardiologists and
medical students, the present work achieves a milestone.

PART I

Basic Cardiovascular Physiology

The heart, with the veins and arteries and the blood they contain, is to be regarded as the beginning and the author, the fountain and original of all things in the body, the primary cause of life.
William Harvey, 1628
Warden, Merton College, Oxford

The heart is an organ of fire.
Michael Ondaatje,
The English Patient, 1992

1

Introductory
Cardiovascular Concepts

*No understanding of the circulatory reactions of the
body is possible unless we start first with the
fundamental properties of the heart muscle itself,
and then find out how these are modified, protected
and controlled under the influence of the
mechanisms—nervous, chemical and mechanical—
which under normal conditions play on the heart
and blood vessels.*

E. H. Starling, 1920

FROM PREHISTORY TO HARVEY

The existence of the heart was well known to the ancient Greeks, who gave it
the name *kardia,* as in cardiac, tachycardia, and bradycardia. Aristotle thought
that the heart was the seat of the soul and the center of man. The Romans modified *kardia* to *cor,* the latter word still surviving as evidenced in *cordial greet-
ings* and in the term "cor pulmonale." The old Teutonic word *herton* also is
derived from cor and gives us "heart" via the medieval English *heorte.*

Galen (about 200 AD), the "father of experimental physiology," knew that the
heart set the blood in motion. He discovered that arteries contained blood and
not air. Yet he thought that there were pores between the left and right side of the
heart and that a "vital spirit" was formed in the lungs by a mixture of blood and
air. Such was Galen's authority that his views on the circulation became dogma,
dispelled only by the careful anatomic dissections of Vesalius (1514–1564), who
worked at Padua in Italy and clearly showed that there were no pores in that part
of the heart (the septum) separating the left and right sides.

The critical point that the circulations of the left and right heart are separate
was grasped by Servetus (1511–1553):

3

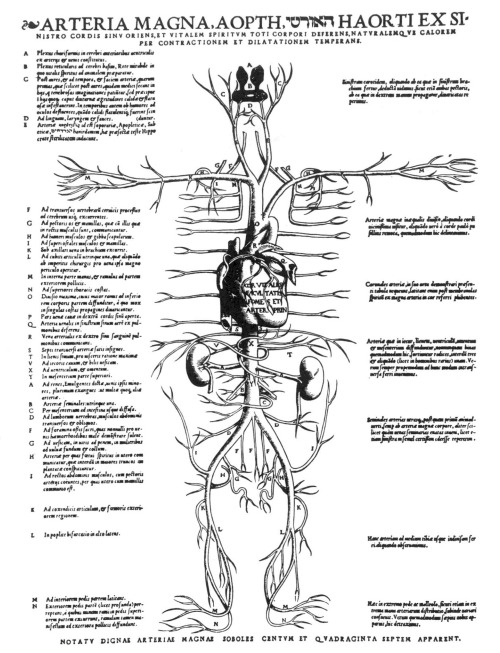

FIG. 1-1. The heart at the center of the circulation, as drawn by Vesalius (1514–1564) in his *Tabulae Anatomicae.*

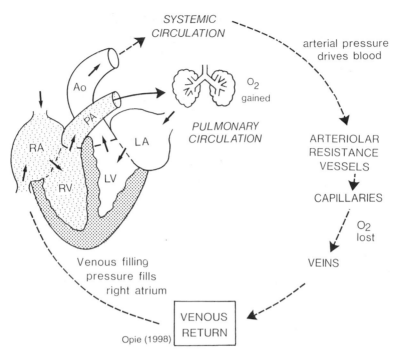

FIG. 1-2. Normal circulation. Harvey wrote in 1628: "These are then the very elements . . . of the passage and circulation of blood, from the right auricle into the right ventricle; from the right ventricle by way of the lungs into the left auricle; thence to the left ventricle and aorta; whence by the arteries at large through the tissues into the veins, and by the veins back again . . . to the base of the heart." Harvey used the term "auricle," which has been replaced by the modern term "atrium." RA, right atrium; RV, right ventricle; PA, pulmonary artery; LA, left atrium; LV, left ventricle; Ao, aorta; O_2, oxygen. The dotted contents of the RA, RV, and PA represent deoxygenated blood.

> The connection between the cavities of the heart is not established through the median partition of the heart; a wonderful track conducts the blood, which flows in a long detour from the right of the heart to the lung and becomes red; at the moment of relaxation it reaches the left cavity of the heart.

Servetus hid this brilliant passage in a book of theology in which he criticized the Trinity, thereby falling foul of the Calvinist rulers of Geneva, who burnt him at the stake. In 1571, an Italian, Cesalpino, described the function of valves:

> Special membranes at the openings of the vessels prevent blood flowing back so that there is perpetual movement of the blood from the vena cava through the heart and lungs into the aorta.

The basis of modern concepts of the circulation was laid by Harvey (1578–1657), who reasoned that the circulation of the blood was caused by pumping of the heart. His *Anatomical Treatise on the Motion of the Heart and Blood in Animals* appeared in 1628 and is probably the most important single volume in the history of cardiology. Born in England and trained in Padua before returning to St. Bartholomew's Hospital in London, he must have been influenced by Vesalius' masterly drawing of the circulation (Fig. 1-1). Thus, it is to Harvey (and his predecessors) that we owe our knowledge of the heart as a mechanical pump. His concepts provide the foundation for our modern understanding of the fundamental facts of the circulation (Fig. 1-2).

BASIC ANATOMY OF THE HEART

Left Side of Heart

In the lungs, venous blood received from the right side of the heart is oxygenated and then flows into the *left atrium* of the heart, which is a thin-walled muscular chamber continuously receiving blood from the lungs. From the left atrium, blood enters the much thicker *left ventricle*. For the left ventricle to fill in this way requires that the valve lying between the left atrium and the left ventricle, namely the *mitral* or *bicuspid valve*, should be open (Fig. 1-3). That only happens when the pressure in the left ventricle is very low, as during its relaxation phase called *diastole* (from the Greek for apart + send). The large anterior and small posterior cusps of this valve are sometimes thought to resemble a bishop's miter, hence the term "mitral." Each cusp is a thin flexible sheath of

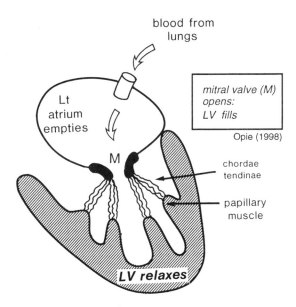

FIG. 1-3. Role of mitral valve in diastole (left ventricular relaxation phase), regulating flow between the left atrium and left ventricle. When the mitral valve is open, during diastole, then blood flows from the left atrium to the left ventricle.

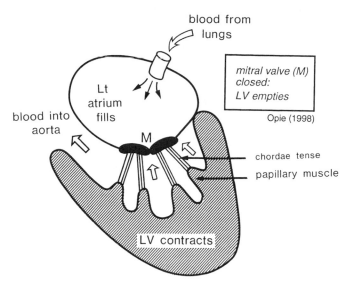

FIG. 1-4. Role of mitral valve in systole (left ventricular contraction phase). LV contraction increases the LV pressure above that in the left atrium and the mitral valve shuts. The chordae tendineae become tense, which prevents the mitral valve from being pushed into the left atrium. The closed mitral valve and the increased pressure in the left ventricle force the blood into the aorta.

connective tissue, secured at its base to the mitral valve annulus. The latter is a ring of connective tissue surrounding the opening between the atrium and the ventricle. The *chordae tendineae* are the thin tendinous structures linking the free ends of the cusp to the *papillary muscles*, which are long muscular projections of the inner wall of the ventricle. During left ventricular contraction or *systole* (from the Greek for contraction) the increased pressure in the left ventricle forces the two cusps of the mitral valve together, which then closes (Fig. 1-4). Thus, blood in the left ventricle is prevented from re-entering the atrium. During systole the papillary muscles also contract to tense the chordae tendineae so that the mitral valve closes properly and is not forced into the atrial cavity.

Left ventricular contraction not only abruptly shuts the mitral valve, but shortly thereafter forces open the *aortic valve*, located at the base of the aorta, so that blood is expelled into the aorta (Ao, Fig. 1-2), from where it travels throughout the circulation to reach all parts of the body.

Transmural Distribution of Fibers in the Left Ventricle. The left ventricular wall, about three times thicker than that of the right ventricle, has its fibers distributed in various layers. The inner and outer layers run longitudinally in the direction from the apex of the heart to the base; the center fibers run circumferentially, and intervening layers have intervening patterns. The result of this change in muscle fiber pattern is that when the left ventricle contracts, it not only squeezes out the blood from the ventricle, but twists and turns toward the chest wall so that the apex of the heart can be felt from the outside as the *apical impulse* (or apex beat). The overall effect of left ventricular contraction can be summarized as a reduction in both length and diameter of this chamber.

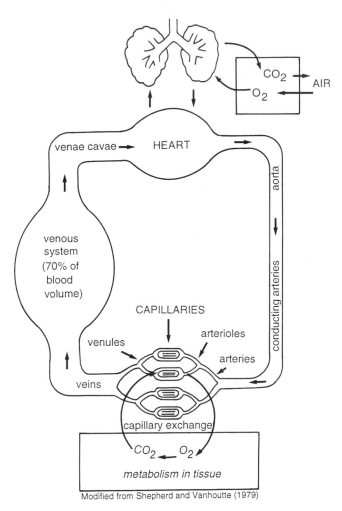

Modified from Shepherd and Vanhoutte (1979)

FIG. 1-5. Role of heart in transport of oxygen. Schematic diagram showing how the pumping heart conveys oxygenated blood to the peripheral circulation. Note the role of the capillaries in allowing rapid gas exchange, with diffusion of oxygen to the various tissues and collection of the carbon dioxide made during metabolism in the tissues. The veins function both as a collecting and as a storage system. For the latter reason, they are called venous capacitance veins. Modified from Shepherd and Vanhoutte (1979).

Right Side of the Heart

The systolic ejection of blood from the left ventricle provides enough force to drive the blood through the branches of the aorta, eventually to reach the minute vessels called the *capillaries*, from where deoxygenated blood is returned by the venous system to the right atrium of the heart (Fig. 1-5). The right atrium, like the left, is a thin-walled muscular chamber that receives the venous return from the large veins of the circulation. The two main veins entering the right atrium are the superior vena cava and the inferior vena cava, which drain the upper and lower limbs, respectively. In addition, the right atrium receives blood from the coronary sinus, which is the main vein draining the heart muscle itself.

Blood flowing into the right atrium must thereafter enter the right ventricle through the *tricuspid valve* (three cusps), which is open during right ventricular diastole, when the right ventricle fills with blood. The tricuspid valve is closed when the right ventricle contracts. (Note the analogy to mitral opening and closing and to left ventricular relaxation and contraction.) The principles of right ventricular contraction are similar to those described for the left ventricle, except that the right ventricle is much thinner because it only has to drive blood into the lungs and not around the whole body as does the left ventricle. Therefore, the right ventricle has to generate less pressure than does the left. The contracting right ventricle forces venous blood to enter the pulmonary vascular tree. This blood is then oxygenated in the capillaries of the lungs, to return to the left atrium and thereby to complete the circulation.

Pericardium

The pericardium is a thin fibrous baglike structure within which the heart lies. The pericardium almost entirely surrounds the heart, except for the sites of entry and exit of the great vessels. The pericardium is composed of two layers: one lies on the outer surface of the heart and the other is in contact with the surrounding lungs and other tissues. The two layers are separated by a small amount of lubricating fluid to allow movement of the heart during contraction and relaxation to occur without disturbance of the surrounding lungs. Normally the pericardium does not interfere with the mechanical function of the heart, but when it is diseased, cardiac filling can be compromised.

Endocardium

The endocardium, which covers the inner surface of the heart, has a large surface area because of the many papillary muscles and the irregular pattern of the inner wall of the left ventricle (Fig. 1-3). Previously thought to be inert, the endocardium is now suspected of being metabolically active and thereby contributing to the regulation of left ventricular contraction. For example, experimental removal of the endocardium alters the pattern of the relaxation phase of the left ventricle.

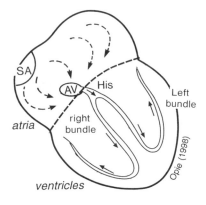

FIG. 1-6. Schematic of conduction system. The spontaneous origin of the electrical impulse is in the sinoatrial (SA) node in the right atrium, from where the impulse travels over the atrial walls to be collected in the atrioventricular (AV) node, thence to pass down the bundle of His and into the left or right bundle before eventually reaching ventricular myocardium. This path is followed during every heart beat.

Conducting System

Each time the heart beats, ventricular contraction is triggered by a wave of electricity that arises spontaneously in a collection of specialized cells in the right atrium (Fig. 1-6). These cells are collectively called the sinoatrial node or sinus node because they are situated near the coronary sinus (into which veins from the heart muscle drain). From the sinoatrial node the electrical impulse spreads rapidly through the left and right atria, to be collected into a second node, the atrioventricular node. The impulse slows down in the atrioventricular node and then again spreads up along a specialized bundle of conducting fibers, the His bundle before dividing into two major branches, the left and right bundles, by which the electrical impulses spread throughout the ventricles, there to trigger ventricular contraction. This series of electrical events is repeated with every heart beat.

ANATOMY OF THE CIRCULATION

There are two anatomically separate vascular beds or circuits through which blood is driven (Fig. 1-2). The left ventricle drives blood through the *systemic circulation*, and the right ventricle drives it through the *pulmonary circulation*. In each case the vessels connecting the ventricle to capillaries of that circulation have to withstand more pressure and are thicker than the vessels leading from the capillaries to the atrium. The former vessels are called *arteries*, the latter *veins*. In the systemic circulation, arteries convey oxygenated blood from the left ventricle to the capillaries, whereas the veins carry the deoxygenated blood from the capillaries to the heart. In the pulmonary circulation, the arteries are again by definition those vessels conveying blood from the right ventricle to the pulmonary capillaries. Because this blood has reached the right ventricle from the systemic veins and is deoxygenated, the blood in the pulmonary arteries is deoxygenated, in contrast to the blood in all the other arteries, which is oxygenated. Similarly, blood leaving the pulmonary capillaries by the pulmonary veins to the heart is oxygenated, in contrast to blood in all the other veins, which is deoxygenated.

Microcirculation.   When blood is ejected from the left ventricle, it enters the aorta, which divides into many arteries, eventually becoming the smaller *arterioles* before reaching the capillaries (Fig. 1-5). In the *capillaries*, which are the exchange vessels, oxygenated blood becomes deoxygenated as the oxygen leaves the red cells and enters the tissue by diffusion. It is also here that nutrients such as glucose and fatty acids (Chapter 10) leave the blood to provide for the energy needs of the tissues of the body, whereas products of metabolism such as carbon dioxide and some waste products leave the tissues. The capillaries are therefore crucially concerned with the metabolism of all organs and tissues of the body. Metabolism includes all those processes whereby the carbon atoms from glucose and fatty acids interact with the oxygen to form carbon dioxide and energy. The importance of the capillaries is underscored as follows:

> The heart and vasculature exist for one fundamental purpose: the delivery of metabolic substrates to the cells of the organism. This delivery takes place across the thin walls of the capillaries, which thus subserve the ultimate function of the cardiovascular system (Levick, 1991).

The deoxygenated venous blood leaving the capillaries enters the veins, which constitute a low-pressure, large-volume system containing most of the blood volume. Taken together, the veins constitute the *venous capacitance system*. From that reservoir, blood reaches the right atrium by the large veins or vena cava. At the start of exercise, blood is forced out of the venous capacitance system by muscular contraction and by nervous influences so that more blood is returned to the right atrium. This increased *venous return* stimulates the heart to contract more forcefully.

Arteriolar Resistance.   Because of the crucial role of the capillaries, it would intuitively be expected that there would be a way in which the rate of blood flowing through these vessels could be carefully controlled. For example, during exercise, more blood must flow through the capillaries to meet the much higher demand of the exercising muscles for oxygen.

Arterioles are small arteries about 30 µm in lumen diameter with relatively thick muscular walls. They constitute the major resistance against which the ventricles pump, and collectively they constitute the *peripheral* or *systemic vascular resistance*. If the arterioles dilate, the vascular resistance decreases and more blood enters the capillaries.

Regulation of the degree of arteriolar dilation or constriction is extremely complex, involving nervous, hormonal, and metabolic control (Chapter 2). When there is excess arteriolar constriction (high systemic vascular resistance), then the pressure inside the arterial tree increases, as in hypertension. Conversely, a number of vasodilator drugs and exercise can reduce the systemic vascular resistance.

Arterial Blood Pressure.   The pressure pattern in the circulation varies from high arterial to low venous values and can be measured invasively at any point by insertion of a needle connected to a pressure transducer. The pressure changes abruptly at the level of the arterioles, site of the major resistance component of the systemic vascular resistance (Fig. 1-7). The aorta has the crucial function of transforming the abrupt increase and decrease of pressure in the left ventricle to a smoother pressure pattern with a much higher diastolic value (Fig. 1-8). This "peak-equalizing" function is crucial because a relatively high diastolic pressure is required to help transfer the blood to various organs, particularly the heart.

The peak pressure in the major arteries is actually higher than in the aorta, partly due to the increasing resistance offered by the decreasing and tapering arterial lumen, and partly due to variations in the transmission velocity of the blood. Clearly, therefore, the arterial blood pressure will vary according to the site of its measurement.

In humans, the standard noninvasive technique involves measurement of the arterial blood pressure in the brachial artery. This pressure is usually simply called the *blood pressure*. By using a cuff that automatically inflates at preset intervals (e.g., every 10 to 20 minutes) and recording the sound electronically, a *24-hour ambulatory blood pressure* can be obtained (Fig. 1-9). The pattern

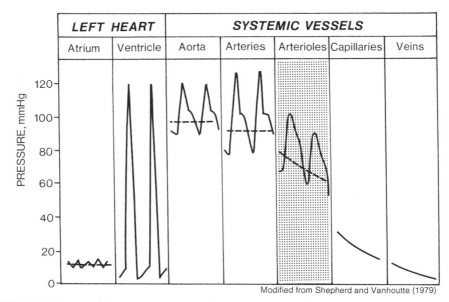

FIG. 1-7. **The arterial pressure pattern** changes quite abruptly at the level of the arterioles, where the systemic peripheral vascular resistance is generated. The pressure then becomes very low in the capillary and veins. Modified from Shepherd and Vanhoutte (1979) with permission.

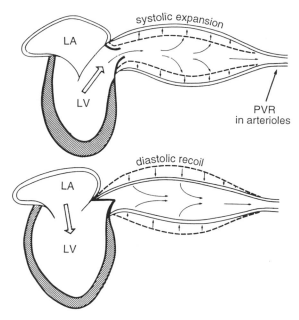

FIG. 1-8. The aorta. The "pressure-equalizing" or "buffering" function of the aorta. During ventricular systole the stroke volume ejected by the ventricle results in some forward capillary flow, but most of the ejected volume is stored in the elastic arteries. During ventricular diastole the elastic recoil of the arterial wall maintains blood flow throughout the remainder of the cardiac cycle. PVR = peripheral (systemic) vascular resistance. Modified from Berne and Levy (1983) with permission.

shows marked diurnal variations and is also influenced by the subject's emotional status and exercise. During the daytime, when stimulatory nervous activity dominates, the blood pressure values are much higher than by night, when inhibitory nervous activity dominates. Changes in the pulse rate accompany those in the blood pressure, so that emotional excitement or the stimulus of waking in the morning leads to an increase in both, whereas at night heart rate and blood pressure both decrease.

SUMMARY

The basic function of the heart is to act as a pump, which ejects blood from the thick-walled left ventricle to be propelled throughout the body, ultimately to reach the peripheral circulation. There, in the capillaries, oxygen is removed to nourish the various organs and tissues of the body. The deoxygenated venous blood flows back to the right side of the heart, to be ejected from the right ventricle to the lungs, once more to be oxygenated and to enter the left atrium and left ventricle.

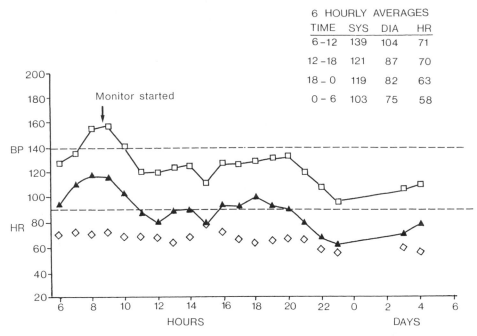

6 HOURLY AVERAGES			
TIME	SYS	DIA	HR
6–12	139	104	71
12–18	121	87	70
18–0	119	82	63
0–6	103	75	58

FIG. 1-9. Diurnal pattern of blood pressure and heart rate. Variation over 24 hours (diurnal, over 24 hours) taken by ambulatory machine. From top to bottom: systolic blood pressure (SYS, □), diastolic blood pressure (DIA, ▲) and heart rate (HR). The dashed lines indicate the conventional upper limits of normality (systolic/diastolic 140/90 mmHg). There is an initial transient hypertensive reaction in response to the psychological stress of visiting the doctor ("white coat hypertension"). Thereafter the blood pressure values are within normal limits.

STUDENT QUESTIONS

1. Describe the function of the valves separating left atrium and left ventricle.
2. Define systole and diastole.
3. Describe the pulmonary circulation.
4. What is the role of the arterioles?
5. Why are capillaries important?

CARDIOLOGIST-IN-TRAINING QUESTIONS

1. When the heart contracts, the left ventricular cavity becomes smaller. Yet systolic contraction be felt on the precordium as the apical impulse. Why?
2. What is the function of the endocardium?
3. Diastolic recoil of the aorta—how does it contribute to the blood pressure?

REFERENCES

1. Berne RM, Levy MN (eds). *Physiology.* Mosby: St Louis, 1983.
2. Levick JR. Vascular smooth muscle. In: *An Introduction to Cardiovascular Physiology.* London: Butterworths, 1991;171–175.
3. Shepherd JT, Vanhoutte PM. In: *The Human Cardiovascular System. Facts and Concepts.* New York: Raven, 1979.
4. Starling EH. On the circulatory changes associated with exercise. *J R Army Med Corps* 1920;34: 258–272.

2

Control of the Circulation

Physiology is the logic of life, and control mechanisms are the key to the regulation of this logic. Such controls may be exerted either at the central nervous system level or at the periphery. In addition to nervous control by the autonomic nervous system, locally produced metabolites convey integrative signals during specific physiologic changes and challenges. Messages that play a major role in regulating the circulation reach the heart from the central nervous system along the *autonomic pathways*, which function independently of the conscious nervous system (hence the name "autonomic"). The two divisions of the autonomic nervous system have opposite functions (Fig. 2-1). First, the *adrenergic* or *sympathetic nervous system* is able to release its excitatory messengers, epinephrine and norepinephrine, in "sympathy with" states of excitation, such as waking up, the start of exercise, or during emotional stress (Fig. 2-2). Second, the *parasympathetic system* acts alongside (*para,* beside) the adrenergic nervous system to release its own transmitter, acetylcholine. Alternate names are the *cholinergic nervous system* or the *vagal nervous system* (Fig. 2-3).

ADRENERGIC AND CHOLINERGIC EFFECTS

Each system has a certain intensity of stimuli flowing down (*neural traffic*) to the terminal nerve fibers or neurons (or *varicosities*), which lie close to the cells of the organ to be controlled. These terminal neurons liberate their primary messengers, or *neurotransmitters*, chiefly norepinephrine or acetylcholine, which travel across the short distance called the *synaptic gap* or *synaptic junction* (*synapse,* join) to the external cell membrane of the heart or of the vascular smooth muscle. These neurotransmitters act on receptors, which are specific sites on the cell membrane. The tight molecular fit between the stimulant molecule (*agonist*) and the receptor gives rise to the *key and lock* model.

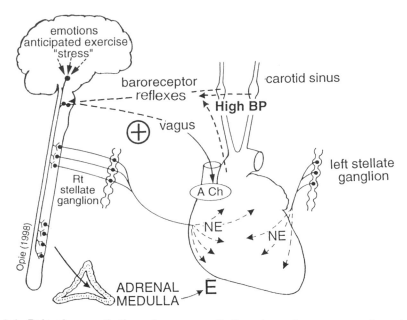

FIG. 2-1. Role of sympathetic and parasympathetic autonomic nervous systems in the control of the heart. Sympathetic adrenergic stimulation is achieved by a combination of (1) neurotransmitter (NE, norepinephrine) released from the terminal neurones (nerve varicosities) of postganglionic fibers running from left or right stellate ganglia; or (2) epinephrine (E) release from adrenal medulla. NE or E act on cardiac β-adrenoceptors, chiefly β_1. The parasympathetic or cholinergic system acts through the vagal nerve to release acetylcholine (ACh), which in general opposes the effects of sympathetic stimulation. To keep the BP within narrow limits, there are baroreflexes (baro, pressure) that respond to changes of pressure in the carotid sinus or the aortic arch, anatomic structures shown in the drawing. If there is acute hypertension, the barore-flexes mediate an increase in vagal tone to decrease heart rate, cardiac output, and peripheral resistance (see Fig. 2-3). Opposing events occur when the arterial tension is too low (hypoten-sion), as in congestive heart failure when baroreflexes mediate adrenergic activation. NE, nor-epinephrine; E, epinephrine.

Receptors

Two major types of such receptors have been defined by the specific nature of the cardiovascular reactions evoked by infused catecholamines. Those receptors concerned with enhanced contractility and heart rate are called *β-adrenergic receptors*, and those concerned with increasing the tone of arterioles are called *α-adrenergic receptors* (Ahlquist, 1948). *Cholinergic receptors* respond to their messenger, *acetylcholine*, and in general have the opposite effect to adrenergic stimulation (Table 2-1). For example, β-adrenergic stimulation increases heart rate, whereas cholinergic stimulation decreases it (Figs. 2-2 and 2-3). Choliner-gic receptors are also called *muscarinic receptors* because they respond to the complex chemical compound, muscarine, derived from certain mushrooms.

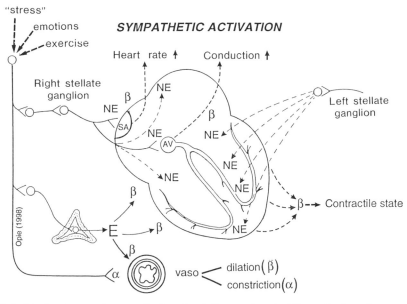

FIG. 2-2. Mechanisms of sympathetic stimulation, acting via (1) a collection of nerve cells (right stellate ganglion) to increase release of norepinephrine (NE) to areas of sinus (SA) and atrioventricular (AV) nodes; (2) another collection of nerve cells, the left stellate ganglion, to increase release of NE to left ventricle; and (3) adrenal medulla to release epinephrine (E) to all parts of the heart. The receptors stimulated are the β-adrenergic receptors. As a consequence, the heart rate increases, as does the rate of conduction of the electrical impulse through the AV node and the conduction system. At the same time, the force of contraction increases.

Effects of Infusion of Catecholamines

The similar chemical structures of *norepinephrine* and *epinephrine* gives rise to the family name of *catecholamines*. Barcroft and Swan (1953) found that an infusion of epinephrine (also called *adrenaline*) increased the heart rate, increased systolic blood pressure (BP), but decreased the diastolic value while augmenting blood flow in the arms and legs (Fig. 2-4). The β-adrenergic receptors can be further separated into those with a cardiac stimulatory effect (*β_1-adrenegic receptors*) and those found chiefly but not exclusively in extracardiac sites such as the arterioles (*β_2-adrenergic receptors*), where they cause vasodilation. During physiologic exercise, such as vigorous cycling, most but not all of the hemodynamic changes can be explained by an increase of plasma epinephrine levels. The increased amount of blood ejected from the heart in systole overrides the arteriolar dilator effect to increase the systolic BP, whereas in diastole the arteriolar dilation tends to decrease the BP (Fig. 2-4). Thus, the mean BP may not increase much. Two of the major effects of epinephrine are an increase in cardiac output and an increase in limb blood flow, the latter as a result of arteriolar vasodilation (Fig. 2-5).

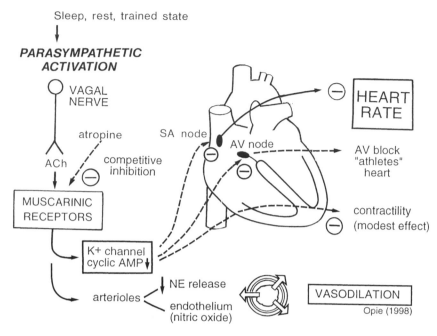

FIG. 2-3. The parasympathetic or cholinergic system, acting via the muscarinic receptors, has inhibitory effects on the heart. The major site of action of parasympathetic control of the heart appears to be the sinoatrial (SA) node, where it reduces the heart rate in contrast to sympathetic stimulation (Fig. 2-2). Other lesser parasympathetic effects include inhibition of the AV node and a mild inhibitory effect on contractile force. In trained athletes, parasympathetic activity increases to slow the heart rate. In overtraining, the AV node can be inhibited to block the conduction of the impulse from the SA node to the ventricles, an example of AV block (see Chapter 5).

Infusion of Norepinephrine

Norepinephrine (also called noradrenaline), like epinephrine, increases the heart rate, but in contrast to epinephrine it reduces limb blood flow and increases both systolic and diastolic BP (Fig. 2-6). The major reason for these differences lies in the dual effect of norepinephrine, stimulating both myocardial β-adrenergic receptors and arteriolar α-adrenergic receptors. The latter, being vasoconstrictory, cause the arterioles to contract, thereby increasing the resistance against which the heart works (Fig. 2-7). Despite the direct β-adrenergic–mediated increase in heart rate as a result of stimulation of the sinoatrial node, the heart rate decreases after an initial transient increase. The explanation for this phenomena is the existence of a pressure-sensitive control mechanism located in the *baroreceptors* (*baro,* pressure), as shown in Fig. 2-1.

TABLE 2-1. *Proposed patterns of receptor stimulation to explain opposite effects of sympathetic adrenergic and parasympathetic cholinergic stimulation on the heart and circulation*

	β-Adrenergic	α-Adrenergic	Cholinergic
Heart			
SA node pacemaker	+	0	–
AV node conduction	+	0	–
His Purkinje system conduction	+	0	–
Myocardial contraction[a]	+	0, +	0, –
Peripheral circulation[b]			
Coronary arterioles	Dilate	Constrict[e]	Dilate
Skeletal muscle	Dilate	Constrict[e]	Dilate
Splanchnic flow	Dilate[d]	Constrict[f]	0
Renal flow[c]	Constrict	Constrict	0
Colon and genitals	Dilate	Constrict	Dilate

[a]Cholinergic effects controversial. See Boyett et al. (1988).
[b]See Shepherd and Vanhoutte (1979), pages 116–124. For modifications, see below.
[c]Werko et al. (1951)
[d]Freyschuss et al. (1986).
[e]During exercise, direct α-mediated vasoconstriction (Taylor et al. 1992) is opposed by β-mediated increased force of myocardial contraction and production of vasodilator metabolites. For β-adrenergic and α-adrenergic receptors, see Figs. 2-4, 2-7, and 2-8.
[f]Splanchnic flow decreases as plasma norepinephrine increases.
+, stimulation; –, inhibition; 0, no effect.
The above patterns are inferred from the known properties of adrenergic and cholinergic receptors in isolated systems and from the effects of infusions into humans of epinephrine (chiefly β-stimulation), norepinephrine (combined cardiac β-stimulation and vascular α-stimulation), and acetylcholine (inhibition of release of norepinephrine from nerve terminals).

INTRAVENOUS EPINEPHRINE

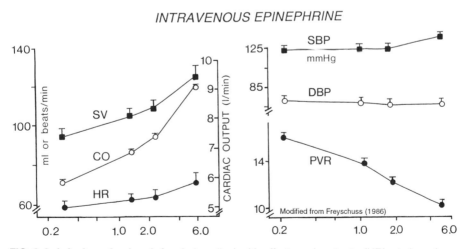

FIG. 2-4. Infusion of epinephrine (adrenaline) with effects on heart rate (HR), stroke volume (SV), cardiac output (CO), systolic blood pressure (SBP), diastolic blood pressure (DBP), and PVR in healthy adults. Modified from Freyschuss et al. (1986) with permission.

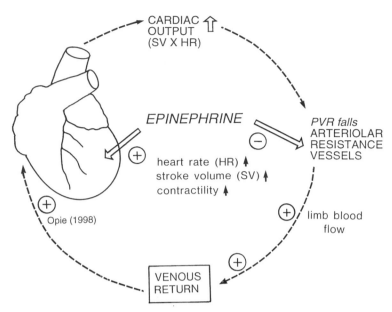

FIG. 2-5. Effects of epinephrine on the circulation. Epinephrine, released from the adrenal gland in response to emotion or exercise, has a stimulatory effect on myocardial β-receptors. Epinephrine reduces systemic vascular resistance by effects on β2-adrenergic receptors. The net result is that the diastolic BP decreases. However, the systolic pressure may increase because of the increased cardiac output.

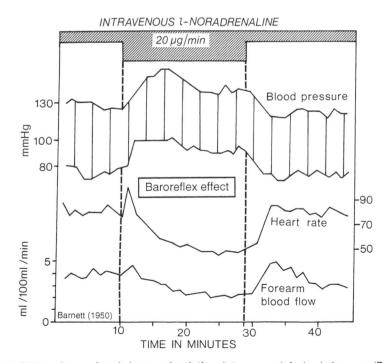

FIG. 2-6. Effect of norepinephrine on circulation. Intravenous infusion in humans (Barnett et al., 1950).

22

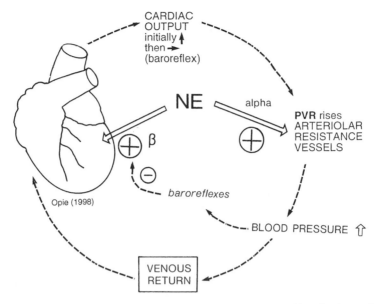

FIG. 2-7. Schema of norepinephrine effects (NE) on the circulation. Note β-adrenergic effects on the myocardium to increase heart rate and contractility, which initially increase cardiac output. In addition, the afterload increases as a result of α-adrenergic-mediated stimulation of arteriolar resistance vessels with increase in peripheral vascular resistance (PVR). The net effect is that the BP increases so that the baroreflexes are stimulated to slow the heart rate. In the end, the cardiac output is unchanged or might even decrease.

Sympathetic Stimulation

When the sympathetic nerves to the heart but not to the peripheral circulation are stimulated, then β-adrenergic effects predominate (Fig. 2-8). There is a marked increase of heart rate, left ventricular pressure, and the index of left ventricular contractile activity. The BP increases abruptly because much greater cardiac output has been ejected into the same vascular bed. During exercise, where such β-adrenergic stimulation of the heart is accompanied by a mixture of peripheral effects, α-adrenergic vasoconstriction tends to be offset by β-adrenergic vasodilation.

SIGNAL SYSTEMS

The opposite effects of sympathetic and parasympathetic stimulation on myocardial contraction and on arteriolar tone can be explained in terms of intracellular signal systems. These signals link receptor occupation to the change in biologic function, such as muscular contraction (Fig. 2-9) or vasoconstriction or vasodilation. When β-adrenergic receptors are occupied, the membrane-bound enzyme adenylate cyclase is stimulated into activity by one of a superfamily of

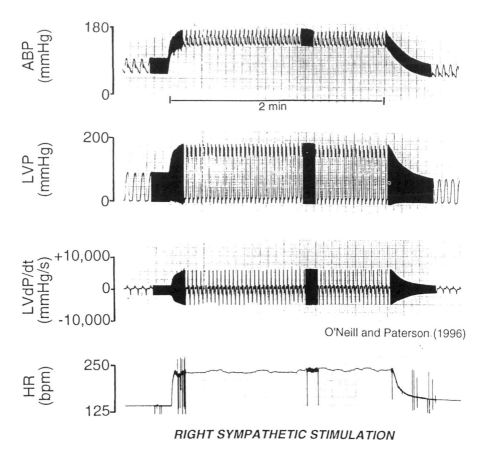

O'Neill and Paterson (1996)

RIGHT SYMPATHETIC STIMULATION

FIG. 2-8. Effect of rapid sympathetic stimulation on the heart, in the absence of changes in PVR. HR, heart rate; LVP, left ventricular pressure; LVdP/dt, left ventricular rate of pressure increase as a function of time; ABP, arterial BP. Courtesy of Dr. David Paterson, University Laboratory of Physiology, Oxford.

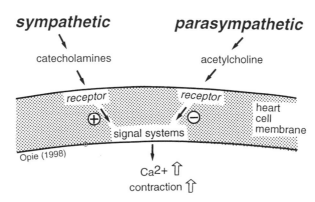

FIG. 2-9. Opposing autonomic effects of sympathetic and parasympathetic systems on cardiac myocytes.

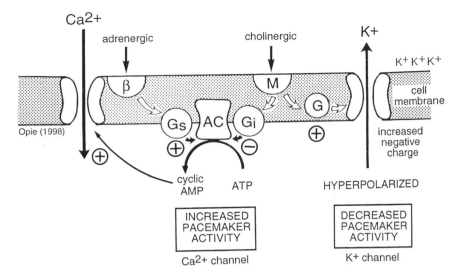

FIG. 2-10. Autonomic effects on sinus (sinoatrial) node. Effects of sympathetic stimulation in increasing pacemaker activity with opposite effects of parasympathetic activity. β, β-adrenergic receptor; G_s, stimulatory G protein; G_i, inhibitory G protein; AC, adenylate cyclase; M, muscarinic receptor.

proteins, the stimulatory G protein G_s (Fig. 2-10). The result is conversion of adenosine triphosphate (ATP) into cyclic adenosine monophosphate (cAMP), the second messenger, which in turn promotes calcium entry into the myocardial cell by increasing the opening of the calcium channel. Next follows enhanced release of stored calcium from the sarcoplasmic reticulum, so that cytosolic calcium increases more as the force of contraction increases.

Parasympathetic stimulation leads to an opposite series of events (Fig. 2-10). Occupation of the muscarinic (M) receptor by the neurotransmitter acetylcholine interacts with the inhibitory G protein, G_i, to decrease activity of adenylate cyclase. The result is less formation of cAMP and a sequence of events opposite to those achieved by β-adrenergic stimulation. The end result is decreased contractile force.

This cholinergic sequence may not be as important as anticipated in ventricular muscle because (1) the muscarinic receptors are relatively sparse and (2) the inhibitory sequence may be most evident when activity of adenylate cyclase is increased by prior β-adrenergic stimulation. Thus cholinergic activity can act as a break to excess to adrenergic stimulation of the myocardium.

Sinus Node Pacemaker Activity

Similar systems work in the case of the sinus (sinoatrial) node (Fig. 2-10), with β-adrenergic stimulation increasing heart rate because cAMP, the second messenger, enhances the rate of spontaneous pacemaking. The latter is a complex event, dependent on at least three currents (see Chapter 5), thereby providing fail-safe mechanisms to prevent sinus arrest, which is one cause of sudden cardiac death. Cholinergic stimulation slows the pacemaker rate by decreasing formation of cAMP. This sequence lessens the degree of increase of heart rate achieved by β-adrenergic stimulation. Yet there must be another mechanism at work. At night, when vagal turn is high and adrenergic tone is low, there is a marked slowing of heart rate. This may be explained in part by two factors decreasing the rate of formation of cAMP, namely lessened activity of G_s and increased activity of G_i. The additional mechanism is as follows.

Cholinergic stimulation of the muscarinic receptor acts via another G protein (Fig. 2-10) to help open a specific type of K^+ channel (technical term K_{ACh}). The result is increased outward flow of K^+ ions, with a relatively greater positive charge outside the cell membrane and a relatively greater negative charge within the membrane of the sinus node cells. That is, the difference between positive and negative charges has increased, which is called hyperpolarization. This is an event that leads to decreased pacemaker activity because, starting from a greater negative charge within the cell, the inward potassium current and other pacemaking currents require more time to reach the threshold at which spontaneous depolarization and firing of the pacemaker takes place.

Vascular Control

Of particular importance is the diameter of the small arteries (arterioles) that control the resistance against which the heart works (the peripheral vascular resistance [PVR]). Control of this site cannot be simplified into opposing effects of the sympathetic and parasympathetic systems. Rather, vasoconstrictors and dilators act in opposing ways (Fig. 2-11). Although norepinephrine acting by α_1-adrenergic receptors causes vasoconstriction, almost paradoxically, circulating norepinephrine and epinephrine cause vasodilation acting through the β_2-receptors, which increase cAMP in vascular smooth muscle. The latter change, for complex reasons, causes vasodilation rather than the expected vasoconstriction. Parasympathetic stimulation causes vasodilation via nitric oxide released from the inner lining of the blood vessels (endothelium), provided that the endothelium is not damaged. Signals emanating from the endothelium play a major role in regulation of vascular tone (see Chapter 9). Such signals include nitric oxide, released not only in response to acetylcholine, but also during exercise. Adenosine is a further vasodilatory local mediator. Control of vascular smooth muscle tone is extremely complex but of great importance because of the role of the PVR in determining the load against which the heart works and in setting the BP.

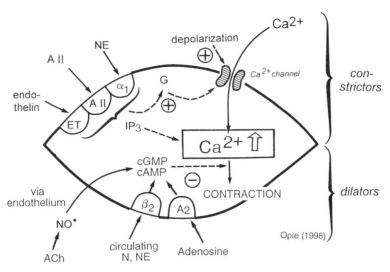

FIG. 2-11. Signal systems in arteriolar smooth muscle cell. When calcium increases sufficiently within the cell, contraction occurs. The entry of calcium is enhanced by activity of the α_1-adrenergic receptors and the angiotensin II receptors, under the influence of locally released norepinephrine (NE). Angiotensin II (AII) and endothelin are also vasoconstrictive (see Chapter 9). Occupation of these receptors therefore causes vasoconstriction. The messenger system for these receptors includes release of IP$_3$ (inositol trisphosphate), which increases intracellular calcium levels. The vascular endothelium liberates the vasodilator nitric oxide (NO), in response to acetylcholine (ACh) release by cholinergic stimulation. Nitric oxide increases cyclic guanosine monophosphate in the vasculator smooth muscle cells which, in turn, decreases the calcium levels. cAMP, formed in response to β-adrenergic or adenosine receptor stimulation, is vasodilatory (see Chapter 9).

Release of Norepinephrine from Terminal Adrenergic Nerves

During the sympathetic adrenergic response, norepinephrine is released from small swellings, the *terminal varicosities*, lying on minute end-branches of the neurons of the adrenergic nervous system (Fig. 2-12). Norepinephrine is synthesized in the varicosities via two compounds called dopa and dopamine, and ultimately from the amino acid tyrosine, which is taken up from the circulation. Such synthesis takes place only in the sympathetic nerve terminals, not in the ordinary myocardial cells. The norepinephrine thus synthesized is stored within the terminals in *storage granules* (or *vesicles*) to be released on stimulation by an adrenergic nervous impulse. Thus, when central stimulation increases during excitement or exercise, an increased number of adrenergic impulses liberate an increased amount of norepinephrine from the terminals. Most of the released norepinephrine is taken up again by the nerve terminal varicosities to re-enter the storage vesicles or to be metabolized. At least some of the released norepinephrine interacts with the specific vascular α-receptors, and another fraction enters

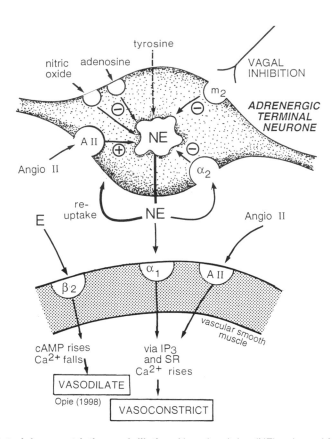

FIG. 2-12. Arteriolar constriction and dilation. Norepinephrine (NE), released from the storage granules of the terminal neurons into the synaptic cleft, has predominantly vasoconstrictive effects acting via postsynaptic α_1-receptors. In addition, presynaptic α_2-receptors are stimulated to allow feedback inhibition of its release to modulate any excess release of NE. Parasympathetic cholinergic stimulation releases acetylcholine (ACh), which stimulates the muscarinic (m_2) receptors to inhibit the release of NE and thereby indirectly to cause vasodilation. Circulating epinephrine (E) stimulates vasodilatory β_2-receptors. Angiotensin II, formed ultimately in response to renin released from the kidneys, is also powerfully vasoconstrictive, acting both by inhibition of NE release and directly on arteriolar receptors. SR, sarcoplasmic reticulum; IP_3, inositol trisphosphate; AII, angiotensin II; VSM, vascular smooth muscle.

the circulation to account for the increased blood norepinephrine levels found during states of excitement or stress or exercise.

Feedback Inhibition of Presynaptic Receptors

There are two types of α-adrenergic receptors. Those situated on the sarcolemma are called *postsynaptic* or *postjunctional receptors*, whereas those situated on the terminal varicosities are called the *presynaptic* or *prejunctional*

TABLE 2-2. *Presynaptic receptors and their effects on release of norepinephrine (NE) from terminal neurons*

Presynaptic receptor	Agonist	Source of agonist	Effect on NE release
m_2	Acetylcholine	Cholinergic	−
α_2	NE	Adrenergic terminal	−
AII	Angiotensin II	Renin–angiotensin system	+

−, inhibits; +, enhance; agonist, messenger or hormone stimulating receptors; m_2, cholinergic cardiac muscarinic; α_2, α_2-adrenergic.

receptors (Fig. 2-12). Norepinephrine can inhibit its own release, acting on the α_2-adrenergic receptors. Anatomically these are presynaptic α-receptors (Table 2-2). *α_1-adrenergic receptors* are situated on the arteriolar sarcolemma and therefore called *postsynaptic receptors* (Table 2-3). It is these receptors that norepinephrine stimulates to cause vasoconstriction.

Neuromodulation

This is the process whereby the release of norepinephrine from the terminal neurones is either increased or decreased. The most powerful neuromodulator stimulating the release of norepinephrine *is angiotensin II*, a circulating vasoconstrictor that helps to control the BP. When the BP decreases, renin is released from the kidneys, ultimately to form circulating angiotensin II and thereby to promote vasoconstriction and to elevate the BP. Angiotensin II also causes vasoconstriction by direct effect on the postsynaptic angiotensin II receptors on the vascular sarcolemma. Negative neuromodulators, decreasing the release of norepinephrine, include the local messengers adenosine and nitric oxide formed during exercise. Norepinephrine release is also lessened when there is increased cholinergic activity, as at night, when the muscarinic presynaptic receptors on the terminal neurones are stimulated (Fig. 2-12).

TABLE 2-3. *Postsynaptic receptors and their proposed effects on cardiac or vascular cytosolic calcium levels (Ca^{2+}) and on cardiovascular (CV) function*

Postsynaptic receptor	Cardiac Ca^{2+}	Vascular Ca^{2+}	Overall CV effect
α_1	(+)	++	SVR ++
β_1	++	(−)	CO ++
β_2	+	−	CO +, SVR −
AII	(+)	++	SVR ++

For receptor agonists, see Fig 2-12.
+, increased; −, decreased; (+) or (−), controversial and/or modest effect; SVR, systemic vascular resistance; CO, cardiac output.

TABLE 2-4. *Effects of adrenergic stimulation by
norepinephrine and epinephrine on vascular tone[a]*

Norepinephrine
Released from terminal neurons
Vasoconstriction throughout vascular bed
Circulating
Vasoconstriction of cutaneous, splanchnic, and renal beds
Venoconstriction
Circulating epinephrine
Predominant β_2 vasodilatory effect
Muscular arterioles (heart and skeletal muscle)
Predominant α-vasoconstrictor effect
Other resistance vessels and veins
Overall effect—vasodilatory[b]

[a]Tone, from Greek *tonos,* "something stretched."
[b]Stratton et al. (1985), Freyschuss et al. (1986).

Overall Adrenergic Effects on the Vascular Bed

Adrenergic stimulation has very complex overall effects on various vascular beds and on the cardiovascular system (Tables 2-1 and 2-4). In vascular smooth muscle, the α_1-mediated vasoconstrictive affects of norepinephrine are opposed by circulating epinephrine, which is simultaneously released (e.g., during exercise) and stimulates vasodilatory β_2-receptors. In arterioles of the splanchic bed, epinephrine also stimulates α_1-adrenergic receptors to cause vasoconstriction, thereby helping to divert blood from nonmuscular to muscular tissues. Although norepinephrine can stimulate the vasodilatory β_2-receptors, the reasons for its overall vasoconstrictory effect are thought to be (1) that the α_1-receptors are anatomically closer than the β_2-receptors to the sites of norepinephrine release from the terminal neurons, and (2) the α_1-adrenergic receptors may be greater in number or activity than the vasodilatory β-receptors. Furthermore, the overall effects of sympathetic stimulation on the arterioles differ from individual to individual. In individuals who are hypertensive or may be prone to develop hypertension, vasoconstrictory effects appear to predominate.

Why does blood flow during exercise increase only in those muscles that are actually used, whereas flow decreases in those that are not being used? Even when the vasodilatory β_2-receptors are experimentally blocked, there is still an increase in muscle blood flow during exercise. Thus, the explanation may lie in the production of vasodilatory local metabolites by the exercising muscles.

BAROREFLEXES

When the BP increases excessively, pressure-sensitive cells in the aortic arch and the carotid artery (in a small dilation called the carotid sinus) respond by conveying impulses to a central coordinating site (the vasomotor center), which then sends out vagal stimuli to decrease heart rate, which in turn will lower the cardiac output so that the BP then decreases to the normal range (Fig. 2-3):

Increased BP → baroceptors → vasomotor center → vagal stimulation → decreased heart rate → decreased cardiac output → BP decreases to appropriate levels.

This sequence explains the *reflex bradycardia* that can be expected during an acute elevation of arterial BP as a result of stimulation of the baroreceptors in response to peripheral α_1-adrenergic vasoconstriction resulting from an infusion of norepinephrine (Fig. 2-6).

An interesting application of the principles of baroreflex control is the use of *carotid sinus massage* in the therapy of some types of tachycardia that originate above the ventricle, i.e., supraventricular tachycardias. External manual stimulation of the mechanoreceptors in the carotid sinus provokes the afferent stimuli, which travel to the vagal nucleus to stimulate the efferent limb so that there is increased vagal inhibition of both sinus and atrioventricular nodes, which in turn helps to terminate the tachycardia.

VASODILATORY LOCAL MESSENGERS

During exercise, adrenergic outflow is increased. Stimulation of the heart by β-receptors leads to an increased frequency and force of contraction (Fig. 2-8), yet simultaneously α-adrenergic stimulation will tend to constrict the resistance arterioles (Fig. 2-7). Therefore, exercise would be associated with an inevitable increase of BP. The reason why this does not happen is as follows: vasodilatory messengers are locally formed during muscle metabolism and act on the arterioles to vasodilate. Together with epinepherine-induced β_2-receptor stimulation, they account for the decrease in PVR during exercise. Similar messengers are thought to account for the increase in coronary blood flow, also occurring during exercise (see Chapter 10). Of particular current interest is the proposed role of a newly defined messenger, *nitric oxide*, manufactured by the vascular endothelium (Fig. 2-13). The stimulus to such release of nitric oxide during exercise is not fully known. Hypothetically, a low tissue oxygen tension, occurring as oxygen is used during exercise, could stimulate the synthesis of nitric oxide. Alternatively, the increased rate of blood flow during exercise causes a mechanical effect on the endothelium (shear stress) that liberates nitric oxide. Another vasodilatory messenger is *adenosine*, a metabolite formed as the rate of breakdown of the high-energy phosphate compound ATP exceeds the rate of its resynthesis during exercise.

NEUROREGULATION BY LOCAL MESSENGERS

Both adenosine and nitric oxide are local messengers, being small molecules that very significantly influence local autonomic control of the arterioles. For example, adenosine is both a direct vasodilator by its actions on the adenosine

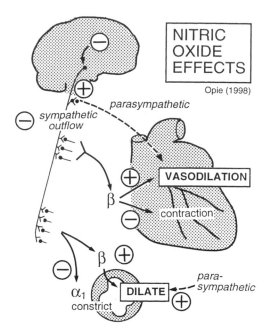

FIG. 2-13. Nitric oxide effects on circulation. Proposed sites at which the local messenger nitric oxide can alter autonomic effects on the cardiovascular system (see also Persson, 1996).

receptor on vascular smooth muscle cells (Fig. 2-11) and it acts as a negative neuromodulator, thereby inhibiting release of norepinephrine (Fig. 2-12).

Nitric oxide not only acts as a local messenger to convey signals from the endothelium to vascular smooth muscle, but it also is a modulator at every known level of neurogenic control. Physiologically, nitric oxide can be synthesized not only in the vascular endothelium, but also in the nerve terminals of the nitric oxide–releasing nerves (*nitroxidergic nerves*), as well as in other sites in the nervous system. Pathologically, nitric oxide can be synthesized in myocardial cells to inhibit contraction in some disease states. In general, nitric oxide acts on the autonomic nervous system at several levels to inhibit sympathic outflow and to lessen the release of norepinephrine from terminal neurones (Fig. 2-13). These are all vasodilatory effects. Nitric oxide also mediates parasympathetic-induced vasodilation because it is released by the normal endothelium in response to acetylcholine.

REDISTRIBUTION OF BLOOD DURING EXERCISE

Apart from the heart and lungs, the internal organs of the body do not require an increased blood flow during exercise. Such organs are the liver, kidneys, stomach, and intestines. In these organs, blood flow actually decreases during exercise, which helps to direct the blood volume to the muscular organs under-going increased metabolic activity, such as the heart and skeletal muscle. The mechanisms of such redistribution of blood are multiple: (1) the absence of vasodilatory metabolites in nonmuscular nonexercising organs, (2) the continued vasoconstrictory effects of norepinephrine in the nonexercising organs, and (3) the capacity of epinephrine to stimulate vasoconstrictory α-receptors rather than vasodilatory β_2-receptors in the arterioles of these organs (Table 2-4).

PERIPHERAL VASCULAR RESISTANCE

The total PVR (also called the systemic vascular resistance) is crucial to the control of the circulation (Fig. 2-14). It is calculated using the following for-mula:

$$BP = CO \times PVR$$

Therefore,

$$CO = BP/PVR$$

and

$$PVR = BP/CO$$

where CO is cardiac output per minute (stroke volume × heart rate). The BP is the difference between the mean pressures in the aorta and in the right ventricle, and the cardiac output is the product of the stroke volume and the heart rate. The stan-dard approach to the measurement of these entities and of the PVR has been the use of invasive catheterization techniques. Noninvasive echocardiographic meth-ods (using ultrasound principles) are being used increasingly, even though they are less accurate. Physiologically, the PVR is low during and just after exercise or

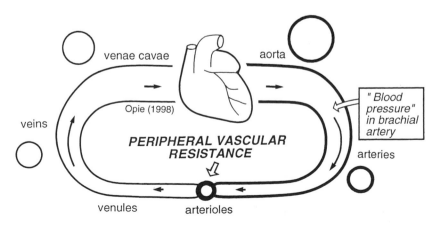

FIG. 2-14. Schematic role of peripheral vascular resistance in the circulation.

when the ambient temperature is high (peripheral vasodilation helps cutaneous heat loss). The PVR is high in the cold or when the body is deprived of fluid and the blood volume is low because there is stimulation of the system that ultimately forms angiotensin II. Three disease states abnormally increase systemic vascular resistance: (1) arterial hypertension; (2) severe congestive heart failure when the heart contracts too feebly to keep up the BP, so that the baroreflexes are stimulated to cause compensatory adrenergic activity; and (3) when the heart develops a shocklike state (cardiogenic shock), as in a massive heart attack with myocardial infarction (see Chapter 19) and intense reflex adrenergic stimulation is evoked.

Blood flow through the arterioles occurs because the pressure gradient at the arterial end is higher than at the capillary end (see Fig. 1-7). Apart from the pressure differences, a crucial factor is the radius of the blood vessel, which is regulated by the balance of vasodilatory and vasoconstrictory effects and, therefore, at least in part by the autonomic nervous system. In idealized conditions with blood flowing smoothly (*laminar flow*) in a rigid tube, resistance to flow through

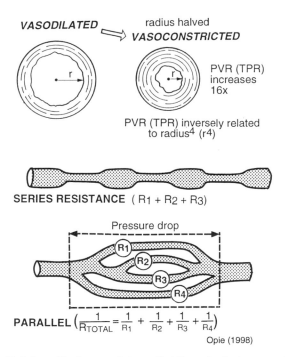

FIG. 2-15. Poiseuille's law. The top panel shows that the major factor governing the resistance of the arterioles is the radius. PVR is inversely related to the fourth power of the radius (r^4). The bottom panel shows that most of the resistance arterioles in the circulation are in parallel and constitute the total peripheral resistance (TPR = PVR). At the level of the arterioles, the resistance is largely governed by the radius in such a way that resistance decreases in proportion to the fourth power of the radius.

that vessel is inversely proportional to the fourth power of the tube's radius (Fig. 2-15). Hence, reduction of the diameter of the arterial lumen is the most powerful determinant of resistance to flow.

Technically the resistance (R) of a rigid tube can be given by *Poiseuille's law*, whereby:

$$R = P/Q = (8 \times \text{viscosity} \times \text{length})/r^4$$

where Q is flow, r is radius, and P is the pressure decease over the length of the tube (Fig. 2-15).

Normally the blood viscosity is not an important variable and the length factor does not change, so it is the radius that is dominant among the factors regulating vascular resistance. In the presence of vascular disease, such as coronary stenosis, turbulent blood flow increases the resistance further.

Altered arteriolar diameter not only regulates the PVR, but changes the pattern of blood flow distal to the arteriole. Because the flow through the arteriole is highly dependent on the radius (according to Poiseuille's equation), more blood reaches the capillaries during vasodilation. Thus, during exercise, increased capillary flow delivers more oxygen to exercising tissues.

THE MICROCIRCULATION

Because arterioles and capillaries act so closely in concert, they constitute what is called the microcirculation (Fig. 2-16).

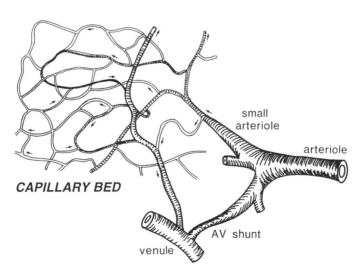

FIG. 2-16. The microcirculation, which includes the arterioles and the capillary bed. Note the existence of arteriolar-venule (AV) shunts, which can open or close to increase the amount of blood actually in the capillary bed.

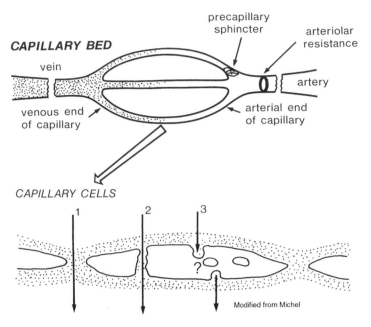

FIG. 2-17. Structure of capillary bed and capillary cells. Blood flow to the capillary bed is regulated by the arteriolar resistance, the activity of precapillary sphincters, and by AV shunts (see Fig. 2-11). The capillary cells have pores between the cells (1) and through the cells (2), and the vesicles may have a role in transferring more complex molecules (3). Capillary cell structure modified from Michel (1988). The dots around the capillary cells represent the glycocalyx.

Structure and Function of Capillaries

To perform its specialized functions, the capillaries have walls only one cell thick (Fig. 2-17). There are three possible modes of exchange across the capillary walls: (1) through pores between cells, (2) through small pores within the cells, and (3) by means of *vesicles*. Gases, such as oxygen and carbon dioxide, readily flow by diffusion through the pores, as do small molecules such as glucose and lactate. Transport of complex molecules, such as fatty acids, may require transport by vesicles. The latter are small pinched-off fragments of the cell membrane that can entrap a large molecule, close up, and hypothetically transport the molecule to the opposite side of the cell, where the vesicle can reopen to release the transferred molecule. However, this proposed role of vesicles is controversial.

Oxygen, diffusing from the capillaries, is used in the mitochondria, which are intracellular organelles (see Chapter 3), where the oxygen is converted by a series of metabolic steps to CO_2 and water, and energy in the form of ATP is produced (Fig. 2-18). This CO_2 diffuses from the mitochondria back to the capillary blood, and the water joins the total body water. For such energy production to occur also requires that the potential fuels for the heart, such as glu-

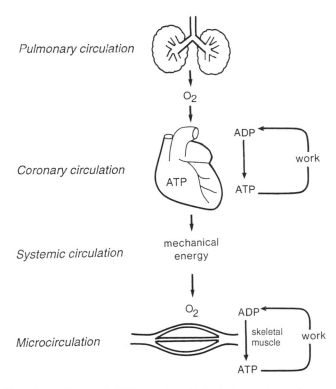

FIG. 2-18. The circulation and ATP transfer. Links between the pulmonary circulation, coronary circulation, systemic circulation, and microcirculation. In essence, ATP made in the myocardium as a result of the oxygen delivered by the coronary circulation is broken down and the power is transferred to mechanical energy, which propels blood through the systemic circulation to deliver oxygen to the capillaries and thence to the tissues, where ATP is formed from adenosine diphosphate (ADP). In that way, the whole circulation acts as an ATP transferral system.

cose and fatty acids, be broken down into much simpler components of only two carbons, which can then enter the mitochondria and participate in energy production.

CORONARY CIRCULATION

Just as the general systemic circulation conveys oxygenated blood to the tissues of the body, so the coronary circulation takes oxygen to the heart muscle. Anatomically, oxygenated blood leaves the aorta just above the aortic valve through two small openings called ostia, from which the left and right coronary arteries convey blood to the heart muscle. The left coronary artery subserves chiefly the large left ventricle, whereas the right serves chiefly the smaller right ventricle, although this pattern is variable. Each artery splits into smaller branches and then into arterioles and capillaries, following the pattern already described for the systemic circulation. From the capillaries run venules into veins, which ultimately collect into the coronary sinus to enter the right atrium. The major coronary arteries run on the surface of the heart, sending branches down so that the arterioles actually lie within the myocardium. During exercise, when the oxygen requirement of the heart increases considerably, the coronary flow rate also increases to deliver the increased oxygen needed. Although the coronary arteries do not have extensive major branches joining up with each other—i.e., there are no large *collaterals* (width, laterally)—at the level of the small arterioles such connections do exist to open up during exercise, thereby increasing the blood flow through the capillary bed.

From the metabolic point of view, the circulation could be regarded as a system for the transfer of energy from the heart to the organs of the periphery (Fig. 2-18). In the heart, the oxygen taken up is used for the oxidation of the major fuels, glucose and fatty acids, with the production of CO_2, H_2O, and energy-rich ATP. Myocardial contraction uses ATP and provides the mechanical energy to drive blood through the circulation and to deliver oxygen to the various tissues.

CONTROL OF CIRCULATION BY LOCAL MESSENGERS

During exercise, more venous blood is returned to the right atrium. The reason is that (1) more blood is squeezed out of the venous capacitance vessels by the contracting skeletal muscle and (2) there is an increase in the *venous tone* (an increase in tension in the muscle walls), induced by autonomic activation (Table 2-2). In addition, the cardiac output increases substantially, so that the venous return must also increase by the same amount. To maintain balance in the circulation, the greater venous return must in some way stimulate the heart to contract (Fig. 2-14). This mechanism was first described by Starling as follows:

> Within physiological limits, the larger the volume of the heart, the greater the energy of its contraction and the amount of chemical change at each contraction.

The latter conclusion was reached in Starling's fundamental lecture on the law of the heart, given at Cambridge, England, in 1915 and published in 1918. He was aware of the longitudinal fibrils constituting muscle and proposed that "lengthening the muscle increases the extent of the active surface," very similar to the modern concept of crossbridge interaction. He also gave an early view on molecular mechanisms in heart failure, proposing that the "concentration of active molecules becomes less," which leads to the modern view that there are abnormalities of the calcium cycle in heart failure.

An important proposal made by Starling was that the heart volume and hence the length of the heart muscle fiber could be increased by an increased venous filling pressure, now often termed the "preload" (see Chapter 12).

ROLE OF KIDNEYS: RENIN–ANGIOTENSIN SYSTEM

If the blood volume decreases excessively, the circulation must fail. On the other hand, if the blood volume is excessive, then the heart will be overloaded by means of the Starling principle. To help regulate the blood volume, there is an important physiologic control mechanism, namely the *renin–angiotensin system*. Renin is an enzyme liberated from the kidneys in response to a low renal perfusion, low blood volume, or low BP. These changes release renin, which stimulates the conversion of a polypeptide called angiotensinogen to angiotensin I in the liver. Angiotensin I circulates and is converted to angiotensin II by the activity of the angiotensin-converting enzyme found in the capillary bed of the lung and elsewhere. Angiotensin II is a powerful vasoconstrictor (Fig. 2-11). Hypothetically, the regulatory role of this system might have evolved as follows. When early hunters lacked water, their blood volume would tend to decrease, with a consequent decrease of BP and stimulation of renin release from the kidneys. The end result would be a compensatory angiotensin II–mediated vasoconstriction that would help rectify the low blood volume. Renin release is also triggered by left ventricular failure.

Left Ventricular Failure

When the left ventricle fails, as after a prolonged pressure overload (see Chapter 16), it sets in motion a similar sequence of events. The failing left ventricle is unable to pump sufficiently strongly to maintain the arterial BP. This tendency to an excessively low BP (arterial hypotension) elicits powerful protective reactions that maintain the BP, including stimulation of the baroreflexes and release of the adrenergic hormones that stimulate the β-adrenergic receptors in the kidneys to release renin and at the same time stimulate the α-adrenergic receptors in the arterioles to constrict. Although these mechanisms help keep up the BP, they decrease the caliber of the arterioles against which the heart must work, thereby actually exaggerating the degree of heart failure.

These concepts show how the function of the heart cannot be separated from the control of the circulation. Starling emphasized that the circulation could control the heart by variations in the load. The heart, in turn, can send biochemical signals to the circulation by means of the baroreflexes, the adrenergic hormones, and the renin–angiotensin system.

SUMMARY

1. *The heart and circulation work in concert.* The activity of the autonomic nervous system links the heart rate and contractile response of the heart to the requirements of the peripheral tissues via the peripheral circulation.
2. *The two major branches of the autonomic nervous system are the adrenergic or stimulatory system and the cholinergic or inhibitory system.* The

adrenergic system liberates two neurotransmitters, epinephrine and norepinephrine, whereas the cholinergic neurotransmitter is acetylcholine.

3. *Each of these neurotransmitters has a different pattern of effect on the heart and circulation.* Epinephrine stimulates β-adrenergic receptors in the heart to increase heart rate and force of contraction. Epinephrine also dilates the arterioles by their β-adrenergic receptors. Although circulating norepinephrine stimulates β-receptors, locally released norepinephrine has a powerful arteriolar vasoconstrictory effect, the result of α_1-adrenergic stimulation.

4. *Acetylcholine, the neurotransmitter of the parasympathetic nervous system,* acts to decrease the heart rate and, to some extent, the force of ventricular contraction. It is an arteriolar vasodilator acting through release of nitric oxide from the intact vascular endothelium.

5. *The baroreflexes link the heart and circulation.* When the arterial pressure is low, then baroreflexes are stimulated to activate adrenergic vasoconstriction and to increase the heart rate. Converse changes occur when the blood pressure is too high, for example, after an experimental infusion of norepinephrine.

6. *During exercise, the activity of the adrenergic autonomic nervous system increases* so that the heart rate increases, contractility increases, and more blood is pumped from the heart (cardiac output increases). This blood is redistributed in the tissues according to the needs during exercise. More blood is required in the myocardium and skeletal muscle, so that the arterioles to these tissues vasodilate during exercise. On the other hand, arterioles serving those organs (such as the kidney) that do not need more blood during exercise are vasoconstricted.

7. *The heart pumps against the peripheral vascular resistance,* caused by the highly muscular small-bore arterioles. It is their constriction or dilation which explains an increase or decrease in the peripheral vascular resistance, because that resistance is inversely related to the fourth power of the radius (Poiseuilles law). Hence, only small changes in arteriolar radius have major consequences.

8. *The PVR is influenced both by the autonomic nervous system and by local messengers.* For example, norepinephrine released from the terminal neurones of the sympathetic nervous system is vasoconstrictory, whereas the local messengers adenosine and nitric oxide are vasodilatory. Formation of these local messengers may account for arteriolar vasodilation during exercise, which allows more blood to be brought to the functioning skeletal muscles, and also helps to reduce the blood pressure, thereby avoiding an excessive hypertensive response during exercise.

STUDENT QUESTIONS

1. What are the divisions of the autonomic nervous system, and which are the associated receptors?

2. What are the major cardiovascular effects of stimulation of each branch of the autonomic nervous system?
3. How do epinephrine and norepinephrine differ in their effects on the circulation?
4. Outline how messenger systems act to decrease or increase heart rate?
5. What is neuromodulation?

CARDIOLOGIST-IN-TRAINING QUESTIONS

1. How does the peripheral vascular resistance respond to autonomic stimuli?
2. What are the signal systems that control (1) arteriolar constriction and (2) arteriolar dilation?
3. Describe the various receptors found on the adrenergic terminal neuron, and how they affect the release of norepinephrine. What are the anticipated changes in the blood pressure in response to stimulation of each of these receptors?
4. What is Pousieuille's law, and what is its relevance to the control of blood pressure?
5. Describe the effects of stimulation of the right sympathetic nerves on the cardiovascular system.

REFERENCES

1. Ahlquist RP. A study of the adrenotropic receptors. *Am J Physiol* 1948;153:586–600.
2. Barcroft H, Swan HJC. In: *Sympathetic Control of Human Blood Vessels.* London: Edward Arnold, 1953.
3. Barnett AJ, Blacket RB, Depoorter AE, Sanderson PH, Wilson GM. The action of noradrenaline in man and its relation to phaeochromocytoma and hypertension. *Clin Sci* 1950;9:151–179.
4. Boyett MR, Kirby MS, Roberts A. The negative inotropic effect of acetylcholine on ferret ventricular myocardium. *J Physiol* 1988;404:613–635.
5. Curry FE. Determinants of capillary permeability: a review of mechanisms based on single capillary studies in the frog. *Circ Res* 1986;59:367–380.
6. Freyschuss U, Hjemdahl P, Juhlin-Dannfelt A. Cardiovascular and metabolic responses to low dose adrenaline infusion: an invasive study in humans. *Clin Sci* 1986;70:199–206.
7. Lund-Johansen P. Central haemodynamic effects of β-blockers in hypertension. A comparison between atenolol, metoprolol, timolol, penbutolol, alprenolol, pindolol and bunitrolol. *Eur Heart J* 1983;4(suppl D):1–12.
8. Michel CC. Capillary permeability and how it may change. *J Physiol* 1988;404:1–29.
9. Park KH, Rubin LE, Gross SS, Levi R. Nitric oxide is a mediator of hypoxic coronary vasodilation. Relation to adenosine and cyclooxygenase-derived metabolites. *Circ Res* 1992;71:992–1001.
10. Persson PB. Modulation of cardiovascular control mechanisms and their interaction. *Physiol Rev* 1996;76:193–244.
11. Rowell LB. In: *Human Circulation, Regulation During Physical Stress.* New York: Oxford University Press, 1986;231–243.
12. Shepherd JT, Vanhoutte PM. In: *The Human Cardiovascular System. Facts and Concepts.* New York: Raven, 1979.
13. Starling EH. In: *The Linacre Lecture on the Law of the Heart.* London: Longmans, Green and Co, 1918.
14. Stratton JR, Pfeifer MA, Ritchie JL, Halter JB. Hemodynamic effects of epinephrine: concentration-effect study in humans. *J Appl Physiol* 1985;58:1199–1206.
15. Taylor J, Hand GA, Johnson DG, Seals DR. Augmented forearm vasoconstriction during dynamic exercise in healthy older men. *Circulation* 1992;86:1789–1799.
16. Werko L, Bucht H, Josephson B, Ek J. The effect of noradrenalin and adrenalin on renal hemodynamics and renal function in man. *Scand J Clin Lab Invest* 1951;3:255–261.

3

Heart Cells and Organelles

Thus far the theme has been developed that myocardial contraction plays a crucial role in the regulation of the circulation by ejection of blood from the left ventricle and that the tone of the peripheral arterioles provides much of the resistance against which the heart works. The emphasis of the present chapter will be on the general organization of myocardial contractile cells and the properties of their supporting cells. Comparisons and contrasts will also be made between myocardial and vascular smooth muscle cells because the peripheral and coronary circulations crucially govern myocardial function.

Most of the heart is made up of contractile muscle cells, also known as *myocytes* or, more specifically, *cardiomyocytes*. The rest consists of pacemaker and conducting tissues (which are concerned with the generation and propagation of the heart's electrical activity), blood vessels, and the extracellular space (Table 3-1). Myocytes constitute about 75% of the total volume of the

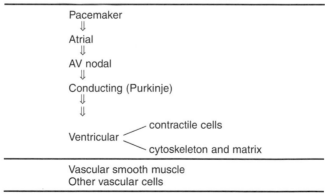

TABLE 3-1. *Cells of the heart*

Pacemaker
⇓
Atrial
⇓
AV nodal
⇓
Conducting (Purkinje)
⇓
⇓

Ventricular ⟨ contractile cells
cytoskeleton and matrix

Vascular smooth muscle
Other vascular cells

Top panel shows the cells concerned with initiation and conduction of the cardiac impulse to the ventricular contractile cells. Cytoskeletal and matrix cells give support. Vascular smooth muscle and other vascular cells regulate the load against which the heart contracts.

myocardium (Brilla et al., 1991). A *myofiber* is composed of a group of myocytes held together by surrounding connective tissue (see frontispiece). Further strands of collagen connect myofibers to each other. The myocytes are filled with bundles of contractile proteins, each bundle called a *myofibril*.

WORKING VENTRICULAR MYOCYTES

Although there are many different cell types in the heart, it is the ventricular myocytes that by their contraction propel the blood throughout the body. These working myocytes are described first, followed by atrial cells and vascular smooth muscle cells.

The individual ventricular myocytes that account for more than half of the heart's weight are roughly cylindrical in shape. Those in the atrium are small, being less than 10 μm in diameter and about 20 μm in length. Relative to the atrial cells, the ventricular myocytes are large, measuring about 10 to 25 μm in diameter and 50 to 100 μm in length (Table 3-2).

Early in life there are vast numbers of myocytes in the heart, possibly as many as 6×10^9 cells. Millions of cells are lost for every year of life, so that the centenarian has only about one third of the original number of cells (Olivetti et al., 1991).

When examined under the light microscope, these cells have cross-striations and are branched. Each myocyte is bounded by an external membrane called the *sarcolemma* (Latin *sarco,* flesh; *lemma,* thin husk), and is filled with rodlike bundles of *myofibrils* (see frontispiece). The latter are the contractile elements. The sarcolemma of the myocyte invaginates to form an extensive tubular network (*T tubules)* that extends the extracellular space into the interior of the cell (see frontispiece). The nucleus, which contains almost all of the cell's genetic

TABLE 3-2. *Microanatomy of contractile and conducting (Purkinje) cells*

	Ventricular myocyte[a,b]	Atrial myocyte[a,c]	Purkinje cells[a,d]
Shape	Long and narrow	Elliptical (oral)	Long and broad
Length (μm)	50–100	About 20	150–200
Diameter (μm)	10–25	5–6	35–40
T tubules	Plentiful	Rare or none	Absent
Intercalated disk and gap junction	Prominent end-to-end transmission	Side-to-side and end-to-end transmission	Very prominent; abundant gap junctions; fast end-to-end transmission
General appearance	Mitochondria and sarcomeres, very abundant; rectangular branching bundles with little interstitial collagen	Bundles of atrial tissue separated by wide areas of collagen	Fewer sarcomeres, paler

Note that the length of isolated myocytes from rat and human ventricles is similar, as is sarcomere length.[e]
[a]Legato. *The Myocardial Cell for the Clinical Cardiologist.* Mount Kisco, NY: Futura, 1973.
[b]Laks et al. *Circ Res* 1967;21:671.
[c]McNutt and Fawcett. *J Cell Biol* 1969;42:46.
[d]Sommer. *J Mol Cell Cardiol* 1982;14(suppl 3):77.
[e]Moody et al. *Circ Res* 1990;67:764.

information, is often centrally located. Some myocytes have several nuclei. Interspersed between the myofibrils and immediately beneath the sarcolemma are many *mitochondria*, the main function of which is to generate the energy in the form of adenosine triphosphate (ATP), needed to maintain the heart's function and viability.

Cytosol

The sarcolemma separates the intracellular and extracellular spaces. Within the sarcolemma, the contractile apparatus and various organelles do not lie loose but are contained in a fluid microenvironment with a specific content of ions, especially potassium, calcium, and sodium. The intracellular fluid, together with the proteins in it, is the *cytoplasm*, also called the *sarcoplasm*. Its fluid component, excluding the proteins, is called the *cytosol*. As is common usage in physiology and medicine, the term "fluid" is used even though "liquid" is strictly correct. It is the much higher intracellular than extracellular concentration of potassium ions that gives cardiac (and other) cells their specific electrical properties, whereby the inner side of the sarcolemma is negatively charged, while the outer side has positive charges, thereby conferring a state of *polarization*. It is also in the cytosol that the concentrations of calcium ions increase and decrease to cause cardiac contraction and relaxation. The proteins of the sarcoplasm contain many specialized molecules, including *enzymes*, that act to accelerate the conversion of one chemical form to another, thereby eventually producing energy. For example, glucose taken up from the circulation by cardiomyocytes is broken down by a series of enzymes to become much smaller molecules that can enter the mitochondria, there to be broken down further with the eventual production of ATP.

Myofibrils and Contractile Proteins

The major function of myocardial myocytes lies in the contraction–relaxation cycle. The two chief contractile proteins, located within the myofibrils, are the thick *myosin filaments* and the thin *actin filaments* (Latin *filament,* delicate thread). During contraction, the filaments slide over each other without the individual molecules of actin or myosin actually shortening (Fig. 3-1). As they slide, they pull together the two ends of the fundamental contractile unit called the *sarcomere* (Latin *mere,* part). On electronmicroscopy (Fig. 3-2), the sarcomere is limited on either side by the *Z line* (abbreviation for German *Zückung,* contraction) to which the actin filaments are attached. These are also called *Z bands* or *Z disks*. Conversely, the myosin filaments extend from the center of the sarcomere in either direction toward but not actually reaching the Z lines. A third major protein, titin, attaches the myosin filaments to the Z lines. *Titin,* a macromolecule of high molecular weight, has expansile properties and contributes to the mechanical stretch capacity of the myocardium.

RELAXATION

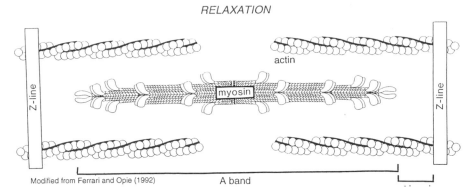

Modified from Ferrari and Opie (1992)　　　A band

FIG. 3-1. Schematic concept of contractile proteins in relaxation phase. Thick myosin filaments stretch to either side from the center, and lie between the thinner actin filaments. The latter extend inward from the Z lines on either side of the myofibril. During cardiac contraction myosin heads interact with actin filaments to move the Z lines closer together. Modified from Ferrari and Opie (1992) with permission.

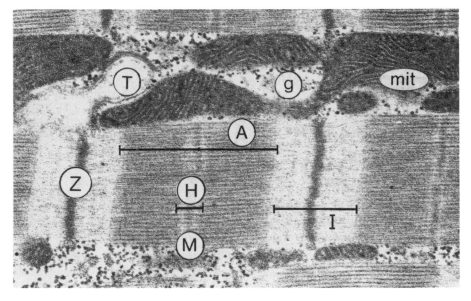

FIG. 3-2. Myofibrils and sarcomeres. Longitudinal section of rat papillary muscle showing regular arrays of myofibrils, divided into sarcomeres (see frontispiece). Note the presence of numerous mitochondria (mit) sandwiched between the myofibrils, and the presence of T tubules (T), which penetrate into the muscle at the level of the Z bands. This two-dimensional picture should not disguise the fact that the Z line is really a "Z disk." For description of A, I, and H zones, see text. M, M-band; g, glycogen granules ×32,000. Courtesy of Dr. J Moravec, Dijon, France.

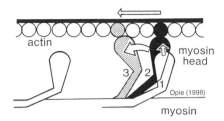

FIG. 3-3. Crossbridge contraction phase. Schematic of interaction between myosin head and actin filament during contraction. The myosin head flexes to interact with one of the actin units (*black*). During flexion, this unit is moved along (new position indicated by dotted circle). Then the myosin head relaxes, thereby being able to restart the cycle. There are many different myosin heads interacting, some in flexion and some in extension, the whole process occurring throughout the period of contraction during the availability of calcium ions.

The site where the myosin and actin filaments overlap is called the *anisotropic (A) band,* which shows up darkly on electronmicroscopy, in contrast to the lighter zones or *isotropic (I) bands* on either side, which contain only actin filaments. These bands have different light-scattering properties, the A bands being more powerful in this regard than the I bands. In the center of each A band there is a relatively clear zone known as the *H zone* (abbreviation for the German *helle,* clear). Here, only myosin is present because the overlapping of the thin and thick filaments falls short of this region. Each H zone contains a central dark region, the *M line,* which contains M-line proteins that appear to extend across the filaments as if to hold them in their correct anatomical position.

Crossbridge cycling is the entire process whereby the myosin heads interact with actin filaments (Fig. 3-3). The cycle is initiated by an increase of cytosolic calcium in response to the wave of electricity that reaches the ventricular myocytes from the conduction system. As the actin filaments move inward toward the center of the sarcomere, drawing the Z lines closer together, the sarcomere shortens. Relaxation takes place when ATP attaches to the myosin head.

Mitochondria

Mitochondria occupy a large proportion (Table 3-3) of each myocyte. They are wedged between the myofibrils, presumably so that the chief source of energy supply is close to the chief site of energy use. Mitochondria are often described as the powerhouses of the cell, producing the energy (such as ATP) that the cells need to survive and function (Fig. 3-4). Much of the molecular machinery that is responsible for producing this energy is located on the inner multifolded membrane containing the *cristae* (Latin *crista,* crest), which occupy a vast membrane area when compared with other cell membranes (Table 3-4). The enzymes located here promote the activity of the citrate cycle, originally described by the

TABLE 3-3. *Cardiac organelles and their function[a]*

Organelle	% of cell volume	Function
Myofibril	About 50[b] About 60 in humans[c]	Interaction of thick and thin filaments during contraction cycle
Mitochondria	16 in neonate[b] 33 in adults[b] 23 in adult men[c]	Provide ATP chiefly for contraction
T system	1[d]	Transmission of electrical signal from sarcolemma to cell interior
Sarcoplasmic reticulum	33 in neonate[b] 2 in adults[b]	Takes up and releases Ca^{2+} during contraction cycle
Terminal cisternae	0.33 in adults[d]	Site of calcium storage and release[e]
Rest of network	Rest of volume	Site of calcium uptake en route to cisternae
Sarcolemma	Very low	Control of ionic gradients. Channels for ions and action potential. Maintenance of cell integrity. Receptors for drugs, hormones, and neurotransmitters.
Nucleus	5	Protein synthesis
Lysosomes	Very low	Intracellular digestion and proteolysis
Sarcoplasm (cytoplasm)	12[d]	Provides cytosol in which increase and decrease of ionized calcium occurs; contains other ions and small molecules.
Sarcoplasm with nuclei	18 in humans[c]	Gene control

Note that the extracellular space occupies about 75% of the total heart volume (Brilla et al., 1991).

[a]Composition and function of rat ventricular heart cell with some data for humans. Modified from Page and McCallister, *Am J Cardiol* 1973;31:172.

[b]David et al. *J Mol Cell Cardiol* 1979;11:631.

[c]Schaper et al. *Circ Res* 1985;56:377.

[d]Page and McCallister. *Am J Cardiol* 1973;31:172.

[e]Page and Surdyk-Droske. *Circ Res* 1979;45:260.

Nobel prizewinner Sir Hans Krebs. The energy that is released during the transfer of these hydrogen atoms to oxygen is harnessed for the synthesis of ATP; hence the term *oxidative phosphorylation.*

Besides generation of ATP, cardiac mitochondria have another important role. They can potentially accumulate calcium. This process helps to prevent the level of calcium in the cytosol from becoming too high in conditions of calcium overload, as during severe lack of oxygen.

TABLE 3-4. *Membrane areas of ventricular cells[a]*

	Area/volume (μm^2 membrane area/μm^3 cell volume)
External sarcolemma	0.3
External sarcolemma plus T tubules	0.4 (or more)[b]
Sarcoplasmic reticulum	1.2
Mitochondrial cristae	11.0

[a]From Page and McCallister. *Am J Cardiol* 1973;31:172.

[b]Other workers estimate that the T tubules increase the area/volume ratio by several times.

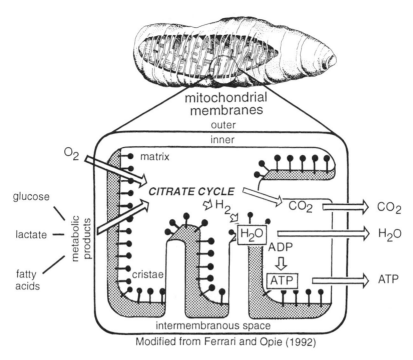

FIG. 3-4. Mitochondrial structure and function. The traditional cocoon mitochondrion is shown here. In the production of ATP, simplified metabolic products derived from the major fuels and oxygen taken up by the myocardium are able to enter the citrate cycle that produces ATP, CO_2, and H_2O. The cristae on the inner surface of the inner mitochondrial membrane are the site of ATP synthesis. Each crista resembles a button projecting from the inner membrane and contains the enzymes concerned with ATP synthesis.

Sarcolemma and Glycocalyx

Because actin and myosin only contract in the presence of calcium, one of the major functions of the sarcolemma is to regulate with precision the intracellular calcium ion concentration. The extracellular concentration of calcium is about 1,000 times higher than the intracellular value, so that the sarcolemma must be impermeable to calcium ions, only allowing the passage of minute amounts required to trigger certain intracellular events concerned with contraction. The sarcolemma also by its pumps and exchangers (Chapter 4) maintains major differences in the ionic composition of intracellular and extracellular fluids. Lying between the sarcolemma and the extracellular space is a "twilight zone," the glycocalyx, which appears to help in the regulation of calcium ion entry into the myocytes.

The *glycocalyx* is the outermost layer of the cell, composed chiefly of complex carbohydrates called polysaccharides, often associated with proteins (glycoproteins). The latter have negative electrical charges that act to trap positively charged ions such as the calcium ions. Experimentally, the glycocalyx can be peeled away from the underlying sarcolemma by completely removing and then reintroducing extracellular calcium (the calcium paradox). Loss of the protective glycocalyx allows a normal concentration of extracellular calcium, otherwise harmless, to flood into the cardiac myocytes, causing massive damage.

The *lipid bilayer* is immediately within the glycocalyx and is usually regarded as the only true component of the sarcolemma (Fig. 3-5). The lipid bilayer is similar in composition to most external cell membranes, so that the general term "plasmalemma" is also used. Chemically, the *phospholipids* are the major constituent of this membrane. These lipids have a phosphate group that joins their *hydrophilic* (water-loving) heads to the *hydrophobic* (water-repelling) fatty acid tails, the latter pointing inward toward each other. Molecules with such opposite charges are called *amphiphiles* (Latin *amphi,* on both sides). When the sarcolemma breaks down in severe ischemia, liberation of amphiphiles can alter the balance of intracellular charges to have potentially toxic effects.

Integral proteins have highly specialized and varied functions. They are tightly held (hence the term "integral") in the sarcolemma by the side chains of their amino acids, which bind to the lipid tails in the center of the bilayer. Integral proteins control the flow of ions across the sarcolemma, some acting as ion channels, others as ion exchangers, and yet others as ion pumps (see Chapter 4).

Calcium binds to external binding sites on the sarcolemma and glycocalyx, both to the complex lipids containing phosphate groups (phospholipids) of the outer layer of the sarcolemmal bilayer and, in a more diffuse fashion, to the

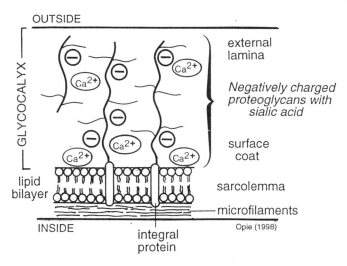

FIG. 3-5. Lipid bilayer and glycocalyx. The predominantly negative charges on the glycocalyx are thought to interact with positively charged calcium ions, thereby buffering the myocardial cells from the much higher external calcium concentration. See also Curry (1986).

negatively charged proteins of the glycocalyx (Fig. 3-5). When Langer (1985) noted that the amount of calcium that could be displaced was proportional to the force generated during contraction, he concluded that during the wave of electrical excitation passing over the sarcolemma, some of this superficially bound calcium could be displaced into the cell to help activate contraction. In some way, not fully understood, the wave of excitation can allow such bound calcium ions to enter through those integral proteins that function as calcium channels.

Channels and Ion Transport

Ion-selective channels are examples of membrane proteins. They open as the wave of electrical excitation travels across the myocardium to allow a controlled and sequential passage of minute amounts of sodium, calcium, and potassium ions across the sarcolemma, which is otherwise relatively impermeable to these ions. Thus, during electrical excitation, the opening of ion-selective channels alters the charges across the sarcolemma. This highly regulated series of changes in electrical charge (or *potential*) is called the *action potential.*

Sodium channels open first, to bring in positively charged sodium ions at a very rapid rate, thereby causing the equally rapid upstroke phase of the action potential. *Calcium channels* are relatively selective for the entry of calcium ions, which occurs somewhat slower and after most of the rapid entry of the sodium ions has ceased. Calcium ion entry accounts for at least part of the flat phase (*plateau*) of the action potential. *Potassium channels* are highly complex in their number and function, but some of them open toward the end of the action plateau phase of the action potential, to carry positive charges across the sarcolemma, thereby terminating the action potential. Although the function of each of these channels is complex, a reasonable simplification would be as follows. Opening of the sodium channel is crucial for the swift conduction of the electrical impulse throughout the heart. By rapidly changing the electrical charge across the sarcolemma, sodium entry creates conditions suitable for onward transmission of the impulse (see Chapter 4). Entry of calcium ions is concerned with the triggering of the contractile cycle (see frontispiece). Outward flow of potassium ions, by restoring the normal electrical charge of the cell membrane, prepares the myocardial cells for the next wave of depolarization.

Transverse Tubular System

The sarcolemma does not just line the outer surface of the cardiac myocyte but penetrates into the intracellular space to form a series of tubelike invaginations (Fig. 3-6). "It is by means of *T tubules* that both intra- and extra cellular domains are in the closest contact possible, short of fusing together" (Ferrari and Opie, 1992).

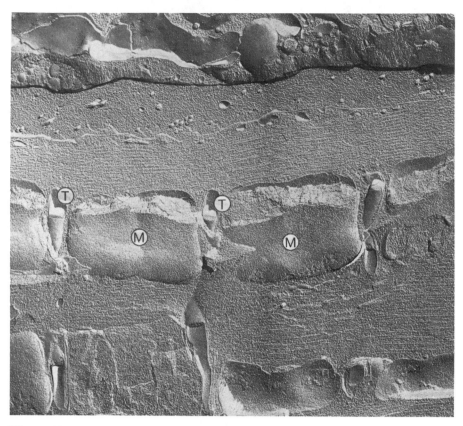

FIG. 3-6. T-tubular system. The extensive network lies between mitochondria (M) and penetrating the rows of sarcomeres at the Z lines, delineated by a freeze-fracture micrograph. The lumen of the T tubules (T) is continuous with the extracellular space and brings the extracellular fluid into the ventricular myocyte. For relation between T tubules and SR, see frontispiece. Original magnification ×31,580. From Scales (1981).

The salient features of the *T tubules* are as follows:

1. Because the T tubules are an extension of and have the same ultrastructure as the cell surface, they increase the surface area of the cell, at least by 30% (Table 3-4) and possibly much more, thereby facilitating the spread of the excitatory stimulus to within the cell.
2. The lumen of the T tubules at the surface of the cell is relatively wide, which ensures that an adequate supply of oxygen and nutrients, contained in the extracellular space, becomes available for transfer to intracellular space. Nonetheless, fluid in the T tubules is not exactly the same in composition as that in the extracellular space because communication is not entirely free.

3. T tubules contain a certain type of calcium channel, the L type, that responds to the wave of electrical excitation by allowing the entry of calcium ions to activate the sarcoplasmic reticulum (SR) to release much more calcium (see ensuing section).

Caveolae (Latin for small caves) are small folds that project inward from the sarcolemma to increase the membrane surface area. During myocardial development, caveolae may evolve into T tubules (Forbes and Sperelakis, 1995).

Sarcoplasmic Reticulum

The SR is crucial for the regulation of calcium ion movements within the cell. Cardiac SR can be sedimented from suitably treated cells by ultracentrifugation. When isolated, the SR takes on the appearance of little vesicles or granules. These still have the capacity for active transport and release of calcium, which is crucial for the regulation of cardiac contraction and relaxation. Calcium ions stored within the SR are released by the entry of a relatively small number of calcium ions from the T tubules. As cytosolic calcium increases, the crossbridge cycle is triggered. Reuptake of calcium ions by the SR lowers the cytosolic calcium ion concentration to cause relaxation. Anatomically, the SR is a fine network (Latin *reticulum,* small network) spreading throughout the myocytes, demarcated by its lipid bilayer, which is similar to that of the sarcolemma. Parts of the SR lie in close apposition to the T tubules (Fig. 3-7). Here the tubules of the SR expand into bulbous swellings, still hollow, which lie along the inner surface of the sarcolemma or are wrapped around the T tubules (Fig. 3-7). These expanded areas of the SR have several names: *subsarcolemmal cisternae* (Latin for baskets) or *junctional components.* Sometimes the cisternae occur in pairs lying astride the T tubule, the three components having the appearance of *triads.* The combination of one cisterna and the T tubule is a *diad.* The function of these units is to release calcium to initiate the contractile cycle (Fig. 3-8). The close physical contact between the cisternae and the sarcolemma is made even more intimate by the development of small *electron-dense feet* found at coupling sites. The *foot structure,* also called the *junctional channel complex,* is thought to facilitate communication between the T tubules and the SR. Thus, the wave of depolarization when it reaches the T tubules has only to send its messenger (calcium) on a short journey across the foot space to the calcium release channel of the SR, from where the calcium that triggers contraction originates.

The second part of the SR, the *longitudinal* or *network SR,* consists of ramifying tubules (see frontispiece) and is concerned with the uptake of calcium from the cytosol to initiate relaxation. At the start of diastole, the calcium pump located on this part of the SR rapidly transfers enough calcium from the cytosol to the interior. Such calcium is then thought to flow along the longitudinal tubules of the SR to reach the cisternae, then again to be released by the next wave of depolarization. (Note that these longitudinal tubules of the SR have a completely different function from those of the T tubules.)

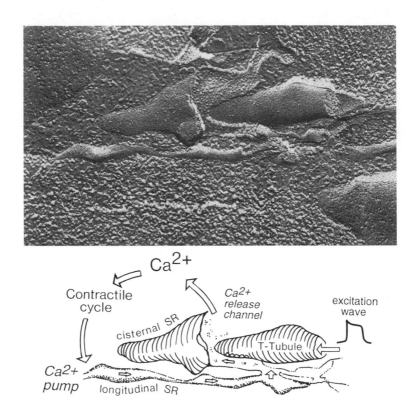

FIG. 3-7. Calcium kinetics and sarcoplasmic reticulum. Release of calcium from the cisternal or junctional component of the SR is rapid. In the heart it is potentiated by entry of calcium from the T tubule, around which the cisternal SR is wrapped. The uptake of calcium, which causes relaxation of the contractile proteins, probably occurs through the tubular network of the SR. Original magnification ×86,400. Freeze-fracture electron micrograph from Scales (1981).

The Nucleus

Cardiac myocytes usually contain only one nucleus, although binucleate and multinucleate cells are also found. Nuclei usually are located near the center of the cell and account for about 5% of the cell's volume. Almost all of the genetic information that is needed for each myocyte to maintain and repair its structure is contained in its nucleus or nuclei. Each nucleus is surrounded by an envelope formed by two membranes that are each about 10 nm thick. The envelope is perforated at frequent intervals, and the pores are believed to be responsible for the selective passage of chemical materials into and out of the nucleus.

The major role of the nucleus is to control the systems responsible for tissue maintenance and repair. The genetic information that is required for this process is stored as sequences of bases in DNA. The actual process of protein synthesis

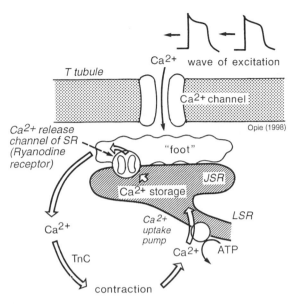

FIG. 3-8. Calcium-induced calcium release. Proposed role of wave of depolarization spreading down T tubule to release calcium ions across the lipid bilayer of the T tubule, and then to release many more calcium ions from the calcium release channel of the SR. See also Jorgensen et al. (1988).

takes place in the cytosol on very small particles called *ribosomes*. There must be a system that allows the coding information stored in the genes to be transferred to the amino acid assembly sites on the ribosomes. This function of information transfer is performed by a special form of ribonucleic acid called *messenger RNA* (mRNA), which leaves the nuclei throughout the nucleus pores, carrying within it the required coding sequence. mRNA is bound to ribosomes free in the cytosol or attached to a netlike system known as the *rough endoplasmic reticulum*. These bound ribosomes are lined up on the outside of the endoplasmic reticulum, giving a rough appearance. (Note the important distinction between the endoplasmic reticulum and the SR.) Hence, mRNA molecules originating in the nucleus alert the ribosomes to the particular amino acid sequences that are required. Another form of RNA, *transfer RNA*, supplies the required amino acids in activated form to the ribosomes, where the amino acids are joined in the sequence dictated by mRNAs. Once assembled, the proteins fold, associate with others, and are distributed throughout the cell.

The *Golgi apparatus* is functionally associated with the endoplasmic reticulum. It is concerned with the processing and completion of those proteins due for secretion from cells or for incorporation into lysosomes or membranes of the cell.

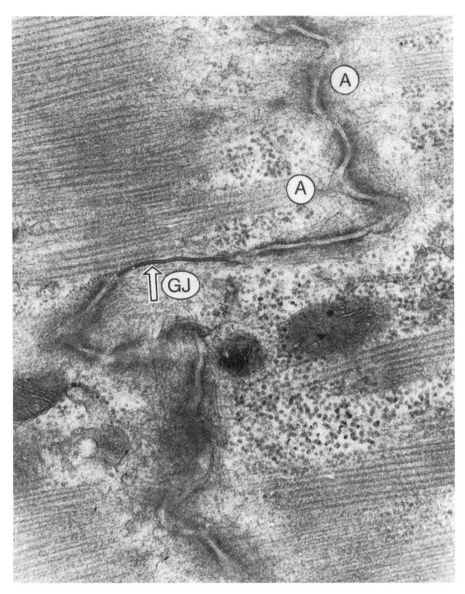

FIG. 3-9. Intercalated disk, which connects adjacent ventricular myocytes. The disk serves to anchor actin filaments, to bind cells to each other, and to communicate between cells. A, actin filaments inserting into fascia adherens; GJ, gap junction (see Fig. 2-6). Original magnification ×43,000. Courtesy of Dr. J. Moravec, Dijon, France.

Communication Between Cardiomyocytes

Where the ends of neighboring cardiac myocytes make contact with one another, the sarcolemma becomes highly specialized and altered in nature to form the *intercalated disk* (Fig. 3-9). The major part of the disk is where the actin filaments are inserted into the *fascia adherens junction* (Latin *fascia,* band; i.e., the adherent band). Some actin filaments actually run through localized micro-areas of the disk, called *spot desmosomes* (Greek *desmo,* band), which occupy about 1/20 of the disk surface. All these structures allow mechanical continuity between cardiac myocytes, thereby linking the force of contraction of one myocyte to that of its neighbors.

Gap junctions are microchannels passing through the intercalated disk to allow physical communication of the cytosol of one cell with that of the next. These structures are also called *nexus junctions* (Latin *nexus,* bond). A small part, perhaps 5% of the disk, occupies the space between the opposing surfaces of the adjacent cells (Fig. 3-10), reduced to only 1 or 2 nm, and microchannels appear within it, as if to connect the facing membranes of the opposing cells. These *connexons* probably transport small molecules and ions from cell to cell and also act as low-resistance electrical pathways. The molecular structures of the gap junction proteins (*connexins*) have now been identified (Kanter et al., 1992). The depolarizing current can spread directly from cell to cell through the connexons, explaining the heart's capacity to function as a group of cells with similar behavior (this is called a *syncytium;* Latin *syn,* together; *cytium,* cell). Connexons are very sensitive to an abnormal increase in cytosolic calcium concentrations as may

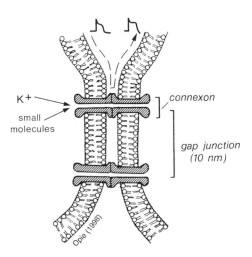

FIG. 3-10. Gap or nexus junction, where the distance between the adjacent cells is reduced to only 1 or 2 nm. Note the proposed connexons or microchannels that allow end-to-end communication between cells and are particularly prominent in Purkinje fibers.

occur in ischemia. Then the connexons close to seal off the damaged cells. Gap junctions also occur laterally between adjacent cardiomyocytes, allowing lateral connection, especially in atrial cells, where side-to-side connections are frequent.

MYOCYTE CYTOSKELETON

The term *cytoskeleton* includes those proteins that connect the contractile system to the cell membrane, connect sarcomeres to each other, and connect cells to the extracellular structures (Table 3-5). The cytoskeleton also includes the microtubular system, in which *tubulin* is found.

Besides actin and myosin, the myocyte contains *intermediate filaments* that are about 10 nm diameter and consist of different proteins including *desmin* (Fig. 3-11). It is organized in a three-dimensional network of interconnecting transverse and longitudinal fibers to form ringlike bands around the myofibrils at the Z-line level, to provide lateral interconnections between the Z bands, and to link the desmosomes. *α-Actinin* links the actin filaments at the site of the insertion into the Z band into a three-dimensional array (Fig. 3-12).

The cell adhesion molecule (*A-CAM*; also called *N-cadherin*) links two adjacent myocytes across the extracellular space because it is an important structural protein of the cell-to-cell adherens junction. *Vinculin* is an elongated molecule, like a balloon on a string, that has binding sites for other vinculin molecules and for α-actinin (Fig. 3-12). Through molecules such as α-actinin, vinculin binds to actin filaments and through other closely related molecules (probably including α-catenin) to N-cadherin in the adherence junction. Thus, vinculin constitutes a riblike network, running underneath the sarcolemma and helping to bind it to the Z line. In ischemia sustained beyond 120 minutes, vinculin is destroyed, a process that probably allows the sarcolemma to rupture more easily, thereby liberating intracellular enzymes and hastening cell death. *Integrin* is the transverse membrane protein that links the contractile system and the Z lines to the extracellular collagen matrix (Fig. 3-13). In transient ischemia followed by reperfusion, another protein of the cytoskeleton, *calspectin* is damaged and may contribute to reperfusion stunning.

CARDIAC CONNECTIVE TISSUE

Although it is clear that the cardiac connective tissue plays an important supportive mechanical role by surrounding the cellular components of the heart and binding them to each other, this network also may have additional and important metabolic functions. The connective tissue, also called the *extracellular matrix*, is produced largely by fibroblastic cells and contains collagen, as well as other important matrix proteins (Table 3-6). *Collagen* is a major determinant of myocardial tissue stiffness, and if it accumulates, it increases stiffness abnormally to alter myocardial function. On boiling, collagen becomes gelatinous, which explains the name (Greek for glue + production). Fibrous tissue formation may

TABLE 3-5. *Major proteins of the cytoskeleton matrix*

Name	Where found	Molecular properties	Proposed function
Desmin[a]	Z lines, myofibrillar attachment to sarcolemma. Major part of intermediate filaments.	MW 55 kDa, relatively flexible, hollow core, 7–11 mm thick	An intermediate filament protein that connects Z lines and prevents sarcomeres from slipping during contraction
Vinculin[a,b]	At attachment of myofibrils to Z lines and intercalated disks; in VSM cells at dense bands	MW 122 kDa; like a balloon on a string, 8 nm globular head, 19 nm tail	Binding sites: vinculin–vinculin, α-actinin, talin
N-cadherin[b]	Fascia adherens	MW 135 kDa, glycoprotein, calcium dependent	Links two adjacent cells across the EC space
Integrin[b]	Transmembrane protein with cell surface adhesion receptors	MW 130–160 kDa; external globular head with ligand binding site; small IC domain with talin binding site	Internal talin binding, external binding to collagen, laminin, and fibronectin
Talin[b]	With integrin	MW 213 kDa, elongated	Links integrin and vinculin to intercalated disks
α-actinin[b]	Z bands; dense bodies and dense bands in VSM cells	MW 95 kDa; rodlike, about 4 nm in diameter and 40 nm in length	Links tails of actin fibers at Z bands and cross-links actin filaments; links actin to dense bodies in VSM
Filamin[c]	Z bands and intercalated disks; close to actin in VSM	MW 270 kDa	Support of actin-intermediate filament system
Calspectin = spectrin[d]	Sarcolemma, intercalated disks, Z bands	α and β subunits; rod-shaped tetramers, each about 240 kDa	Links desmin to cell membrane

VSM, vascular smooth muscle; EC, extracellular; IC, intracellular; MW, molecular weight.

[a]Schaper et al. *Circulation* 1991;83:504.
[b]Ganote and Armstrong. *Cardiovasc Res* 1993;27:1387.
[c]Hüttner et al. In: Camilleri (ed). *Diseases of the Arterial Wall*. London: Springer-Verlag, 1989;3.
[d]Yoshida et al. *Circ Res* 1995;77:603.

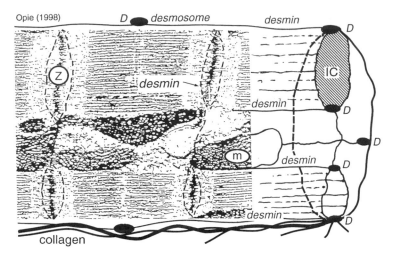

FIG. 3-11. Desmin in cardiomyocyte cytoskeleton. Note desmosomes (D), joined by desmin, that link cell membranes along intercalated (IC) disks. Desmin joins both longitudinally, running between the myofiber and transversely to encircle myofibers at the Z bands. M, mitochondria.

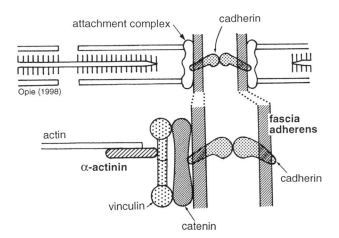

FIG. 3-12. Proteins of the fascia adherens joining the ends of cardiac myocytes. N-cadherin (A-CAM, adherens junction cell adhesion molecule) is calcium dependent and links the two adjacent intercalated disks. Vinculin binds other vinculin molecules (and a closely related protein, α-catenin), α-actinin, and talin, thereby anchoring the actin filaments to the fascia adherens.

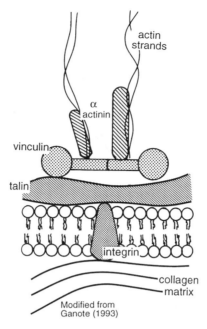

actin
strands

α
actinin

vinculin

talin

integrin

collagen
matrix

Modified from
Ganote (1993)

FIG. 3-13. Proteins of the cell-to-matrix junctions. Integrin, the transmembrane protein, links vinculin and talin to the collagen matrix. Modified from Ganote and Armstrong (1993) with permission.

TABLE 3-6. *Major proteins of the extracellular matrix*

Name	Where found	Molecular properties	Proposed function
Collagen[a]	Collagen matrix (Fig. 3-11)	MW 95–180 kDa, helical structure of three polypeptide chains, each of about 1,000 amino acids Type I: thick fibers; major part of collagen Type III: thinner fibers, 10% of total	Links myocytes, prevents excess stretch, transmits force from myofilaments to ventricular or vascular wall. Provides elasticity to aorta. In excess, causes myocardial fibrosis and contractile dysfunction. Determines stiffness of myocardium.
Fibronectin[b]	EC matrix	Two large chains linked by disulfide bonds; MW of each, 220 kDa	Essential meshwork for organization of other matrix proteins including collagen[d]
Elastin[c]	Vessel walls; subendocardial myocardium	MW about 140 kDa with elastic links between subunits	Major source of elasticity of arterial matrix. In atheroma, lipid content increases.

VSM, vascular smooth muscle; EC, extracellular; MW, molecular weight.
[a]Weber et al. *J Mol Cell Cardiol* 1994;26:279.
[b]Coller. In: Fossard et al. (eds). *The Heart and Cardiovascular System.* 2nd ed. New York: Raven, 1991;226.
[c]Robert and Birenbaut. In: Camilleri (ed). *Diseases of the Arterial Wall.* London: Springer-Verlag, 1989;46.
[d]Knowlton et al. *J Clin Invest* 1992;89:1060.

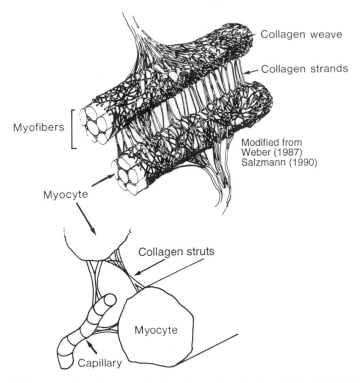

FIG. 3-14. Collagen matrix of the normal left ventricle. Groups of myocytes held together by the collagen weave are termed "myofibers." Myofibers are connected to one another by strands of collagen, whereas those between myocytes and their adjacent capillaries are by struts of collagen. Collagen is a basic protein of white fibrous material. On boiling, collagen becomes gelatinous, which explains the name (collagen = glue + production, from the Greek). Modified from Weber et al. (1987) and Salzmann et al. (1990).

be regulated by the renin–angiotensin–aldosterone system, which includes the possibility of local production of angiotension II (Weber et al., 1995). Collagen is organized into *collagen fibers* that are present in the extracellular space and lie close to the surface of the myocytes, forming an important part of the extracellular matrix within which the myocytes lie (Fig. 3-14). Collagen fibers extend from the surface of the cells to the tissue skeleton, as well as from cell to cell. These fine fibers and filaments act as struts to hold the myofibrils in position so that the pattern of contraction is orderly. The collagen matrix probably limits the amount by which the heart can be dilated in diseased states. The major types of cardiac collagen fibers are collagens I and III. Collagen I is organized into thick bundles and is strong enough to resist tensile stretch, even in the volume-overloaded heart. Collagen III cross-links with collagen I. Another type of collagen, type IV, is a major component of *basement membranes*, where it attaches to the glycoproteins fibronectin and laminin. Hypothetically, the increased collagen and greater severity of fibrosis in diseased states is linked to a marked increase in myocardial stiffness and depressed systolic as well as diastolic function (Conrad et al., 1995).

Elastic fibers containing *elastin* (Table 3-6) are found in close proximity to collagen, for example, around the collagen skeleton, on the surface of capillaries, and around the myocytes. These elastic fibers have properties similar to those of polymeric rubber, accounting in part for the elasticity of the myocardium. Another component of the elasticity resides in the crossbridges so that the myocardium becomes less elastic as the crossbridges interact during systole. A third elastic component lies in the titan molecules that link myosin filaments to the Z lines.

Glycoproteins, also called the *proteoglycans*, are proteins of one or more attached short sugar chains, such as chondroitin and heparan sulfate, as well as fibronectin and laminin. Also present are various growth factors, including insulin growth factor, fibroblast growth factor, transforming growth factor β, and platelet-derived growth factor. *Fibronectin* is a glycoprotein that influences cellular properties, including growth and hormonal repair, through an interaction with fibronectin cell surface receptors. Hence, fibronectin increases after experimental myocardial infarction, possibly the result of synthesis by cardiac fibroblast. *Cardiac fibroblasts* are mesenchymal cells that potentially produce components of the extracellular matrix, including collagen and fibronectin, in response to simulation by growth factors and/or angiotensin II. *Laminin* is a glycoprotein of the basement membrane that has a molecular weight almost double that of fibronectin and is composed of three subunits linked by disulfide bonds.

The *matrix metalloproteins* include the various enzymes that break down all the types of collagen (*collagenases*) as well as other components of the extracellular matrix, including laminin, fibronectin, and other glycoproteins. The balance between synthesis of extracellular matrix collagen by growth factors, angiotensin II, and aldosterone versus degradation by the metalloproteinases has important implications for the mechanical properties and hence the function of the myocardium.

ATRIAL CELLS

Atrial contraction helps to fill the left ventricle during the relaxation phase (see Fig. 1-2). The force of contraction that must be developed is low because the left ventricular diastolic pressure is just above zero. Thus, in contrast to ventricular myocytes, atrial cells do not have prominent myofibrils, and other specialized structures concerned with contraction such as T tubules are rare. Atrial cells are smaller than ventricular cells and are elliptical rather than rodlike in shape (Table 3-1). There is also a prominent collagen matrix that may help to avoid overdistension of the atria. To help spread the electrical impulse rapidly throughout the atria, there are side-to-side as well as end-to-end junctions between the cells. Whether there are, in addition, specialized conduction pathways in the atria is still controversial.

VASCULAR SMOOTH MUSCLE CELLS

The major function of these cells is to maintain vascular tone and hence to regulate the peripheral vascular resistance. There are two types of contraction, namely phasic and tonic, the latter being sustained. Vascular smooth muscular cells differ from myocardial cells in several major ways (Fig. 3-15). First, they are approximately fusiform in shape, which allows them to form the muscular tube of the arteries. In length, these cells are 100 to 500 μm and in diameter about 5 to 6 μm thick. There is a very large surface-to-volume ratio, made even larger (about 70%) by the appearance of numerous prominent surface vesicles (*caveolae*). These caveolae probably have a function similar to that of T tubules in myocardial cells, conveying surface electrical charges to the SR. A second difference from myocardial cells is that vascular muscle cells do not need to respond rapidly to a wave of depolarization because contraction and relaxation are so much slower. Thus, the SR is relatively poorly developed. Nonetheless, it remains the chief organelle concerned with the regulation of cytosolic calcium concentrations. The arrangements of other organelles and the contractile filaments are also different. Organelles such as the Golgi apparatus, mitochondria, and lysosomes are situated chiefly in the *sarcoplasmic core* where they surround the nucleus (Forbes, 1995).

The *myofilaments* lie in the more peripheral part of the cell, away from the central organelles. In this peripheral myoplasm, there is no clear pattern of cross-striations, as in cardiomyocytes. Although, in general, the myofilaments lie in

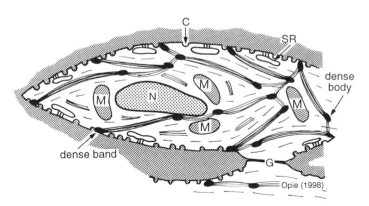

FIG. 3-15. Structure of vascular smooth muscle cell. Note the absence of well-defined muscular striations, with prominent caveolae (C), the relative absence of mitochondria (M), the dense bands or bodies (DB), and the gap junctions (G) between adjacent cells.

the same longitudinal direction as do the vascular muscle cells, the exact pattern has not yet been determined. The myofilaments are composed of three types of filaments: thin (actin), thick (myosin), and intermediate. Actin filaments 5 to 8 nm in diameter are interspersed with myosin filaments 15 to 20 nm in diameter. *Intermediate filaments*, about 10 nm in diameter, consist largely of a protein called *vimentin*. Hypothetically, such filaments contribute to the cytoskeleton of vascular muscle cells.

Myofilaments are often grouped into bundles that insert into dense bodies, the equivalent of the Z line in cardiac myocytes. Some dense bodies are free floating in the cytosol, whereas others are subsarcolemmal in site, when they are often called dense bands. Forced transmission from the contractile myofilaments to the cell surface takes place by insertion of actin filaments into the subsarcolemmal dense bands. Dense bands and bodies contain *α-actinin* that helps to cross-link the actin filaments as in the Z lines of striated muscle. Not all actin filaments are myosin linked and attached to dense bodies and bands. Some are held together by cross-linking intermediate proteins. The role of these noncontractile actin fibers is not clear. One possibility is that they could be fixed at any length by cross-linking filaments to permit *tonic contractions*. Another proposal is that the actin fibers could be organized into bundles in response to activation of a signal system involving protein kinase C (see Chapter 9) to cause a calcium-independent contraction. In contrast, in response to depolarization, cytosolic calcium increases to activate the calcium-binding protein calmodulin, thereby allowing interaction of actin and myosin, which may explain *phasic vascular contractions*. The molecular mechanisms underlying phasic and tonic contractions are not yet clearly understood.

From the electrophysiologic point of view, the shape of the action potential is different from that of myocardial cells. Starting from a less negative voltage, the upstroke is much slower because the sodium channel that is associated with rapid conduction in cardiac cells is so low in its activity in vascular muscle cells. The plateau of the action potential is not sustained, in part because the opening of the calcium channel is brief. Outward depolarizing potassium currents play a major role in terminating the action potential and in maintaining the resting potential, as in cardiac cells. The depolarizing calcium current can be opened not only by voltage, but by occupation of several receptors that respond to vasoconstrictive agonists such as α_1-adrenergic stimulation or to angiotensin II.

Besides their contractile function, vascular smooth muscle cells can have an important synthetic role. In normal adult vascular muscle cells, this system is quiescent, yet it can be activated to play an important role in the pathologic growth of vascular cells that occurs in atheroma formation and in restenosis. These muscle cells contain prominent nuclei and retain the capacity both to reproduce themselves by hyperplasia and to grow larger by hypertrophy in response, for example, to a sustained intra-arterial pressure as in systemic hypertension. They can manufacture all the principal components of the vascular matrix and its connective tissue, including collagen and the elastic fibers. This function is especially evident during periods of growth and development, when there is an evident organelle system (including an extensive rough endoplasmic reticulum and Golgi complex) that secretes the required macromolecules.

SUMMARY

1. *The basic unit of the contracting myocardial cell is the myocyte,* consisting chiefly of the contractile proteins. Z lines terminate the myocyte on either side. Thin actin filaments extend inward from the Z lines and interdigitate with the thicker and much larger myosin filaments. The latter extend from the center of the myofibril toward the Z lines without touching them. Myosin fibers are indirectly linked to the Z lines by large titan elastic molecules. When contraction is initiated by the arrival of calcium ions, the myosin heads flex to move the actin fibers in such a way that the Z lines come closer together.

2. *To regulate the intracellular concentration of calcium ions requires a series of interacting events.* The external cell membrane or sarcolemma has embedded in its lipid bilayer specialized proteins that act as channels. The calcium channels allow the entry of relatively small amounts of calcium ions during each wave of electrical excitation. The electrical impulses are conveyed into the interior of the myocytes by invaginations of the sarcolemma called T tubules. These lie in close proximity to that part of the sarcoplasmic reticulum (the cisternae or junctional component) that stores calcium ions. The sarcoplasmic reticulum and the adjoining T tubules are physically linked by specialized structures called feet, which are thought to guide calcium ions entering the myocyte through the T tubule to the specific receptor that releases calcium from the sarcoplasmic reticulum. This increase in internal cytosolic calcium concentration triggers contraction.

3. *Relaxation of the contractile proteins is achieved by the uptake of calcium ions into the longitudinal component of the SR,* in which the calcium ions travel back to the storage sites on the cisternae to await the arrival of the next excitation wave.

4. *Communication between myocytes occurs at the gap junctions at the ends and sides of the cells,* by minute conducting channels called connexons. These regulate the passage of ions and small molecules from one cell to the next. Also, the electrical impulses pass preferentially along the gap junctions.

5. *Within each cardiac myocyte is a cytoskeleton that supports the contractile proteins and links them to the Z lines.* Other parts of the cytoskeleton link the myocytes to the extracellular matrix.

6. *The supporting connective tissue cells of the matrix bind groups of myofibers together and provide a framework for the contracting cells.* Furthermore, this extracellular matrix is metabolically active. When fibrous tissue is abnormally increased in amount, myocardial contraction and relaxation are impaired.

7. *Atrial cells differ ultrastructurally from ventricular cells,* being smaller, with smaller T tubules and less prominent sarcomeres. Atrial cells also have

prominent side-to-side gap junctions. These differences from ventricular myocytes may explain the lesser force of atrial contraction and the far more rapid conduction of the electrical impulse through atrial than through ventricular contractile cells.

8. *Vascular smooth muscle cells are different in shape, ultrastructure, and function from striated myocardial cells.* These cells are adapted to much slower rates of contraction and relaxation and to the maintenance of sustained tonic contractions. Thereby they help to regulate the resistance against which the heart pumps out blood.

9. *The cardiac conduction system is composed of cells that have poorly developed contractile structures* and are adapted to rapid conduction (Table 3-2).

STUDENT QUESTIONS

1. Describe the major features of the ultrastructure of the myofiber.
2. Describe in outline form the interaction between the thick and thin filaments during contraction.
3. What are T tubules? Do they have any role in the contractile cycle?
4. Describe in outline form the major functions of the sarcoplasmic reticulum.
5. How do conducting cells differ in their ultrastructure from ordinary contracting myocardial cells? What are these conducting cells called?
6. How do atrial cells differ in their ultrastructure from ventricular cells? Are there any explanations for these differences?

CARDIOLOGIST-IN-TRAINING QUESTIONS

1. How does the sarcolemma protect the cardiac myocyte from cytosolic calcium overload? Is there any special role for the glycocalyx?
2. T tubules: what role do they play in initiating cardiac contraction?
3. What is the anatomy and function of the sarcoplasmic reticulum?
4. How do atrial and ventricular cells differ?
5. How do cardiac and vascular myocytes differ in their ultrastructure?

REFERENCES

1. Brilla C, Janicki JS, Weber KT. Impaired diastolic function and coronary reserve in genetic hypertension. Role of interstitial fibrosis and medial thickening of intramyocardial coronary arteries. *Circ Res* 1991;69:107–115.
2. Conrad CH, Brookes WW, Hayes JA, et al. Myocardial fibrosis and stiffness with hypertrophy and heart failure in the spontaneously hypertensive rat. *Circulation* 1995;91:161–170.
3. Curry FE. Determinants of capillary permeability: a review of mechanisms based on single capillary studies in the frog. *Circ Res* 1986;59:367–380.
4. Ferrari R, Opie LH. In: *Atlas of the Myocardium.* New York: Raven, 1992;60.
5. Forbes MS. Vascular smooth muscle cells and other periendothelial cells of mammalian heart. In: Sperelakis N (ed). *Physiology and Pathophysiology of the Heart.* Boston: Kluwer Academic, 1995;803–826.

6. Forbes MS, Sperelakis N. Ultrastructure of mammalian cardiac muscle. In: Sperelakis N (ed). *Physiology and Pathophysiology of the Heart.* Boston: Kluwer Academic, 1995;1–35.
7. Ganote C, Armstrong S. Ischaemia and the myocyte cytoskeleton: review and speculation. *Cardiovasc Res* 1993;27:1387–1403.
8. Jorgensen AO, Broderick R, Somlyo AP, Somlyo AV. Two structurally distinct calcium storage sites in rat cardiac sarcoplasmic reticulum: an electron microprobe analysis study. *Circ Res* 1988;63: 1060–1069.
9. Kanter HL, Saffitz JE, Beyer EC. Cardiac myocytes express multiple gap junction proteins. *Circ Res* 1992;70:438–444.
10. Langer GA. The effect of pH on cellular and membrane calcium binding and contraction of myocardium. A possible role for sarcolemmal phospholipid in EC coupling. *Circ Res* 1985;57:374–382.
11. Olivetti G, Melissari M, Capasso JM, Anversa P. Cardiomyopathy of the aging human heart. Myocyte loss and cellular hypertrophy. *Circ Res* 1991;68:1560–1568.
12. Salzmann JL, Labopin M, Belichard P, et al. Collagen remodelling in cardiac hypertrophy. In: Swynghedauw B (ed). *Research in Cardiac Hypertrophy and Failure.* London: INSERM/John Libbey Eurotext, 1990;293–306.
13. Scales DJ. Aspects of the mammalian cardiac sarcotubular system revealed by freeze-fracture electron microscopy. *J Mol Cell Cardiol* 1981;13:373–380.
14. Weber KT, Clark WA, Janicki JS, Shroff SG. Physiologic versus pathologic hypertrophy and the pressure-overloaded myocardium. *J Cardiovasc Pharmacol* 1987;10(suppl 6):47–49.
15. Weber KT, Sun Y, Katwa LC, Cleutjens JP. Connective tissue: a metabolic entity? *J Mol Cell Cardiol* 1995;27:107–120.

PART II

Electrophysiology and Electrocardiogram

4

Channels, Pumps, and Exchangers

The crucial two qualities of the sarcolemma are (1) the capacity to maintain vast gradients of ions and enzymes between the intracellular and extracellular environments (Fig. 4-1) and (2) the capacity to respond to the wave of depolarization by the brief opening and closing of highly specific ion channels. Several consequences follow, including triggering of the contractile mechanism in the case of cardiomyocytes.

When the electrical charge is not flowing, during diastole, the inside of the cell is negatively charged and the outside of the cell is positively charged so that the sarcolemma is *polarized*. This polarity is lost and reversed during the ionic movements that accompany the wave of electrical excitation, a process called *depolarization*. The juxtaposition of the depolarized and polarized cells allows current to flow between these cells with differing polarities so that the current spreads further and other adjacent cells become depolarized (see Chapter 5). The initial phase of depolarization, by changing the membrane potential from its resting negative value, allows the opening of *voltage-gated channels* for sodium and calcium ions that carry positive charges to within the cell, which explains the temporary reversal of polarity. Thereafter, the outward flow of potassium ions is the major factor causing *repolarization*. This sequence of electrical changes during the cardiac action potential can be divided into five arbitrary phases: phases 0, 1, 2, 3, and 4 (Fig. 4-2). There are substantial differences between Purkinje cells, adapted for fast conduction of the cardiac impulse, and ventricular cells, adapted to generate pressure. During the rapid phase of initial depolarization (phase 0), the Purkinje cells reach a greater positive value and then repolarize much more rapidly (phase 1) before the plateau phase (phase 2) is reached. The whole duration of the action potential is shorter in Purkinje fibers, so that repolarization (phase 3) is relatively more rapid in these fibers. Looking at the underlying currents (bottom panel, Fig. 4-2), the sodium channel plays a more prominent role in Purkinje fibers and the calcium channel in ventricular myocytes.

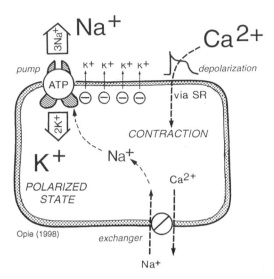

FIG. 4-1. Ionic balance in a cardiomyocyte. The potassium concentration is much higher within than without the cell, whereas sodium is much higher outside than inside the cell. These differential concentrations are maintained by the activity of the sodium–potassium pump using energy in the form of ATP. A high internal potassium concentration in turn promotes outward transsarcolemmal diffusion of a relative minute number of potassium ions thereby creating a negative charge within the sarcolemma and thereby the polarized state. Note calcium ion entry during the action potential leading to contraction, and outward transport of the calcium ions that have entered the cell by the sodium–calcium exchanger.

This difference is understandable because the main task of Purkinje fibers is to rapidly conduct the wave of excitation, and the main task of ventricular cells is to contract and to generate pressure (Fig. 4-3).

It should be stressed that the ionic movements accompanying the waves of excitation involve only minute numbers of ions across the sarcolemma, whereas the overall cell content of these ions remains virtually unchanged. Thus, the opening of sodium and calcium channels during depolarization leads to a small net gain of these ions. To restore ionic balance, calcium ions leave the cardiomyocyte as sodium ions enter through the sodium–calcium exchanger. Sodium ions are therefore gained both by the sodium channel and by this exchange system. Activity of the sodium–potassium pump is then required to pump sodium out of the cell against a concentration gradient (Fig. 4-4).

RESTING MEMBRANE POTENTIAL

Starting with a hypothetical resting cell with equal concentrations of the principal charge-bearing ions (Na^+, K^+, Cl^-) on either side of the sarcolemma, it is interesting to see how the resting membrane potential could be generated. The calcium ion can be left out of consideration because its permeability is so low.

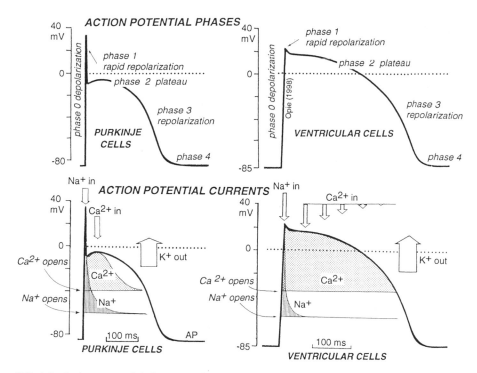

FIG. 4-2. Action potential phases and currents. The four phases of the cardiac action potential (top) and the underlying currents (bottom) with Purkinje cells on the left and ventricular cells on the right. The rapid entry of sodium ions accounts for the initial phase of rapid depolarization of the action potential. Calcium ions enter chiefly by the slow calcium channel. After entry of positively charged sodium and calcium ions, the cell is fully depolarized. Then potassium channels open. The outward flow of positively charged potassium ions largely explains repolarization. Finally the cell re-enters the state of polarization. Purkinje cells, adapted for fast conduction of the cardiac impulse, have a phase 0 that is relatively more prominent than in ventricular cells. The latter, adapted for contraction, have a more prominent plateau phase with more prolonged calcium ion entry.

The sodium–potassium pump, localized to the sarcolemmal membrane (Table 4-1), actively transfers potassium ions inward to give a high intracellular potassium concentration. As potassium accumulates in high concentrations on the inner surface, some of the ions start to move back again to the outer surface because the sarcolemma is normally relatively highly permeable to potassium ions, that is, the *conductance* to K^+ is high. As these K^+ ions cross the sarcolemma, they leave behind unbalanced negative charges so that the cell becomes polarized with a resting membrane potential of about −85 mV in the case of the ventricular myocyte. Only a small fraction of the total cell K^+ ions are involved in the generation of the resting membrane potential. To depolarize fully requires less than 1 µmole/kg of electrically unbalanced K^+ movement compared with the ventricular content of 70 mmole/kg (Table 4-2). The appar-

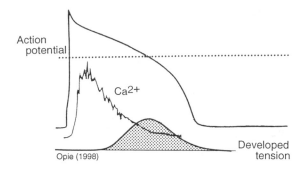

FIG. 4-3. Ventricular action potential, cytosolic calcium, and developed tension. Note that in this guinea pig papillary muscle preparation there is a small delay between phase 0 (rapid depolarization, Fig. 4-2) and the start of the calcium transient, because the sodium channel opens before the calcium channel. The delay between the peak of the calcium transient and the peak of muscle contraction (developed tension) is because the calcium ion concentration must increase to a certain critical value to trigger the actin–myosin interaction.

ent paradox is that the high internal concentration of potassium, a positively charged ion within the cell, is associated with a negative internal charge at the inner layer of the sarcolemma as just described.

By contrast, sodium ions pumped out of the cell accumulate on the outer surface of the sarcolemma and tend to diffuse inward (Fig. 4-4). The latter process is much slower than the outward diffusion of potassium ions because the sarcolemma is so much less permeable to sodium than to potassium. Therefore, sodium ions contribute little to the resting membrane potential.

The activity of the sodium–potassium pump also helps to generate the resting membrane potential. A theoretical example may be given. Let 400,000 Na^+ and K^+ ions be pumped per millisecond per unit area (Woodbury, 1963). Suppose that of the 400,000 K^+ ions pumped inward, 200 K^+ ions will diffuse outward. By contrast, supposing that only 4 Na^+ ions diffuse inward due to the much lower conductance than that of potassium (Fig. 4-4), there would now be a charge difference of 196 negative ions on the inside of the sarcolemma. It is this difference in charges that causes the electrical potential. The actual contribution of potassium to this potential can be calculated using the *Nernst equation*:

$$E_m = -61.5 \log K_i/K_o$$

where K_o is the external potassium ion concentration, K_i is the internal potassium ion concentration (Table 4-2), and E_m is the electrical potential. If the external potassium were 4 mmol/L and the internal value 140 mmol/L, the calculated *equilibrium potential* for potassium would be −93 mV; 80 mmol/L is a better value for the active intracellular K^+ concentration (K^+ *activity*), so the calculated equilibrium potential is in reality about −78 mV. Up to −10 mV can be generated by the electrogenic nature of the sodium–potassium pump, which pumps in 2 K^+ ions for 3 Na^+ ions extruded (Fig. 4-4). The sum total of −88 mV is close to the

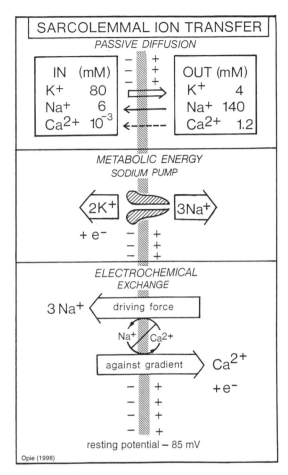

FIG. 4-4. Non-channel ion transfer across the sarcolemma. Note roles of passive diffusion, Na/Ca exchange, and sodium–potassium pump (sodium pump). The intracellular concentrations are an approximation for those free to act, i.e., the activities. The Na/Ca exchange can reverse according to the transmembrane potential and the relative concentrations of each ion on each side of the membrane. For transfer of ions by channel opening and closing during action potential, see Fig. 4-2.

measured value of −85 mV. Nonetheless, to be exact, sodium and chloride ions also contribute, and their permeability is also considered by the far more evolved *Goldman field equation* (Goldman, 1943).

In the idealized, simplified cell just described, it is assumed that intracellular ions are distributed uniformly throughout the cell. In reality, the apparent *concentration* of an ion in the heart cell must be distinguished from its *activity* (Table 4-2). When a ventricular biopsy is taken, the apparent concentration or *content* of the ion is the value per unit mass. To correct the content to the intra-

TABLE 4-1. *Approximate density of channels, pumps, and receptors in ventricular sarcolemmal membrane*

	Per μm^2 of sarcolemma
Sodium–potassium pump	About 400
Sodium channel	16
Calcium channel (DHP binding sites)[a]	25
Calcium channel (L-type)[b]	1.2
Calcium channel (T-type)[b]	0.1
Potassium channels	
ATP sensitive[c]	10
I$_{k1}$ (inward rectifier)[d]	1
I$_k$ (delayed rectifier)[d]	1
β-adrenergic receptor	2
Muscarinic receptor	6

[a]Aiba and Creazzo. *Circ Res* 1993;72:396–402; Wibo et al. *Circ Res* 1991;68:662–673.
[b]Rose. *J Physiol* 1992;456:267–284.
[c]Nichols and Lederer. *J Physiol* 1990;423:91–110.
[d]Coetzee. *Cardiovasc Drugs Ther* 1992;6:201–208.
Other data from Reuter (1984) and Colvin et al. (1983).

cellular concentration requires allowance for that component of the ion that is in the *extracellular* space, which in the case of sodium is considerable. Thus, the limits of the extracellular space must be defined to allow correction for those ions outside the cell. Of more importance, therefore, is the *activity* of the ion—the actual concentration that is in a free state in cytosolic water and is physiologically active. Measurements of the activities of sodium and potassium by microelectrodes show that only a part of the cellular value of each ion is electrically active, so that the gradient across the sarcolemma for both sodium and

TABLE 4-2. *Intracellular and extracellular concentrations of ions in normal heart*

Ion	Extracellular concentration		Apparent ventricular content (mmol/kg wet wt)	Activity or intracellular concentration ionized in cytosol (mmol/L)	References
	Total (mmol/L)	Ionized (mmol/L)			
Na$^+$	140	140	40	About 6	a
K$^+$	4	4	70	About 80	a
Mg^{2+}	1.20	0.60	8	About 0.6–0.9	b,c
Ca^{2+}	2.50	1.25	0.6	0.0003–0.001	d
Cl$^-$	140	140	25	About 25	e

[a]Dalby et al. *Cardiovasc Res* 1981;15:588. Values refer to activities. See Lee and Fozzard, *J Gen Physiol* 1975;65:695.
[b]Page and Polimeni. *J Physiol* 1972;224:221.
[c]Steenbergen et al. *Circulation* 1989;80(suppl II):19.
[d]Jennings and Shen. *Myocardiology* 1972;1:639.
[e]Desilets et al. *Circ Res* 1994;75:862–869.

potassium is about 20-fold. For calcium, the intracellular ionized concentration in diastole is very low, about 10,000 times below the extracellular value.

CURRENT FLOW THROUGH CHANNELS

Ions will only permeate the membrane by some type of carrier, such as a channel, exchanger, or pump. If through a channel, this occurs only when the channel is in the open state. Ion movement through open channels is governed by two factors: (1) the potential (electrical driving force) across the membrane and (2) the concentration gradient across the membrane for that particular ion. These two factors provide the *net driving force*. The current-carrying capacity of the sarcolemma is influenced by three factors:

$$I = N \times i \times p$$

where I = total current (over the whole sarcolemma), N = number of open channels, i = current through each of the channels, and p = probability of channel opening.

The word *potential* is derived from potent, meaning power. The resting membrane potential is the electrical driving force across the membrane resulting from the charge differences.

Current literally means running in Latin. An electrical current is a flow of electricity due to the difference in potential between two points or poles. This difference is measured in volts. The actual amount of current flow depends not only on the voltage but on the resistance to flow and is measured in *amperes*. One ampere is defined as 1 volt acting through a *resistance* of 1 ohm. The *voltage* is the electrical force resulting from the differences in potential across the sarcolemma. It is the voltage that actually causes the current to flow, as, for example, when sodium ions enter the cell (Fig. 4-2). During the passage of the electrical wave, as the inner layer of the sarcolemma becomes depolarized, the sodium channel is opened by the process of *voltage activation*.

STRUCTURE OF CHANNELS

Ion channels are pore-forming membrane proteins that span the lipid bilayer to allow a highly selective pathway into the cell when the channel changes from a *closed* to an *open state*. A simplified model of how channels open and close during the voltage changes associated with the action potential was initially evolved from electrophysiologic considerations, and is the basis of the present molecular proposal. Hypothetically, each channel is guarded by two or more *gates* that control its opening and closing (Fig. 4-5). Ions can pass through the channel only when both gates are open, a process that responds to changes in the voltage, both being *voltage-operated gates*. When both activation and inactivation gates are open, the inward flow of sodium or calcium ions through their respective channels produces the sodium and calcium inward currents.

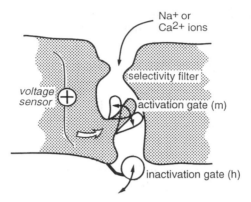

FIG. 4-5. Channel pore model, showing activation and inactivation gates. The selectivity filter allows a specific ion to enter. The voltage sensor is a highly charged segment (helix) of the membrane-spanning domain (see Fig. 4-6) responding to the voltage changes during depolarization and repolarization. The sensor "tells" the activation and inactivation gates to open and close.

Molecular Structure of Ion Channels. Modern techniques of molecular biology and immunology have allowed cloning and sequencing of channel proteins (Tomaselli et al., 1993). From the evolutionary point of view, perhaps a very simple potassium channel served as the basis from which more complex channels evolved (Fig. 4-6). There is a striking molecular similarity between the sodium and calcium channels. This conservation of structure is probably common to all voltage-gated ion channels and suggests that there is a gene superfamily. Both sodium and calcium channels have in their major α_1-subunit four repeating transmembrane domains, very similar to each other in structure. When antibodies are directed against these domains, the channel is inactivated (Grant, 1990), suggesting that crucial properties such as voltage sensitivity are located within these structures. In addition to the major α_1-subunit, both sodium and calcium channels contain a number of other subunits of ill-defined function, such as the β-subunit.

Each of the four transmembrane domains is made up of six helices. In each domain, one specific helical segment, called S4, is rich in amino acids and highly positively charged and may act as the voltage sensor (Fig. 4-6). As the wave of depolarization reaches the ion channel, the charges on the *voltage sensor* respond and include conformational changes in the channel pore that admits the ions and is thought to be formed by the four domains that make one α_1-subunit; these domains are folded in on each other, somewhat like four beer cans placed next to each other to form the channel pore between them (Fig. 4-7). Technically, one functioning sodium or calcium pore is formed by the union of four H5 or P loops, each lying between helices S5 and S6 of each of the four domains that make one α_1-subunit (Tomaselli et al., 1993). In the case of the voltage-operated potassium channel K_v, there are four separate subunits, each with six segments, that make up one pore (Fig. 4-6).

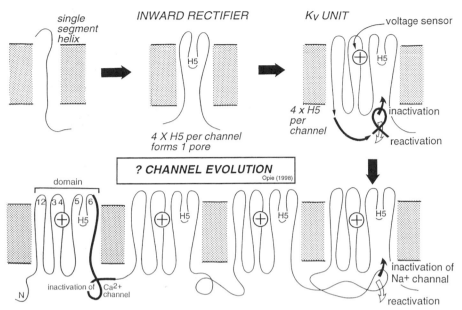

FIG. 4-6. Possible channel evolution. Hypothetically, primitive cells required potassium entry to act as a molecular signal. The simplest structure is with a single transmembrane helix (span) previously thought to be a channel and called K_{MIN}. It cannot function on its own. Next came the inward rectifier, with two spans and one H5 loop; four of these are required to function. Potassium channel structure became progressively more complex until evolving into the voltage-dependent potassium channel K_V. Even this cannot function on its own but requires four pore-forming subunits with four pore (P or H5) loops to make one functioning channel, i.e., 4×6 spans = 24 spans. Sodium and calcium channels are more highly evolved, serving functions such as conduction (sodium) and contraction (calcium). Both consist of a long polypeptide chain, with four transmembrane domains. Each domain consists of six helices or spans with a total of 24 spans. Helix S4, the fourth span, is highly charged (+) and thought to be the voltage sensor that activates the pore that transmits the ions (see Fig. 4-5).

Gating Kinetics. Functionally, the Hodgkin-Huxley hypothesis proposes that channels pass through three sequences: resting, active, and inactivated (Katz, 1993). In the *resting state*, the activation gate is shut, and the inactivation gate is open. In the *active state* early during depolarization, both gates are open (Fig. 4-5), and the current flows. With increasing depolarization, the inactivation gate shuts, the current ceases to flow, and the channel becomes inactivated. Next, the channel is reactivated (h gate opens) to resume the resting state. Each of these states is thought to be interchangeable in response to voltage (resting to active state and vice versa) or continued depolarization (conversion to inactivated state) or repolarization (reconversion to resting state). More complex models may be more accurate (Bennet et al., 1995).

The movement of an ion across these gates at any given instant depends on (1) the voltage and (2) the time after the onset of depolarization. In technical

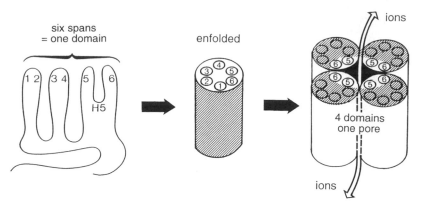

FIG. 4-7. Ion channel structure and function. The basic structure is that of six transmembrane spans and one pore-forming loop, H5. Four of these domains, when enfolded, make one channel pore, each contributing their S5 and S6 spans with linking H5 loops. The resultant functional pore allows the transmission of ions. For sodium and calcium channels, four domains are joined by linker loops to make one α_1-subunit (see Fig. 4-6), whereas for potassium, each six-span domain is a separate subunit (see Fig. 4-15).

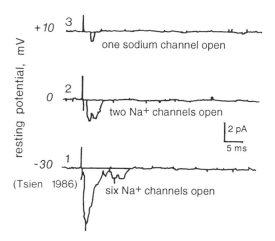

FIG. 4-8. Sodium current in single channels. The patch recordings are the summated values of single channels. The membrane potential just before depolarization (holding potential, V_m) was made progressively more positive in relation to the resting potential (1 = –30 mV; 2 = 0 mV; 3 = +10 mV). The I_{Na} generated in single channels was recorded when the cell depolarized to a value 40 mV above the resting membrane potential (RP). Straight and noisy lines indicate average baseline and single-channel current levels, respectively. As the holding potential was made less negative, the number of sodium channels that opened in response to the test depolarization decreased (from six to two to one). From Tsien (1986) with permission.

terms, this process is both *voltage gated* and *time dependent*. The time factor is of considerable importance because the calcium channels only start to open fully by the time the majority of the sodium channels has already closed. It is thought that only a small percentage of the potentially active channels operate at any one time.

In a single myocyte, there are many thousands of each type of ion channel, constituting a *multichannel preparation* that behaves in a complex way, being a summation of the behavior of the many thousands of individual channels in that cell. Each individual channel is, at any given time and at any given voltage, either open or closed (Figs. 4-8 and 4-9). Opening takes place in bursts (Fig. 4-9). When depolarization is initiated, the individual sodium channels are more likely to be in the open state, so that there is an increased *probability of*

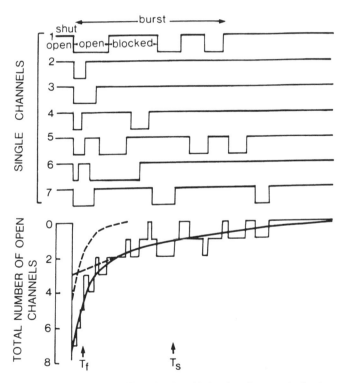

FIG. 4-9. Channels open in bursts. The simulated behavior of seven single channels is shown in the upper panel. All seven opened (downward deflection) nearly synchronously in response to stimulation at zero time. Each channel had a different degree of block, and each produced only one burst of openings before it finally shut. For example, channel 1 had two blockages and three openings before it shut, whereas channel 2 had only one opening. The lower panel shows the sum of all seven individual records. The initial decline was rapid (time constant T_f) as open channels became blocked, but the current thereafter declined more slowly (time constant T_s). The continuous line, which would be recorded from a multichannel preparation of all seven channels, is the sum of two exponential curves. Modified from Colquhoun and Hawkes (1983).

channel opening. Then as depolarization proceeds and the membrane potential approaches zero and then becomes positive, the individual sodium channels are more likely to be closed (Figs. 4-8 and 4-9).

Incorporated into models of the channel are *selectivity filters* that govern the specificity for ions. The calcium channel is far more selective for calcium ions than is the sodium channel for sodium ions. In reality, selectivity depends on the properties of specific amino acids such as glutamate that make up the lining of the channel pore (Jan and Jan, 1994).

Molecular Mechanisms for Gating.   The *voltage-gated* sodium, calcium, and potassium currents, which pass through channels that respond to voltage changes, stand in contrast to the *ligand-operated channels.* Ligands (Latin *ligare,* bind) bind to the cell membrane at receptor sites and then convey the signal to the channel gate usually by a specialized protein, crucial to the process of intracellular signaling, called the G protein. Examples are ligand-gated and G-dependent potassium channels (Table 4-3).

Voltage-gated channels (such as those for sodium, calcium, and some potassium currents) have two molecular gates. The *voltage sensor,* located on the S4 span, responds to changes in voltage to open the pore and may explain the *activation gate,* traditionally called the *m gate.* In the case of the sodium channel, the *inactivation gate* (*h gate*) may open and close according to the ball-and-socket model. Inactivation can be localized to only three amino acids that link domains III and IV (Bennett et al., 1995). In the case of the calcium channel, inactivation is associated with the sixth transmembrane–spanning segment (S6) of the first domain (Fig. 4-6), so that the mechanism of inactivation is not ball and chain (Zhang et al., 1994), but might rather involve a molecular conformational reshuffle of the channel. In the case of the potassium channel, the amino-terminal region of the channel protein may serve to plug the channel from within (Jan and Jan, 1994).

TABLE 4-3. *Control of cardiac ionic channels*

Voltage-gated
   Sodium channel
   Calcium channel
   Potassium channels
Ligand-gated (G-dependent)
   Acetylcholine-sensitive K channel
   Adenosine-sensitive K channel
   ATP-sensitive K channel
Stretch-activated channels
   (mechanoreceptors)
   Nonselective channels[a]
   Specific channels (e.g., swelling-operated Cl^- channel)

---

[a]Suleymanian et al. *J Mol Cell Cardiol* 1995;27:721–728.

SODIUM CHANNEL

One of the first events in response to the onset of depolarization of phase 0 of the action potential is opening of the sodium channel (Figs. 4-2 and 4-7) when the voltage reaches −70 to −60 mV, which is its *threshold of activation* (Table 4-4). The sodium current flows inward very rapidly during the first millisecond of depolarization (Fig. 4-9). The inactivation gates (probably intracellular amino acids) turn off the current flow more slowly and have two time constants. The first time constant is less than 1 msec, switching off the sodium current very rapidly. The second component is much slower (Grant, 1990), at about 4 seconds and may account for the continued but constantly decreasing sodium inflow during the later stages of the action potential (current $I_{Na(s)}$). The sodium channel can exist in any of three hypothetical states: resting, activated, and inactivated (Fig. 4-10). Depolarization changes the resting to the activated state. The conductance increases and sodium ions flow inward.

Sodium Conductance Versus Current. The conductance is a measure of the permeability of the membrane to an ion and helps to determine the rate of current flow. Thus,

$$I_{Na} = gNa(V_m - E_{Na})$$

TABLE 4-4. *Contrasting properties of sodium and calcium channels*

Property	Sodium channel	Calcium channel
Ion specificity	Sodium	Calcium
Inhibitors	Tetrodotoxin; lidocaine, quinidine and other Class I antiarrhythmics	Ca^{2+}-antagonists (L channel); nickel, mibefradil (T channel)
Physiologic occurrence	Atrial, Purkinje and ventricular tissue	Nodal and vascular tissue; as component of normal atrial, Purkinje or ventricular action potential
Effect of β-adrenergic receptor stimulation[a]	Increases (controversial)	Enhances Ca^{2-} entry by opening channels
Threshold of activation	−70 to −60 mV	−60 to −30 mV (−60 mV, T-type channel in SA node; −30 mV, L-type channel in ventricles)
Time constant of		
activation	<1 msec (fast)	10–20 msec
inactivation	4 msec (slow)[b]	50–500 msec
Overshoot	+20 to +35 mV	0 to +15 mV
Maximal rate of depolarization	100–1,000 V/sec (phase 0)	1–10 V/sec
Type of conduction	Fast (0.3 to 3.0 msec)	Slower (0.01 to 0.10 msec)
Role in arrhythmias	Ventricular tachyarrhythmias; ectopic activity; possibly in ischemia as inhibited fast responses	Slow conduction predisposes to re-entry; role in early ischemic or reperfusion arrhythmias

For L and T calcium channels, see Table 4-5.
Electrophysiologic data modified from Singh et al. (1980), Zipes (1988), and Coetzee (1988).
G_s, stimulatory component of G protein; SA, sinoatrial.
[a]By increasing internal sodium, Na/Ca exchange increases with a positive inotropic effect.
[b]Antoni et al. (1988); this value refers to membrane potentials more positive than −20 mV, with even longer times reported by other investigators.

where I_{Na} is sodium current flow, gNa is sodium conductance, V_m is voltage across the membrane, and E_{Na} is the sodium equilibrium or reversal potential. The latter depends on the concentration of ions on either side of the sarcolemma. In the resting state, between depolarizations, the *reversal potential* is +40 mV for sodium. At the start of phase 0 depolarization I_{Na} is large because the conductance is high and the voltage across the sodium channel is also large. I_{Na} decreases as depolarization proceeds (Fig. 4-8) because (1) the voltage across the sodium channel V_m decreases, and therefore the potential approaches E_{Na}, the reversal potential for sodium, and (2) the inactivation gates start to shut, thereby decreasing sodium conductance (Fig. 4-11). Hence, the driving force decreases,

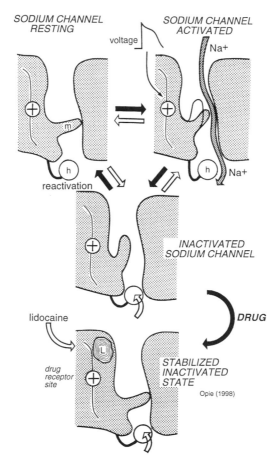

FIG. 4-10. Resting, activated, and inactivated sodium channels. Hypothetically, the sodium channel can exist in any of three states. The activation gates (m gates) open upon activation, whereas the inactivation gate (h gate) closes to form the inactivated state. According to one model (Katz, 1993), the inactivated state undergoes reactivation to enter the resting state. Each of the above arrows is reversible; the change from the resting to the activated state and from the inactivated to the resting state occurs during the normal cardiac cycle. A sodium channel inhibitory drug such as lidocaine keeps the channel in the inactivated state, so that the channel activation is largely inhibited. These proposed concepts are based on the Hodgkin-Huxley model.

and the flow of sodium ions slows and then stops. In the meantime, the calcium conductance has increased.

Clinical Applications.   Antiarrhythmic agents that inhibit the sodium channel are known as *class I antiarrhythmics* and include lidocaine, quinidine, and others (Fig. 4-10). Lidocaine probably acts on the inactivation gate, to prolong the inactive state (Bennett et al., 1995). *Tetrodotoxin* (TTX) is a highly toxic experimental inhibitor of the sodium channel. More physiologically, the sodium channel can be totally inhibited by increasing the extracellular potassium to depolarizing *hyperkalemic* values, which remove the potential difference from within to without the cell. The result is inhibition of cardiac contraction with cardiac arrest (*cardioplegia*).

Ionophores.   Ionophores are compounds that enhance the flow of ions along their electrochemical gradient. They enter membranes to act as pathways for ions. For example, *monensin* is a sodium ionophore, and *nigericin* is a potassium ionophore. Although such compounds are not used in clinical practice, they have important physiologic and pharmacologic implications. For example, an unex-

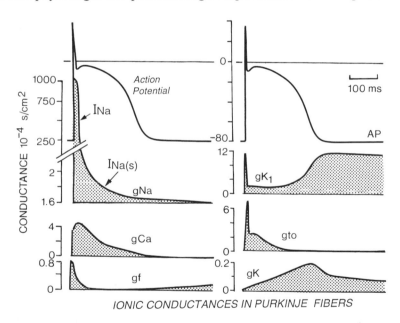

IONIC CONDUCTANCES IN PURKINJE FIBERS

FIG. 4-11. Ionic conductances during action potential. How changing conductances contribute to shape of cardiac action potential of Purkinje fibers. Computed action potential and ionic conductances (g) per unit of membrane surface. Note the extremely large initial peak of Na conductance (gNa) about 250 times that of Ca conductance (gCa). The initial peak corresponds to the fast phase of the inward sodium current, I_{Na}. Thereafter follows a slower phase, $I_{Na(s)}$. g_f is the conductance for current I_f found in Purkinje and pacemaker cells (see Chapter 5). g_{k1} is the conductance of the inward rectifier potassium current, i.e., the background K conductance that decreases during depolarization. g_{to} is the conductance giving rise to the transient outward potassium current, I_{to}, is; in atria and in Purkinje fibers (see Fig. 4-2) and causes prominent phase 1. g_k is the conductance of the voltage-gated delayed rectifier, I_{kv}. Modified from unpublished data of A. Coulombe and from data of Professor E. Coraboeuf, Paris.

pected effect of monensin is to promote release of atrial natriuretic peptide from the atria.

CALCIUM CHANNEL

Although the calcium ion concentration in the extracellular space outside the heart cell is very much higher than inside, a large concentration gradient is main-

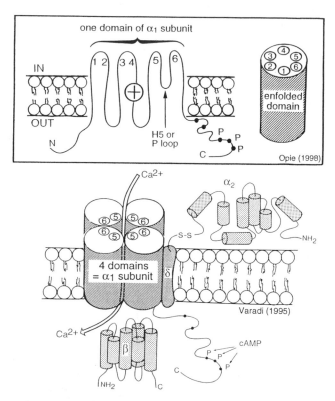

FIG. 4-12. Calcium channel structure. The molecular structure of one domain of the α_1 subunit of the calcium channel is shown in the upper panel. Note voltage sensor on segment S4, and the pore-forming loop, H5 or P, between S5 and S6, as for the sodium channel (see Fig. 4-6). Four enfolded domains (top right) arranged around the channel pore make up one α_1-subunit (lower panel). The major differences from the sodium channel lies in the nature of the C-terminal chain, in the phosphorylation (P) sites on the C-terminal chain, the mechanism of inactivation, and the existence of a large β-subunit. The latter binds to the α_1-subunit to change its properties and to increase sensitivity to calcium antagonist drugs. The functions of the α_2-subunit and the delta subunit are not known. The gamma subunit, present in skeletal muscle, is absent in heart and vascular smooth muscle. During β-adrenergic stimulation, cAMP phosphorylates (P) several sites on the C-terminal chain of the α_1-subunit to increase the probability of calcium channel opening (see Fig. 4-13). Lower panel modified from Varadi et al., *Trends Pharmacol Sci* 1995;16:43, with permission of the authors and Elsevier Science Ltd.

tained because the sarcolemma is virtually impermeable to calcium. Achieving the correct voltage required to open the calcium channel calls for a greater degree of depolarization than to open the sodium channel. Some calcium also enters through reversal of the sodium–calcium exchange system, especially during the early phase of the plateau of the action potential (see section on Sodium–Calcium Exchange).

Molecular Structure of Calcium Channel.   There are four subunits of the cardiac calcium channel (α_1, α_2, β, and δ), with a combined molecular weight of 220 kDa. In the α_1-subunit (molecular weight 165 kDa), there are four repeating domains, each of six helices, which is very similar to that of the sodium channel, and suggests a common gene (Figs. 4-6 and 4-12). The major evident difference from the sodium channel lies in the established phosphorylation sites of the calcium channel protein, almost all located on the C-terminal tail. In addition, there are critical differences between sodium and calcium channels in the amino acid structure of the channel pores, probably in the descending loop located between helices S5 and S6 of each domain. Thus, the presence or absence of glutamate residues in the structure of the channel pore can determine specificity for calcium ions (Yatani et al., 1994). The β-subunit of the calcium channel appears to interact with the α_1-subunit to make more binding sites available for calcium antagonist drugs (Pragnell et al., 1994).

Calcium Permeation.   The major functional property of the calcium channel is to regulate the entry of calcium ions. This process is inhibited when calcium antagonist drugs (calcium channel blockers) bind to their binding sites on the calcium channel protein. One model for the physiologic function of the calcium channel (Fig. 4-13) proposes that the channel is opened as depolarization reaches a critical threshold potential that converts the resting channel to the active state, when both the activation gate (m) and the inactivation gate (h) are open. At this time, the hypothetical gates have a greater probability of being in the open rather than in the closed state. It should be remembered that they are opening and shutting continuously in bursts of activity. The calcium ions flow during a certain time (time-dependent) and until a certain voltage is reached (voltage-dependent) during the depolarization process. Then most of the gates come to be in the shut state, and the channel is inactivated.

Receptor Sites for Calcium Channel Antagonist Drugs.   The transmembrane-spanning helices are probably the site to which the calcium antagonist drugs bind. There are three chief categories of such drugs: those resembling nifedipine (dihydropyridines), verapamil and diltiazem, giving rise to the N, V, and D binding sites. Some properties of these drugs are similar, whereas others differ. There are additional binding sites to which other new calcium antagonist drugs such as amlodipine also may bind. It is likely that the drug-binding sites differ somewhat from organ to organ. For example, certain calcium channel antagonist drugs act

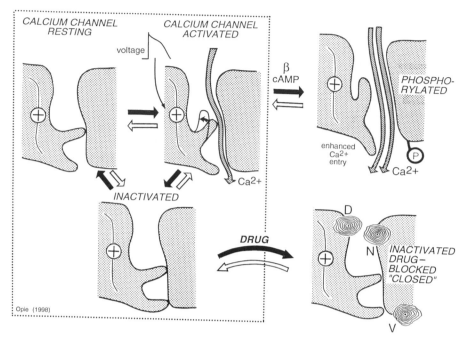

FIG. 4-13. States of the calcium channel. The channel can go through the same cycle and state changes as in Fig. 4-11, changing from the resting to the activated and inactivated states in response to voltage. Calcium antagonist drugs (N, nifedipine and other dihydropyridines; D, diltiazem; V, verapamil) can bind to various schematic sites to induce the drug-blocked inactivated state. β-adrenergic (β) activation by formation of cAMP promotes calcium channel phosphorylation (P) and probability of the open state.

more specifically on the vascular tissue than on the myocardium, which is important in hypertension when peripheral arteriolar dilation is a crucial property.

Calcium Channel Phosphorylation. The α_1-subunit (organ-specific subunit) of the calcium channel can be phosphorylated, especially in the C-terminal tail (Fig. 4-12). This process occurs in response to catecholamine stimulation, which increases internal cyclic adenosine monophosphate (cAMP) to activate a kinase enzyme that transfers a phosphate group from ATP to the calcium channel. Thereby, the electrical charges near the inner mouth of the nearby pores are altered to induce changes in the molecular conformation of the pores. Ultimately there is an increased probability of opening of the calcium channel, of importance in helping to cause an enhanced inotropic response during β-adrenergic stimulation. One of two mechanisms may explain what is happening. Either the time that the channel remains in the open state is increased so that more calcium ions flow with the same degree of voltage activation, or phosphorylation may bring into play calcium channels that were otherwise inactive.

T- and L-type Calcium Channels. There are two major subpopulations of calcium channels relevant to the cardiovascular system, namely the T channels and the L channels. A third population of N channels is found in nervous tissue. The *T (transient) channels* open at a more negative voltage (Fig. 4-14), have shorter bursts of opening, and do not interact with calcium antagonists. Because they open at a more negative voltage than the L channels, the T channels presumably account for the earlier phase of the opening of the calcium channel, which also may give them a special role in the early electrical depolarization of the sinoatrial node and hence of initiation of the heart beat (see Chapter 5). Although T channels are found in atrial cells (Bean, 1985), their existence in normal ventricular cells is still controversial (Table 4-5). By contrast, T channels are found in cells from hearts with left ventricular hypertrophy. T channels are also of considerable importance in the initiation of contraction in vascular smooth muscle.

The *L (long-lasting) channels* open at a less negative voltage (Table 4-5), thus accounting for the later phases of calcium channel opening. The L channels have two patterns in which their gates work (modes of gating). Mode 1 has short bursts of opening, and mode 2 has longer periods of opening. Calcium antagonist drugs change the mode of opening of L channels to a preponderance of mode 1, so that the amount of calcium entering through the channel is reduced.

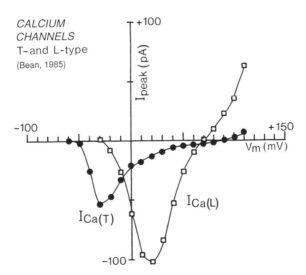

FIG. 4-14. Calcium channel subtypes. Contrasts between the transient calcium channel, I$_{Ca(T)}$, and the long-lasting calcium channel, I$_{Ca(L)}$. Voltage-current relationship is shown for the dog atrial cells exposed to an external calcium concentration of 5 mM. Note that the transient channel opens a more negative voltage than the long-lasting channel and therefore opens first during the depolarization process. The transient channel also starts to close earlier and reaches a lesser peak current flow. Modified from Bean with permission.

TABLE 4-5. *Contrasting properties of T- and L-calcium channels*

	T–type	L–type
Activation threshold: SA node[a]	–60 to –50 mV	–40 mV
Activation threshold: atria[b]	–50 mV	–30 mV
Activation threshold: ventricles[c]	Absent except in LVH (-40 mV)[f]	–30 to –35 mV
Channel conductance (pS)[d]	7–8	20–25
Mean open time	Short 1–2 msec	Very short, <1 msec
Inactivation kinetics[e]	Rapid	Slow
Channel blockers	Nickel, amiloride, mibefradil[g]	Classical calcium antagonists, such as verapamil, nifedipine, and diltiazem
β-receptor stimulation[b]	No effect	Major effect
Calcium agonist (Bay K 8644)	No effect	Channel opens

[a]Guinea pig sinoatrial node cells. Hagiwara et al. *J Physiol* 1988;395:233–253.
[b]Dog atrial myocytes. Bean (1985).
[c]Guinea pig ventricular myocytes. Doerr et al. (1990).
[d]pS, picosiemens; 1 siemen = 1 mho. Flockerzi and Hofmann. In: Sperelakis N (ed). *Physiology and Pathophysiology of the Heart*. 3rd ed. Boston: Kluwer, 1995;91–99.
[e]Activation and inactivation voltages and kinetics depend on surface potential and hence on concentration and type of external divalent ions. For other circumstances and values. See Hess in: Zipes DP, Jaliffe J (eds). *Cardiac Electrophysiology. From Cell to Bedside*. Philadelphia: Saunders, 1990;10–17.
[f]Nuss and Hauser. *Circ Res* 1993;73:777–782; T channels in left ventricular hypertrophy (LVH).
[g]Mishra and Hermsmeyer. *Circ Res* 1994;75:144–148.

POTASSIUM CHANNELS

Potassium channels can now be grouped within two distinct molecular families, namely the voltage-gated (or voltage-operated) channels and the inward rectifier channels (Deal et al., 1996). These are currently designated K_v and K_{ir}, respectively, although they often are still called the K and K_1 channels (Table 4-6). Both families of potassium channels help to control the outward flow of potassium ions, especially during repolarization (K_v) and in the maintenance of the resting membrane potential (K_{ir}).

Why Are There So Many Potassium Channels?   Seen from an evolutionary perspective, a very simple K^+ channel, probably with only two transmembrane helices (spans), might first have come into existence to generate the resting membrane potential of primitive cells (Fig. 4-6). This simple structure is now called the inward rectifier, K_{ir}. Another member of this family, the ATP-sensitive K^+ channel, $K_{(ATP)}$, evolved to stop the potassium leak induced by hypoxic damage. When the beating heart emerged, the K_v superfamily (Fig. 4-15) came into existence with its voltage sensor on an adjacent transmembrane span (S4). Hypothetically, transmembrane segments (or spans) S2 and S3 evolved to protect the charge bearing S4 from the charges of the lipid bilayer. Members of the K_{ir} family evolved into another superfamily (Fig. 4-16), including K_{ACh} and

TABLE 4-6. *Currents associated with normal cardiac action potential*

Current	Abbreviation	Qualities
Fast inward sodium current	I_{Na}	Responsible for upstroke of action potential; abolished by tetrodotoxin; inhibited by class I antiarrhythmic agents; four units each of six transmembrane spans.
Slower inward calcium current	I_{Ca}, I_{si}	Important for plateau phase of cardiac action potential; involved in excitation–contraction coupling; increased by β-stimulation; four units each of six transmembrane spans.
Subtype T channel	$I_{Ca(T)}$	Transient calcium current, opening at low voltages; may be important in sinus node depolarization.
Subtype L channel	$I_{Ca(L)}$	Long-duration calcium current, admitting major calcium ion flow, inhibited by standard calcium antagonists.
Potassium currents		
Background K current (inward or anomalous rectifier)	I_{k1} or I_{kir}	Helps to regulate resting membrane potential (RMP) and contributes to late phase 3 repolarization; above RMP, outward potassium current; below RMP, strong inward current with rectification that augments flow; depolarization shuts channel, current flows again during repolarization to help end action potential; not a pacemaker current.
Voltage-gated K current (delayed rectifier)	I_k or I_{kv} includes rapid (K_r) and slow (K_s) phases	Outward potassium current chiefly responsible for repolarization; voltage-gated; enhanced by increased internal calcium[a] activated by depolarization (fully active at +10 mV) and deactivated by full repolarization; time-dependent; promotes spontaneous depolarization as it decays; six transmembrane spans. Two phases K_r (rapid) and K_s (slow); HERG[b] is molecular basis of K_r, K_s structure not known,[c] includes previous K_{min}.
Early transient outward K current	I_{to}	Prominent in Purkinje cells, in atrial cells, and in epicardial ventricular cells; causes obvious phase 1; shortens action potential duration.
Other currents		
Diastolic pacemaker current in SA node or Purkinje fibers	I_f	Inward "funny" sodium (and potassium) current; increased by β-stimulation; causes automaticity in SA node or injured Purkinje fibers.
Sodium–calcium exchange	$I_{Na/Ca}$	Contributes to late phase of cardiac action potential plateau (Na^+ inward).
Chloride current	I_{Cl}	Inward negative current activated by cAMP; shortens action potential duration during adrenergic activation.

[a]Nitta et al. *Circ Res* 1994;74:96–104.
[b]Kiehn et al. *Circulation* 1996;94:2572.
[c]Attali. *Nature* 1996;384:24.

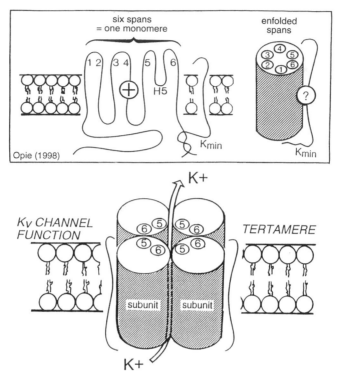

FIG. 4-15. Structure of voltage-operated potassium channel. This channel (K_v) consists of four unlinked subunits. Each of these potassium channel subunits is composed of a transmembrane domain with a positively charged S4 helix, similar to the voltage sensor of sodium or calcium channels (see Fig. 4-6). Four subunits, each a monomomere, make a functional voltage-sensitive potassium channel (heterotetramere = combination of four different subunits) with one functional pore. The single transmembrane span, K_{MIN}, interacts with the last of the other six spans to produce one subunit, in the case of the slow component of K_V.

K_{ADO}, that helps to decrease the heart rate by responding to acetylcholine and adenosine, respectively. To achieve a functioning potassium channel pore requires the combination of multiple subunits, that is, either four subunits each of six spans or the combination of four units each of only two spans (Figs. 4-15 and 4-16). Such variable combinations mean that a great molecular diversity of potassium channels is possible.

Voltage-Operated K^+ Channel, K_v or K (Including K_r and K_s). This channel, also called the delayed rectifier, conducts the current I_k that physiologically makes a major contribution to repolarization (Table 4-6). By analogy with Na^+ or Ca^{2+} channel structures, one would expect an α_1-subunit with four repeat domains each of six transmembrane helices. It would also be anticipated that all four domains would contribute to the single pore per channel protein. In the case

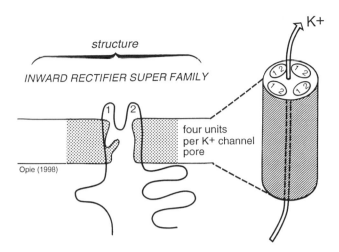

FIG. 4-16. Inward rectifier superfamily, basically having only two transmembrane spans (1 and 2) and the loop (H5) that participates in the pore. The drawing on the right shows that four of these simple structures are required to make one functioning channel pore that passes potassium ions. See Jan and Jan (1994).

of K_v, the above plan is modified as follows. The α-subunit of each channel has only six helices, therefore being about one fourth the molecular size of the α_1-subunit of the Na^+ or Ca^{2+} channels (Jan and Jan, 1994). To make one single potassium pore, four of these α-subunits combine, so that as in the case of the Na^+ or Ca^{2+} channel, there is one pore per 24 helices. Other molecular properties more directly resemble those of the Na^+ and Ca^{2+} channel. For example, the highly conserved H5 loop folds back into the membranes and constitutes part of the lining of the water-filled pore, through which the potassium ions cross the channel. Also, the S4 segment has a specific sequence of amino acids with positive charges that is thought to act as the voltage sensor that responds to the changes in membrane voltage, i.e., confers the property of voltage gating.

The superfamily that includes this channel is sometimes called the *Shaker family* because the delayed rectifier was first cloned in a mutant of the fruitfly, drosophila. When this channel is genetically absent from the fruitfly, exposure to ether provokes spasms of muscular shaking.

The molecular structure of K_r and K_s, the rapid and slow components, respectively, is important for the understanding of an inherited human disorder called the long QT syndrome that predisposes to certain potentially fatal arrhythmias (see Chapter 20).

The Transient Outward Potassium Current (I_{to}). This voltage-gated potassium current chiefly contributes to the very early repolarization after the peak of the upstroke of the action potential. This current is especially prominent in atrial,

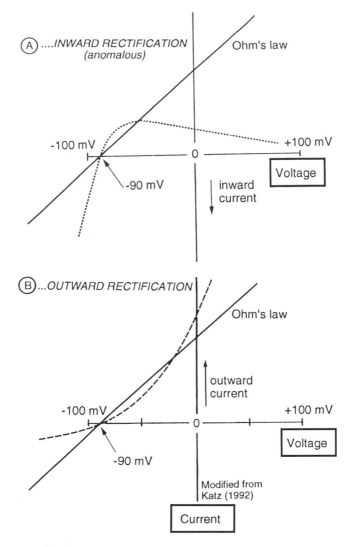

FIG. 4-17. Inward versus outward rectification. Current–voltage relationships showing the effects of changing membrane potential (abscissa) on the ionic currents (ordinate) generated by three different types of potassium channels. Inward currents are downward; outward currents are upward. All potassium currents are zero at about 90mV, the equilibrium potential for potassium. An ohmic current (A) is a linear function of membrane voltage because resistance is constant. Inward (anomalous) rectification (**A**) occurs when depolarization causes potassium channels to close, thereby decreasing outward current. Outward rectification (**B**) occurs when depolarization opens potassium channels and so increases outward current. Thus, outward rectification favors outward current, whereas inward rectification favors inward current. Modified from Katz (1992) with permission.

Purkinje, and subepicardial ventricular cells (Fig. 4-2), giving the typical spike-and-dome appearance (Sicouri and Antzelevitch, 1991). The notch created by I_{to} resets the action potential to the early phase of the plateau. I_{to} also contributes to phase 2 repolarization because the action potential duration is prolonged when this current is inhibited. The molecular correlate for this current in the human heart is the K_v 4.3 potassium channel gene (Dixon et al., 1996).

The Inward Rectifier Superfamily, K_{ir}. Potassium channels of this family set the resting membrane potential of cardiac myocytes. Structurally, this is an extremely simple channel with only two transmembrane helices and one pore (Fig. 4-16). K_{ir} passes an *outward current* when the membrane potential is above the potassium equilibrium potential (E_k) to contribute to the repolarization phase of the action potential and thereby to help end the action potential, thereby regaining the resting membrane potential (Fig. 4-17). Conversely, this same channel potentially passes a large *inward* K^+ current, when the cell membrane is hyperpolarized (i.e., when the resting membrane potential is below -85 mV), and this inward current helps to maintain the high internal K^+ activity and hence the membrane polarity. The unusual nature of the current flow, which is much larger in one direction, has given rise to the name *anomalous rectifier*. Hypothetically, Mg^{2+} ions can plug the inner side of the pore when the K^+ flux is directed outward, to reverse the direction of current flow. Conversely, the Mg^{2+} ions can be pushed away to unplug the channel when K^+ flows inward (Quast, 1995).

ATP-Sensitive Potassium Channel. This channel represents a hybrid between the K_{ir} superfamily and the totally different ABC (ATP-binding cassette) family (Fig. 4-18). The latter provides two binding sites, one the SUR (sulfonylureas,

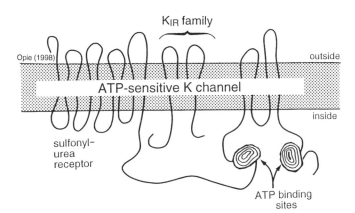

FIG. 4-18. Hybrid composition of ATP-sensitive potassium channel, which represents a union between a member of the inward rectifier K_{iR} family and the ABC superfamily (ABC, ATP-binding cassette). On the left is the sulfonylurea receptor (SUR) and on the right the ATP-binding sites. The actual channel pore is composed of four K_{iR} subunits.

epitomized by the oral antidiabetic agent, glibenclamide) and the other for ATP. Because the K_{ir} component of the channel is controlled by the binding of internal ATP, it is called the K_{ATP} *channel.* Technically, the inward rectifier concerned is K_{ir} 6.2, (Philipson, 1995). In general, this channel is closed in physiologic conditions when ATP is high. As ATP breaks down during ischemia with formation of ADP and adenosine, opening of this K^+ channel is promoted (Ferrero et al., 1996). The K_{ir} component of the channel forms the channel pore as a heteromultimer of four subunits, each of only two helices (Ashford et al., 1994). Also participating in this functioning channel pore are four peripore structures, each constituted by the two transmembrane spanning domains (the SUR component and the ATP-binding site component).

There appears to be no physiologic role for K_{ATP} in cardiac myocytes. Pathophysiologically, one hypothesis is that as ATP breaks down in response to severe ischemia, the outward passage of K^+ ions and their accumulation on the outside of the cell causes loss of normal membrane polarization with a decreased contractile response and an induced state of inactivity or rest.

The function of K_{ATP} *in vascular smooth muscle* is much more clear. There, in response to the formation of adenosine, this channel opens and participates in coronary vasodilation. Adenosine formed during myocardial hypoxia or during vigorous work is thought to diffuse from the cardiac myocyte to the K_{ATP} channel on vascular smooth muscle cells, to relieve the inhibition by ATP and to allow channel opening. The egress of potassium ions opening causes hyperpolarization that, in turn, leads to vasodilation by inactivation of the calcium channels. (This vasodilatory mechanism is distinct from the interaction of adenosine with I_{kADO}, described in the next section of this chapter, although both mechanisms lead to hyperpolarization.)

The clinical implications of the inhibition K_{ATP} *by sulfonylureas* relate to their use as oral agents in the therapy of maturity onset diabetes mellitus. These drugs, such as glibenclamide, inhibit K_{ATP} and promote coronary vasoconstriction. They also lessen ischemic loss of potassium and early ischemic arrhythmias (Kantor et al., 1990). They inhibit the protective phenomenon of preconditioning (see Chapter 19). Other drugs known as *potassium channel openers*, such as pinacidil, cromakalim, minoxidil, diaxozide, and the mixed nitrate-potassium opener nicorandil, all induce coronary dilation by promoting K_{ATP} opening. By mechanisms not fully understood, these drugs protect ischemic myocardial cells.

Ligand-Operated Members of the K_{ir} Superfamily. Ligand-operated channels, also part of the K_{ir} superfamily (Krapivinsky et al., 1995), include the muscarinic and adenosine-operated channels found in nodal tissue and in the atrium (Table 4-7). The muscarinic-operated channel, operated by the M_2 receptor, is linked to the channel by the inhibitory G protein, G_i (Fig. 4-19). Hence, this K^+ channel is also called GIRK$_1$ (G protein–activated inward rectifying K_1 current). The current conducted is sensitive to acetylcholine, I_{kACh}.

TABLE 4-7. *Ligand-operated and additional potassium currents*

Current	Abbreviation	Qualities
Ligand-operated G protein–gated K channels (inward rectifier family)		
Acetylcholine-sensitive	I_{kACh}	Activated by acetylcholine muscarinic receptors (m_2) in nodal, Purkinje, and atrial cells. Not in ventricles. Time-independent. When current switched on in nodal cells, spontaneous depolarization is delayed. Heteromultimer of two distinct inwardly rectifying subunits.[a]
Adenosine-sensitive	I_{kADO}	Probably same as I_{kACh}. Adenosine stimulates time-independent potassium current.
ATP-regulated	I_{kATP}	ATP inhibits physiologic concentrations. Decrease of ATP/ADP ratio and adenosine activate. Inhibited by sulphonylureas, activated by K-channel activators. Structure part of inward rectifier family.[b]
Additional K currents		
Calcium-activated	Ik_{Ca} or BK_{Ca}	Important in vascular smooth muscle, to hyperpolarize and thereby to inhibit calcium channel; vasorelaxation; large conductance ("big" channel).
Sodium-activated[c]	I_{kNa}	Activated when internal sodium increases as in ischemia or during sodium pump inhibition.
Fatty acid-activated[c]	I_{kFFA}	Activated by increased internal free fatty acids (FFA) during sustained ischemia.

[a]Krapivinsky et al. *Nature* 1995;374:135–141.
[b]Ashford et al. *Nature* 1994;370:456–459.
[c]For further details, see Carmeliet (1992).

LIGAND OPERATED K+ CHANNEL

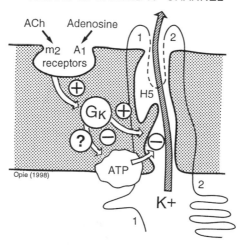

FIG. 4-19. Ligand-gated potassium channels. These channels are part of the inward rectifier superfamily. This drawing shows the proposed control mechanisms in response to acetylcholine (ACh) and adenosine, both of which slow the heart rate. M₂, muscarinic receptor subtype 2; A₁, adenosine receptor subtype 1; Gₖ, G protein controlling activity of this potassium channel.

The adenosine-sensitive K^+ current, I_{kADO}, probably identical to I_{kACh}, responds to the adenosine receptor A_1 rather than to the muscarinic receptor, and is also linked to the channel by means of G_i. Both of these currents function to increase outward potassium flow in nodal tissue and, therefore, to hyperpolarize. Thus, the membrane potential is moved away from the threshold for spontaneous firing, so that the discharge rate of nodal tissue slows and the heart rate decreases.

The Smallest Known Potassium Channel Structure, K_{min}.   Previously thought to be an extremely primitive channel, K_{min} is a single strand of only one helix with 130 amino acids and is now known to be a regulator of the slow component of the delayed rectifier current, K_{vs} (Fig. 4-15). From the molecular point of view, K_{min} is coexpressed with one functioning six-membrane spanning standard potassium K_v channel (Attali, 1996).

The Largest Known Potassium Channel, BK_{ca}.   This calcium-activated potassium channel, part of the K_v superfamily, is probably of major importance in vascular smooth muscle. The concept is that calcium building up during the opening of the vascular calcium channels opens this channel. The result is a large efflux of potassium ions, so that the vascular cell hyperpolarizes and the calcium channel closes. This channel has by far the largest conductance for potassium, meaning that when the channel is open, much more potassium can flow through it than in the case of the other potassium channels.

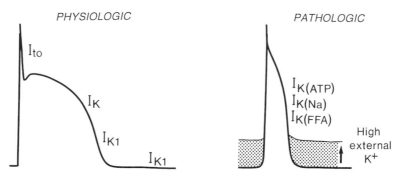

FIG. 4-20. Physiologic versus pathologic potassium channels. Note contribution of potassium channels to the repolarization process. In physiologic conditions (left, Purkinje cell), I_{to} causes the early phase of repolarization, I_k and I_{k1} contribute to repolarization, and I_{k1} maintains the negative resting potential. In anoxic conditions (right), the action potential duration is markedly shortened by I_{kATP} with contributions from I_{kNa}, I_{kFFA}, and I_{kCa}. See Aksnes (1992). In contrast, vascular smooth muscle, $I_{k(ATP)}$ has a physiologic role.

Ischemia-Induced Potassium Current Flow. In ischemia, not only is it the ATP-sensitive potassium channel that opens, but several other new channels may come into operation (Fig. 4-20). A *sodium-activated potassium current,* responding to an increase in internal sodium, may become important in ischemia, when internal sodium is known to increase (Bertrand et al., 1989). Its existence remains controversial. Likewise, the *fatty acid–activated potassium channel* also appears to respond to changes in ischemia when there is a buildup of fatty acid metabolites (Carmeliet, 1992).

CHLORIDE CHANNELS

In the past, chloride currents were thought to play an insignificant electrophysiologic role in the heart, especially because one of the proposed chloride currents, I_{to}, was more correctly identified as a potassium current. There are no less than five distinct cardiac chloride currents (Ackerman and Clapham, 1993). The most important seems to be $I_{Cl(cAMP)}$ the chloride current activated by catecholamines (Fig. 4-21). This shortening of the action potential duration is crucial during β-adrenergic stimulation, when the whole heart "speeds up." By promoting influx of chloride ions with negative charges, there is in effect an outward current that helps to shorten the action potential duration (Table 4-8). Without this chloride current, β-adrenergic stimulation would widen the action potential by enhanced opening of the calcium channel.

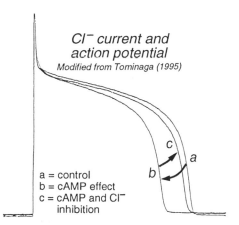

Cl^- current and
action potential
Modified from Tominaga (1995)

a = control
b = cAMP effect
c = cAMP and Cl^-
    inhibition

FIG. 4-21. Inward chloride (Cl^-) current. Role in shortening action potential duration during catecholamine β-adrenergic stimulation. In response to cAMP, the action potential duration shortens from a to b. When the chloride current is blocked, the action potential duration widens from b to c. This abbreviation of the action potential is especially important during β-adrenergic stimulation, when the heart rate increases and the duration of the cardiac cycle shortens. For further details, see Tominaga et al., *Circ Res* 1995;77:417–423.

TABLE 4-8. *Currents terminating action potential plateau*

Increased outward positive currents
   Delayed rectifier potassium current I_{kv} or I_k, including rapid (I_{kr}) and
   slow phases (I_{ks}) (to lesser extent the inward rectifier, I_{kir} or I_{k1})
Decrease of inward positive currents
   L calcium current
   Na/Ca exchange current (sodium entry)
   Slow decay phase of sodium current
Increase of inward negative current
   Chloride current $I_{Cl(cAMP)}$

VENTRICULAR ACTION POTENTIAL

The characteristic appearance of the ventricular action potential can now be interpreted in greater detail in terms of opening and closing of sodium, calcium, and potassium channels that have just been discussed. Data obtained by computer modeling (Fig. 4-22) help to define the contribution of each of these channels.

The rapid phase of depolarization of the action potential (*phase 0*) is the result of opening of the sodium channels. Sodium conductance first increases very rapidly, as does the flow of the inward current (I_{Na}), to peak within 1 msec and then falls off equally rapidly (Fig. 4-2). This flash of inward sodium movement, carrying positive charges, fully depolarizes the cell causing the rapid upstroke, or phase 0.

In the meantime, the much slower L calcium channels have already started to open, at about −20 mV (Table 4-5). As the sodium current fades away, it is replaced by flow of the L-type calcium current (I_{Ca} or I_{si}, slow inward current), which forms most of the plateau. From the peak of depolarization, the overshoot is lost (*phase 1*), and in the case of atrial and Purkinje tissue and subepicardial ventricular cells, the transient outward potassium current, I_{to}, flows at this stage. In the remaining ventricular myocardium, I_{to} is not so strong. Therefore, phase 1 is much better defined in atrial and Purkinje fibers than in the ventricular myocardium (exception: epicardial cells, Fig. 4-23). As soon as phase 1 has passed, a relatively flat plateau forms (*phase 2*), which merges into the phase of rapid repolarization (*phase 3*).

Phase 3 is complex in origin. It determines the action potential duration (Table 4-8). One of the major proposals is that as a result of the initial depolarization (phase 0), potassium currents are activated after a delay (I_k and I_{k1}), thereby terminating the action potential. A second proposal is that the calcium channel closes in response to a raised internal calcium, so that there is no more influx of calcium. Third, the inward current generated by sodium–calcium exchange ceases and becomes an outward current (see subsequent section). Fourth, an inward flow of negatively charged chloride ions might contribute, especially during catecholamine stimulation (Fig. 4-21). Once the action potential is over, the resting membrane potential is restored and maintained (*phase 4*).

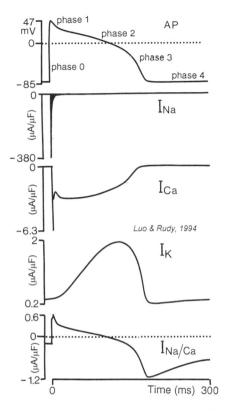

FIG. 4-22. Computed currents and ventricular action potential. Note extreme speed of inward sodium current, I_{Na}. I_{Ca}, calcium current; I_K, voltage-dependent delayed rectifier potassium current; Na/Ca, Na^+/Ca^{2+} exchange. Note that the sodium current base is slightly enlarged from the original trace to allow visibility; in the original it is a straight line. AP, action potential. Units for currents: microamps per 1 microfarad of membrane capacitance. Modified from Luo and Rudy: A dynamic model of the cardiac ventricular action potential. I. Simulations of ionic currents and concentration changes. *Circ Res* 1994;74:1071–1096, with permission of the authors and the American Heart Association.

During this diastolic phase of electrical rest, the activity of the sodium–potassium pump and the various exchange systems restores any remaining ionic balance across the sarcolemma. In atrial and ventricular cells, once the resting membrane potential has been regained, it remains stable throughout diastole, so that these cells cannot fire spontaneously. In injured Purkinje cells and in the sinoatrial and atrioventricular nodes, spontaneous diastolic depolarization can occur (phase 4) by complex mechanisms to be described in Chapter 5. Such depolarization is known as *phase 4 depolarization* and is a very slow process when compared with the rapid depolarization of phase 0.

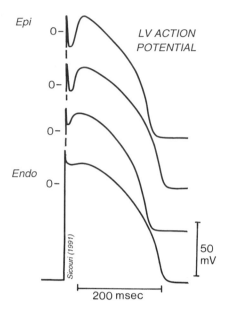

FIG. 4-23. Epicardial versus endocardial action potential patterns. Note prominent spike-and-dome pattern in epicardial (Epi) cells, the result of activity of the early repolarizing potassium current, I_{to}. Endo, endocardial. For technical details, see Sicouri and Antzelevitch, *Circ Res* 1991;68:1729–1741.

Purkinje Action Potential

To *recapitulate*, the action potential of the Purkinje fibers differs substantially from that of endocardial ventricular cells (Fig. 4-2). The patterns of current activation and inactivation are described as follows (Fig 4-24). Phase 0, the first event is voltage-induced activation of the sodium current. Next follows activation of the calcium current. Inactivation of the sodium current occurs near the peak of phase 0. At about the same time, the transient outward current, I_{to}, is activated to form phase 1 and soon thereafter inactivated. Termination of the action potential plateau (phase 2) occurs through a combination of activation of the potassium current, I_K and in activation of the calcium current. About this time, the background potassium current, I_{K1}, is activated to help contribute to rapid repolarization (phase 3).

SODIUM–CALCIUM EXCHANGE

Recent intense investigations have delineated an important role for sodium–calcium exchange both in the normal cardiac action potential and in excitation–contraction coupling (Gilbert et al., 1991). The bulk of evidence suggests that three sodium ions are exchanged with one calcium ion through a process not

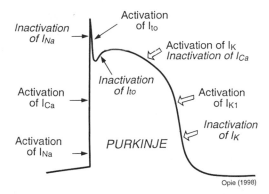

Opie (1998)

FIG. 4-24. Patterns of activation and inactivation in Purkinje fibers. The currents associated with the Purkinje fiber action potential are as follows: I_{Na}, sodium current; I_{Ca}, calcium current; I_{to}, transient outward current; I_K, voltage-gated or delayed rectifier potassium current; I_{K1}, background potassium current or anomalous rectifier. For further details, see Hauswirth and Singh (1979).

requiring energy but responsive to the membrane potential and the concentration of sodium and calcium ions on either side of the membrane. Because three Na^+ ions exchange with one Ca^{2+} ion, the exchange is *electrogenic* in the direction of sodium transport.

Any lingering doubt about the existence of the exchanger has been put to rest by Nicoll (1990), who has cloned its structure. There are 970 amino acids, with a molecular weight of 108 kDa, and part of the structure has homology to the sodium pump. There is a large cytoplasmic domain of 520 amino acids to which calmodulin binds. The meaning of this potential control mechanism is still unclear. There is now a specific peptide inhibitor (XIP, exchange inhibitor peptide) (Chin et al., 1993).

Because sodium and calcium ions can move either inward or outward, in part in response to the membrane potential (Fig. 4-25), there must be a specific membrane potential at which the ions are so distributed that they can move as easily one way as the other. This *reversal potential* ($E_{Na/Ca}$) could theoretically be calculated from the concentrations of sodium and calcium ions on either side of the membrane. Yet the subsarcolemmal sodium and calcium ion concentrations (more correctly the activities) are not known. The reversal potential may be about halfway between the resting membrane potential and the depolarized state (Bers, 1991). Changing the membrane potential from the resting value of, say, -85 mV to $+20$ mV in the phase of rapid depolarization affects the sodium–calcium exchange in such a way that sodium ions tend to exit, sometimes called "reverse mode Na/Ca exchange." Predisposing to this early outward movement of sodium ions is the internal accumulation of those sodium ions carried in through the sodium channel in a small subsarcolemmal space (see "fuzzy space," later in this section). During this early phase, calcium ions may be entering both by the exchange mechanism and through the calcium channel.

Consequently, the rapid accumulation of calcium ions within the subsarcolemmal space changes the balance of charges in such a way that the tendency is for calcium ions to leave and for sodium ions to enter. Therefore, during the late phase of the action potential plateau, it is postulated that the exchanger operates in the "forward mode" (or inward mode) to promote an inward sodium current, thereby contributing to the late phase of the action potential duration (Doerr et al., 1990).

It should be appreciated that the above simplified scheme of sodium and calcium ion movements during the action potential is derived from indirect evidence. The scheme does not reflect hard experimental data apart from the changes in the membrane potential during the action potential pattern development and the internal overall cytosolic calcium ion concentration. Other factors must be extrapolated or calculated from computer models.

The driving force of the exchanger is:

$$V_m - E_{Na/Ca}$$

where V_m is the membrane potential and $E_{Na/Ca}$ is the reversal potential for the current carried by the sodium–calcium exchanger. This reversal potential is:

$$3E_{Na} - 2E_{Ca}$$

which, in turn, depends on the voltage differentials and transmembrane activities of sodium and calcium ions, all of which are constantly changing. When E_m is more positive than $E_{Na/Ca}$, then sodium ions tend to be driven out, and when I_m is more negative than $E_{Na/Ca}$, then calcium ions tend to to be driven out (Fig. 4-25).

Postulated Role of Exchanger in Arrhythmias. Repetitive rhythmic activity of the sodium–calcium exchanger may explain certain arrhythmias (see triggered arrhythmias, Chapter 20). Calcium excess will be associated with egress of calcium ions and electrogenic entry of sodium ions. The further postulate is that there should be recycling of the excess of cytosolic calcium ions in and out of the sarcoplasmic reticulum, which would cause a rhythmic inward current, the *transient inward current*. There is good evidence for the activity of this current in digitalis-induced ventricular arrhythmias, and some evidence for its role in ischemic and reperfusion arrhythmias.

RESTITUTION OF IONIC BALANCE

Sodium and Calcium. As a direct result of the rapid opening of the sodium channel followed by the slower opening of the calcium channel, each action potential will lead to an early gain of sodium ions and a later gain of calcium

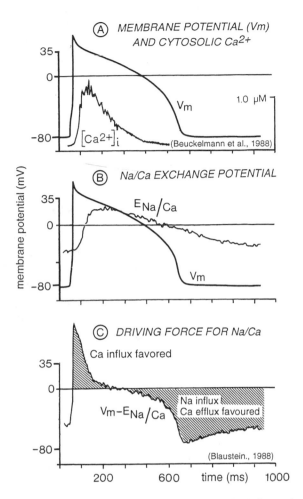

FIG. 4-25. Na/Ca exchanger and action potential. Proposed role during various phases of the cardiac ventricular action potential. **(A)** Relationship between action potential and internal calcium. **(B)** Potential for the Na/Ca exchanger ($E_{Na/Ca}$). Note that early, soon after the onset of rapid depolarization, conditions are such that Ca^{2+} influx is favored **(C)**, whereas later during phase 3 of the action potential (Fig. 4-2) conditions favor Ca^{2+} efflux and, therefore, Na^+ influx. Because three sodium ions are exchanged for one calcium ion, there is a net inward current flow, which contributes to the late phase of the action potential. Modified from Blaustein et al. (1988) with permission.

ions. Both of these ionic imbalances, theoretically, can be corrected by the sodium–calcium exchanger. Early activity of the exchanger, soon after sodium influx through the sodium channel, will theoretically help extrude the sodium ions just gained. Later operation of the sodium–calcium exchange in the "forward mode" will help extrude the calcium ions already gained. There is at present no proof that these neat hypothetical balancing acts actually occur, yet the concept is attractive. Noble's computer calculations show that Na/Ca exchange virtually ceases as soon as the cell is fully repolarized, provided that certain assumptions are made about the activation of the exchange process by calcium. Thus, it might be supposed that the sodium–calcium exchanger acts *during* the action potential itself adequately to restitute the ionic imbalances created by the sequential opening of the sodium and channels.

Potassium. During the repolarization phase of the action potential there is a net but albeit small loss of potassium ions. To pump these ions back into the cell against a large concentration gradient requires the activity of the sodium pump.

SODIUM–PROTON EXCHANGE AND ACID–BASE HOMEOSTASIS

The *internal pH*, pH_i, is more alkaline than can be expected if protons (H^+) were passively distributed across the cardiac cell membrane, (Lazdunski et al, 1985). Therefore protons must be transported out of the myocyte. Such transport is achieved by the electroneutral 1-for-1 exchange of Na^+ and H^+ (Fig. 4-26). The activity of this exchanger (also called an *antiporter*) is driven by the gradient of sodium ions, much higher outside than inside the myocyte (Fig. 4-4). The function of the exchanger can be defined by a number of inhibitors, including the diuretic *amiloride* and the novel specific inhibitor HOE 694.

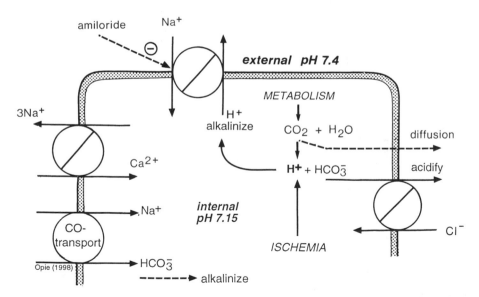

FIG. 4-26. Intracellular acid–base homeostasis. Proposed role of Na/H exchanger and interaction with Na/Ca exchanger. The Na/HCO₃ cotransporter and Cl/HCO₃ exchanger act to alkalinize and acidify, respectively.

This exchanger corrects an acid load during ischemia and acidosis by transporting protons (H^+) out of the cell while transporting Na^+ into the cell. The resultant increase of internal sodium can be dealt with either by the operation of the sodium–calcium exchanger or by the sodium–potassium pump (Piwnica-Worms et al., 1986). Alternatively, the exchanger may later operate in the reverse direction to extrude sodium from the cells. Physiologically, Na^+/H^+ exchange also may play a role in the regulation of protein synthesis.

SODIUM–POTASSIUM PUMP

To *recapitulate*, the resting heart cell sarcolemma is relatively impermeable to sodium ions but becomes highly permeable with the opening of the sodium gate initiated by depolarization. Even more sodium ions enter during the later phase of the action potential plateau by sodium–calcium exchange. All such sodium ions must eventually be returned to the extracellular space, or else the cell will be overloaded with sodium, with the further threat of absorption of water by osmosis, which could burst the overloaded cells. Most of this influx of sodium across the sarcolemma is corrected by the activity of the sodium–potassium pump. A lesser component is linked to the sodium–calcium exchange system when it transiently functions to extrude sodium from the cell during the early phase of the action potential (Fig. 4-25).

The *sodium–potassium pump* uses energy to extrude sodium out of the cell and potassium into the cell against the electrochemical gradients (Fig. 4-27). Although commonly called the *sodium pump*, more accurate names are the sodium–potassium pump or the Na^+/K^+-ATPase. The pump is activated by internal sodium or external potassium and uses energy in the form of ATP complexed to magnesium. Binding sites for ATP, Na^+, K^+, and digitalis have been identified.

$$3 \, (Na^+) \text{ in} \rightarrow 3 \, (Na^+) \text{ out}$$

$$2 \, (K^+) \text{ out} \rightarrow 2 \, (K^+) \text{ in}$$

$$MgATP^{2+} \rightarrow MgADP^{1-} + P_i^{2-} + H^+$$

One ATP molecule is used per transport cycle. The ions are first secluded within the pump protein, then extruded to either side. One positive charge must leave the cell for each three sodium ions exported because only two potassium ions are imported. Thus, the pump is electrogenic because an unbalanced negative charge is left behind, tending to make the inside of the cell negatively charged.

Sodium Pump Activation by Ions. The sodium–potassium pump is asymmetrically situated in the sarcolemma so that sodium activation sites are located on the internal surface and most of the potassium activation sites on the external surface (Fig. 4-27). The pump is activated as the internal sodium increases, for example, after repetitive openings of the sodium channel. According to the fluid

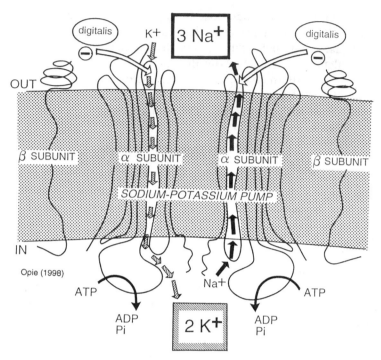

FIG. 4-27. Sodium pump function and structure. The sodium pump (also called the Na⁺/K⁺ ATPase) transports three sodium ions outward and two potassium ions inward. In structure, the pump is thought to consist of two α-subunits, each with a molecular weight of about 112,000, and of two surrounding β-subunits, with a molecular weight of about 35,000. The ionic channel is located in the α domain, which also has (1) the external digitalis binding site, (2) the external potassium binding site, (3) the internal sodium binding site, and (4) the ATP hydrolysis site. Note that external potassium inhibits the binding of digitalis.

mosaic model of the cell membrane, the lipid bilayer is interspersed with globular proteins, some of which penetrate the membrane. The sodium–potassium pump is probably such a protein. When K⁺ binds to the outside or Na⁺ to the inside surface, the enzyme undergoes a change in molecular configuration, which is transmitted to other subunits of the sodium pump, which also change their configuration to the active form. ATP binds to the enzyme to form a phosphorylated intermediate that breaks down to provide the energy required for transport of sodium and potassium ions against a concentration gradient. Thus, the pump is activated, and 3 Na⁺ exchanged for 2 K⁺ ions.

Molecular Structure of the Sodium Pump. The α-subunit consists of a long polypeptide chain, with N and C terminal units, and a molecular weight of about 112 kDa. There are at least six and possibly eight transmembrane spanning units (Fig. 4-27). External digitalis and potassium binding sites are located on the external hinges between the transmembrane units, whereas sodium binds to an inner hinge. The hydrolytic site for ATP is also defined. The significance of the phosphorylation site remains unknown.

Significance of Digitalis Effect.   Digitalis-type compounds, including digoxin and ouabain, inhibit the sodium–potassium pump to increase internal sodium. Thereby, they promote sodium–calcium exchange with an increase in internal calcium and a positive inotropic effect. The significance is twofold. First, digoxin is often used in the therapy of patients with heart failure to improve the contractile state of the myocardium. Second, digitalis compounds are frequently used in physiologic experiments to eliminate the effects of this pump, thereby better uncovering the role of the activity of the exchange systems.

CALCIUM PUMPS

Energy in the form of ATP is required to transport calcium ions against the large concentration gradients that exist between the relatively low calcium ion concentrations in the cytosol and the much higher values in the sarcoplasmic reticulum or the extracellular space. The sarcoplasmic reticulum is no less than a battery of calcium pumps. These pumps are switched on by a membrane protein called phospholamban (Greek *phospho*, phosphate; *lamban*, receptor), which requires a phosphate group for its maximal activity. Such phosphorylation is achieved either by (1) catecholamine β-adrenergic stimulation or (2) an increased cytosolic calcium ion concentration. Therefore, the increase of calcium ions associated with systole will stimulate the uptake of calcium into the sarcoplasmic reticulum to help initiate diastole. Catecholamine stimulation will further accelerate the uptake of calcium ions into the sarcoplasmic reticulum to shorten diastole and to accelerate relaxation, so that the left ventricle can fill better.

MAGNESIUM

Magnesium is an important constituent of the cytosol and is essential for numerous enzymatic reactions (including the sodium pump, myosin ATPase, oxidative phosphorylation, and various enzymes of glycolysis). The vital functions of ATP and other adenine nucleotides are performed in their ionized forms chelated with magnesium. The total magnesium in the cell is about 8 mmole/kg wet weight with a calculated overall intracellular content of 17 mmol/L (Page et al, 1972). Of this, about 10 mmol/L should be bound to adenine nucleotides and a small proportion to mitochondria (12% of total) and myofibrils (2% of total). To measure the true intracellular magnesium concentration is difficult. The activity might be about 0.6 mmol/L (Table 4-1), although the values are controversial (Garfinkel et al., 1986; Kirkels et al., 1989). This value may increase to 10 times during severe ischemia, probably because of breakdown of magnesium bound to ATP as total ATP decreases. This ischemia-induced increase of magnesium is of importance because it helps to sensitize the ATP-operated potassium channel to open even when there is only a relatively small decrease in the total ATP level (Lederer et al., 1989).

The mechanisms regulating magnesium transport in and out of the heart cell are still obscure; an exchanger may be involved (Romani et al., 1993). Presently available data suggest that magnesium is not involved in the beat-to-beat regulation of contraction, although it is an important controller of the activity of certain key enzymes.

NONSPECIFIC STRETCH CHANNELS

Unsolved are the potential links between stretch of the myocardium, as during sustained heavy heart work, and protein synthesis, which is required to produce compensatory hypertrophy (see Chapter 16). Several types of nonmyocardial cells, varying from simple protozoa to hair cells of the ear, have the capacity to translate mechanical cell deformation into activation of an ion channel and to allow the gated entry of ions. Such channels respond to stimulation of *mechanoreceptors*. In the myocardium, such stretch-activated channels (SACs) act as mechanoreceptors and admit calcium ions (Suleymanian et al., 1995). During acute cardiac stretch, SACs may help to increase the force of cardiac contraction (see Anrep effect, Chapter 13).

ENERGY FOR ION FLUXES

Whenever an ion is transported against a concentration gradient, energy is required. To estimate how much ATP is expended on maintenance of ionic gradients is not easy and requires a number of assumptions. It is simplest to take the case of potassium ion flux. The transport of 0.7 μmol K^+/g/min requires 0.35 μmol ATP/g/min or about 4 μL O_2/g/min. This contrasts with the oxygen uptake of the human heart in basal conditions of about 100 μL/g/min. Thus, roughly up to 4% of the energy needs of the heart might be expended on potassium movements by the sodium–potassium pump. The same pump is ultimately responsible for balancing sodium ion movements. When based on the requirements to pump out the sodium that has entered, much higher estimates for energy needs, up to 15%, are obtained (Table 4-9). Only about 2% of the total ATP production is required for sodium entry by the fast sodium channel.

Estimates suggest that the entry and exit of calcium ions across the sarcolemma requires relatively little energy, not more than 3% of the myocardial ATP usage (Table 4-9). Intracellular calcium ion movements also need energy. Calcium uptake by the sarcoplasmic reticulum in diastole requires 1 mole of ATP for 2 moles of calcium. Such use of energy can concentrate calcium by 1,000 to 5,000 times within the sarcoplasmic reticulum. A significant percentage of the total oxygen uptake (up to 20%) of the heart is required for the calcium uptake associated with the process of relaxation.

TABLE 4-9. *Estimated ATP requirements for ion fluxes and phases of cardiac action potential*

	Effect of increasing beating rate[b]			
Ion	K$^+$-arrested heart[a] (μmol/g wet wt/min)	75 beats/ min[b] μmol/g/min	150 beats/ min[a] μmol/g/min	330 beats/ min[a] μmol/g/min
Total sodium flux	Up to 0.1	3.1	6.2	13.6
Fast channel (I$_{Na}$)	—	0.4	0.8	1.7
Potassium flux	Included in above	Included in above	Included in above	Included in above
Calcium flux				
Slow channel[c] (I$_{si}$)	—	0.1–0.5	0.2–1.0	0.4–2.2
Contractile Ca^{2+} flux				
for 50% tension	About 1.2	About 2.4	—	—
for peak tension	—	—	—	About 30
Total ATP needed	10	23	41	152
Percentage breakdown				
Na$^+$ flux	Up to 1%	15%	15%	9%
I$_{Na}$	—	2%	2%	1%
I$_{si}$	—	0.4–2.2%	0.5–2.4%	0.3–1.5%
Average internal Ca^{2+} flux	—	5%	6%	—
Peak internal Ca^{2+} flux	—	—	—	20%

[a]Isolated rat heart.
[b]Dog heart.
Data based on Table 4-5 of Opie. *The Heart. Physiology, Metabolism, Pharmacology and Therapy.* 1st ed. Orlando, FL: Grune & Stratton, 1984.

SUMMARY

1. *The myocardial cell takes up potassium and ejects sodium ions* to produce the resting negative membrane potential. This process is achieved by activity of the sodium pump (sodium–potassium ATPase) which stretches across the cell membranes.

2. *As the wave of electrical excitation arrives, it initiates depolarization,* which causes a current to flow that opens the voltage-activated gates of the sodium channel to allow the very rapid entry of positively charged sodium ions (phase 0 of the action potential). As depolarization proceeds, the calcium channel opens because it is activated by a less negative voltage than the sodium channel. After depolarization ceases, there is a brief period of rapid repolarization (phase 1) before the pattern of the action potential levels off to form the plateau phase (phase 2). It is the continued inflow of calcium ions that causes the action potential plateau.

3. *There are two major types of potassium channels:* those that are voltage-gated and those that are ligand-gated. It is the voltage-operated channels that respond to depolarization in an orderly time-dependent way.

4. *During diastole, potassium ions leave the cell* as a background current, which maintains the resting membrane potential. During repolarization, the potassium current starts to flow again as the rectifying current that helps to terminate the action potential plateau (phase 3), so that the resting potential is regained (phase 4).

These descriptions apply to contractile myocardial cells and conducting Purkinje fibers, not to spontaneously firing nodal tissue, which is considered in the next chapter.

ACKNOWLEDGEMENT

Professor E. Carmeliet, Leuven, Belgium, kindly reviewed this chapter.

STUDENT QUESTIONS

1. What is a voltage-dependent ion channel?
2. Describe the two types of calcium channels.
3. What are the two major mechanisms for regulation of potassium. Give the name and function of four specific potassium channels and the principles of their regulation.
4. What are the phases of the action potential and how is the action potential plateau regulated?
5. Briefly describe sodium–calcium exchange and its physiologic function.

CARDIOLOGIST-IN-TRAINING QUESTIONS

1. The resting membrane potential of ventricular cells is aboiut −85 mV. Which are the crucial ions involved and what governs their transmembrane distribution?
2. What is a current and what is a channel? Describe the currents that explain the phases of the cardiac ventricular action potential.
3. How is a sodium channel pore formed? Which commonly used antiarrhythmic drug alters the probability of sodium channel opening? Give one hypothesis for its mode of action.
4. Calcium channel opening is enhanced by β-adrenergic stimulation and decreased by calcium antagonist drugs. Explain each of these changes.
5. Outline the major differences between each of the following potassium currents: delayed rectifier and its component HERG, inward rectifier, transient outward current, ATP-regulated current.
6. How do acetylcholine and adenosine cause the sinus node discharge rate to slow?
7. Which are the changes in the action potential that occur in anoxia, and how are they explained?
8. What is the physiological role of the sodium-calcium exchanger? How does it contribute to the cardiac action potential?

REFERENCES

1. Ackerman MJ, Clapham DE. Cardiac chloride channels. *Trends Cardiovasc Med* 1993;3:23–28.

2. Aksnes G. Why do ischemic and hypoxic myocardium lose potassium. *J Mol Cell Cardiol* 1992;24:323–331.
3. Ashford MJL, Bond CT, Blair TA, Adelman JP. Cloning and functional expression of a rate heart K_{ATP} channel. *Nature* 1994;370:456–459.
4. Attali B. A new wave for heart rhythms. *Nature* 1996;384:24–25.
5. Bean BP. Two kinds of calcium channels in canine atrial cells. Differences in kinetics, selectivity and pharmacology. *J Gen Physiol* 1985;86:1–30.
6. Bennett PB, Valenzuela C, Chen L, Kallen RG. On the molecular nature of the lidocaine receptor of cardiac Na^+ channels. Modification of block by alterations in the α-subunit III–IV interdomain. *Circ Res* 1995;77:584–592.
7. Bers DM. In: *Excitation-Contraction Coupling and Cardiac Contractile Force.* Boston: Kluwer Academic, 1991.
8. Bertrand D, Bader CR, Berheim L, Haimann C. K_{Na}. A sodium-activated potassium current. *Pflugers Arch* 1989;414(suppl 1):76–79.
9. Blaustein MP. Sodium/calcium exchange and the control of contractility in cardiac muscle and vascular smooth muscle. *J Cardiovasc Pharmacol* 1988;12(suppl 5):56–58.
10. Carmeliet E. Potassium channels in cardiac cells. *Cardiovasc Drugs Ther* 1992;6:305–312.
11. Chin TK, Spitzer KW, Phillipson KD, Bridge JHB. The effect of exchanger inhibitory peptide (XIP) on sodium–calcium exchange current in guinea-pig ventricular cells. *Circ Res* 1993;72:497–503.
12. Coetzee WA. Channel-mediated calcium current in the heart. *Cardiovasc Drugs Ther* 1988;1: 447–459.
13. Colquhoun D, Hawkes AG. The principles of the stochastic interpretation of ion-channel mechanisms. In: Sakmann B, Neher E (eds). *Single-Channel Recording.* New York: Plenum, 1983;135–175.
14. Colvin RA, Ashavaid TF, Katz AM, Herbette LG. Estimation of receptor densities in canine cardiac sarcolemmal vesicles [Abstract]. *Circulation* 1983;68(suppl III):399.
15. Deal KK, England SK, Tamkun MM. Molecular physiology of cardiac potassium channels. *Physiol Rev* 1996;76:49–67.
16. Dixon JE, Shi W, Wang H-S, et al. Role of the Kv4.3 K^+ channel in ventricular muscle. A molecular correlate for the transient outward current. *Circ Res* 1996;79:659–668.
17. Doerr T, Denger A, Doerr A, Trautwein W. Ionic currents contributing to the action potential in single ventricular myocytes of the guinea-pig studied with action potential clamp. *Pflugers Arch* 1990;416:230–237.
18. Ferrero JM Jr, Saiz J, Ferrero JM, Thakor NV. Simulation of action potentials from metabolically impaired cardiac myocytes. Role of ATP-sensitive K^+ current. *Circ Res* 1996;79:208–221.
19. Garfinkel L, Altschuld RA, Garfinkel D. Magnesium in cardiac energy metabolism. *J Mol Cell Cardiol* 1986;18:1003–1013.
20. Gilbert JC, Shirayama T, Pappano AJ. Inositol triphosphate promotes Na/Ca exchange current by releasing calcium from sarcoplasmic reticulum in cardiac myocytes. *Circ Res* 1991;69:1632–1639.
21. Goldman DE. Potential, impedance and rectification in membranes. *J Gen Physiol* 1943;27:37–60.
22. Grant AO. Evolving concepts of cardiac sodium channel function. *J Cardiovasc Electrophysiol* 1990;1:53–67.
23. Hauswirth O, Singh BN. Ionic mechanisms in heart muscle in relation to the genesis and the pharmacological control of cardiac arrhythmias. *Pharm Rev* 1979;30:5–63.
24. Jan LY, Jan YN. Potassium channels and their evolving gates. *Nature* 1994;371:119–122.
25. Kantor PF, Coetzee WA, Carmeliet EE, et al. Reduction of ischemic K loss and arrhythmias in rat hearts. Effect of glibenclamide, a sulfonylurea. *Circ Res* 1990;66:478–485.
26. Katz AM. In: *Physiology of the Heart.* 2nd ed. New York: Raven, 1992;453.
27. Katz AM. Cardiac ion channels. *N Engl J Med* 1993;328:1244–1251.
28. Kirkels JH, van Echteld CJA, Ruigrok TJC. Intracellular magnesium during myocardial ischemia and reperfusion: possible consequences for postischemic recovery. *J Mol Cell Cardiol* 1989;21:1209–1218.
29. Krapivinsky G, Gordon EA, Wickman K, et al. The G-protein–gated atrial K^+ channel I_{kACh} is a heteromultimer of two inwardly rectifying K^+-channel proteins. *Nature* 1995;374:135–141.
30. Lazdunski M, Frelin C, Vigne P. The sodium/hydrogen exchange system in cardiac cells: Its biochemical and pharmacological properties and its role in regulating internal concentrations of sodium and internal pH. *J Mol Cell Cardiol* 1985;17:1029–1042.
31. Lederer WJ, Nichols CG. Nucleotide modulation of the activity of rat heart ATP-sensitive K channels in isolated membrane patches. *J Physiol* 1989;419:193–211.

32. Luo CH, Rudy Y. A dynamic model of the cardiac ventricular action potential. I. Simulations of ionic currents and concentration changes. *Circ Res*, 1994;74:1071–1096.
33. Matsuda JJ, Lee HC, Shibata EF. Acetylcholine reversal of isoproterenol-stimulated sodium currents in rabbit ventricular myocytes. *Circ Res* 1993;72:517–525.
34. Nicoll DA, Longoni S, Philipson KD. Molecular cloning and functional expression of the cardiac sarcolemmal Na$^+$-Ca^{2+} exchanger. *Science* 1990;250:562–565.
35. Noble D, Noble SJ, Bett CL et al. The role of sodium-calcium exchange during the cardiac action potential . *Ann NY Acad Sci* 1991;639:334–353.
36. Page E, Polimeni PI. Magnesium exchange in rat ventricle. *J Physiol* 1972;224:121–139.
37. Philipson LH. ATP-sensitive K$^+$ channels: Paradigm lost, paradigm regained. *Science* 1995;270:1159.
38. Piwnica-Worms D, Jacob R, Shigeto N, et al. Na/H exchange in cultured chick heart cells: Secondary stimulation of electrogenic transport during recovery from intracellular acidosis. *J Mol Cell Cardiol* 1986;18:1109–1116.
39. Pragnell M, Waard MD, Mori Y. Calcium channel beta-subunit binds to a conserved motif in the I–II cytoplasmic linker of the alpha$_1$-subunit. *Nature* 1994;368:67–70.
40. Quast U, Glocker S. Vascular pathology and the K$_{ATP}$ channel. In: Yellon DM, Gross GJ (eds). *Myocardial Protection and the K$_{ATP}$ Channel*. Boston: Kluwer Academic, 1995;31–50.
41. Reuter H. Electrophysiology of calcium channels in the heart. In: Opie LH (ed). *Calcium-Antagonists and Cardiovascular Disease*. New York: Raven, 1984;43–51.
42. Romani A, Marfella C, Scarpa A. Regulation of magnesium uptake and release in the heart and in isolated ventricular myocytes. *Circ Res* 1993;72:1139–1148.
43. Sicouri S, Antzelevitch C. A subpopulation of cells with unique electrophysical properties in the deep subepicardium of the canine ventricle. The M cell. *Circ Res* 1991;68:1729–1741.
44. Singh BN, Collett JT, Chew CYC. New perspectives in the pharmacologic therapy of cardiac arrhythmias. *Prog Cardiovasc Dis* 1980;22:243–301.
45. Suleymanian MA, Clemo HF, Cohen NM, Baumgarten CM. Stretch-activated channel blockers modulate cell volume in cardiac ventricular myocytes. *J Mol Cell Cardiol* 1995;27:721–728.
46. Tomaselli GF, Backx PH, Marban E. Molecular basis of permeation in voltage-gated ion channels. *Circ Res* 1993;72:491–496.
47. Tsien R. Excitable tissues: the heart. In: Andreoli T, Hoffman JF, Fanestil DD, Schulz SG (eds). *Physiology of Membrane Disorders.* New York: Plenum, 1986;475.
48. Woodbury JW. Interrelationships between ion transport mechanisms and excitatory events. *Fed Proc* 1963;22:31–35.
49. Yatani A, Bahinski A, Mikala G. Single amino acid substitutions within the ion permeation pathway alter single-channel conductance of the human L-type cardiac Ca^{2+} channel. *Circ Res* 1994;75:315–323.
50. Zhang J, Ellinor PT, Aldrich RQ, Tsien RW. Molecular determinants of voltage-dependent inactivation in calcium channels. *Nature* 1994;372:97–100.
51. Zipes DP. Genesis of cardiac arrhythmias: electrophysiological considerations. In: Braunwald E (ed). *Heart Disease.* Philadelphia: Saunders, 1988;581–620.

5

Pacemakers, Conduction System, and Electrocardiogram

No one ionic current alone is responsible for SA node pacemaking.

Irisawa et al., 1993

The cardiac electrical impulse is generated in the sinoatrial (SA) node, rapidly conducted through the atria to the atrioventricular (AV) node, where it undergoes filtration and delay. Then follows another phase of rapid conduction through the His bundle and bundle branches, finally leading to excitation–contraction coupling in the ventricular myocyte. The whole sequence can be monitored by the electrocardiogram (ECG) (Fig. 5-1). The initiator of these events lies in the automatic pacemaker activity of the SA node, in which there is spontaneous diastolic depolarization.

SINOATRIAL NODE AUTOMATICITY

How does the *internal time clock* of the SA node know to undergo regular diastolic depolarization at a regular interval and thereby satisfactorily to initiate the heart beat? The explanation for the pacemaker current that underlies automaticity in the SA node has swung away from the idea that an outward potassium current is the dominant factor to emphasize the additional and more important role of inward currents (Table 5-1). Nonetheless, the exact regulation of the repetitive spontaneous firing of the SA node, essential for the pumping action of the heart and hence for human and animal life, is still not fully understood.

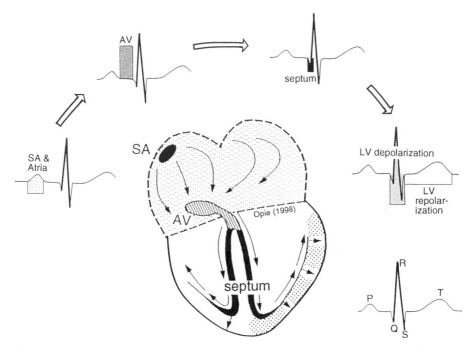

FIG. 5-1. Cardiac impulse and ECG patterns. From the pacemaker situated in the SA node, the wave of electrical depolarization spreads throughout both atria, causing the greater part of the P wave of the ECG. Conduction slows down considerably through the AV node, causing the interval between the P and Q waves. Then conduction accelerates through the His-Purkinje system and immediately reaches the cardiac septum, where it causes the small Q wave. Later, it reaches the left ventricle to cause the QRS deflection in the bottom ECG. Thereafter, ventricular repolarization follows until the end of the T wave. In the bottom right ECG trace, the conventional letters defining the waves (P, QRS, T) of the normal complex are shown.

TABLE 5-1. *The four pacemaker currents in sinoatrial node*

Current	Qualities	Proposed role
Outward decaying current, I_k	Initial activation at −50 mV, fully activated at −10 mV[a]	Depolarization inactivates so that inward currents take over
Inward background current, I_p or I_b	Ill-defined; not inhibited by β- or Ca²⁺ blockers	May initiate first half of spontaneous depolarization
Inward calcium currents, I_{Ca-T} and I_{Ca-L}	I_{Ca-T} activated at −60 to −50 mV[b] I_{Ca-L} activated at −30 mV; inhibited by Ca²⁺ blockers	Second half of diastolic depolarization Steep upstroke of action potential
Inward current I_f I_f (Na⁺ and K⁺)	Initially activated at hyperpolarizing voltages; range −90 to −50 mV[c]; β-response	May initiate spontaneous depolarization, especially during β stimulation

β, β-adrenergic; Ca²⁺ blockers, calcium antagonist drugs.
[a]Irisawa and Noma. *J Mol Cell Cardiol* 1984;16:777–781.
[b]Hagiwara et al. *J Physiol* 1988;395:233–253.
[c]Brown and DiFrancesco. *J Physiol* 1980;308:331–351.

Structure of the Sinoatrial Node

Anatomically, the human SA node is spindle shaped and measures about 20 × 3 × 1 mm. It contains clusters of cells, poor in contractile filaments, where the automatic activity mostly resides in the *pacemaker* or *P cells* (Fig. 5-2). In contrast are *transitional cells*, which lie near the periphery of the node. It is probably the gradual change from P cells to peripheral T cells that explains the different patterns of action potential obtained in central and peripheral sites.

Each cluster of P cells is enveloped by a basement membrane, and junctions between P cells are largely undifferentiated. P cells connect with each other by simple apposition of plasma membranes. The coordination is good enough for the transmembrane potential to change almost simultaneously in all P cells in one cluster. Synchronization between clusters of P cells occurs by conductance from a dominant pacemaker site that shifts in response to physiologic stimuli, such as adrenergic or parasympathetic discharge (Opthof, 1988). Thus, the site of predominant pacemaker discharge can move as the dominant autonomic tone changes from sympathetic to parasympathetic or vice versa. For example, parasympathetic stimulation seems to cause a shift to slower firing, more peripheral cells. Because the autonomic nervous innervation is more dense in the SA node than in the AV node, variations in autonomic tone have more influence on the activity of the pacemaker (SA node) rather than that of the filter (AV node).

Patterns of Depolarization

The crucial characteristic of SA tissue is the spontaneous diastolic depolarization in phase 4 of the action potential (Fig. 5-3). This depolarization starts at

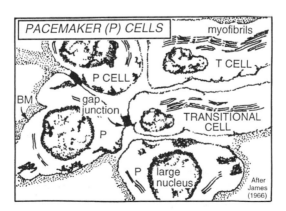

FIG. 5-2. P (pacemaker) cells of the SA node, where the heart beat originates. These cells have a very low content of myofibrils and a large prominent nucleus, and there are occasional gap junctions between the P cells. Transitional T cells, closer to normal myocardial cells in histology, help to conduct the impulse away from the P cells. BM, basement membrane. (Modified with permission of American Heart Association, from James et al. *Circulation* 1966;34:139).

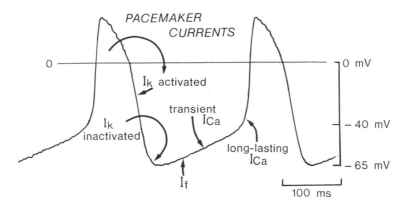

FIG. 5-3. Pacemaker currents in SA node. There are four proposed different pacemaker currents. The repolarizing potassium current, I_k, is activated by full depolarization. Then, as the voltage decreases, it becomes inactivated and decays. At that time inward currents begin to flow, namely I_b (nonspecific background current, not shown), and probably I_f (inward current evoked by hyperpolarization). Later the voltage range for activation of the transient inward calcium current I_{Ca-T} is reached, and even later, the threshold for activation of the action potential itself is attained so that there is rapid depolarization, typical of the upstroke of the action potential of the SA node, involving I_{Ca-L}. For details of individual currents, see Table 5-1 and Fig. 5-4.

about −65 mV. When the *activation threshold* of the cell is reached at about −40 mV, the nodal cell fires and rapid depolarization initiates the nodal action potential. The pattern of this action potential differs markedly from that described in the previous chapter. There is virtually no plateau, because of the rapid onset of potassium-dependent depolarization, achieved by the activation of "delayed rectifier" potassium current, I_k (see Table 4-6).

Delayed Rectifier Potassium Current and Background Current

The major potassium current in pacemaker cells is the delayed rectifier I_k, whereas I_{k1} does not exist (Irisawa et al., 1993). Alterations in the rate of flow of this potassium current, I_k, are important in governing the pattern of the action potential of the SA node (Fig. 5-3). This current is activated by the full depolarization threshold reached at the apex of the action potential, so that it contributes to repolarization, and with time (it is time dependent), it decays to allow inward currents to take over and to initiate the next wave of depolarization. This phenomenon explains why the decaying potassium current is often emphasized in descriptions of SA automaticity. One estimate is that a decaying I_k can make its presence felt for approximately the first half of the phase of spontaneous depolarization of SA pacemaker cells (Hagiwara et al., 1988). The second half is predominantly caused by calcium currents, which start to flow at about −60 to −50 mV.

There also appears to be a constant *background inward current* that remains when all others are blocked. Sometimes this current is called I_p (p = pacemaker) or I_b (b = background). The driving force is likely to be the spontaneous inward movement of sodium ions along their concentration gradient. The activity of this background inward current may explain why as the outward potassium current decays, the nodal cells start spontaneously to undergo depolarization (Irisawa et al., 1993).

Slow Inward Nodal Calcium Currents

The slow inward calcium current (I_{Ca}) explains the latter half of the distinctive, slowly increasing depolarization phase (Hagiwara et al., 1988). When normal ventricular muscle has the fast phase eliminated by tetrodotoxin (TTX) or by a sodium-free and calcium-rich perfusion solution, the nature of the resultant slow current resembles that found in nodal tissue. The inward current in nodal tissue is blocked by lowering the external calcium ion concentration to zero or by the calcium antagonist agents verapamil and diltiazem. Verapamil depresses the sinus pacemaker so as to increase the cycle time for spontaneous firing. This effect is opposed by β-adrenergic receptor agonists, which are thought to open calcium channels to enhance the long-lasting calcium current I_{Ca-L}.

Of the two types of calcium channels (see Table 4-5), it is the transient T-type that opens first because its activity is initiated at a more negative voltage than that of the longer lasting channels. The T current is predominantly responsible for the early phase of the second half of slow diastolic depolarization (Fig. 5-3). Voltage clamp studies on the SA cells show that the calcium current can be separated into the transient component, with a threshold potential of about −60 to −50 mV, and the long-lasting component, with a threshold of about −30 mV. The early transient calcium current (I_{Ca-T}) of the SA node is inhibited neither by standard calcium antagonists nor by β-adrenergic blockers. Experimentally, when the transient channels are fully blocked, a slow diastolic depolarization can still occur (Hagiwara et al., 1988), slower than normal because the L channels open more readily at a less negative voltage (i.e., closer to zero).

Inward Current, I_f

Voltage-clamp studies on the SA node also have identified an inward current that operates best in a voltage range more negative than that usually found in centrally located SA cells. Because of its unexpected and *funny* properties, the new current is called I_f. The range of activation of this current (−90 to −50 mV) overlaps with but does not coincide with the normal diastolic voltage range of the spontaneously beating SA node, so I_f may be fully operative only when the SA node is hyperpolarized. The role of I_f as a potential pacemaker current remains highly controversial. One view is that the activation threshold for I_f in SA cells may be only −35 to −45 mV, hence this current becomes physiologically

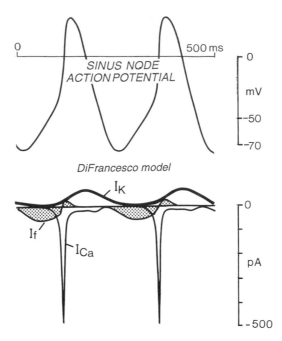

FIG. 5-4. Model of DiFrancesco (1991). The three major pacemaking currents are (1) decaying I_K, (2) I_f, and (3) I_{Ca}. I_{Ca} includes transient (I_{Ca-T}) and long-lasting (I_{Ca-L}) components. Note, however, that in this recording the diastolic membrane potential falls below −75 mV, i.e., more than in the model shown in Fig. 5-3, where the diastolic potential is −65 mV. Hence, DiFrancesco might have studied more peripheral and hence more depolarized nodal cells in which I_f would be more active. Modified from DiFrancesco (1991) with permission.

important (Fig. 5-4). Alternatively, I_f may play a more major role when β-adrenergic stimulation shifts the pacemaker focus from the dominant P cells of the SA node to the peripheral transitional cells, which have a lower negative resting membrane potential, more like that of the atrial cells. β-adrenergic stimulation also shifts the activation range of I_f to a more positive potential (Chang et al., 1990). Similar pacemaker shifts may occur when the dominant pacemaker cells are injured by ischemia or inhibited by drugs. Another name for the inward current activated during hyperpolarization is I_h (h = hyperpolarization). This is the same as I_f. Probably both sodium and potassium ions can carry the I_f pacemaker current, although sodium ions are thought to play a dominant role.

Safety Factors in the Sinoatrial Node

In the SA node, the existence of at least three pacemaking currents (I_k, I_{Ca}, and I_f), as well as the background inward current as a fourth, provides a safety factor so that inhibition of any one current still leaves at least two others to perform the vital depolarizing function (Fig. 5-1). Which of the these pacemaker currents is most important? Irisawa's group (1995) proposed that all four currents play a role. First there is the decay of the outward K^+ current, I_K, previously activated by the preceding nodal action potential. Then the background inward current depolarizes to the threshold for spontaneous firing. I_f also contributes, as does I_{Ca} in the later phase. There are many safety factors built into SA pacemaking: when one pacemaking node fails, there is another waiting in the wings to take over (Irisawa et al., 1993). An alternate view is that I_f could be the major pacemaking current, its contribution often being overlooked (DiFrancesco, 1991).

AUTONOMIC CONTROL OF THE SINOATRIAL NODE

The tachycardia of exercise or emotional excitement results from the combination of sympathetic stimulation and withdrawal of inhibitory parasympathetic (vagal) activity. Because vagal activity promotes bradycardia and adrenergic activity promotes tachycardia, it would be logical to suppose that these two contrasting effects on heart rate could be explained by opposite effects on the SA node.

Vagal Stimulation: The Acetylcholine-Regulated Potassium Channel

Acetylcholine, the messenger of vagal stimulation, reduces the amplitude, rate of increase, and duration of the action potential of the SA node. During physiologic vagal stimulation, the SA node does not arrest. Rather, pacemaker function may shift to those cells that fire at a slower rate. Additionally, acetylcholine helps to open certain potassium channels so that the outward potassium current I_{KACh} flows (see Fig. 4-9). The channel involved is the *acetylcholine-activated potassium channel* (see Table 4-7), which by definition opens in response to parasympathetic vagal stimulation. This channel is also called the *muscarinic acetylcholine-gated potassium channel* because it is the activity of the muscarinic receptor that responds to liberated acetylcholine. By opening this specific potassium channel, the potential of the membrane of the SA node is driven toward the hyperpolarizing direction as the positively charged potassium ions leave the inner side of the sarcolemma. This acetylcholine-induced hyperpolarization decreases the rate at which the activation threshold is reached because of the more negative initial hyperpolarized voltage (Fig. 5-5A). In addition, acetylcholine inhibits the long-lasting calcium current, I_{Ca-L}.

The intracellular signals involved in the effects of acetylcholine are more fully considered in Chapter 7. In brief, the specific G protein, G_k, transmits the signal from the acetylcholine muscarinic receptor to the activation gate of the channel (see Fig. 4-19), so that the current I_{KACh} flows more readily. In addition, stimulation of muscarinic receptors inhibits formation of cyclic adenosine monophosphate (cAMP), the messenger of β-adrenergic activity. An important proposal is that muscarinic stimulation also activates nitric oxide synthase (NOS), which stimulates the formation of cyclic guanosine monophosphate (cGMP) to oppose the

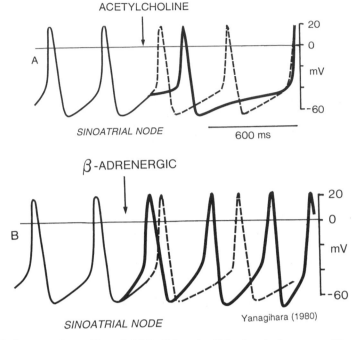

FIG. 5-5. A: Increased vagal tone inhibits SA node. At the terminal neurons of the vagal system, acetylcholine (ACh) is released, which acts on the muscarinic receptor to stimulate the intracellular protein G_K, which in turn opens the activation gate of I_{KACh} (see Fig. 4-17). The result is outward flow of potassium ions and hyperpolarization, so that a longer time is needed to reach the activation threshold for spontaneous firing of the nodal action potential. The heart rate slows (sinus bradycardia). **B: Adrenergic stimulation of SA node.** β-adrenergic stimulation accelerates the cardiac pacemaker and increases its rate of firing (sinus tachycardia). By steps still not fully understood, β-receptor occupancy leads to hyperpolarization. Possibly, the dominant pacemaker zone moves to the peripheral parts of the SA node where cells are more transitional and more polarized than are the central zones. When the diastolic membrane potential is low enough, the current I_f is fired. This current responds to β-adrenergic but not to vagal stimulation. Firing of this current rapidly leads to a loss of membrane polarity to reach the normal activation threshold that allows I_{Ca-L} to become more active and to enhance the depolarization process. The earlier depolarization leads to earlier activation of I_K with a greater rate of repolarization. The total extent of depolarization is greater, as a result of the combined activity of these two currents. For original computer calculations, see Yanagihara et al. (1980).

ehancing effect of cAMP on the calcium current, I_{Ca-L}. Hence, the inward calcium current flow is also reduced by vagal stimulation. Through all of these processes, it becomes more difficult for the depolarizing inward currents to act, and the rate of discharge of the SA node is decreased.

Sympathetic Adrenergic Effects on the Sinoatrial Node

The effects of β-adrenergic stimulation are even more complex (Fig. 5-5B). First, adrenergic stimulation hyperpolarizes the SA node, which may cause a *pacemaker shift* from the normal dominant focus of the P cells, with their characteristic pacemaker action potential, to a pattern more closely resembling atrial tissue and, therefore, more polarized in diastole. The mechanism of the hyperpolarization associated with β-adrenergic stimulation is controversial but totally different from that caused by acetylcholine. Probably β-adrenergic stimulation increases the activity of the electrogenic sodium–potassium pump. The consequent hyperpolarization changes the pacemaker potential in early diastole into the zone required for activity of the I_f current, so that activation of the impulse occurs earlier, and less time is required to reach the normal activation threshold at which the inward calcium current starts to flow. A similar hyperpolarization induced by acetylcholine during vagal stimulation does not cause I_f to flow, and the proposal is that acetylcholine can directly inhibit I_f (DiFrancesco and Tromba, 1987).

Second, β-adrenergic stimulation acting via its second messenger, cAMP, increases the probability of opening of the long-lasting inward calcium current (I_{Ca-L}), although the transient component (I_{Ca-T}) is unaffected (Hagiwara et al., 1988). The combination of the early operation of I_f and the later operation of the long-lasting calcium currents causes the rate of diastolic depolarization to increase with more rapid SA node pacemaker firing. These multiple mechanisms acting through the β-adrenergic receptors explain how adrenergic stimulation during exercise creates the tachycardia required to increase the cardiac output.

Intrinsic Heart Rate

The intrinsic heart rate is uncovered when autonomic control is removed by the combined pharmacologic blockade of sympathetic β-adrenergic and parasympathetic vagal activity (Jose, 1996). In normal subjects, the intrinsic rate can be up to 50% higher than the resting rate, showing that normally vagal inhibition is more powerful than adrenergic stimulation. In the presence of heart failure, the resting rate is increased because of the increased adrenergic tone required to maintain the blood pressure (see Chapter 16). The limited ability of the heart rate to increase in heart failure means that, with exercise, the cardiac output cannot increase to the levels required for adequate muscle perfusion, and fatigue sets in.

Overdrive Suppression

Overdrive suppression is the phenomenon whereby the sinus node overrides the activity of other potential pacemaker cells, as found in the AV node and elsewhere (Wanzhen et al., 1991). *Postpacing inhibition* is a closely related event whereby pacemaker activity is slow to resume when an induced tachycardia is terminated. When the sinus node is diseased, as in the *sick sinus syndrome* of the elderly, the sinus node recovery time is pathologically prolonged.

The mechanism of overdrive suppression usually is studied in isolated Purkinje fibers rather than in the SA node. During overdrive suppression induced by tachycardia, the slope of diastolic depolarization is decreased, and the voltage required to reach threshold is more positive. Hence, it is more difficult to initiate the action potential. A proposed mechanism is that the high heart rate causes repetitive entry of sodium ions with each action potential. Internal sodium activity increases. The activity of the sodium pump is enhanced, sodium ions are extruded, and the electrogenic current is increased, so that there is hyperpolarization and the net inward pacemaker current is less.

PROPAGATION OF IMPULSE

Once the impulse has formed in the SA node, it spreads rapidly throughout the atrium to reach the AV node. In atrial tissue, there is a new pattern of the action potential that is dominated by a fast sodium channel (Fig. 5-6). The action poten-

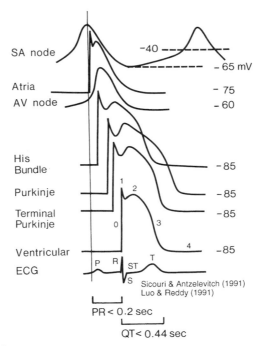

FIG. 5-6. Patterns of action potential from the SA node to the ventricle. The values on the right indicate the resting membrane potential (for data on atria, AV node, and ventricles, see Wang et al. *Circ Res* 1996;78:697). For details of SA node, see Fig. 5-3. For details of ECG see Fig. 5-11. For human atrial action potential see Carmeliet. *Cardiovasc Drug Ther* 1992;6:305. For ventricular action potential pattern, see Sicouri and Antzelevitch. *Circ Res* 1991;68:1729; and Luo and Reddy. *Circ Res* 1991;68:1501. PR, PR interval of ECG; QT, QT interval of ECG.

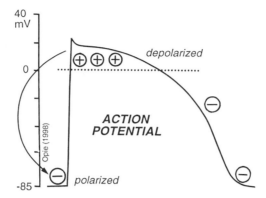

FIG. 5-7. Mechanism for spread of electrical impulse in relation to ventricular action potential. After depolarization, a current will flow from positive to negative charges, thereby opening the sodium channel of the adjacent previously polarized tissue, and spreading the impulse rapidly.

tial duration of atrial tissue is short (when measured at 50% of the peak amplitude), especially when compared with that of the ventricles, which may mean that the inward flow of calcium ions through the calcium channel is less, which in turn would link with the lesser force of contraction developed in the atrium rather than in the ventricle and the relatively lower activity of L-type calcium channels. The basic processes involved in depolarization and spread of the wave of excitation should be recalled at this stage. When the electrical impulse arrives at the sarcolemma, it opens the sodium activation gate to cause depolarization to a less negative voltage, which in turn opens the calcium gate. Sodium and calcium ions enter, causing an internal microzone of positive changes within the

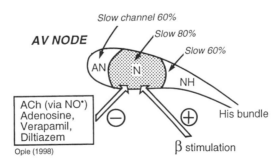

FIG. 5-8. Role of slow calcium channel in AV node. Note possible contributions of slow calcium and fast sodium channels to the three parts of the AV node: the atrionodal zone (AN), middle zone of true nodal cells (N), and nodal-His (NH) zone. For fast sodium channel in AV node, see Irisawa et al. (1995). Note the effect of the inhibitory factors, such as acetylcholine (ACh), adenosine, or calcium antagonists (verapamil, diltiazem), which slow conduction through the AV node. Conversely, β-agonists enhance conduction. NO, nitric oxide. See Fig. 5-9.

cell. The crucial aspect of the spread of the wave of excitation is that positive ions will now be attracted to the negative zone on the outside of the sarcolemma (Fig. 5-7). There are opposite changes on the inner side. Thus, as in a battery, current can flow from positively to negatively charged cells (it should be recognized that in strict terms, the current is actually a flow of electrons from the negative to the positive pole, not vice versa). Thus, by these processes, the surrounding sarcolemma tends to lose its polarity, which opens more of the surrounding sodium channels. A self-perpetuating process occurs, and the impulse readily spreads throughout the sarcolemma of a single heart cell. The greater the rate of depolarization, the more rapid the development of the charge differences between depolarized and polarized tissue, and the more rapid the rate of conduction from cell to cell. Thus, conduction of the wave of depolarization is rapid through tissues where the upstroke of the action potential is also rapid (considerable fast sodium channel activity), whereas conduction is slower through the AV node, where there is chiefly calcium channel activity with a slower rate of depolarization (Fig. 5-8). *Conduction between myocardial cells* may be explained by low-resistance *gap* or *nexus junctions* between cells through which the current can flow (see Fig. 3-10).

ATRIAL CONDUCTION

Are there specialized conducting fibers carrying the impulse through the atria from the sinus to the AV node? Three *internodal tracts* have been thought to serve as pathways that preferentially conduct the cardiac impulse through the atria. Histologically, they consist of cells somewhat similar to those of the Purkinje system. Physiologically, these cells are highly resistant to an increased extracellular potassium concentration, a property that resembles that of the sinus node. The pattern of atrial activation has been studied and displayed in the form of isochrones (Scher et al., 1979). *Isochrones* look like weather charts and display wavy lines that link sites of simultaneous excitation. The pattern of movement of isochrones shows how the impulse spreads. Such studies show that from the functional point of view, there are no narrow specialized atrial tracts. Rather, the entire atrial septum functions as a conduction system to take waves from the sinus to the AV node. According to this view, those atrial cells with specialized functional properties (resistance to high potassium, spontaneous diastolic depolarization) are not necessarily found in the three internodal tracts. Nonetheless, cardiac surgeons provide evidence for the importance of intranodal pathways that, when damaged at operation, can promote atrial rhythm abnormalities (Tamiya et al., 1992).

ATRIOVENTRICULAR NODE

Atrial impulses cannot travel directly to the ventricles because of the connective tissue that separates the two chambers of the heart. Hence, the electrical impulse is collected in the AV node (Fig. 5-8), which is located in the right atrium just above the origin of the tricuspid valve. From this node, the impulse continues along the His bundle through the connective tissue separating atria and ventricles. The AV node may be divided into three regions—atrionodal, nodal, and nodal-His—on the basis of striking differences in the shape of the action potential rather than on anatomic grounds. Most of the cells of the AV node are slender transitional cells, similar to the T cells of the SA node. These are a few simple rounded cells identical to P cells of the sinus node, and at the margin of the node are ordinary working myocardial cells. As the AV node becomes transformed into the His bundle and conduction system, the cells become more linearly arranged, and their properties correspond more and more closely to fast conduction tissue.

Electrophysiologic Properties of the AV Node

Many of the electrophysiologic properties of the AV node closely resemble those of the sinus node. In particular, there is a spontaneous slow diastolic depolarization with a slow upstroke, which is normally overridden by the sinus node. However, the AV node can serve as a subsidiary pacemaker when the main pacemaker in the sinus node fails to function. A second function of the AV node is to delay the rate at which the electrical impulse reaches the ventricles to ensure that the ventricles are relaxed at the time of atrial contraction (P wave), which therefore can help to fill the ventricles. A third function of the AV node is that it acts to control the number and order of supraventricular impulses.

The AV node responds in a highly complex way to the rate and type of electrical activation (Scher and Spah, 1979). Like other cardiac tissue, there is a built-in recovery time: the time lag before the next impulse can be processed. In addition, short cycles, as when the heart rate is fast, advance the recovery time (facilitation); in contrast, sustained very fast impulses slow conduction (fatigue). All three properties are required to explain the great variation in the responses of the AV node, including the phenomenon of AV block (described later in this chapter).

Autonomic Control of the Atrioventricular Node

The space just behind the AV node (*retronodal space*) is richly supplied with autonomic nerves. Here, adrenergic nerves deliver stimulatory sympathetic stimuli to the AV node to increase the rate of conduction (*positive dromotropic effect*), whereas vagal cholinergic nerves deliver inhibitory stimuli (*negative dromotropic effect*). These opposing effects are mediated by adrenergic stimulation and cholinergic inhibition of the L-type calcium current. When there is vagal stimulation of the muscarinic M_2 receptor, several mechanisms combine ultimately to inhibit the calcium current. First, as in the case of the SA node (see Fig. 2-11), interaction with G proteins inhibits the formation of cAMP and opens the K^+ channel, both of

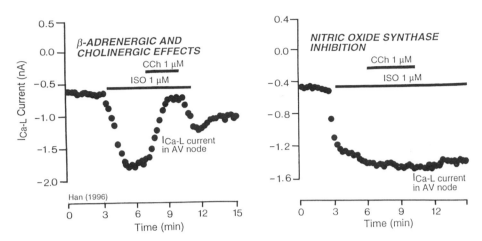

FIG. 5-9. Nitric oxide (NO) mediates cholinergic effects on AV node. Acetylcholine (mimicked by carbamylcholine, CCh) acts on the muscarinic M_2 receptor to stimulate NOS in SA node (see Kelly et al. *Circ Res* 1996;79:363), which in turn promotes formation of cGMP, the nucleotide that inhibits the calcium current (I_{Ca-L}). Hence, β-adrenergic stimulation of the calcium current, here achieved by isoproterenol (ISO), is opposed by cholinergic stimulation (CCh), and this inhibition is removed when synthesis of NO is inhibited (right panel). Modified from Han et al. *Circ Res* 1996;78:998, with permission of American Heart Association.

which tend to close the calcium channels. But an obligatory event, as in the case of the SA node, is the stimulation of NOS to form nitric oxide, which in turn promotes the formation of cGMP by the enzyme guanylate cyclase (Fig. 5-9). cGMP tends to close calcium channels. These inhibitory vagal mechanisms are most active when there is concurrent adrenergic stimulation.

Inhibition of the Atrioventricular Node by Calcium Antagonists

The contribution of the long-lasting calcium current to the action potential is most in the central nodal zone (Fig. 5-8), where automaticity is absent and where the upstroke of the action potential increases most slowly. Of the calcium antagonists, verapamil and diltiazem are most inhibitory on the AV node. These agents promote calcium channel closure (see Fig. 4-13). For complex reasons, drugs of the nifedipine family do not inhibit the AV node sufficiently to have clinical effects. Automaticity of this node may depend in part on sodium channel activity and in part on the T-type calcium channels that are insensitive to conventional verapamil and diltiazem.

Inhibition of the Atrioventricular Node by Adenosine

Adenosine, a breakdown product of adenosine triphosphate, both inhibits the L-type calcium current and hyperpolarizes the cell, the latter via the adenosine-sensitive potassium channel (see Table 4-7). These effects, similar to those of acetylcholine, inhibit the AV node (Fig. 5-10), which explains its pharmacologic effect in interrupting re-entry pathways that travel through this node to cause a type of supraventricular arrhythmia.

Changes in Acute Myocardial Infarction

Sensory receptors in the AV nodal area are thought to convey different afferent stimuli to central vasomotor regulatory centers, effecting reflexes involving efferent vagal stimulation with symptoms such as bradycardia, AV conduction delay, and nausea. Such reflex vagal effects may be precipitated by a certain type of acute cardiac damage, as in acute myocardial infarction involving the nodal area (inferoposterior infarction). Regarding adenosine, if it were carried to the AV node cells from other neighboring acutely ischemic cells, there would be transient AV conduction disturbances in the early phase of acute myocardial infarction. An interesting prediction has been made and proven experimentally: methylxanthines, which prevent adenosine from interacting with its cell receptor, could be useful in combating AV heart block.

His BUNDLE AND ITS BRANCHES: PURKINJE FIBERS

The His bundle, which divides into left and right bundles, runs from the AV node. It penetrates the connecting tissue dividing atria and ventricles and is the only muscular connection between these chambers. The cells found in the common bundle and bundle branches are the characteristic Purkinje cells (see Chapter 3). They are adapted to the rapid conduction of the electrical impulse as fol-

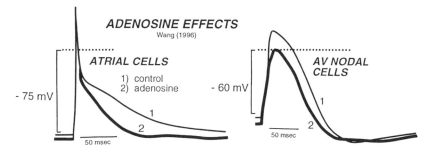

FIG. 5-10. Adenosine inhibits AV node and atria. In atrial tissue (left) adenosine shortens action potential (AP) duration and modestly hyperpolarizes. In the AV node, as shown in the right panel, adenosine had similar effects and also decreased the action potential amplitude and the rate of increase of the action potential. In ventricular cells, adenosine had no effects. The inhibitory effects of adenosine on the AV node account for its therapeutic use in certain fast heart rates (supraventricular tachycardias) in which there is re-entry through the AV node. Modified from Wang et al. *Circ Res* 1996;78:697, with permission of the American Heart Association.

lows. First, these cells are about three times wider than the standard ventricular myocytes (see Table 3-1), the principle being that the resistance to electrical conduction decreases as the cellular diameter increases. Second, the sparseness of myofibrils and T-tubules decreases the resistance to internal conduction. Third, Purkinje cells are packed tightly together so that the diameter effectively available for conduction is that of the entire bundle rather than of the individual components. Finally, there are numerous end-to-end gap junctions that facilitate faster conduction between cells. It is all these properties that confer on Purkinje cells the ability to conduct electrical impulses quickly enough (200 cm/sec) to enable all the cells of the ventricles to be excited almost simultaneously.

Although Purkinje cells have the potential for spontaneous diastolic depolarization, two factors keep them from doing so. First, the rate of spontaneous firing is much slower than that of nodal tissue, being only about 30 per minute. Thus, the potential automaticity is overdriven by that of both the sinus and the AV nodes. Second, although the Purkinje pacemaker current I_f operates at a negative voltage range as found in normally polarized Purkinje fibers, such fibers have a high resting potassium conductance, so the outward potassium current more than neutralizes the inward current carried by I_f. However, when the Purkinje fibers are damaged as may occur in ischemia, the resting voltage range moves into that appropriate for firing of I_f, with risk of spontaneous depolarization and ectopic beats.

The His bundle has a dual blood supply, from both left anterior and posterior descending coronary arteries, so ischemic damage is unusual. In contrast, the bundle branches run into the ventricles, where coronary artery disease is common and can cause ischemia of the bundles with risk of bundle branch block.

THE ELECTROCARDIOGRAM

A big gap exists between the origin of the heart beat in the specialized cells of the sinus node and the contraction of the ventricular myofibril. That gap is bridged first by the rapid conduction of the electrical impulse through the atria, so as to fire the AV node, which in turn sends another impulse down the specialized His bundle and Purkinje fibers. The terminal branches (*arborization of the Purkinje system*) spread the impulse throughout the ventricles, eventually traveling along the sarcolemma of the myocytes, whence the process of *excitation–contraction coupling* links the wave of depolarization on the cell surface to the contractile system. This whole sequence can be followed relatively simply by the use of the body surface electrocardiogram (ECG) (Fig. 5-11). The normal ECG complex consists of the P wave, the PR interval, the QRS wave, the ST segment, and the T wave. The P wave of the normal ECG trace reflects the spread of the impulse through the atria (Fig. 5-1). From the SA node, most of the PR interval indicates the slower rate of conduction through the AV node (strictly, it should be the PQ interval), whereas the small Q wave shows that the ventricular impulse is spreading through the septum in the direction opposite to the site

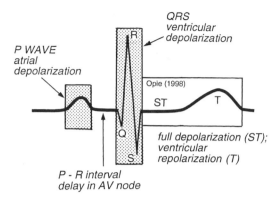

FIG. 5-11. Normal ECG. This shows the normal ECG pattern of a limb lead, such as lead II, and the basic events that each component represents. See also Fig. 5-1.

where the body surface electrode is placed. The large QR wave represents fast depolarization with rapid conduction toward the electrode (hence a positive wave), followed by a stage when the whole ventricle is fully depolarized, corresponding to the plateau phase of the ventricular action potential. Because there is no current flowing at that stage, the body surface registers this absence of flow

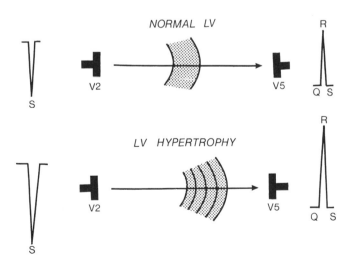

FIG. 5-12. Two fundamental laws. As the electrical impulse approaches the surface ECG electrode, a positive wave develops (upward deflection, right panel). Conversely, a negative wave indicates current flow away from the ECG electrode (downward deflection, left panel). Second, when the mass of muscle underlying the electrode is thicker and closer to the electrode, then the current flow is greater and the voltage deflection also greater. The second law is a simplification of the solid angle theory (Holland and Arnsdorf, 1977).

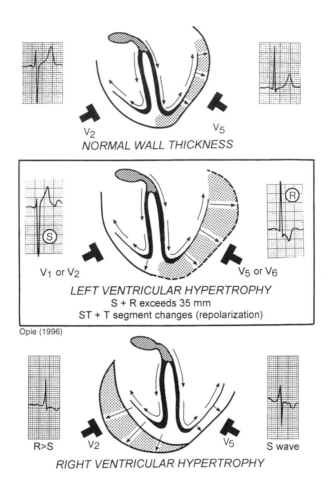

NORMAL WALL THICKNESS

LEFT VENTRICULAR HYPERTROPHY
S + R exceeds 35 mm
ST + T segment changes (repolarization)

Opie (1996)

RIGHT VENTRICULAR HYPERTROPHY

FIG. 5-13. ECG in ventricular hypertrophy. Thickening of the ventricular wall (hypertrophy) changes the ECG pattern (Molloy et al., 1992). The normal ECG deflections in lead V_5, facing the left ventricle, and V_2, looking at the LV from the other side, are shown in the top panel. In the presence of left ventricular hypertrophy (LVH, middle panel), there is a greater positive voltage deflection in the electrodes facing the left ventricle, such as leads II, V_5, and V_6, and a greater negative voltage in leads facing the ventricle from the other direction, such as V_2. Hence, the S wave in V_1 or V_2 is increased as is the R wave in V_5 or V_6. The bottom panel shows similar principles applied to right ventricular hypertrophy (RVH). In reality, the ECG diagnosis of LVH is not too precise. Some criteria are that LVH exists when (1) the sum of RS in V_2 and QR in V_5 exceeds 35 mm; (2) there is some widening of the QRS (conduction delay); and (3) there are repolarization changes in the ST segment and T wave. A product of the QRS voltage in all 12 standard leads and the QRS duration may be one of the more accurate ECG indices of LVH. RVH exists when QR exceeds RS in V_1 and the axis in the limb leads shows right axis deviation. For axis, see Fig. 5-15.

as an isoelectric (Greek *iso,* the same) state. The RS wave represents the return from the charged to the isoelectric state, and the ST segment the duration of the isoelectric state. Finally, the myocardium repolarizes, and the ensuing T wave is in the same direction as the QRS wave. Hence, the surface ECG makes it possible to follow the wave of conduction from the SA node, through the atria, to the AV node, and ultimately to the ventricles.

There are two simple rules. An electrode (lead) facing an approaching wave of depolarization records a positive potential, which inscribes an upright deflec-

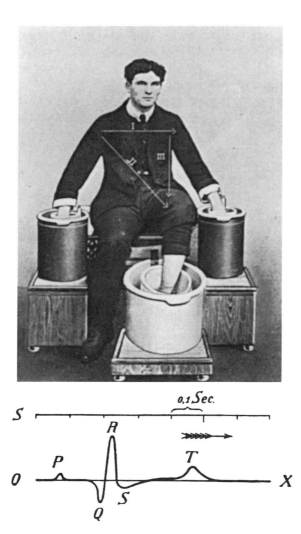

FIG. 5-14. Einthoven's ECG. The apparatus used to obtain this ECG in 1913 is taken from the book of Sir Thomas Lewis, *Clinical Electrocardiography.* Note, in white, the Einthoven triangle on the subject's chest. See also Fig. 5-15.

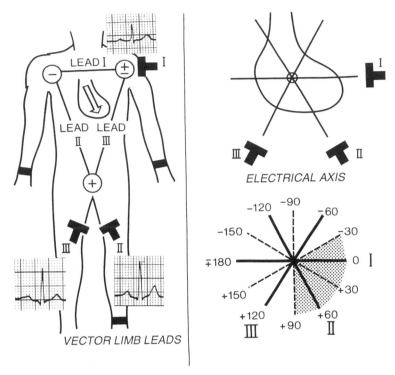

FIG. 5-15. Limb leads and electrical axis. Limb leads I, II, and III of the body surface ECG. When the axis is normal (between –30 degrees and +90 degrees, shaded), then the ECG deflection is usually positive in all three leads as shown. To derive the electrical axis, Einthoven's triangle (on body, left) is transposed to the frontal plane hexaxial (six axes) system derived from leads I, II, and III. The peak amplitude of leads I and III is plotted on its respective axis (seven little blocks for lead I, 12 for lead III), and perpendicular lines are dropped. Where these lines cross is connected to the hub of the system to give the electrical axis, in this case about +70 degrees, i.e., normal. An axis situated from –30 degrees to –90 degrees represents left axis deviation and an axis from +90 degrees to +180 degrees represents right axis deviation (the latter is often found in right ventricular hypertrophy).

tion in the ECG, positive potentials conventionally being recorded as upward deflections (Fig. 5-12). If the wave of depolarization moves away from the recording electrode, a downward deflection is written. Second, the greater the mass of tissue that the electrode faces, the greater the positive deflection as the wave approaches (Fig. 5-13).

Twelve Conventional ECG Leads

The rhythmic repetitive spread of the electrical impulse throughout the heart from the SA node to ventricular myocytes that has just been described can be

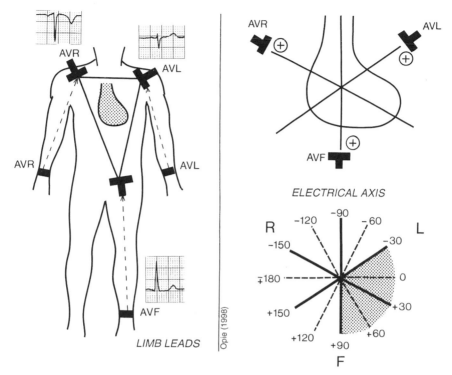

FIG. 5-16. Augmented vector limb leads. These are augmented vectors for the right arm (aVR), left arm (aVL), and left foot (aVF) with their contributions to the hexaxial system. The axis also can be calculated from these leads. For example, in the traces shown, aVF has a positive deflection of 12 small squares, and aVR a negative deflection of 12 small squares. Using the same principles as in Fig. 5-15, the axis can be calculated to be +60 degrees, again within normal limits.

monitored by the body surface ECG. The original ECG recorded by Einthoven (Fig. 5-14) had huge immersion electrodes into which were placed the left arm, the right arm, and the left leg, whereas the right leg was used as the earth. These electrodes recorded the difference of electrical potential between each of these limbs. The electrodes were primitive and their sensitivity low, so the traces were poor and difficult to interpret. With modern suction electrodes and high fidelity transducers and the aid of amplification, it is possible to achieve excellent recordings of the body surface ECG.

The bipolar standard leads—leads I, II, and III—are the same as those used by Einthoven (Fig. 5-15). In addition, the unipolar limb leads record the electrical potential at only one of the limbs (Fig. 5-16). Because the deflections recorded need further augmentation to give clearly visible traces, the letter "a" for "augmented" is added to the letter "V" for "vector." Thus, the unipolar recording from each point is called aVR from the right arm, aVL from the left

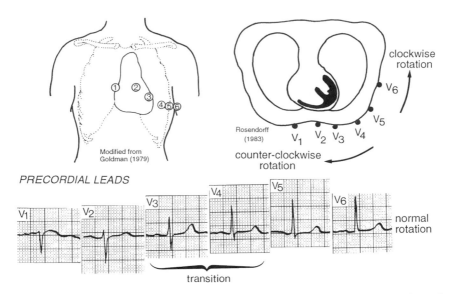

FIG. 5-17. Precordial electrodes. Standard anatomic situation of the precordial electrodes agreed upon by the American Heart Association and the British Cardiac Society. The positions are:

V_1 = 4th right intercostal space at sternal edge

V_2 = 4th left intercostal space at sternal edge

V_3 = halfway between V_2 and V_4

V_4 = 5th left intercostal space in the midclavicular line

V_5 = anterior axilliary line, same plane as V_4

V_6 = mid-axilliary line, same plane as V_5

With a normal situation of the heart (normal rotation), the ECG complexes change from RV in type (precordial RS wave dominant) to LV in type (dominant QR) at V_3 to V_4. With clockwise rotation, RV complexes are found in V_5 or even V_6, and with counterclockwise rotation, QR complexes dominate in V_3 and even V_2.

arm, and aVF from the left foot. Each unipolar lead is recorded against a combination of leads, which is empirically known to produce a continuous zero potential. Thus, for example, aVR records the ECG deflection from the right arm versus the zero produced by the combined electrical input of aVR, aVL, and aVF. Leads V_1 to V_6 represent unipolar precordial chest leads, working on a similar principle to the augmented limb leads. Each V lead is taken from a specific site on the chest wall (Fig. 5-17).

SINOATRIAL RATE

A simple rule to derive the rate of sinus node discharge (heart rate) is to count the number of R-R intervals per 3 seconds of ECG tracing and to multiply by 20. At the standard ECG paper speed of 25 mm/sec, every 15th square (3 seconds) has a vertical line above it. Conventionally, if the rate exceeds 100 per minute (R-R less than three large squares) and the beat originates in the sinus node, that is a sinus tachycardia (Greek *tachys,* fast). Conversely, if the R-R interval exceeds five large squares and the sinus rate is below 60 per minute, that is a sinus bradycardia (Greek *bradys,* slow). In the normal subject, the heart rate may vary between a sinus tachycardia (exercise, emotion) and a sinus bradycardia, as during sleep.

Sinus Arrhythmia

Normally during inspiration there is a reflex mechanism that transiently increases the heart rate (Fig. 5-18). In some individuals, this reflex (the *Hering-Breuer reflex*) seems highly active, so that the inspiratory-expiratory cycle produces a marked change in heart rate. This physiologic variation is only an apparent irregularity, called sinus arrhythmia (*a* = not; i.e., not a normal rhythm). It must be distinguished from serious pathologic arrhythmias, the latter usually the result of organic heart disease (see Chapter 20).

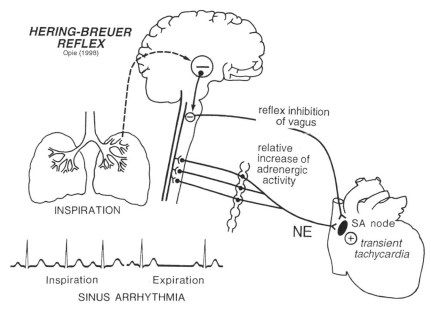

FIG. 5-18. Sinus arrhythmia. This is one of the most common physiologic irregularities of the rhythm. It reflects varying rates of discharge of the sinus node. During inspiration, the Hering-Breuer reflex is stimulated to inhibit the vagal center. The latter normally depresses the sinus rate, and its inhibition results in a relative increase of adrenergic activity. Consequently, there is a transient tachycardia. NE, norepinephrine.

TABLE 5-2. *Physiologic or pharmacologic procedures or agents that increase the discharge rate of the sinoatrial node and the heart rate*

Procedure or agent	Presumed mechanism
Acute exercise, emotional stimuli	β-adrenergic discharge
β-adrenergic receptor agonists	Increased opening probability of L-calcium channels via formation of cAMP and L-channel phosphorylation; also increased I_f in sinus node
Atropine	Competitive inhibition of acetylcholine at muscarinic cholinergic receptors
Congestive heart failure	Compensatory reflex increase in adrenergic tone required to maintain blood pressure

Sinus Tachycardia and Bradycardia

Sinus tachycardia, the most common of the supraventricular tachycardia, occurs when the sinus rate exceeds an arbitrary value of 100 beats/min, as typically occurs in response to acute exercise or emotional stimuli as a result of increased activity of the adrenergic system (Table 5-2). Drugs or disease also can cause a sinus tachycardia.

When the sinus node discharges below a certain arbitrary rate, usually below 60 beats/min, the condition is called sinus bradycardia. Physiologically, athletes have slow heart rates because aerobic training increases the parasympathetic tone relative to that of the sympathetic adrenergic system (Table 5-3). The longer diastolic interval of the athlete's heart allows a greater end-diastolic fiber length and a greater stroke volume according to Starling's law (see Chapter 12), so that the cardiac output is maintained at normal despite the slower heart rate. Another physiologic cause of bradycardia is sleep, when the high vagal tone causes the heart rate to decrease. Pharmacologically, sinus bradycardia is typical of treatment by β-adrenergic antagonist drugs (Table 5-3).

TABLE 5-3. *Physiologic or pharmacologic procedures or agents that inhibit the sinoatrial node and decrease the heart rate*

Procedure or agent	Presumed mechanism
Athletic training	Increased vagal activity and decreased adrenergic effects
Sleep	Increased vagal and decreased adrenergic effects
Vagal stimulation	Release of acetylcholine and stimulation of I_{KACh} and hyperpolarization; also decreases L-calcium channel activity by inhibition of formation of cAMP; also inhibits β-adrenergic increase of I_f
β-adrenergic receptor	Inhibition of formation of cAMP with lesser probability of L-calcium antagonists channels being in open state; also indirect inhibition of I_f
Calcium antagonists (verapamil, diltiazem)	Inhibition of L-calcium channel current
Digitalis	Vagal stimulation
Adenosine	Stimulation of adenosine-operated potassium channel resulting in hyperpolarization

In the *sick sinus syndrome*, the SA node intermittently and progressively fails to fire, with risk of *sinus arrest*. This disease characteristically occurs in the older age group, frequently a result of coronary artery disease or idiopathic fibrosis (see also Pacing by Suppression).

ATRIOVENTRICULAR NODAL DISEASE AND HEART BLOCK

First, the physiologic function of the AV node should be recalled. The depolarization of ventricular cells starts about 80 msec after the impulse leaves atrial tissue (Scher et al., 1959). This is the time taken for the impulse to traverse the AV node, His bundle, and bundle branches. Electrocardiographically, this interval corresponds to the *PR interval* (beginning of P wave to beginning of R wave, normal upper limit 0.20 seconds) most of which reflects delays within the AV node (Fig. 5-19). The importance of this delay is that the atrial booster contraction, occurring with the P wave, has sufficient time to complete the process of finally filling the ventricle before ventricular contraction starts. However, the delay within the AV node can be excessive when this node is damaged by disease such as in ischemia or myocarditis (an inflammatory disease). Also, excess AV delay occurs in some overtrained athletes. This condition is termed *AV nodal block*, or often simply *heart block* (Fig. 5-20).

When the only abnormality on the ECG is the prolonged PR interval, there is *first-degree heart block*. Besides its occurrence in ischemia, myocarditis, or overtraining, it also can be caused by a variety of drugs inhibiting the AV node. Not surprisingly, the calcium channel antagonists verapamil and diltiazem inhibit the AV node. This inhibition reflects the prominent role of the L-type cal-

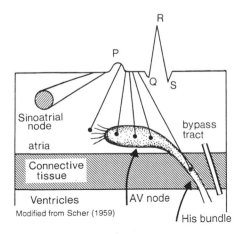

FIG. 5-19. PR interval of ECG. Components of the conduction system and their contribution to the PR interval of the ECG. For significance of the bypass tract in production of arrhythmias, see Chapter 20. Modified from Scher et al. (1959).

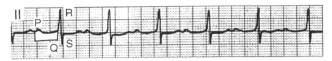

AV BLOCK   1st degree   PR=0.36sec

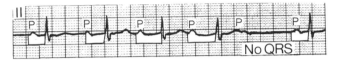

AV BLOCK   2nd degree   Wenckebach

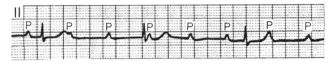

AV BLOCK   3rd degree   AV dissociation

FIG. 5-20. Atrioventricular block. In first-degree AV block, in the top panel, the PR interval is prolonged beyond 0.2 seconds. In second-degree AV block, in the middle panel, some of the atrial impulses (P) fail to reach the ventricles, so that there are dropped beats (no QRS complexes). In third-degree AV block (bottom panel), there is complete AV dissociation, so that P and QRS waves bear no relation to each other. Second-degree heart block has many different varieties. The type shown in the middle panel is also called the Wenckebach phenomenon, (Talajic et al., 1991) where progressive lengthening of the PR interval leads to dropped QRS complexes. First- and second-degree block may not be pathologic and also can occur physiologically in athletes (see Fig. 2-3).

cium channel in AV nodal conduction (Fig. 5-8). Another inhibitory drug is digitalis, which stimulates the vagus in addition to inhibiting the sodium pump (see Fig. 4-27).

When the conduction between the atria and ventricles is severely inhibited, usually as a result of disease of the AV node and His bundle, the P wave intermittently fails in its efforts to reach the ventricles (*second-degree heart block*), or there is a total block between atria and ventricles (*third-degree* or *complete heart block*). In the latter instance, ventricular asystole occurs, and death is inevitable unless a subsidiary pacemaker takes over. Such an *idioventricular rhythm* usually arises in the Purkinje fibers of the His bundle or upper bundle branches and fires at a much lower spontaneous rate than the sinus node. When there is sudden development of complete heart block, the idioventricular rhythm may take some time to develop. During the period of asystole, there is risk of cerebral ischemia and syncope may develop (*Stokes-Adams attack*).

Subsidiary Pacemakers

Physiologically, only the sinus node functions as a pacemaker. When it fails, the AV node can take over at 36 to 60 depolarizations per minute (*nodal rhythm*). When the AV node itself is blocked or injured, a new even slower pacemaker site may form at the junction of the AV node and His bundle (*junctional escape rhythm*). When this site is also inhibited, then the Purkinje fibers in the His bundle or below may fire at about 30 per minute (*idioventricular rhythm*).

Bundle Branch Block

In coronary artery disease, the blood supply to one of the two main His bundles may be blocked with characteristic ECG changes. In *left bundle branch block*, there is typically a bifid widened QRS complex (*bifid* means a double deflection divided by a notch) in leads facing the left ventricle such as V_4 to V_6 (Fig. 5-21). In *right bundle branch block*, a similar bifid pattern holds in leads facing the right ventricle, that is, V_1 and V_2 (Fig. 5-22).

Each of the two branches of the left bundle may be independently blocked. It needs emphasis that these are functional not anatomic branches. In *left anterior hemiblock*, also called left anterior fascicular block (Latin *fasciculus,* bundle), there is an electrically silent zone of the heart in the territory of this bundle. The result is that the initial phase of left ventricular depolarization occurs by the posterior rather than the anterior bundle. The result is an initial R wave in the leads facing the left ventricle, such as leads II and V_6. Because of the electrical silence of the territory of the left anterior bundle, the normal full development of the positive deflection of the QRS wave is impaired. Rather, there is a net wave away

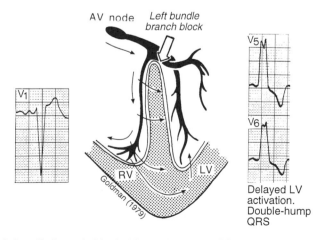

FIG. 5-21. Left bundle branch block. Mechanism and ECG traces. Modified from Goldman (1979) with permission.

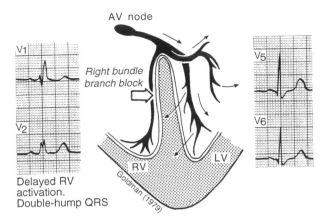

FIG. 5-22. Right bundle branch block. Mechanism and ECG traces. Modified from Goldman (1979) with permission.

from the left ventricular leads, that is, an S wave. As a rough rule, if the R wave amplitude equals or exceeds the S wave in lead II, one cause is left anterior hemiblock (Fig. 5-23).

In *left posterior hemiblock* there is an electrically silent part of the heart in the territory of the left posterior bundle, which serves the left ventricular side of the

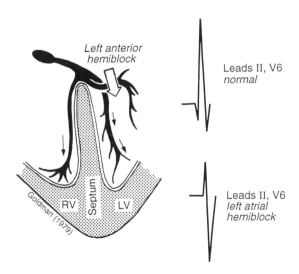

FIG. 5-23. Left anterior hemiblock (left anterior fasicular block). Mechanism and ECG traces. Hypothetically, there is an electrically "silent" area in the left anterior part of the left ventricle, so that the leads facing the left ventricle, such as II and V6 (see Figs. 5-15 and 5-17), display a greater amplitude of negative than of positive deflection. That is because the major current flow is away from the lead. There is thus left axis deviation. Modified from Goldman (1979) with permission.

septum and the posterior wall of the left ventricle. This is a rare condition, apart from acute myocardial infarction. aVL, normally showing a positive QRS deflection as the electrical wave moves toward it, becomes negative as the wave moves away from it, and the QRS has a downward pattern.

One important complication of bundle branch block is in the presence of coronary artery disease. If a patient with acute myocardial infarction has a block of two of the three bundles (*bifascicular block*), then the fear is that extension of the infarction will block all three bundles with complete heart block and threat of cardiac arrest. Hence, in a patient with acute myocardial infarction, special attention is paid to the management of bifascicular block; a temporary cardiac pacemaker may be inserted until the outlook improves.

SUMMARY

1. *The spontaneous heart rate is chiefly governed by the rate of diastolic depolarization of the pacemaker (P) cells of the sinus node,* the mechanism of which is still not completely understood. There are at least three pacemaker currents: the decaying potassium current, I_k, the calcium current, I_{Ca}, and the inward current, I_f. A background inward current is the fourth pacemaking current. These currents respond to adrenergic or cholinergic stimulation to increase or decrease the heart rate, for example, during exercise or at night, respectively.

2. *The electrical impulse travels from the sinus node to the AV node.* Conduction through the AV node is normally slow. Conduction through the His bundle and down the bundle branches to the ventricular endocardium is by Purkinje cells, which in some ways are primitive and in other ways are highly specialized, with a very rapid rate of conduction. The cardiac impulse has now arrived at the sarcolemma of the ventricular myocyte, and the next step is excitation–contraction coupling, whereby depolarization leads to the contraction process.

3. *These processes can be monitored by the body surface ECG* in which the P wave represents atrial depolarization, the PR interval the delay in the AV node, and the QRS wave the phase of rapid ventricular depolarization. The ST segment represents the fully depolarized ventricle, corresponding to the plateau of the action potential. The T wave reflects the process of repolarization. Although it would be expected that the T wave would be negative, it is normally positive, that is, in the same direction as the QRS wave.

4. *The ECG allows precise determination of the heart rate.* There are also characteristic ECG changes of ventricular hypertrophy and of heart block when conduction from the atria to the ventricles is impaired.

STUDENT QUESTIONS

1. Enumerate the chief pacemaker currents of the sinoatrial node and describe the proposed function of each.

2. What are the effects of the autonomic nervous system on the sinoatrial node? Describe the currents involved.
3. Describe the spread of the cardiac impulse from the sinoatrial node to the surface of the contractile myocardium.
4. Describe a typical normal ECG complex from a limb lead. How is the heart rate derived? What basic electrophysiologic events does each component of the ECG complex reflect?
5. What is Einthoven's triangle?
6. Which are the physiologic events that increase the heart rate? Which events decrease the heart rate? What is sinus arrhythmia?

CARDIOLOGIST-IN-TRAINING QUESTIONS

1. Describe the action potential of the sinoatrial node, and the participation of each of the pacemaker currents.
2. Why do the calcium antagonist drugs verapmil and diltiazem slow but not arrest the sinoatrial node?
3. Explain the proposed cellular basis of overdrive suppression.
4. Describe the mechanism whereby adenosine inhibits the atrioventricular node. How does this differ from the mechanism involved in the inhibitory effects of verapamil or diltiazem?
5. Explain the origin of the PR interval of the ECG.
6. Explain the characteristic electrocardiographic changes of left ventricular hypertrophy.
7. How many types of conduction block do you recognize?

REFERENCES

1. Chang F, Gao J, Tromba C, Cohen I, DiFrancesco D. Acetylcholine reverses effects of beta-agonists on pacemaker current in canine cardiac Purkinje fibres but has no direct action. A difference between primary and secondary pacemakers. *Circ Res* 1990;66:633–636.
2. DiFrancesco D. The contribution of the "pacemaker" current (I_f) to generation of spontaneous activity in rabbit sinoatrial node myocytes. *J Physiol* 1991;434:23–40.
3. DiFrancesco D, Tromba C. Acetylcholine inhibits activation of the cardiac hyperpolarizing-activated current If. *Pflugers Arch* 1987;410:139–142.
4. Goldman MJ. In: *Principles of Clinical Electrocardiography*. 10th ed. Los Altos, CA: Lange Medical Publications, 1979.
5. Hagiwara N, Irisawa H, Kameyama M. Contribution of two types of calcium currents to the pacemaker potentials of rabbit sinoatrial node cells. *J Physiol* 1988;395:233–253.
6. Han X, Shimoni Y, Giles WR. A cellular mechanism for nitric oxide-mediated cholinergic control of mammalian heart rate. *J Gen Physiol* 1995;106:45–65.
7. Holland RP, Arnsdorff MF. Solid angle theory and the electrocardiogram: Physiologic and quantative interpretations. *Prog Cardiovasc Dis* 1977;19:431–457.
8. Irisawa H, Brown HF, Giles W. Cardiac pacemaking in the sinoatrial node. *Physiol Rev* 1993;73:197–227.
9. Irisawa H, Noma A, Matsuda H. Electrogenesis of the pacemaker potential as revealed by atrioventricular nodal experiments. In: Sperelakis N (ed). *Physiology and Pathophysiology of the Heart*. 3rd ed. Boston: Kluwer Academic, 1995;137–151.
10. Jose AD. Effect of combined sympathetic and parasympathetic blockade on heart rate and cardiac function in man. *Am J Cardiol* 1966;18:476–478.

11. Molloy TJ, Okin PM, Devereux RB, Kligfield P. Electrocardiographic detection of left ventricular hypertrophy by the simple QRS voltage-duration product. *J Am Coll Cardiol* 1992;20:1180–1186.
12. Opthof T. The mammalian sinoatrial node. *Cardiovasc Drug Ther* 1988;1:573–597.
13. Scher AM, Rodriquez MI, Liikane J, Young AC. The mechanism of atrioventricular conduction. *Circ Res* 1959;7:54–61.
14. Scher AM, Spah MS. Cardiac depolarization and repolarization and the electrocardiogram. In: Berne RM (ed). *Handbook of Physiology. The Cardiovascular System.* Bethesda: American Physiological Society, 1979;357–392.
15. Talajic M, Papadatos D, Villemaire C, et al. A unified model of atrioventricular nodal conduction predicts dynamic changes in Wenckebach periodicity. *Circ Res* 1991;68:1280–1293.
16. Tamiya T, Yamashiro T, Hata A, Kuge K, et al. Electrophysiologic study of dysrhythmias after atrial operations in dogs. *Ann Thorac Surg* 1992;54:717–724.
17. Wanzhen Z, Glass L, Shier A. Evolution of rhythms during periodic stimulation of embryonic chick heart cell aggregates. *Circ Res* 1991;69:1022–1033.
18. Yanagihara K, Noma A, Irisawa H. Reconstruction of sino-atrial node pacemaker potential based on the voltage clamp experiments. *Jpn J Physiol* 1980;30:841–857.

PART III

Calcium and Contraction:
Receptors and Signals

6

Excitation–Contraction Coupling and Calcium

Phospholamban: a prominent regulator of myocardial contractility.
Koss and Kranias, 1996

The rapid propagation of the cardiac impulse from the pacemaker cells of the sinus node to the ventricular cells is largely dependent on the activity of the fast sodium channel. Once the impulse has reached the ventricular cells, the next event of critical importance is the voltage-induced increased opening of the calcium channels of contractile cells of the ventricles, followed by a series of intracellular movements of calcium ions, leading to myocardial contraction and relaxation. Contraction must be followed by relaxation, which results from uptake of calcium ions into the sarcoplasmic reticulum (SR). Only small amounts of calcium ions actually enter and leave the cell with each cardiac cycle. The majority of calcium ion movements are from the intracellular calcium stores to the cytosol and back again (Fig. 6-1). The sarcolemma maintains a vast gradient of calcium ion concentration from the extracellular value of about 1 mmol/L (10^{-3} mol/L) to intracellular values, which increase from diastolic values of about 10^{-7} mol/L up to systolic values of 10^{-5} mol/L during maximal contraction (Fig. 6-2).

This chapter concentrates on those calcium ion fluxes that link the wave of excitation to contraction by the process of excitation–contraction coupling. The chapters that follow explain the role of the adrenergic system, its β-adrenergic receptor, and the second messenger, cyclic adenosine monophosphate (cAMP), in the control of cellular calcium ion movements and the calcium-dependent contractile mechanism of the myocardium.

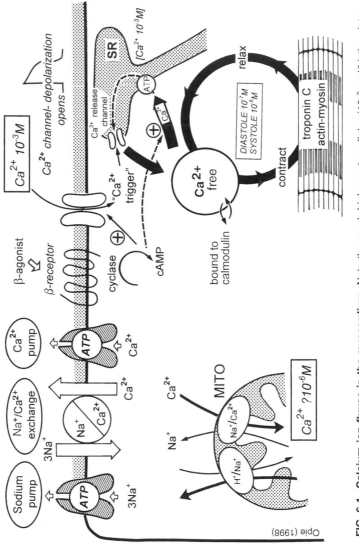

FIG. 6-1. Calcium ion fluxes in the myocardium. Note the much higher extracellular (10^{-3} mol/L) than intracellular value and a hypothetical mitochondrial value of about 10^{-6} mol/L. The mitochondria could act as a buffer against excessive changes in the free cytosolic calcium concentration. MITO, mitochondria.

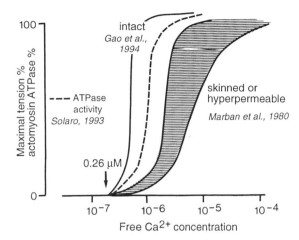

FIG. 6-2. Relationship of free ionized calcium concentration to tension development. The resting diastolic value is about 0.26 μmol/L, increasing to 10^{-5} mol/L at maximal tension development. For details, see Marban et al. *Nature* 1980;286:845; Solaro et al. *Circulation* 1993;87(suppl VI):38; and Gao et al. *Circ Res* 1994;76:720.

CALCIUM ION MOVEMENTS

The overall pattern of calcium ion movements associated with the contraction cycle is not yet fully clarified. The key event in the generally accepted model is calcium-induced release from the SR as follows. The major intracellular calcium store is probably in the SR (Fig. 6-3). It is from here that relatively large amounts of calcium ions are liberated by the small but varying amounts of calcium entering the cell during the opening of the L-type calcium channels induced by depolarization. The result is an increasing interaction of calcium ions with the contractile protein troponin-C. When the ambient calcium concentration is low, troponin-C has a molecular structure that inhibits the interaction between actin and myosin. As the cytosolic calcium increases, the molecular structure of troponin-C changes, and this inhibition is removed. (Details will be described in Chapter 8.) The interaction of actin and myosin is facilitated and contraction takes place. When the release of calcium ions from the SR ceases, then the increase of cytosolic calcium comes to an end and contraction ceases. To initiate relaxation, the cytosolic calcium is rapidly taken up by the calcium pump of the SR. This hypothesis has received strong support from the molecular characterization of the receptor on the SR that releases calcium (Berridge, 1993). A lesser amount of calcium is moved out of the cell. As the cytosolic calcium concentration decreases, relaxation is initiated as troponin-C starts to inhibit actin and myosin once more.

To balance the small amount of calcium entering the heart cell with each depolarization, a similar quantity of calcium ions leaves the cell by one of two processes (Fig. 6-3). First, internal calcium can be exchanged for external

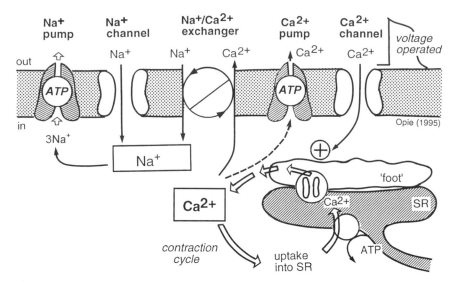

FIG. 6-3. Regulation of calcium balance in cardiac myocyte. There is a balance between the Ca^{2+} ions entering upon depolarization (right) and those leaving the cell by the Na$^+$/Ca^{2+} exchange mechanism. A smaller number of Ca^{2+} ions leave by an ATP-dependent sarcolemmal Ca^{2+} pump. Ion gradients for Na$^+$ and K$^+$ are maintained by the operation of the sodium pump (Na$^+$/K$^+$-ATPase). An increased internal Ca^{2+} after Ca^{2+} release from the SR is reduced by competition among one of three routes: uptake into the SR, Na$^+$/Ca^{2+} exchange, and outward pumping by the membrane Ca^{2+}-ATPase. The dominant uptake mechanism is into the SR, followed by the exchanger, followed by the membrane pump.

sodium ions by Na$^+$/Ca^{2+} exchange (Table 6-1). Second, and of lesser importance, a sarcolemmal calcium pump that is adenosine triphosphate (ATP) consuming can transfer calcium outward into the extracellular space against a concentration gradient. The exchange between mitochondrial and cytosolic calcium is relatively slow when compared with that between the SR and the cytosol. Hence, mitochondria do not participate in the beat-to-beat control of calcium ion movements. Nevertheless, during conditions of cellular cytosolic calcium over-

TABLE 6-1. *Mechanisms for lowering cytosolic Ca^{2+} concentration in myocardial cells[a]*

	% of total uptake of calcium from cytosol[b]
SR	
Phospholamban-modulated Ca^{2+} pump	88
Sarcolemma	
Na$^+$-Ca^{2+} exchange	5
Ca^{2+} pump	1
Mitochondria	6

[a]From Carafoli. *Membrane Transport of Calcium.* New York: Academic, 1982;134.
[b]Relative contribution at 1 µmol/L Ca^{2+} and 1–3 mmol/L Mg^{2+}.

load, to be discussed later in this chapter, mitochondria may help to protect the cell by storing some of the excess calcium.

Calcium Transients

The cyclic variations in the concentration of cytosolic calcium ions are also called calcium transients. Recent refinements in techniques for measuring internal calcium suggest a diastolic level of about 10^{-7} mol/L, and the systolic peak can be up to 10^{-5} mol/L, depending on the contractile state of the myocardium (Fig. 6-2). Calcium transients are increased in amplitude by β-adrenergic stimulation. It might be supposed that there would be a simple relationship between the calcium transients and the events of the contraction–relaxation cycle because the contractile proteins are directly sensitive to the prevailing internal calcium concentration (see Chapter 8). However, when calcium transients are measured by the calcium-sensitive dye *aequorin*, the calcium transient decreases before contractile force increases (Fig. 6-4), an apparently unexpected finding. An important technical point is as follows. The aequorin signal may be especially sensitive to a cytosolic subcompartment of calcium that is concerned predominantly with the release and uptake of calcium by the SR, and aequorin may be

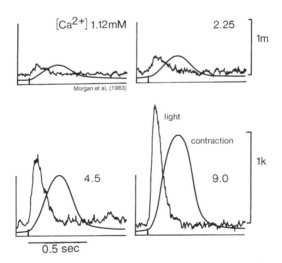

FIG. 6-4. Intracellular calcium and tension development. Influence of increasing extracellular calcium ion concentration on the aequorin signals for papillary muscle (in millinewtons [mN]). The calcium concentrations are given in the individual panels (in mmol/L). The symbol k donates thousands of photon counts per second and is a reflection of the calcium ion concentration that activates the aequorin signal. The contractile activity is shown as the smooth continuous line. The exact relationship in time between the intracellular free calcium and contractile force needs further study. One possibility is that aequorin reflects changes in a superficial calcium compartment. Modified from Morgan et al. *Circ Res* 1983;52(suppl 1):47 with permission from the American Heart Association and the authors.

sensing the increase and decrease of cytosolic calcium closer to the cell surface than in the contractile apparatus. Nonetheless, it seems highly likely that calcium transients similar to those already measured govern the contraction–relaxation cycle of the contractile cardiac cells. On the basis of indirect evidence, it is currently postulated that there are intracellular gradients for calcium ions, with more marked changes in the concentration in the subsarcolemmal space than in the cytosol as a whole (Callewaert, 1992). Thus, it is highly likely that the calcium concentration at the mouth of the open calcium channel is considerably higher than that in the cytosol as a whole (Wier et al., 1994).

CRUCIAL ROLE OF SARCOPLASMIC RETICULUM IN THE CONTRACTILE CYCLE

There is convincing evidence that the cardiac SR plays an indispensable role in the contraction–relaxation sequence (Callewaert, 1992). First, the anatomic proximity of the L-type calcium channels of the T-tubules and the specialized parts of the SR concerned with calcium release provide the anatomic framework for the links between calcium ions entering via the sarcolemmal channels and the release of calcium from the SR. The proposal is that one L channel activates a small group, possibly four, adjacent calcium release channels (Cannell et al., 1994). Second, there is good concordance between the duration of opening of the sarcolemmal L-type calcium channels and release of calcium from the SR (Bouchard et al., 1995). The *calcium release channel* of the SR is part of a complex molecular structure known as the *ryanodine receptor*, which binds the potent insecticide ryanodine (Berridge, 1993). Part of the ryanodine receptor extends from the membrane of the SR to the T-tubule to constitute the "foot" region (Fig. 6-5). The arrival of calcium ions from the L calcium channels of the adjacent T-tubule of the sarcolemma is thought to induce a change in the molecular configuration of the foot, which then sends a further molecular signal that "opens" the calcium release channel of the SR. The proposal is that when one L channel opens, the subsarcolemmal local calcium ion concentration increases by about 100-fold, activating several adjacent ryanodine receptors (Santana et al., 1996). Thus, sufficient calcium is released from the SR to increase the cytosolic calcium concentration to values that trigger contraction (Bootman and Berridge, 1995; Kentish et al., 1990).

Relaxation of the contractile proteins occurs in response to a decrease of the cytosolic calcium level. The calcium ions are taken up by the energy-requiring pump located in the membrane of the SR, the calcium-pumping ATPase, also called the calcium uptake pump. The high cytosolic calcium concentration stimulates the activity of the pump. The calcium pump also responds to β-adrenergic stimulation by phosphorylation of a specific regulatory protein, located in the membrane of the SR, called phospholamban. The overall effect of this sequence is that at any given level of cytosolic calcium, β-adrenergic stimulation causes calcium ions to be taken up more rapidly, so that the relaxation phase is faster.

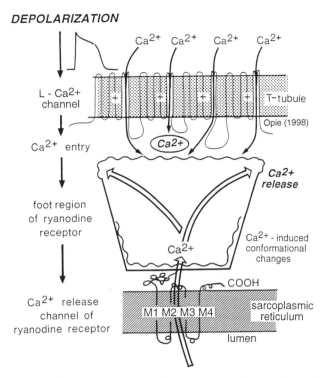

DEPOLARIZATION

FIG. 6-5. Role of ryanodine receptor in calcium-induced calcium release. This process is crucial to the links between the T tubule, the feet, and calcium release channel of the SR in excitation–contraction coupling. Depolarization stimulates the dihydropyridine receptor of the T tubule to allow calcium ion entry, which interacts with the foot region of the ryanodine receptor to cause molecular conformational changes that eventually result in calcium release from the SR.

Thus, the mechanisms of control of the calcium release channel and the uptake pump of the SR are directly relevant to the control of the contractile state.

EXCITATION–CONTRACTION COUPLING

It is now widely accepted that the wave of depolarization during electrical excitation is coupled to contraction by calcium-induced calcium release from the SR by a sequence of events initiated by the entry of calcium ions through the calcium channel. This whole process occurs rapidly. Each L-type channel opens only briefly, perhaps for 0.2 msec (Wier et al., 1994). The overall time between the initial stimulus that opens the L channels and the increase of cytosolic calcium is only about 4 msec, of which much less (< 2 msec) is the interval between the time of activation of the calcium channel and the release of calcium from the SR (Cheng et al., 1994).

Role of L-Type Calcium Channel of the Sarcolemma

The essential role of the L-type calcium channel of the T-tubule in the process of calcium release from the sarcoplasmic reticulum is underscored by the physical linkage of the two by means of the feet (Caswell, 1989). Furthermore, the very rapid removal of calcium from the extracellular space shows that the influx of calcium through the L-type calcium channel is essential for the coupling of depolarization to the release of calcium from the sarcoplasmic reticulum (Nabauer, 1989). Thus, the L-type calcium channel of the T-tubule acts as a voltage sensor that communicates with the calcium release channel of the sarcoplasmic reticulum to promote calcium release (Fig 6-5). An alternate theory is that it is the changes in electrical charges associated with voltage depolarization that cause molecular changes in the "foot" region eventually to "open" the calcium release channel. Of these two possibilities (calcium current versus electrical charge), it is the former that is presently strongly favored (Callewaert, 1992; Nabauer, 1989).

Reversal of Sodium–Calcium Exchange and Other Routes for Calcium Ion Influx

An important question is whether calcium ions entering through the L-type channels are the only trigger for the release of calcium from the SR that causes contraction. Besides the highly gated entry of calcium ions by the L calcium channel, calcium ions probably enter the cytosol by a reversal of the exchange mechanism used for calcium efflux (Kohmoto et al., 1994). Thus, sodium–calcium exchange, which normally operates to expel calcium from the cell, can at depolarized voltages reverse transiently to admit calcium, as may happen shortly after the opening of the sodium channel. The proposal is that sodium ions, having entered by the fast channel, accumulate in a microzone just within the sarcolemma, the "fuzzy space" (Callewaert, 1992; Lederer et al., 1990). Hypothetically, this localized accumulation of sodium then can transiently activate the sodium–calcium exchange in the direction of calcium entry (reverse mode) so that even more calcium ions enter the myocardial cell (Fig. 6-6). Hence, even more calcium ions are released from the SR and the contractile process is enhanced (Kohmoto et al., 1994).

Second, calcium ions already released from the SR may diffuse locally to stimulate neighboring calcium release channels, thereby to release more calcium and providing a positive feedback mechanism (Callewaert, 1992).

Third, direct evidence for this view is that the sodium current can trigger release of calcium from the SR. When such release is blocked by ryanodine, there is still a small residual calcium transient (Lipp and Niggli, 1994), caused by Na^+/Ca^{2+} exchange. The further proposal is that the sodium-induced release of calcium from the SR results in a more rapid and greater rate of release of calcium into the cytosol (Lipp and Niggli, 1994). Thereafter, activity of the inward calcium current through the L-type channel of the sarcolemma helps to sustain calcium release from the SR.

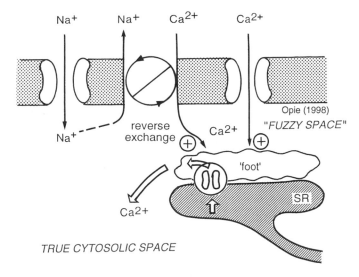

FIG. 6-6. Reverse mode sodium–calcium exchange. Proposal for role of sodium–calcium exchange in the direction of calcium entry after accumulation of sodium ions in the "fuzzy space" to play a role in the liberation of calcium involved in the cardiac contractile cycle.

RELEASE OF CALCIUM FROM SARCOPLASMIC RETICULUM

Crucial evidence favoring the role of calcium-induced calcium release has been obtained with chemically skinned muscle fiber, in which the lipid bilayer of the sarcolemma has been removed. Calcium added to such skinned cells still reacts with the SR to release more calcium. Such release is a graded effect, being greater when the SR is preloaded with calcium or when the concentration of triggering calcium is greater (Callewaert, 1992; Fabiato, 1982). It follows that β-adrenergic stimulation by preloading the SR with more calcium will indirectly enhance subsequent calcium-triggered release of calcium, and the contraction phase of the contractile cycle will be stimulated.

The most direct evidence favoring the role of release of calcium from the SR has been obtained in intact cardiac cells in which the cytosolic calcium has been increased by the flash-sensitive loading compound nitro-5, which has the unusual property of releasing calcium ions in response to illumination at a certain wavelength. Thus, a flash of light can increase internal calcium in cells loaded with nitro-5 and, simultaneously, produce a cardiac contraction (Kentish et al., 1990). Because the amount of calcium required to produce a contraction can be calculated and the amount added with nitro-5 is known, it can be concluded that the flash illumination must be releasing calcium from some intracellular store, such as the SR.

Calcium Sparks

Calcium sparks are the small amounts of calcium that can be spontaneously and locally released from the SR even in the absence of L channel opening. Hypothetically, the spark represents the spontaneous opening of one or, at most, a few calcium release channels, which are termed *elementary release units* of the SR (Bootman and Berridge, 1995). There is so little calcium diffusing away from a spark that it fails to activate the neighboring calcium release channels, and contraction is not initiated. According to one view, it is the synchronous activation of a large number of elementary release units that leads to the normal calcium transient that triggers excitation–contraction coupling. This model predicts that the graded response in calcium release can be explained by both an increased number of channels that are opened and an increased amount of calcium released by each channel (Santana et al., 1996). When the SR is overloaded with calcium as in pathologic conditions such as catecholamine toxicity or during early reperfusion, then calcium sparks can lead to propagated calcium waves with risk of serious arrhythmias or impaired contractile activity.

Calcium Release Channel and Ryanodine

The calcium release channel of the SR has been analyzed by cloning and sequencing the complementary DNA (Takeshima et al., 1989). The predicted structure is that of a large protein comprising over 5,000 amino acids, with two major components. The larger part is the foot, which links the T-tubules and the SR, and the smaller structure is the C-terminal channel region, which constitutes the actual calcium release channel of the SR (Fig. 6-5). The experimental agent ryanodine interacts with the ryanodine receptor in a biphasic manner (Table 6-2).

High concentrations of ryanodine interact with a low-affinity binding site to lock the channel in the closed position to inhibit calcium release from the SR with a negative inotropic effect. At lower concentrations, when ryanodine interacts with a high-affinity binding site, it locks the calcium release channel in the semi-open position, with an early rapid release of calcium, until the SR becomes calcium depleted. An initial positive inotropic effect would be expected (Lewartowski et al., 1994). The proposed explanation for the unexpected negative inotropic effect of low concentrations of ryanodine, is as follows. Once the release channels of the SR have been opened by ryanodine, the calcium release into the subsarcolemmal fuzzy space is then directed outward by the sarcolemmal sodium–calcium exchanger (a reverse of the process shown in Fig. 6-6).

Thapsigargin. A provocative finding is that the addition of thapsigargin, the specific inhibitor of the calcium uptake pump, unexpectedly restores the depressed contractility caused by ryanodine. Hypothetically, the additional block of the calcium uptake pump by thapsigargin could direct calcium coming in through the sarcolemmal L channels straight to the contractile proteins, to restore the contractile

TABLE 6-2. *Effects of drugs on the sarcoplasmic reticulum*

Substance/agent	Ca²⁺ accumulation in the SR	Ca²⁺ release from the SR
Catecholamines, β-adrenergic	Increased. Uptake pump stimulated (increased phosphorylation of phospholamban)	Indirectly increased by greater opening of L-calcium channels, hence greater Ca^{2+} influx
Catecholamines, α-adrenergic	No direct effect	Increased release via second messenger IP₃, which acts on the IP₃ receptor of SR
Caffeine, low doses	Delayed release[a,b]	No effect
Caffeine, high doses, 5 mmol/L	No direct effect	Opens release channel; sensitizes to Ca^{2+}-induced Ca^{2+} release[b,c,d]
Local anesthetic (procaine)	No direct effect	Inhibits[c]
Ca²⁺ antagonists	No direct effect	Indirect decrease. Less Ca^{2+} entry by the L-Ca^{2+} channel with less Ca^{2+}-induced Ca^{2+} release
Ryanodine (low dose)	No direct effect	Increases by locking release channel in open mode[e]
Ryanodine (high dose)	No direct effect	Decreases by locking channel in closed mode
Thapsigargin[f]	Inhibition	No effect
Cyclopiazonic acid[f]	Inhibition	No effect
Heparin	No direct effect	Inhibits IP₃ receptor and activates ryanodine receptor[g]

[a]Weber. *J Gen Physiol* 1968;52:760.
[b]Rasmussen et al. *Circ Res* 1987;60:495.
[c]Hunter et al. *Circ Res* 1982;51:363.
[d]Sitsapesan and Williams. *J Physiol* 1990;423:425.
[e]Rousseau et al. *Am J Physiol* 1987;253:C364–C368.
[f]Du Toit and Opie. *J Cardiovasc Pharmacol* 1994;24:678–684.
[g]Ehrlich et al. *TIPS* 1994;15:145.

state. These data support those workers who hold that calcium entering by the sarcolemmal L channels may play some direct role in excitation–contraction coupling, independently of the SR. In contrast, other data with combined blockade show that when the SR is thus disabled, contraction cannot occur (Kohmoto et al., 1994).

Effects of Caffeine

Caffeine has the property of emptying the SR of its calcium and, therefore, of also interrupting the calcium cycle. The molecular site of action of caffeine also seems to be the ryanodine receptor (Sitapesan and Williams, 1990). However, caffeine seems to act more like calcium itself in its pattern of opening the release channel. In contrast, ryanodine locks the channel and fundamentally alters its molecular configuration (Rousseau et al., 1987). In high concentrations, caffeine is able to increase the opening probability of the sarcoplasmic calcium release channel, without any effect on the conductance of individual calcium release channels. Caffeine is therefore also able to interrupt those arrhythmias resulting from excess calcium recycling. However, caffeine being a methylxanthine also inhibits phosphodiesterase, the enzyme breaking down cAMP, and the tissue levels of cAMP increase. Thus, there may be a greater entry of calcium into the myocardial cell because of enhanced phosphorylation of the calcium channels. The latter action is likely to be positively inotropic and arrhythmogenic in contrast to the direct effects of caffeine on the SR.

IP3-Induced Release of Calcium from the Sarcoplasmic Reticulum

In addition to the ryanodine receptor, there is a second receptor, that for inositol trisphosphate (IP_3). This IP_3 receptor (Fig. 6-7) is only about half the size of the ryanodine receptor but has a high degree of molecular homology with the ryanodine receptor in its transmembrane spanning and C-terminal domains. IP_3

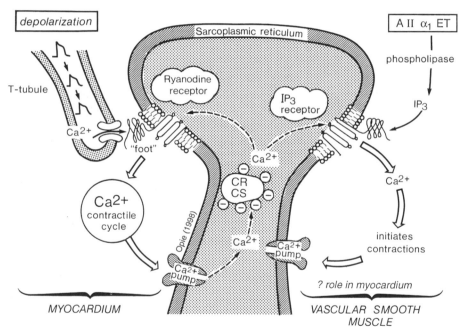

FIG. 6-7. Contrasts between myocardium and vascular smooth muscle in calcium release mechanisms. In the myocardium (left), calcium is released from the SR via the calcium release channel (part of the ryanodine receptor), chiefly in response to calcium that has entered during voltage depolarization. Calcium is taken up again by the calcium pump of the longitudinal SR to interact with the storage proteins calsequestrin (CS) and calrectulin (CR), thence to be released again. In contrast, in vascular smooth muscle, stimulation of vasoconstrictor receptors (see Fig. 9-14) leads to release of inositol trisphosphate (IP_3), which acts on its receptor to release calcium from the SR. Whether the IP_3 path for calcium release operates in the normal myocardium is controversial; in congestive heart failure or in the postischemic myocardium it may be upgraded relative to the ryanodine receptor. AII, angiotensin II; α_1, alpha$_1$-adrenergic activity; ET, endothelin.

is one of the messengers of the pathway initiated when phosphatidylinositol is cleaved by the action of the enzyme phospholipase C, in response to stimulation by certain sarcolemmal receptors such as those for α_1-adrenergic activity, angiotensin II, or endothelin (Berridge, 1993). Although the physiologic role of these agonists in stimulating the myocardium is still in question, they are all established vasoconstrictors. Phospholipase C may be voltage sensitive so that the wave of depolarization actually releases IP_3, a proposal much better worked out for skeletal muscle than for the heart. The IP_3 messenger system is of fundamental importance in regulating calcium release from the SR in vascular smooth muscle (see Chapter 9), which is not surprising because the agonists of the system are strong vasoconstrictors. In cardiac muscle, stimulation by such vasoconstrictor agonists involving the IP_3 path is controversial. Although IP_3 can induce calcium release from the cardiac SR and initiate contraction (Kentish et al., 1990), it seems that the IP_3 receptor plays a lesser role than the ryanodine receptor (Zhu and Nosek, 1991). An attractive hypothesis is that in human heart failure, the ryanodine receptor is downgraded, whereas the IP_3 receptor is upgraded, thereby possibly providing an alternate support pathway for maintenance of calcium transients (Go et al., 1994).

Cyclic ADP Ribose. This compound is formed from NAD (see Chapter 11) and stimulates the ryanodine receptor of isolated SR to release calcium, a process that could be positively inotropic. In reality, after much controversy, it seems as if cyclic ADP ribose plays little or no physiologic role in controlling calcium release in intact cardiac myocytes (Guo et al., 1996).

SARCOPLASMIC RETICULUM AND CALCIUM UPTAKE PUMP (SERCA)

The larger fraction of calcium released from the SR is returned to its site of origin by the activity of the ATP-consuming pump, the *calcium-pumping ATPase*. This pump is also called the sarco(endo)plasmic reticulum calcium-ATPase (*SERCA*), which occurs in several isoforms of which SERCA 2 is the one found in cardiac muscle (Lompre et al., 1994). Studies in which fragments of the reticulum have been isolated (as tiny vesicles) show that the calcium-accumulating activity of the SR requires ATP. The calcium uptake pump of the SR, now isolated and characterized, constitutes nearly 40% of the protein component of the SR and is the major mechanism for reducing the cytosolic calcium ion level to initiate diastole (Table 6-1). It has a molecular weight of about 115 kDa and is distributed asymmetrically across the membrane in such a way that part of it actually protrudes into the cytosol (Fig. 6-8). Probably it consists of dimers of a single polypeptide. For each mole of ATP that is hydrolyzed by this enzyme, two calcium ions are accumulated within the reticulum. This ATPase of the SR differs in many ways from that of the sarcolemma, despite their common capacity to pump calcium. In particular, only the pump of the SR

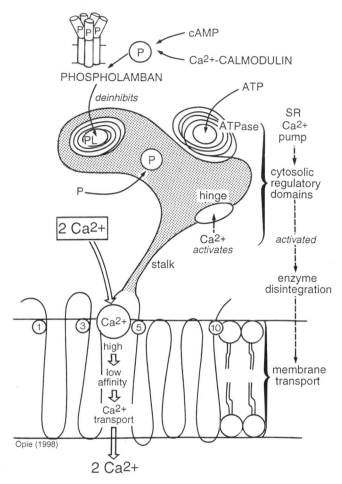

FIG. 6-8. Regulation of calcium uptake pump (SERCA) by phospholamban. The diagram shows the cytosolic regulatory domains of the calcium uptake pump, SERCA, with activation by (1) removal of the phospholamban inhibitory brake, and (2) calcium ions at two sites. There are cytosolic binding sites for ATP, phospholamban (PL), and a nearby phosphorylation site. ATP has two essential functions: it is required both for energy to drive the pump and for phosphorylation. For the effect of phospholamban on cell permeability, see Fig. 6-10.

is modulated by phospholamban, and only this pump is crucial for diastolic relaxation to occur.

Phospholamban Inhibits Calcium Accumulation by the Sarcoplasmic Reticulum

The activity of the calcium pump of the SR is normally inhibited by *phospholamban* (literally, "phosphate receptor") (Tada and Katz, 1982). Phospholamban is a 52–amino acid pentamer, consisting of five subunits each of molecular weight 6 kDa (Fig. 6-9). Phospholamban is an integral part of the membrane proteins of the longitudinal SR and colocalizes in a 1:1 molar ratio with the metabolic pump that provides the energy for the transport of calcium. β-adrenergic stimulation phosphorylates phospholamban to relieve this inhibition, so that calcium uptake is stimulated. Another important stimulus to phosphorylation of phospholamban is an increased intracellular calcium level, acting via calmodulin and the calmodulin-dependent kinase. Calcium also acts directly on the molecular configuration of the calcium pump to enhance its activity (Fig. 6-8). Thus, calcium and cAMP phosphorylate at two different sites on phospholamban, and calcium acts directly on the calcium uptake pump, all these changes increasing the pump activity (Lompre et al., 1994; Voss et al., 1994). The present proposals are (1) that phosphorylation of phospholamban changes the physical nature of the calcium pump from a substantial population of large immobile

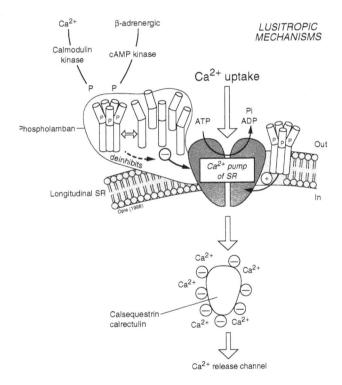

FIG. 6-9. Proposed molecular structure of calcium uptake pump. Phospholamban can be phosphorylated (P) to remove the inhibition exerted by its unphosphorylated form (positive charges) on the calcium uptake pump of the SR. Thereby, calcium uptake is increased either in response to an enhanced cytosolic calcium or in response to β-adrenergic stimulation. Thus, there are two phosphorylations activating phospholamban at two different sites, and their effects are additive. An increase rate of calcium uptake into the SR enhances the rate of relaxation (lusitropic effect) followed by increased release of calcium (positive inotropic effect).

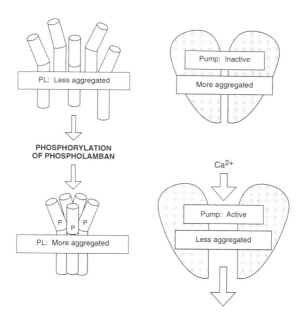

FIG. 6-10. Molecular model for enhanced calcium uptake pump activity by phosphory-lated phospholamban. Hypothetically, phosphorylation of phospholamban (PL) changes the molecular form of PL from a less aggregated, predominantly monomer form to a more aggre-gated structure. This change decreases the intramembranous concentration of inhibitory phos-pholamban monomeres so that the calcium pump becomes less aggregated and more perme-able to calcium. For details see Cornea et al. (*Biochemistry* 1997;36:2960). For other models see Koss and Kranias (1996) and McLeod et al. (1991).

aggregates to more mobile oligomers and monomers (Fig. 6-10); or that (2) five phosphorylated phospholamban molecules form a calcium-permeable ion pore (Koss and Kranias, 1996).

There are additional modes of phosphorylation, of little physiologic importance in heart muscle, namely by protein kinase C or by cGMP (Lompre et al., 1994). The latter path may be more important in blood vessels to explain part of the vasodilatory effects of cGMP, produced for example by the action of nitric oxide.

The *physiologic significance* of these relatively complex controls is as follows. β-adrenergic stimulation phosphorylates phospholamban to relieve its normal inhibition of the calcium uptake pump of the SR, which thereby becomes loaded to release more calcium during subsequent depolarizations. Consequently, the increased cytosolic calcium further phosphorylates phospholamban at a second site, so that there is an added stimulation of the calcium uptake pump, to further increase the rate of relaxation, and thus the SR is even more "loaded" with more calcium to allow a greater release in response to the next wave of depolarization. Hence, phosphorylation of phospholamban promotes the rate of relaxation (lusitropic effect) and indirectly the positive inotropic response, as shown in stud-ies with transgenic mice deficient in phospholamban (Luo et al., 1994). Thus, with justification, phospholamban is called a critical repressor of myocardial contractility (Koss and Kranias, 1996). In response to β-adrenergic stimulation, as in the fight or flight response, the phospholamban brake is released, with a rapid increase in both contraction and relaxation (Koss and Kranias, 1996).

Calcium Storage by Calsequestrin and Calrectulin

The calcium taken up into the SR by the calcium uptake pump needs to be stored in anticipation of further release by the next wave of depolarization (Fig. 6-9). Such storage occurs at the highly charged storage protein, *calsequestrin*. The latter is a 55-kDa protein, not found in the network component of the SR but in the other parts including the cisternal component which lies near the T-tubules (McLeod et al., 1991). Such calcium stored in association with calsequestrin can then be released when the calcium release channel of the SR is stimulated to open by the next wave of depolarization. *Calrectulin* is another storage protein, similar in structure and function to calsequestrin.

Uptake Versus Release of Calcium by the Sarcoplasmic Reticulum

How does the SR "know" when to take up calcium from the cytoplasm and when to release it? Fabiato (1985) proposed that the SR has its release channel opened by an increasing concentration of external calcium (the *free calcium trigger*), and as the calcium continues to increase to a supraoptimal concentration, the channel comes to be inactivated. This proposal has been questioned because the SR release channel maintains its activity at calcium ion concentrations as high as 100 µmol/L (10^{-4} mol/L), values not often reached in the cytosol. Yet the subsarcolemmal fuzzy space allows for such higher localized calcium ion concentrations (Fig. 6-6). The molecular mechanism whereby a high calcium ion concentration could inhibit the release channel appears to involve calcium–calmodulin. Thus, the current proposal is that the subsarcolemmal calcium ion concentrations reached during systole can reach high enough values to inhibit the release channel.

How is a *graded calcium signal* obtained? When the degree of L channel opening is high, then the cytosolic calcium increase is also high, with a lesser increase when the stimulus is less. Although each individual calcium release channel works in an all-or-none manner (i.e., is physiologically closed or open), the greater the stimulus, the larger the number of channels that are recruited. According to one proposal, the graded response may involve the upgrading of sparks into proper openings of the ryanodine release channels (Bootman and Berridge, 1995).

CALCIUM ION EFFLUX FROM CELL

To avoid the myocardial cells from becoming overloaded with calcium requires the ejection of a small number of calcium ions, equivalent to those entering with each wave of depolarization, and there are two exit pathways. The major route for calcium ion efflux is the subsarcolemmal *sodium–calcium exchange* mechanism (Fig. 6-3), which is designed to eject calcium ions whenever the cytosolic calcium ion concentration exceeds a certain critical value, and when the voltage conditions are favorable (see Fig. 4-25), as probably occurs in the latter part of the action potential plateau. Anatomically, this exchanger is located chiefly in the T-tubules near the cisternae of the SR so that it is ideally suited either to bring in calcium that can act on the calcium release channel of the SR, or the exchanger can eject excess calcium ions when the subsarcolemmal space is overloaded with calcium, as when the action potential is over.

The *sarcolemmal calcium pump* is a backup calcium ejection system that uses ATP and pumps calcium ions outward. The chief function of the calcium pump may be as follows. The pump is just active enough to respond to the low cytosolic calcium ion concentration normally found in diastole (0.3×10^{-6} mol/L) (Fig. 6-2). Thus, the pump responds to any higher value to help maintain the diastolic-cytosolic calcium concentration. The protein of this calcium pump can be phosphorylated either by calmodulin or by cAMP. When calcium is high or during catecholamine stimulation, the pump is switched on to function more actively, without being fast enough to cope with all the calcium ions requiring removal from the cytosol in diastole.

CALMODULIN

The previous sections have described how an increase in the cytosolic calcium concentration promotes the activity of at least three processes that remove calcium from the cytosol: the uptake of calcium by the SR, the extrusion of calcium through the sarcolemmal calcium pump, and the activity of the sodium–calcium exchanger. It is not too fanciful to suppose that calcium ions self-regulate their concentration in the cytosol, an important concept because when self-regulation fails, calcium overload ensues, and lethal cellular damage can follow. The calcium regulator protein calmodulin is thought to play a critical role by being the intracellular calcium sensor.

Calmodulin is a small but ubiquitously distributed protein consisting of a single polypeptide chain with a molecular weight of 16,700 daltons (Cheung, 1980) and a high affinity for calcium. It has four calcium-binding domains within its structure, with varying dissociation constants that lie neatly between the diastolic calcium concentration of 10^{-7} mol/L and the systolic value of 10^{-5} mol/L. When calcium is absent, the four binding sites are occupied by magnesium ions. It is thought that the increase in free calcium that accompanies excitation–contraction coupling displaces all the magnesium from three sites, but only a small fraction of magnesium from the fourth site. Thus, the active form is Ca_3Mg_1-calmodulin. As calcium binds, the molecular form of calmodulin changes, and it becomes able to regulate the activity of certain enzymes. For example, calcium–calmodulin stimulates the activity of the calcium pumps of both the SR and the sarcolemma, increasing the rate at which calcium leaves the cytosol when calcium is high. Additionally, calcium–calmodulin inhibits the calcium release channel of the cardiac SR by directly reducing the opening time of the channels (Smith et al., 1989). Structurally, calmodulin binds to the N-terminal chain of the ryanodine receptor (Berridge, 1993). Thus, when the cytosolic calcium is too high, calcium release from the SR will lessen or cease.

The effects of calmodulin are inhibited by the *phenothiazine* compounds. This effect may explain the antipsychotic properties of chlorpromazine. Normally, calmodulin stimulates the phosphodiesterase of the brain to reduce cAMP levels. Phenothiazines may reverse this effect to increase cAMP levels, thereby having the same ultimate effect as other antipsychotic agents that increase cerebral release of catecholamines. In the case of the heart, chlorpromazine seems to have an anti-ischemic effect acting only in part by calmodulin inhibition and possibly also by other modes, such as membrane stabilization (Edoute et al., 1983).

POSITIVE INOTROPIC AND RELAXANT EFFECTS OF β-ADRENERGIC STIMULATION

β-adrenergic stimulation enhances the force of contraction (*positive inotropic* effect) and the rate of relaxation (relaxant or *lusitropic effect*; Greek *lusi,* relaxation). These effects are achieved by an increase in the inward calcium current (I_{ca}), a greater rate of release of calcium ions from the SR, and accelerated reuptake of calcium into the SR (Callewaert, 1992). The phosphorylation of phospholamban is particularly important in the β-adrenergic response (Luo et al., 1994). Many but not all of these changes are achieved by the formation of the second messenger, cAMP. Thus, an increased rate of both contraction and relaxation is ultimately achieved in response to β-adrenergic stimulation, and the increased peak cytosolic calcium transient ensures that the force of contraction is likewise increased (see Fig. 7-17).

CALCIUM OVERLOAD

An important concept in cardiac pathology is that of calcium overload, first emphasized by Fleckenstein (1971). He described how experimental myocardial necrosis occurred in response to high doses of catecholamines, with a greatly increased uptake of calcium by the myocardium. The whole process was inhibited by calcium channel antagonists, such as verapamil and nifedipine. It is thought that cytosolic calcium overload may occur in response to myocardial ischemia, reperfusion, and excess catecholamine stimulation. He proposed that calcium overload could damage myocardial cells by excessive splitting of ATP as a result of the increased activity of the contractile mechanism in response to calcium. It is now known that calcium overload can occur even while the myocardial levels of ATP are normal, so that other mechanisms must also be involved. First, as the mitochondria tend to buffer the cytosolic calcium, they become overloaded with calcium and waste ATP in the process, thereby demanding more oxygen and extending the severity of ischemia. Second, excess calcium may stimulate the phospholipase enzymes, which break down cell membranes. Third, calcium overload may cause the development of contracture, which is a state of sustained excess contraction (Steenbergen et al., 1990). Fourth, excess calcium cycling in and out of the SR may explain certain arrhythmias. Fifth, calcium overload early in the reperfusion period after ischemia may predispose to certain aspects of reperfusion injury, such as reperfusion arrhythmias and reperfusion stunning.

Because of the phasic nature of the increase and decrease in internal calcium in response to the initial wave of depolarization, it would be possible to picture a situation where calcium does not return rapidly to a static diastolic level at the end of relaxation. Rather, there could be spontaneous oscillations as the cytosolic calcium gradually came down to the normal low diastolic level (Meissner and Morgan, 1995). Studies directly localizing internal ionized calcium by a new imaging technique show that internal calcium may increase focally within calcium overloaded cells rather than uniformly (Berlin et al., 1989). Thus, abnormal calcium-induced currents may form at irregular sites throughout the calcium overloaded cell with risk of arrhythmias. As ischemia proceeds, there is eventually an increase of internal calcium occurring concurrently with the development of ischemic contracture, an irreversible event.

SARCOPLASMIC RETICULUM IN PATHOLOGIC CONDITIONS

In *ischemia and reperfusion*, the calcium uptake pump of the SR is damaged, which might contribute to poor contractility (stunning) in the reperfusion period (Zucchi et al., 1994).

Some *arrhythmias* of ischemia and reperfusion appear to be calcium based. When cytosolic calcium is too high, excess oscillations can give rise to *afterdepolarizations* or oscillatory aftercontractions, which involve recycling of calcium through the SR. Arrhythmias dependent on such oscillations should be, and are, stopped by agents that inhibit calcium uptake into the SR (ryanodine) or by inhibitors of the calcium uptake pump, thapsigargin and cyclopiazonic acid (du Toit and Opie, 1994).

In *heart failure*, the force of cardiac contraction is reduced and there is an abnormal delayed pattern of cardiac relaxation. Because the SR is so intimately concerned in both phases of the contractile cycle, it is not surprising that abnormalities at this site may play a fundamental role in heart failure. The messenger RNA (mRNA) levels of proteins regulating calcium uptake and release are decreased in end-stage human heart failure. Specifically, the mRNA for the ryanodine receptor, the calcium uptake pump, and phospholamban are all abnormally low (Arai et al., 1994). Ryanodine receptors are downgraded in relation to IP_3 receptors, the latter perhaps becoming an alternate mechanism for stimulation of the calcium release channel (Go et al., 1994). The hypothesis proposed is that abnormal calcium handling by the SR of the failing myocardium is due to impaired expression of the genes encoding these specific SR proteins (Arai et al., 1994). In contrast, during the early stages of pressure hypertrophy, these genes are upregulated (Arai et al., 1996).

SUMMARY

1. *Cardiac contraction and relaxation is explained by an intracellular calcium cycle.* During depolarization, the small amount of calcium that enters the heart cell is thought to trigger the release of more calcium from the sarcoplasmic reticulum by the process of calcium-induced calcium release.
2. *The proposal is that the wave of depolarization sweeping along the T-tubule* opens the calcium channel of the tubular membrane to allow calcium ions to penetrate. The latter then act on the foot region of the ryanodine receptor to cause molecular configurational changes. The end result is the opening of the calcium release channel of the ryanodine receptor. The cytosolic calcium increases, and contraction occurs.
3. *The increase of cytosolic calcium acts on the sarcoplasmic reticulum* to phosphorylate the regulatory protein phospholamban to increase activity of the ATP-requiring calcium uptake pump of the sarcoplasmic reticulum. When thus phosphorylated, phospholamban removes the normal inhibition on the calcium pump of the sarcoplasmic reticulum. Thereby, calcium uptake into the sarcoplasmic reticulum is promoted and relaxation occurs.
4. *β-adrenergic stimulation via formation of cAMP also phosphorylates phospholamban* by acting at a different site. Thus, calcium pumping is increased. Cytosolic calcium decreases at a greater rate, so that diastolic relaxation is enhanced.
5. *Clinically important events* such as enhanced myocyte necrosis, shortening of the action potential duration, and potentially fatal arrhythmias can occur when the control mechanisms regulating the cytosolic calcium concentration fail, and cytosolic calcium overload develops.
6. *Function of the sarcoplasmic reticulum is impaired in severe ischemia, reperfusion, and heart failure.* Such changes may contribute to the impaired contractility found in these conditions.

STUDENT QUESTIONS

1. How does cytosolic calcium increase at the start of systole?
2. How does cytosolic calcium decrease at the start of diastole?
3. What is the function of phospholamban?
4. Describe the physiologic role of the ryanodine receptor.
5. What is calmodulin? How does it influence the contractile process?

CARDIOLOGIST-IN-TRAINING QUESTIONS

1. Describe the sequence of events involved in excitation-contraction coupling.
2. What is the ryanodine receptor? Why is its "foot" region so important? What common drug acts on this receptor?
3. Phospholamban is described as a prominent regulator of myocardial contractility. Why?
4. What is SERCA? How is it related to a positive lusitropic effect?
5. How is cytosolic calcium overload normally avoided? What are some clinically applied consequences of calcium overload?

REFERENCES

1. Arai M, Matsui H, Periasamy M. Sarcoplasmic reticulum gene expression in cardiac hypertrophy and heart failure. *Circ Res* 1994;74:555–564.
2. Arai M, Suzuki T, Nagai R. Sarcoplasmic reticulum genes are upregulated in mild cardiac hypertrophy but downregulated in severe cardiac hypertrophy induced by pressure overload. *Mol Cell Cardiol* 1996;28:1583–1590.
3. Berlin JR, Cannel MB, Lederer WJ. Cellular origins of the transient inward current in cardiac myocytes. Role of fluctuations and waves of elevated intracellular calcium. *Circ Res* 1989;65: 115–126.
4. Berridge MJ. Inositol triphosphate and calcium signaling. *Nature* 1993;361:315–325.
5. Bootman MD, Berridge MJ. The elemental principles of calcium signaling. *Cell* 1995;83:675–678.
6. Bouchard RA, Clark RB, Giles WR. Effects of action potential duration on excitation–contraction coupling in rat ventricular myocytes. *Circ Res* 1995;76:790–801.
7. Callewaert G. Excitation–contraction coupling in mammalian cardiac cells. *Cardiovasc Res* 1992;26:923–932.
8. Cannell MB, Cheng H, Lederer WJ. Spatial non-uniformities in $[Ca^{2+}]_i$ during excitation–contraction coupling in cardiac myocytes. *Biophys J* 1994;67:1942–1956.
9. Caswell AH, Brandt NR. Does muscle activation occur by direct mechanical coupling of transverse tubules to sarcoplasmic reticulum. *TIBS* 1989;14:161–165.
10. Cheng H, Cannell MB, Lederer WJ. Propagation of excitation–contraction coupling into ventricular myocytes. *Pflugers Arch* 1994;428:415–417.
11. Cheung WY. Calmodulin plays a pivotal role in cellular regulation. *Science* 1980;207:19–27.
12. du Toit EF, Opie LH. Inhibitors of Ca^{2+}-ATPase pump of sarcoplasmic reticulum attenuate reperfusion stunning in isolated rat heart. *J Cardiovasc Pharmacol* 1994;24:678–684.
13. Edoute Y, van der Merwe EL, Sanan D. Normothermic ischemic cardiac arrest and reperfusion of the isolated working heart: effect of chlorpromazine on functional, metabolic and morphological recovery. *J Mol Cell Cardiol* 1983;15:603–620.
14. Fabiato A. Calcium release in skinned cardiac cells: variations with species, tissues and development. *Fed Proc* 1982;41:2238–2244.
15. Fabiato A. Calcium-induced release of calcium from the sarcoplasmic reticulum. *J Gen Physiol* 1985;85:189–320.
16. Fleckenstein A. Specific inhibitors and promoters of calcium action in the excitation–contraction coupling of heart muscle and their role in the prevention or production of myocardial lesions. In: Harris P, Opie LH (eds). *Calcium and the Heart.* New York: Academic, 1971;135–188.
17. Go LO, Moschella MC, Handa KK, et al. Differential regulation of two types of intracellular calcium-release channels during end-stage human heart failure [Abstract]. *Circulation* 1994;90:I–L.
18. Guo X, Laflamme MA, Becker PL. Cyclic ADP-ribose does not regulate sarcoplasmic reticulum Ca^{2+} release in intact cardiac myocytes. *Circ Res* 1996;79:147–151.
19. Kentish JC, Barsotti R, Lea TJ, et al. Calcium release from cardiac sarcoplasmic reticulum induced by photorelease of calcium or Ins (1, 4, 5)P₃. *Am J Physiol* 1990;258:H610–H615.
20. Kohmoto O, Levi AJ, Bridge JH. Relation between reverse sodium–calcium exchange and sarcoplasmic reticulum calcium release in guinea pig ventricular cells. *Circ Res* 1994;74:550–554.

21. Koss KL, Kranias EG. Phospholamban: a prominent regulator of myocardial contractility. *Circ Res* 1996;79:1059–1063.
22. Lederer WJ, Niggli E, Hadley RW. Sodium–calcium exchange in excitable cells: fuzzy space. *Science* 1990;248:283.
23. Lewartowski B, Rozycka M, Janiak R. Effects of thapsigargin in normal and pretreated with ryanodine guinea pig cardiomyocytes. *Am J Physiol* 1994;266:H1829–H1839.
24. Lipp P, Niggli E. Modulation of Ca^{2+} release in cultured neonatal rat cardiac myocytes. Insight from subcellular release patterns revealed by confocal microscopy. *Circ Res* 1994;74:979–990.
25. Lompre A-M, Anger M, Levitsky D. Sarco(endo)plasmic reticulum calcium pumps in the cardiovascular system: function and gene expression. *J Mol Cell Cardiol* 1994;26:1109–1121.
26. Luo W, Grupp IL, Harrer J, et al. Targeted ablation of the phospholamban gene is associated with markedly enhanced myocardial contractility and loss of beta-agonist stimulation. *Circ Res* 1994; 75:401–409.
27. McLeod AG, Shen ACY, Campbell KP, et al. Frog cardiac calsequestrin. Identification, characterization, and subcellular distribution in two structurally distinct regions of peripheral sarcoplasmic reticulum in frog ventricular myocardium. *Circ Res* 1991;69:344–359.
28. Meissner A, Morgan JP. Contractile dysfunction and abnormal Ca^{2+} modulation during postischemic reperfusion in rat heart. *Am J Physiol* 1995;268:H100–H111.
29. Nabauer M, Callewaert G, Cleemann L, Morad M. Regulation of calcium release is gated by calcium current, not gating charge, in cardiac myocytes. *Science* 1989;244:800–803.
30. Rousseau E, Smith JS, Meissner G. Ryanodine modifies conductance and gating behavior of single Ca^{2+} release channel. *Am J Physiol* 1987;253:C364–C368.
31. Santana LF, Cheng H, Gomez AM, et al. Relation between with sarcolemmal Ca^{2+} current and Ca^{2+} sparks and local control theories for cardiac excitation–contraction coupling. *Circ Res* 1996;78: 166–171.
32. Sitsapesan R, Williams AJ. Mechanisms of caffeine activation of single calcium release channels of sheep cardiac sarcoplasmic reticulum. *J Physiol* 1990;423:425–439.
33. Smith JS, Rousseau E, Meissner G. Calmodulin modulation of single sarcoplasmic reticulum Ca^{2+}-release channels from cardiac and skeletal muscle. *Circ Res* 1989;64:352–359.
34. Steenbergen C, Murphy E, Watts JA, London RE. Correlation between cytosolic free calcium, contracture, ATP, and irreversible ischemic injury in perfused rat heart. *Circ Res* 1990;66:135–146.
35. Tada M, Katz AM. Phosphorylation of the sarcoplasmic reticulum and sarcolemma. *Annu Rev Physiol* 1982;44:401–423.
36. Takeshima H, Nishimura S, Matsumoto T, et al. Primary structure and expression from complementary DNA of skeletal muscle ryanodine receptor. *Nature* 1989;339:439–445.
37. Voss J, Jones LR, Thomas DD. The physical mechanism of calcium pump regulation in the heart. *Biophys J* 1994;67:190–195.
38. Wier WG, Egan TM, Lopez-Lopez JR, Balke CW. Local control of excitation–contraction coupling in rat heart cells. *J Physiol* 1994;474:463–471.
39. Zhu Y, Nosek TM. Inositol trisphosphate enhances Ca^{2+} oscillations but not Ca^{2+}-induced Ca^{2+} release from cardiac sarcoplasmic reticulum. *Pflugers Arch* 1991;418:1–6.
40. Zucchi R, Ronca-Testoni S, Yu G, Galbani P. Effect of ischemia and reperfusion on cardiac ryanodine receptors-sarcoplasmic reticulum Ca^{2+} channels. *Circ Res* 1994;74:271–280.

REVIEWS

Cannell MB, Lederer WJ. The control of calcium release in heart muscle. *Science* 1995;268:1045–1049.
Opie LH. Mechanism of cardiac contraction and relaxation. In: Braunwald E (ed.) *Heart Disease.* 5th ed. Philadelphia: Saunders, 1997;360–393.

7

Receptors and Signal Transduction

*. . . bustling communication networks within and
between clans of signaling proteins.*
H.R. Bourne, 1995

The calcium cycles described in the preceding chapters are crucial for the regulation of cardiac contraction and of the heart rate. These two key physiologic activities are stimulated by exercise or emotional stimulation and are decreased during sleep. The relevant calcium cycles need to respond to control by the autonomic nervous system, which emits either stimulatory adrenergic or inhibitory cholinergic messages. These do not communicate directly with cell calcium but require an intermediary system of cellular signals. When the primary autonomic messenger (e.g., epinephrine/norepinephrine or acetylcholine) binds to the adrenergic or cholinergic receptor on the sarcolemma, it initiates a series of molecular signals that eventually result in a corresponding increase or decrease of cell calcium. Such signals cause the heart rate and force of contraction either to increase or decrease. *Signal transduction can be defined as the sum total of these processes converting an extracellular stimulus to an intracellular regulator such as cytosolic calcium, usually starting with an agonist binding to a receptor site and ending in a physiologic event such as a contraction* (Fig. 7-1).

The *first* of the four major types of signal systems that regulate cardiovascular function leads from β-adrenergic stimulation to an increase in cell calcium (Fig. 7-2). Adrenergic stimulation releases the first messenger (epinephrine from the adrenal gland or norepinephrine from the adrenergic nerve terminals), which occupies the β-adrenergic receptor. Then the sarcolemmal G proteins pass on the signal from the receptor to the next step to activate an enzyme called adenylyl cyclase, which produces the second messenger, cyclic adenosine monophosphate (cAMP). The latter unleashes a further series of intracellular signals that

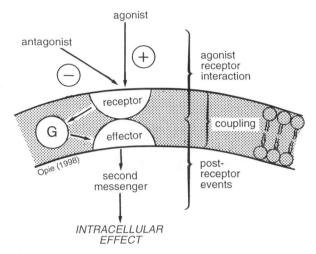

FIG. 7-1. General receptor pattern for interaction of hormone or other agonist with membrane-bound receptor.

eventually increase cytosolic calcium transients, so that the heart rate increases and the force of myocardial contraction increases. The coupling proteins belong to the super family of G proteins (G, guanine nucleotide binding), specific members of which can either stimulate (G_s) or inhibit (G_i) adenylyl cyclase. For example, cholinergic stimulation of the muscarinic receptor, by coupling to G_i

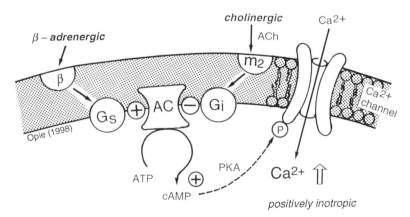

FIG. 7-2. Two major receptors. These are the β-adrenergic receptor (β) and the cholinergic muscarinic (M_2) receptor, the latter for acetylcholine (ACh). The β-adrenergic receptor is coupled to adenylyl cyclase via the activated stimulatory G protein G_s (see Fig. 7-8). Consequent formation of cAMP activates protein kinase A (PKA) to phosphorylate the calcium channel to increase calcium entry. Activity of adenylyl cyclase can be decreased by the inhibitory subunits of the ACh-associated inhibitory G protein G_i.

rather than to G_s, exerts inhibitory influences on the heart at least in part by decreasing the rate of formation of cAMP.

The *second* signal system leads from α-adrenergic stimulation to an increased cytosolic calcium in vascular smooth muscle. Release of norepinephrine from the adrenergic nerve terminals in the blood vessels is followed by occupation of the α-adrenergic receptors that link to another G protein–coupled enzyme. The latter activates the sarcolemmal enzyme phospholipase C to produce two messengers, inositol trisphosphate and diacylglycerol, both of which by different mechanisms increase cytosolic calcium in vascular smooth muscle cells to cause vascular contraction (vasoconstriction). The result is that the peripheral vascular resistance increases and the blood pressure tends to increase.

The *third* signal system causes vasodilation. Nitric oxide, the messenger of this system, is formed in the inner endothelial layers of the blood vessels, in response to several stimuli, including an increase in blood flow as occurs in exercise. Nitric oxide then diffuses to the vascular smooth muscle cells to stimulate the formation of its second messenger, cyclic guanosine monophosphate (cGMP), which lowers the calcium level and causes relaxation. These two opposing messenger systems in vascular smooth muscle, by promoting vasoconstriction (α-adrenergic) and vasodilation (nitric oxide), are able to regulate the peripheral vascular resistance and hence the blood pressure and the load against which the heart works. Similar signal systems also occur in the myocardium to increase or decrease the force of contraction, but are probably of lesser importance than the β-adrenergic and cholinergic systems.

The *fourth* group of signaling systems stands in contrast to the above three signal sequences that link neurotransmitters and hormones to cell calcium and hence to contraction. This fourth system ultimately regulates *cell growth*. Growth stimuli such as insulin and insulin growth factors act on tyrosine kinases to connect with an important internal factor called Ras that in turn links to mitogen-activated protein (MAP) kinases to promote growth. This signal sequence is described in Chapter 13.

The first part of this chapter will emphasize the signals involved in converting adrenergic stimulation of the β-adrenergic receptors to an increased force of contraction (positive inotropic effect) and to an increased rate of relaxation (lusitropic effect).

PROPERTIES OF RECEPTORS

In 1905, Langley made the fundamental proposal that agents released at the nerve endings did not interact directly with the adjacent muscle cells. Rather, receptors were involved, as described by Ehrlich in 1913 to designate the hypothetical specific chemical groupings of the cell that reacted with chemotherapeutic drugs. It is this concept of receptors that is fundamental to modern cardiovascular pharmacology and hence to clinical cardiology (Table 7-1). Ahlquist

TABLE 7-1. *Classification of cardiac receptors, including vascular and myocardial sites*

Broad types and agonists	Subtypes	Comments
Classic neurotransmitters		
Adrenergic	α_1, α_2	Chiefly vascular
	β_1	Chiefly cardiac, also vascular
	β_2	Chiefly vascular, also cardiac
Cholinergic (muscarinic)	M_2	Heart and coronary arteries
	M_3	Endothelial, NO-linked
Adrenergic-related receptors		
Histamine	H_1	Chiefly vascular
	H_2	Chiefly myocardial
Glucagon	—	Adenylate cyclase-linked
Dopamine[a]	DA_1	Postsynaptic; cyclase-linked; vasodilatory
Dopamine	DA_2	Presynaptic; inhibits NE release
Adenosine	A_1	Inhibits myocardial cAMP; role in preconditioning
Vascular receptors (other than adrenergic-cholinergic)		
Adenosine[b]	A_2	Vascular cAMP↑
Angiotensin II	AT_1	Phospholipase C-linked
Endothelin[c]	ET_A	Phospholipase C-linked
Thromboxane	—	Vascular Ca^{2+} influx↑
Prostacyclin	—	Vascular cAMP↑
Purinergic	P_1	Adenosine-sensitive
	P_2	ATP-sensitive, vascular
Peptidergic including	—	Vasoactive
Neuropeptide Y[d]	—	Inactive on coronary artery
Vasoactive intestinal peptide[e]	—	Co-released with ACh
CGRP[d]	—	Vascular cAMP↑
Substance P[d]	—	Endothelial, NO-linked
Enzymes		
Digitalis	—	Sodium-potasium pump
Other hormonal receptors		
Insulin	—	Tyrosine-kinase linked
Steroid	—	—

CGRP = Calcitonin-gene related peptide; NO, nitric oxide; NE, norepinephrine; ACh, acetylcholine.

[a]Murphy and Vaughan. In: Messerli FH (ed). *Cardiovascular Drug Therapy.* Philadelphia: Saunders, 1996;1162.

[b]Jenkins and Belarindelli. *Circ Res* 1988;63:97.

[c]Rosendorff. *Cardiovasc Drugs Ther* 1996;10:795–807.

[d]Gulbenkian. *Circ Res* 1993;73:579.

[e]Chang. *Circ Res* 1994;74:157.

(1948) proposed that sympathetic adrenergic stimulation interacted with two types of adrenergic receptors, α-adrenergic and β-adrenergic.

The term "receptor" refers to a molecule (or molecular complex) that can recognize and selectively interact with the agonist agent, and which, after binding it, can generate some signal that initiates the chain of events leading to the biologic response (Kahn, 1976).

The biologic response is generated by a functionally separate *effector unit* (Fig. 7-1). Generally, the receptor is a specialized part of the external layer of the sarcolemma, sometimes extending through the sarcolemma, whereas the effector is a specialized part of the internal layer. Communication between the two is called coupling. Structurally, many receptors appear to be integral membrane proteins that require strong detergents to break the hydrophobic bonds holding them to the membrane. Sometimes, as in the case of thyroid hormone, the receptors are located within the cell so that the hormone has to cross the sarcolemma to reach the receptor. Especially in the case of drugs, the receptors are ill defined and nonspecific. Thus, the term "receptor" is not always as definite as might be imagined. In other cases, techniques of molecular biology have shown highly specific details of the receptor molecule, often pinning down the actual receptor site to a small number of amino acids. Such a close molecular fit can be compared with a lock-and-key pattern, where the agonist molecule is the key and the receptor molecule the lock. The key turns the lock to produce an intracellular effect, mediated by a second messenger.

The interaction between receptor sites and antagonists may be reversible or irreversible. Reversible agonists and antagonists compete for the same receptor site, and the degree of effectiveness of each depends on the concentration at the receptor site. Irreversible agonists and antagonists bind irreversibly, and no amount of increased concentration of an agonist can overcome the blockade of the receptor site by the antagonist.

Dose-Response Curves

The classic way of relating the concentration of a drug or hormone to its effect is by a dose-response curve (Fig. 7-3). The dose causing 50% of the maximal effect is known as the ED_{50} (effective dose). When the effect is inhibition, the concentration of the agent causing 50% of the maximal inhibition is the IC_{50} (inhibitory concentration). Determination of the ED_{50} or IC_{50} can show whether a drug or hormone is very active in producing its effect (low ED_{50} or IC_{50}) or not so active (high ED_{50} or IC_{50}). When a low concentration of a drug initiates a marked response, it has high intrinsic activity because the drug is assumed to bind to its receptor in such way that a maximal signal is elicited. For example, the circulating concentrations of the catecholamines are normally very low, being about 10^{-10} mol/L or 10^{-9} mol/L. The concentration actually reaching the receptors in the space between the terminal neurons and the receptors (the synaptic clefts) must be higher, possibly by 10-fold, because norepinephrine is released into that space.

In the presence of the β-adrenergic receptor blocking agent *propranolol*, the dose-response curve is shifted to the right, and a much higher concentration of the artificial catecholamine isoproterenol is required to increase the heart rate (Fig. 7-3). With excess propranolol (*β-blockade toxicity*), a suprapharmacologic

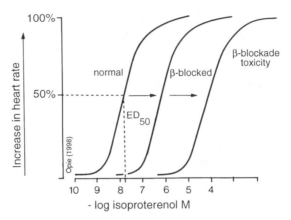

FIG. 7-3. Competitive antagonism between the pharmacologic β-adrenergic agonist isoproterenol and a β-adrenergic receptor antagonist, propranolol. These estimates are based on (1) a high plasma catecholamine concentration of 10^{-9} mol/L; (2) an agonist concentration of 10^{-7} mol/L, which might be needed to displace propranolol from the β-adrenergic receptor; and (3) the much higher doses of propranolol required for toxicity. Thus, β-blockade moves the ED_{50} to the right.

concentration of isoproterenol is required to increase the heart rate. These are the characteristics of competitive antagonism.

The receptor concept allows understanding of two important characteristics of effective drug–tissue interaction: high affinity and marked specificity. High affinity explains why a low concentration of a drug can be so effective, and marked specificity explains why only a small change in molecular structure can decisively change the properties of that drug.

β-ADRENERGIC RECEPTORS

There are two major receptor subtypes. Cardiac β-adrenergic receptors are chiefly the *β₁-adrenergic receptor subtype*, whereas most noncardiac receptors are of the $β_2$ subtype (Lands et al., 1967). Evidence for the existence of different receptors rests on molecular and immunologic studies that allow an exact differentiation of the distribution of β-adrenergic receptor subtypes, varying from 100% β₁-adrenergic receptors in the dog ventricle to 100% β₂-adrenergic receptors in the liver. In humans, there is a substantial population of *β₂-receptors in the atria*, with perhaps about 20% β₂-receptors in the left ventricle (del Monte et al., 1993). Both receptor subtypes can coexist in the same ventricular cell (Del Monte, 1993), and both are involved in positive inotropic responses, although the signal systems may differ (see Physiologic β-Adrenergic Effects, this chapter). The major clinical significance of the subtype difference is in relation to cardioselective *β₁-adrenergic blocking agents* (Fig. 7-4). There is a greater density of β₁-adrenergic receptors in the ventricular myocardium and β₂-adrenergic

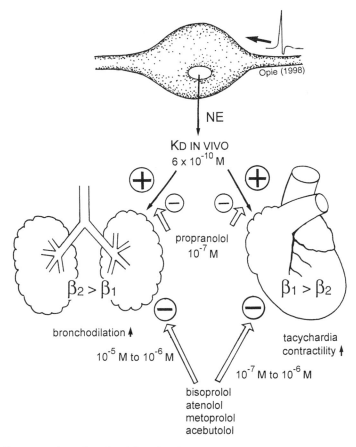

FIG. 7-4. Concept of cardioselectivity, showing the role of comparative density of β_1 and β_2 receptors in the normal heart (80% β_1) and bronchi (chiefly β_2). Note the low concentration of norepinephrine (NE) released in the synaptic cleft, which may, however, be concentrated by several orders of magnitude if the NE stays in the limited space of the cleft. The nonselective β-blocker propranolol inhibits both β_1 and β_2 receptors. The cardioselective β-blockers are more selective for the heart, but at higher concentrations they have an effect on the bronchi. K_D, apparent dissociation constant.

receptors in the lung, so these drugs are preferred if there is lung disease. It must be emphasized that the β_1- and β_2-adrenergic receptors still have some molecular similarity despite their functional differences; β_1-blockers are only relatively selective, and at high doses, selectivity is lost. Molecular proof of differences in receptor subtypes is now available (Kobilka, 1991).

β_1-adrenergic receptor density varies throughout the heart, and the sinus node has about seven to eight times more receptors than does the surrounding atrial muscle or atrioventricular node. The next highest concentration of receptors is found in the ventricles. It seems likely that differences in β-adrenergic receptor density are one factor determining the magnitude of the tissue response to β-adrenergic stimulation. To explain why some β_1-agonist drugs, such as dobutamine, have a more marked inotropic than chronotropic effect, it should be recalled that the ventricles contain chiefly β_1-adrenergic receptors, whereas the sinus nodal tissue contains both subtypes. Hence, β_2-stimulants also cause tachycardia as well as an inotropic response, whereas β_1-agonists, such as dobutamine, may have an apparently dominant inotropic selectivity.

β_3-adrenergic receptors also have been described and cloned. Their chief function is in adipose tissue, where they help to regulate the rate of breakdown of fat.

Molecular Structure of the β-Adrenergic Receptor. The β-adrenergic receptor site is highly stereospecific, and the best fit among catecholamines is obtained with the pharmacologic agent isoproterenol rather than with the natu-

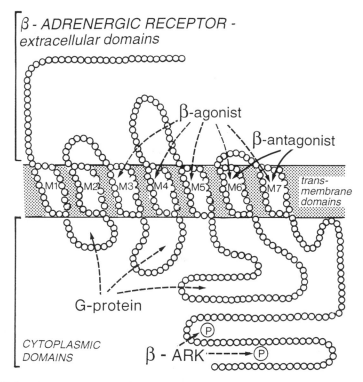

FIG. 7-5. Molecular structure of β_2-adrenergic receptor. Note the three types of domain. The transmembrane domains act as a ligand-binding pocket, with domains M6 and M7 more specific for β-antagonists. β-agonist binding is more diffuse but must also involve M6 and M7. Cytoplasmic domains can interact with G proteins and kinases, such as β-ARK. The latter can phosphorylate and desensitize the receptor by lessening the interaction with G proteins (see Fig. 7-6). Modified from Raymond et al. (1990) with permission.

rally occurring catecholamines norepinephrine and epinephrine. The β_2-adrenergic receptor has been cloned. It and the cholinergic receptor share substantial structural similarities (homology), with the highest homology residing in the membrane spanning domains (Raymond et al., 1990). The transmembrane domains appear to be the site of agonist and antagonist binding, whereas the cytoplasmic domain is where G protein interacts and the terminal COOH tail is the location of one of the phosphorylation sites (Fig. 7-5). Phosphorylation may be involved in the process of desensitization (see next section).

Receptor Desensitization and Downregulation.   Not all the factors governing the chain of events between agonist and tissue response are well understood. Among the most difficult to understand is the way in which receptor numbers and activity can change. The activity of the receptors is not fixed but may be enhanced by the process of receptor sensitization or decreased by receptor desensitization. The number of receptors per unit area of the sarcolemma (the *receptor density*) is also not fixed but can increase or decrease in response to certain physiologic or pathophysiologic circumstances. These changes are called upregulation and downregulation.

Even the meaning of the term *receptor downregulation* is controversial and there are somewhat different models. Some authors use the term "receptor desensitization" whenever there are fewer active receptors available, although the total number of receptors and, therefore, the overall density would be unchanged (Fig. 7-6). A true decrease in receptor numbers and therefore downregulation could result from (1) internalization with destruction by lysosomes, (2) decreased rates of receptor synthesis, and (3) increased rates of receptor degradation by nonlysosomal mechanisms. Presumably changes in the activity of genes encoding receptors play an important role in regulating receptor density and hence contributing to receptor upregulation or downregulation. In general, it is still true to say that "the structural basis for receptor downregulation is poorly understood" (Raymond et al., 1990).

Even short-term exposure of cardiomyocytes to catecholamine leads to a state of refractoriness (desensitization) to continued stimulation (Fig. 7-6). Uncoupling of the excessively stimulated β-receptor from adenylyl cyclase may be explained as follows. The β-receptor is situated in the bilayer and normally coupled by the stimulatory G protein to the activity of adenylyl cyclase to produce intracellular cAMP. During prolonged β-agonist stimulation, an unknown mechanism leads to the transfer of a phosphate group to the β-adrenergic receptor. The enzyme involved is a *kinase* (an enzyme moving a chemical group, in this case the phosphate group). Lefkowitz's group (1995) has termed this enzyme *β-agonist receptor kinase* (β-ARK). It must be translocated from cytosol to sarcolemma to become active (Koch et al., 1996). β-agonist stimulation leads to increased activity of β-ARK, which is followed by a "bite" as the modified receptor becomes uncoupled from G_s (Koch et al., 1996). Phosphorylation of the cytoplasmic domain sites of the β-receptor by β-ARK (and protein kinase A)

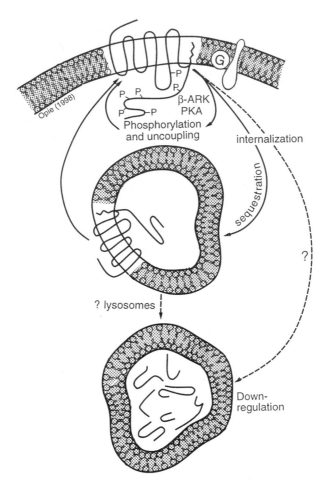

FIG. 7-6. Three types of β-adrenergic receptor desensitization. Uncoupling is initiated by β-receptor stimulation, which leads to activation of the β-ARK. This kinase phosphorylates the β-adrenergic receptor to functionally uncouple it from G_s. The receptor can become resensitized by the activity of phosphatase, which splits off the phosphate group. Alternatively, the receptor can become internalized through one of two processes. In sequestration, an internal vesicle forms that can be reincorporated into the cell membrane. In true downregulation, the receptor numbers decrease because there is degradation of the receptor, possibly by a lysosomal pathway. Downregulation results from exposure to high concentrations of agonist.

appears to change the molecular configuration in such a way that the G protein cannot interact optimally with the receptor (Fig. 7-6). The receptor may then be resensitized if the phosphate group is split off the receptor molecule by a phosphatase and is then once more able to be linked to G_s. This process is aided by the fact that after the β-agonist stimulation is over, β-ARK ceases to be active.

Internalization of receptors may be a self-protective mechanism. Because calcium overload has harmful effects on myocardial cells and because catecholamine β stimulation ultimately acts to increase available cytosolic calcium, it is possible that internalization is one of nature's ways of helping to protect the myocardium from calcium overload. Conversely, externalization of receptors means that the receptors become more sensitive to the prevailing level of catecholamines, as, for example, in acute myocardial ischemia. At a molecular level, one of the mechanisms of sensitization of the β-receptor could be by phospholipid N-methylation, which uncovers the receptor by making the lipid bilayer more fluid (Taira et al., 1990).

β₁- Versus β₂-Selective Downregulation. The above schemas relate chiefly to β₂- and not β₁-adrenergic receptors, for obscure reasons that may involve molecular differences (Muntz et al., 1994). For example, within 24 hours of chronic β-receptor stimulation, only half of the β₁-receptor population is downregulated, in contrast to 80% of the β₂ population. Conversely, in severe heart failure, it is chiefly the β₁-receptors that are downgraded.

Spare Receptors. It must not be assumed that an altered number of receptors automatically leads to a corresponding alteration in the activity of the system. Not all receptors are always in use; those present but out of use are spare receptors. Variations in the proportions of spare receptors mean that even with an unchanged total number of receptors, the response to a given concentration of agonist can vary. What makes receptors spare or fully used is not known but includes the concept of the internal–external cycle.

Drug Therapy and β-Receptor Activity. In the case of certain cardiac drugs that act as positive inotropic agents via *β-receptor stimulation*, such as dobutamine, continued use may lead to a decrease in clinical response, an example of drug *tolerance*. The presumed molecular mechanism is by β-adrenergic receptor desensitization. Although the time scale involved is not well delineated, there appears to be an initial rapid component measured in minutes, perhaps corresponding to uncoupling and/or sequestration. Then follows a delayed decrease in clinical response, measured in hours or days, probably corresponding to true receptor downregulation.

When a *β-receptor antagonist*, such as propranolol, is used long-term, then the β-receptors increase their sensitivity as a result of externalization. If the therapy then is stopped abruptly, the potentially enhanced sensitivity of the β-receptor system can lead to excess stimulation by circulating catecholamines (which also are increased) and aggravation of myocardial ischemia. Thus, these drugs must not be abruptly stopped.

ADENYLYL CYCLASE AND G PROTEINS

To recapitulate, the β-adrenergic receptor is situated on the outer surface of the sarcolemma and is coupled to adenylyl (adenyl or adenylate) cyclase by the stimulatory G protein, G_s. Adenylyl cyclase is the only enzyme system producing cAMP and specifically requires low concentrations of adenosine triphosphate (ATP) (and magnesium) as substrate. The concentration of cAMP in the cell is about 1,000 times lower than the overall cell content of ATP. Thus, activity of adenylyl cyclase is unlikely to be limited by decreases in the cell ATP level (even in ischemia or hypoxia), nor is the conversion of ATP to cAMP by adenylyl cyclase an important route of ATP use in the cell. Adenylyl cyclase in broken cell preparations generally responds to the same hormones that are effective in the intact heart, and this evidence is particularly good for catecholamine stimulation. Only recently has the structure of adenylyl cyclase yielded to cloning technology. Surprisingly, the proposed molecular structure (typography) resembles certain channel proteins, such as that of the calcium channel. However, most of the protein is located on the cytoplasmic side (Schofield and Abbott, 1989), the presumed site of interaction with the G protein.

G Proteins and Signal Transduction

G proteins are a family of guanosine triphosphate (GTP)-binding proteins, crucial in linking the primary event, receptor occupancy, by the first messenger, to the activity of adenylyl cyclase, which is increased by G_s and inhibited by G_i. These G proteins act as on-off switches to adenylyl cyclase (Lefkowitz, 1995). In the resting state, guanosine diphosphate (GDP) is tightly bound to the α subunit, in the off position. The arrival of the β-adrenergic first messenger at its receptor activates the system by displacing GDP by GTP. The stimulatory α subunit of G_s (α_s) now combines with GTP and then separates off from the other two subunits to promote activity of adenylyl cyclase and formation of cAMP (Fig. 7-7). The whole GTP complex also includes the β and γ subunits, which appear to be linked structurally and in function. The α_s subunit also may directly activate the calcium channel. Between these effects, it is possible to explain both positive inotropic and relaxant (lusitropic) effects of catecholamines on contractile cells (Fig. 7-8).

In contrast, a second GTP-binding protein, G_i, is responsible for inhibition of adenylyl cyclase. During cholinergic signaling, the muscarinic receptor is stimulated and GTP binds to the inhibitory α subunit, α_i. The latter then dissociates from the other two components of the G-protein complex, which are the β–γ subunits. The latter seem to play an important role as follows (Fig. 7-9). By stimulating GTPase, they break down the active α_s subunit (α_s-GTP), so that the activity of adenylyl cyclase in response to a β-agonist becomes less (Fig. 7-7). In addition, the α_i subunit activates the potassium channel (Kim et al., 1989) through an unknown mechanism. The latter event contributes to the reduction in heart rate upon cholinergic stimulation.

Two G proteins, the newly described G_h and another G protein called G_q, link myocardial α-adrenergic receptors to the membrane-associated enzyme, phos-

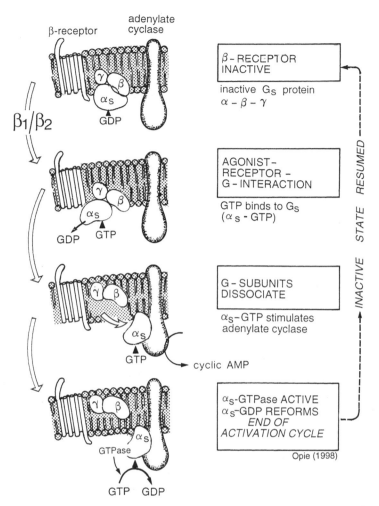

FIG. 7-7. G-protein cycle during activation by β-adrenergic receptor stimulation. In the unliganded state (receptor unoccupied), the G protein consists of three associated units, α, β, and γ. The latter two act as one functional subunit. The α subunit can either stimulate (α_s) or inhibit (α_i), the effector corresponding to the G proteins G_s or G_i. The subunit α_s stimulates adenylyl cyclase when it is activated by binding with GTP at the time of β-agonist occupation of its receptor site. α_s-GTP then interacts with adenylyl cyclase, which produces cAMP. The inherent GTPase activity of the α_i subunit breaks down GTP to GDP, and the initial resting (unliganded) state reforms.

pholipase-C (Hwang et al., 1996). It is not presently clear which G protein works when (Graham et al., 1996).

Other G proteins help to gate ion channels. For example, β-adrenergic stimulation may increase calcium channel activity independently of the formation of cAMP, presumably by direct stimulation of this channel by a G protein.

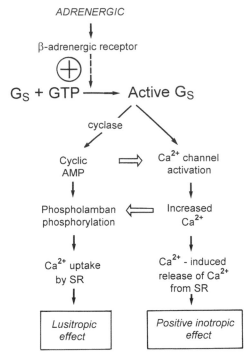

FIG. 7-8. β-adrenergic signal system, with proposed role of G_s protein. Ultimately, there is a calcium-dependent effect in increasing contractile activity (positive inotropic effect) and a phospholamban-dependent increase in the rate of relaxation (lusitropic effect). For further details of inotropic and lusitropic changes, see Fig. 7-16.

At present, the G proteins are subject to intense investigation for their role in cardiovascular responses and in disease states. For example, in dilated poorly contracting and failing hearts, an increase in G_i and a decrease in G_h is found (Hwang et al., 1996). The mechanism and significance of such changes is not currently clear (for details, see Chapter 16).

THE SECOND AND THIRD MESSENGER CONCEPT

The general hypothesis that cAMP, formed from ATP under the influence of activated adenylyl cyclase (Fig. 7-10), is the second messenger of catecholamine β-adrenergic stimulation has gained wide acceptance. A further concept is that calcium is the third messenger of β stimulation, brought into play by several intermediate steps (Fig. 7-11). Another cyclic nucleotide, cGMP, acts as a second messenger for some aspects of vagal activity in heart muscle. In vascular smooth muscle, cGMP is the second messenger of the nitric oxide messenger system.

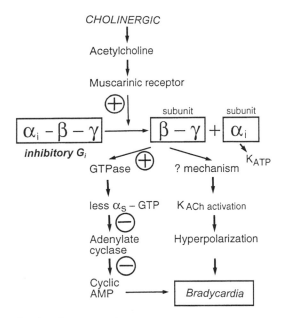

FIG. 7-9. Cholinergic signal system. Proposed role of G protein (α_i-β-γ) in the inhibitory effects of cholinergic stimulation on the heart. In response to occupancy of the muscarinic (M2) receptor by acetylcholine, GTP binds to the inhibitory α subunit (α_i), which dissociates from the rest of the G-protein complex (β-γ). The latter unit has at least two identified functions: (1) to stimulate GTPase to break down GTP, thereby decreasing adenylyl cyclase activity; and (2) to help open the acetylcholine-operated potassium channel. In addition, α_i-GTP also may open the ATP-dependent potassium channel.

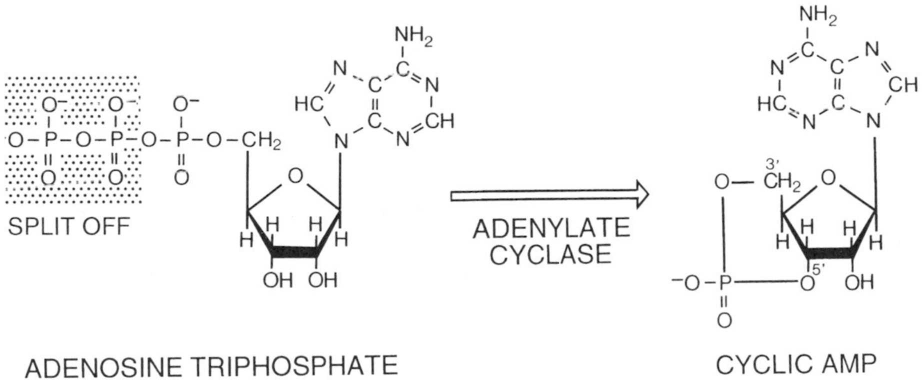

ADENOSINE TRIPHOSPHATE

CYCLIC AMP

FIG. 7-10. Cyclic AMP, the second messenger of β-adrenergic stimulation, is formed from ATP by the activity of activated adenylyl cyclase.

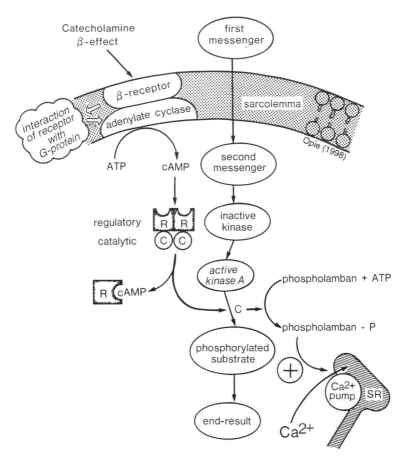

FIG. 7-11. β-adrenergic messenger system. Between the first messenger and the end result is a complex sequence of events. Thus, catecholamine stimulation of adenylyl cyclase eventually enhances calcium uptake by the sarcoplasmic reticulum (SR). Similar principles apply to other end results. R, regulatory; C, catalytic subunits of protein kinase A.

All of these messenger chemicals are present in the heart cell in minute concentrations, about 10^{-10} mol/L for cAMP and about 10^{-11} mol/L for cGMP. The real concentrations in the cytosol are somewhat higher because 80% of the cell is water. A basic feature of the concept of cAMP as second messenger is its rapid turnover as a result of a constant dynamic balance between its formation by adenylyl cyclase and removal by another enzyme, phosphodiesterase. In general, changes in the tissue content of cAMP can be related to the effects of catecholamines in stimulating the contractile activity of the heart (Tables 7-2 and 7-3).

cAMP Compartmentation. There is more involved in responses to adrenergic stimulation than changes in the overall tissue levels of cAMP. When cate-

TABLE 7-2. *Effects of elevated intracellular levels of cAMP on the heart*

Target	Effect
Sinus node	Accelerated discharge
AV node	Accelerated conduction
Purkinje fibers	Accelerated conduction
Normal action potential	Increased slow channel activity (increased Ca^{2+})
Blocked action potential	Provocation of slow responses
Troponin-I	Decreased sensitivity of ATPase to Ca^{2+}
Sarcoplasmic reticulum	Phosphorylation of phospholamban with increased activity of calcium pump
Sarcolemma	Phosphorylation of L-channel with increased entry of calcium
Glycogen	Synthase kinase stimulated; glycogen synthase *b* formed; less glycogen synthesis. Phosphorylase kinase stimulated; increased conversion of phosphorylase *b* to *a*; increased glycogenolysis.
Lipases	Stimulation of lipolysis with provision of energy

cholamines are bound covalently to glass beads, which severely limits the amount of contact that the catecholamines have with the cell surface, maximum contraction of papillary muscles can be achieved without a measurable change in tissue cAMP concentrations (Venter et al., 1975). This may be an example of β-agonism acting through only a small percentage of receptors, according to the spare receptor concept. Second, at any given level of cAMP, it is the degree of stimulation of various protein kinases by cAMP that is of ultimate importance. Theoretically, changes in the activity of specific protein kinases (Fig. 7-11) could occur in response to small localized changes in compartmentalized cAMP. Conversely, certain agents stimulating adenylyl cyclase, such as forskolin, can achieve large increases in myocardial cAMP levels without corresponding changes in the inotropic state. Such noticeable exceptions between the degree of increase of cAMP and the expected consequences show that some degree of compartmentation of cAMP probably takes place in the heart, with only a specific compartment available to increase contractile activity (Hohl and Li, 1991).

TABLE 7-3. *Pharmacologically active agents that alter myocardial levels of cAMP and contractile activity of the heart*

Agent	Mechanism	Effect on cyclic nucleotide	Effect on contractile activity
Epinephrine/ norepinephrine	Stimulate adenylate cyclase via β receptor	↑cAMP	↑
Glucagon/ histamine	Stimulate adenylate cyclase via non-β receptor	↑cAMP	↑
Forskolin	Directly stimulates adenylate cyclase	↑cAMP	↑
β-adrenergic blocking agents	Antagonize effects of β-stimulating catecholamines	↓cAMP	↓
Adenosine	Inhibits adenylate cyclase	↓cAMP	↓

↑, increased; ↓, decreased.

cAMP in Vascular Smooth Muscle.   Although cAMP increases the contractile activity of the heart, it causes relaxation of vascular smooth muscle (see Chapter 9). Hence, β-adrenergic stimulation both increases cardiac contraction and causes vasodilation (see Fig. 2-5).

Other Agents Stimulating Formation of cAMP

Glucagon is a naturally occurring hormone secreted by the pancreas when the blood sugar is low. It stimulates the formation of cAMP in liver cells to break down liver glycogen, thereby replenishing the blood sugar. In the heart, its receptor is coupled by G_s to adenylyl cyclase with formation of cAMP. Glucagon therefore increases the heart rate and contractile activity. These stimulatory effects bypass the β-receptor (Fig. 7-12), and glucagon is used in the therapy of overdoses of β-blocking agents.

Thyroid hormone also can activate adenylyl cyclase independently of the β-adrenergic receptor. A membrane-bound thyroid receptor is by no means the only receptor involved in the explanation of thyroid effects. Formation of cAMP is not likely to be the sole or even the chief effect of thyroid hormone on the heart. The basic site of thyroid action is probably the nuclear receptor for tri-iodothyronine, which stimulates the formation of a diversity of messenger RNA (mRNA) complexes in the presence of this hormone.

Adenosine, formed by the breakdown of ATP, for example, in hypoxia, couples to G_i, inhibiting contraction and heart rate. In addition, adenosine also opens the potassium channel to cause hyperpolarization, thereby directly inhibiting calcium ion entry.

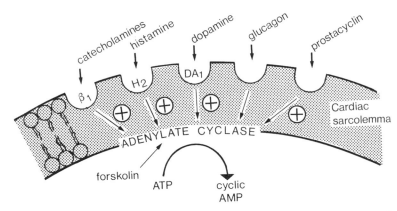

FIG. 7-12. Other receptors linked to cAMP. In addition to the β-adrenergic receptor, there are several other receptors potentially coupled to adenylyl (adenylate) cyclase and hence promoting the formation of cAMP.

Prostacyclin (PGI₂) is a vasodilatory prostaglandin released from the vascular endothelium. It couples to adenylyl cyclase via G_s to promote the formation of cAMP. Although the vasodilatory effect is thought to have physiologic significance, the positive effects on contraction and heart rate appear to be more of a laboratory phenomenon.

Calcitonin gene-related peptide (CGRP) is a vasoactive neurotransmitter. It is found in the nervous system, blood vessels, and heart. It is coupled by its receptor to G_s and hence activates adenylyl cyclase to form cAMP, which is vasodilatory. Experimentally, it also stimulates the contractile activity of the atria but not of the ventricles. The physiologic role of this peptide is still unknown.

Forskolin directly stimulates cardiac adenylyl cyclase. Forskolin is a diterpene isolated from the roots of *Coleus forskohlii*. Even a low concentration of forskolin increases the formation of cAMP and usually stimulates contractile activity. To explain why forskolin can sometimes increase cAMP formation so substantially and yet not have the expected end-organ results, it is now postulated that it is the formation of compartmentalized cAMP that is stimulated by forskolin (Worthington and Opie, 1992).

Dopamine is a natural catecholamine neurotransmitter, also used pharmacologically. It stimulates both pre- and postsynaptic dopamine receptors to vasodilate and to increase contractile activity.

Phosphodiesterase inhibitors are pharmacologic agents that increase cAMP by inhibiting its breakdown. The net effect is similar to that of β stimulation: increased contractile activity, increased rate of relaxation, and increased heart rate.

Organelles Influenced by cAMP

To recapitulate, cAMP itself is unable to alter the cytosolic level of calcium, the third messenger. The intermediate step is activation of the enzyme moving (kinase) a phosphate group from ATP to a specific target protein, which is then said to be phosphorylated (Fig. 7-13). Thus, contraction and relaxation are both enhanced by phosphorylation of a sarcolemmal protein of the calcium channel, of phospholamban of the sarcoplasmic reticulum, and of troponin-I. Of these effects, that on the calcium channel of the sarcolemma and on phospholamban in the sarcoplasmic reticulum have already been discussed in detail. Phosphorylation of the inhibitory subunit of troponin-I decreases the sensitivity of the contractile system to calcium, and promotes the rate of crossbridge detachment (Strang et al., 1994), thereby enhancing cardiac relaxation.

Protein Kinases: Next in the Signal System

At a subcellular level, most if not all of the effects of cAMP are ultimately mediated by protein kinases that phosphorylate various important proteins and enzymes. Each protein kinase is composed of two subunits, regulatory (R) and catalytic (C). When cAMP interacts with protein kinases, it binds to the R sub-

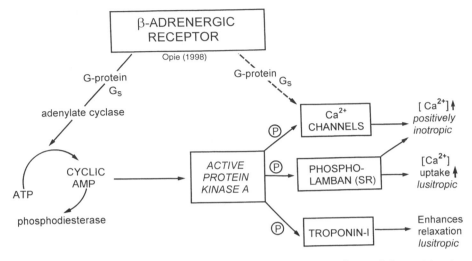

FIG. 7-13. Role of protein kinase A. The major intracellular effects of β-agonist cate-cholamines are by formation of cAMP, which increases the activity of the cAMP-dependent pro-tein kinase A. The latter phosphorylates various proteins concerned with contraction. SR, sar-coplasmic reticulum. For inotropic and lusitropic, see Fig. 7-8.

unit to liberate the C subunit (Fig. 7-11). The inactive kinase, composed of both R and C subunits, is split by cAMP so that active kinase (C) forms.

$$(R_2 + C_2) + 2cAMP \rightarrow 2RcAMP + 2C$$

The ratio of the active protein kinase to the inactive form is called the protein kinase activity ratio. The activity ratio increases in direct relation to the increase of intracellular cAMP levels during stimulation by a variety of agents increasing cAMP, such as epinephrine, glucagon, and phosphodiesterase inhibition. The acti-vated kinase in turn acts as the trigger for a variety of physiologic effects because it switches on or switches off several different enzymes concerned with the regu-lation of calcium ion movements and the breakdown of glycogen and lipid. There are at least eight phosphorylations mediated by the active form of the cAMP-dependent protein kinase. Phosphorylation, the donation of a phosphate group to the enzyme concerned, is therefore a fundamental metabolic switch that can func-tion as a cascade to produce extensive amplification of a signal.

At a molecular level, the basic action of the cAMP-dependent protein kinase is to catalyze the transfer of the terminal phosphate of ATP to serine and threo-nine residues of the protein substrates, leading to a modification of the proper-ties of the proteins concerned. This then leads to further key reactions.

Protein kinase A, activated by cAMP, with its many diverse intracellular sub-strates, occurs in different cells in two forms, with different but similar regula-tor subunits. The type called protein kinase II predominates in cardiac cells. The aim of current work is to determine the order of phosphorylation of the various

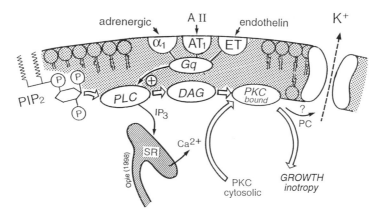

FIG. 7-14. PKC-linked receptors. For example, the α_1-agonist signaling system is coupled via a G protein to phospholipase C (PLC), which breaks down phosphatidylinositol (PIP$_2$) to 1,2-diacylglycerol (DAG) and IP$_3$ (inositol trisphosphate). DAG is thought to translocate PKC from cytosol to the sarcolemma, thereby activating PKC. Signals beyond PKC are not clear. It may phosphorylate ion channels and be concerned with growth regulation. IP$_3$ releases calcium from the sarcoplasmic reticulum to initiate contraction in vascular smooth muscle. Other vasoconstrictors such as angiotensin-II and endothelin act by the same signal system. In the myocardium, a complimentary inotropic system operates via the α_1-receptors to stimulate formation of IP$_3$ with a relatively small contractile response.

proteins that occurs in response to a given cAMP signal within heart cells because this pecking order may determine the order of the ultimate physiologic response.

Protein kinase C is chief in importance among other protein kinases. It is thought to play an important role in transmitting the effects of several agonists linked to phospholipase C and the phosphatidyl inositol system (Fig. 7-14). An example is the effects of α-adrenergic stimulation of vascular cells, which increases contractile activity in arterioles. This kinase also occurs in the myocardium, where it has several isoforms and it may be crucial in preconditioning (see Chapter 19).

If phosphorylation of various critical cellular proteins by kinases is so important in the regulation of heart cell function, it follows that the phosphoprotein *phosphatase* enzymes catalyzing the breakdown of the phosphorylated proteins are equally important in regulation. For example, in vascular smooth muscle, a specific phosphatase dephosphorylates the P light chain of myosin to decrease actin–myosin interaction and to cause vascular relaxation.

PHYSIOLOGIC β-ADRENERGIC EFFECTS

The sequence of molecular signals already described results in certain responses that can be traced out in the whole heart. Thus, β_1-adrenergic stimulation is followed by an increase of tissue cAMP, then the active kinase A increases,

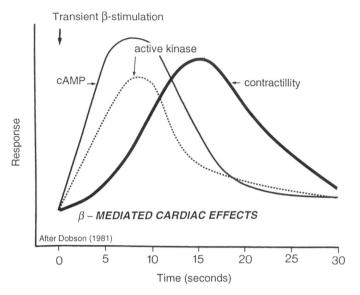

FIG. 7-15. β-adrenergic mediated cardiac effects. After stimulation of the heart by a bolus injection of epinephrine at zero time, cAMP increases before protein kinase is activated. Thereafter, an index of contractility (dP/dt) increases. Only thereafter is there a metabolic response (phosphorylase breaks down glycogen). From Dobson. In: Delius W, Gerlach E, Grobecker H, Kubler W (eds). *Catecholamines and the Heart.* Berlin: Springer-Verlag, 1981;128–141.

and thereafter there is increased contractility, the whole sequence taking about 15 seconds (Fig. 7-15). The overall effect of β_1-adrenergic stimulation on the heart includes the positive inotropic effect, the relaxant effect, the chronotropic effect, and the dromotropic effect. Each will now be considered in turn.

1. Positive Inotropic Effect.   When β_1-adrenergic stimulation increases the rate of contraction and the force developed, then it is said to induce a positive inotropic response, also called increased contractility. The definition of these terms is given in Chapter 13. At present, the probable sequence of events describing the inotropic effects of catecholamines (Fig. 7-16) is as follows:

Catecholamine stimulation → β-receptor → molecular changes → binding of G_s to GTP → catalytic subunit of adenylyl cyclase → formation of cAMP from ATP → activation of protein kinase(s) → phosphorylation of a sarcolemmal protein → increased entry of calcium ion through the cell membrane → calcium-induced calcium release → increase of intracellular free calcium ion concentration → increased splitting of ATP by myosin ATPase, to increase rate of development of contractile force and increase deinhibition of actin and myosin by interaction of calcium with troponin C, to increase total force developed.

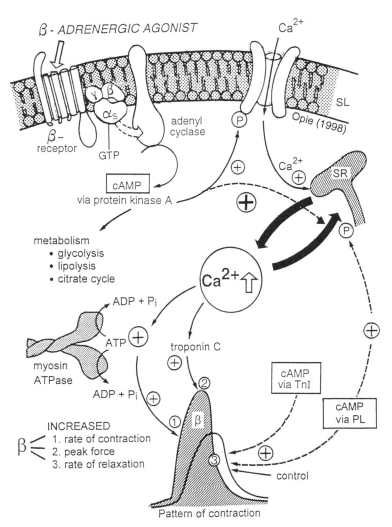

FIG. 7-16. **β-adrenergic signal systems** leading to an increased rate of contraction, increased peak force of contraction, and increased rate of relaxation. SL, sarcolemma; SR, sarcoplasmic reticulum.

An interesting aspect of the catecholamine-induced inotropic response is that it passes off rapidly, within minutes, even though the catecholamine stimulation is maintained. One reason for this *turn-off of the inotropic response* is that the tissue level of cAMP increases much more initially than later. When cAMP increases in the myocardial cell, the enhanced cytosolic calcium concentration activates calmodulin, which in turn enhances the activity of phosphodiesterase, so that the rate of cAMP breakdown is increased. Also, the intense stimulation of the β-adrenergic receptor leads to activation of β-ARK and downregulation (Ungerer et al., 1996) (Fig. 7-6).

2. Relaxant or Lusitropic Effect. This effect, which Katz (1987) has termed the lusitropic response (Greek *lusi,* relaxation), can be explained at a subcellular level by (1) increased activity of the calcium pump of the sarcoplasmic reticulum in response to phosphorylation of phospholamban by cAMP and (2) the effect of an increased internal calcium, as a result of cAMP-induced calcium channel phosphorylation, with the increased calcium also leading to enhanced phosphorylation of phospholamban (see Fig. 6-4). In addition, protein kinase A also phosphorylates troponin-I to increase the rate of crossbridge detachment and relaxation (Strang et al., 1994).

3. Chronotropic Effect. The beating rate of the heart also increases during catecholamine stimulation. This is the positive chronotropic (Greek *chrono,* time) effect that results from the stimulation of the pacemaker (see Fig. 5-5).

4. Dromotropic Effect. Not only does β_1 stimulation cause the positive inotropic and chronotropic effects, but the impulse is conducted more rapidly down the atrioventricular node, His bundle, and Purkinje fibers. This is the positive dromotropic (Greek *dromo,* running) effect. Conduction velocity through the atrioventricular node is enhanced, probably as a result of stimulation of the slow calcium channel in atrioventricular nodal cells. Clinically, the result is shortening of the PR interval on the electrocardiogram (see Chapter 5).

β_2-Adrenergic Effects

It is controversial whether these receptors are linked, like their β_1 brothers, to the adenylyl cyclase–cAMP–protein kinase A signal system. For example, in canine myocytes, a β_2-positive inotropic effect can be found without any increase in overall levels of cAMP despite an increase in cytosolic calcium (Altschuld et al., 1995). Hypothetically, this receptor could be linked directly to the calcium channel by a G protein.

α-ADRENERGIC RECEPTORS

α-adrenergic receptors may help mediate the influx of calcium in cardiac and, especially, vascular smooth muscle. In general, the cardiac effects are usually not prominent, whereas those on the arterioles are substantial (Table 7-4). Pharmacologically, an α-adrenergic receptor mediates the response in which the effects resemble those of the pharmacologic agent, phenylephrine. Among catecholamines, the α-agonist potencies are norepinephrine > epinephrine > isoproterenol (Ahlquist, 1948). Physiologically, it is norepinephrine liberated from nerve terminals that is the chief stimulus to vascular α-adrenergic activity. The antago-

TABLE 7-4. *Comparative cardiovascular effects of α- and β-adrenergic receptor stimulation*

	α-mediated	β-mediated
Electrophysiologic effects	±	++ Conduction Pacemaker Heart rate
Myocardial mechanics	±	++ Contractility Stroke volume Cardiac output
Myocardial metabolism	± Glycolysis	++ O_2 uptake ATP
Coronary arterioles	++ Constriction	+ Direct dilation +++ Indirect dilation (metabolic)
Peripheral arterioles	+++ Constriction SVR BP	+ Dilation

SVR, systemic vascular resistance; BP, blood pressure.

nist properties are mediated by α-blocking agents, such as phentolamine, at low concentrations. Subdivisions of the α-adrenergic receptor are complex. The basic division is into the postsynaptic α_1-adrenergic receptor (inhibited by prazosin) and the presynaptic α_2-adrenergic receptors (inhibited by yohimbine). In the heart, postsynaptic α_1-receptors, when stimulated, usually cause a modest inotropic effect by increased cytosolic calcium. Although several α_1-adrenergic receptor subtypes exist, their differentiation is still incomplete (Graham et al., 1996).

Coupling of α_1-Receptor by G Proteins. When an agonist occupies the α_1-receptor, one of the G protein family, G_h, couples the receptor to the activity of the sarcolemmal enzyme system, phospholipase C (Hwang et al., 1996). The exact steps involved are not as well understood as coupling of the β-receptor to adenylyl cyclase (Deckmyn et al., 1993). Another G protein, G_q, may also link to the α_1-receptor (Graham et al., 1996).

Phosphatidyl Inositol System. After activation of phospholipase C by the G protein, the compound phosphatidyl inositol, part of the membrane phospholipid system (lipid compounds containing phosphate groups), is split into two components: inositol trisphosphate (IP_3) and 1,2-diacylglycerol (Fig. 7-14). IP_3 is one of the second messengers of this system and stimulates the release of calcium from the sarcoplasmic reticulum, which explains why α-receptor stimulation can cause vascular smooth muscle to contract without any entry of calcium from the outside. Berridge has proposed a general role for inositol phosphates in regulating oscillations of cytosolic calcium. Although IP_3 travels to the sarcoplasmic reticulum to liberate calcium, 1,2-diacylglycerol stays in the cell membrane, being highly lipophilic. It stimulates into activity another protein kinase, protein kinase C, by promoting its translocation from cytosol to sarcolemma.

The experimental agents, the *phorbol esters*, are able directly to stimulate protein kinase C and, therefore, to mimic some of the effects of α_1-adrenergic stimulation. In the myocardium, phorbol ester stimulation increases the contractile force.

Positive Inotropic Effect of α_1 Stimulation.   This effect is not thought to be of major importance in the normal myocardium, when the prime regulation of contraction is through the β-adrenergic system. Nonetheless, there is a small positive inotropic effect associated with the formation of IP_3 (Otani et al., 1988). In advanced heart failure, when the β-adrenergic receptor system undergoes desensitization and downregulation, it might be that the α-adrenergic system could come into play as a supportive positive inotropic mechanism. Yet its coupling system is also downgraded (Hwang et al., 1996).

Other Inositol Phosphates.   Besides IP_3, at least two other similar compounds, IP_4 and IP_5, may form in response to α-adrenergic stimulation. These compounds presumably are messengers whose full function is still unknown. A current hypothesis for skeletal muscle is that IP_4 can increase calcium influx across the sarcolemma. Such calcium is then able, together with IP_3, to release calcium from the sarcoplasmic reticulum.

Non–α-Adrenergic Receptors Coupled to Phospholipase C.   Several other receptors couple to phospholipase C. Angiotensin II receptors in the myocardium and in vascular smooth muscle are thus coupled to the phospholipase C system (Allen et al., 1988). Formation of protein kinase C may explain the growth-stimulating properties of angiotensin II. In blood vessels, angiotensin II is strongly vasoconstrictive, acting via IP_3 to release calcium from the sarcoplasmic reticulum. The newly identified endothelial-derived vasoconstrictor peptide, endothelin, also is coupled to the phospholipase C system in the myocardium, as well as in vascular smooth muscle. Endothelin may contribute to the release of atrial natriuretic peptide (see Fig. 16-12).

Negative Inotropic Effects of Phospholipase C.   Unexpectedly, a number of inhibitory effects on cardiac contraction have been found as a result of agonists linked to phospholipase C. For example, α_1-stimulation may have negative rather than positive inotropic effects at high levels of internal calcium (Capogrossi et al., 1991). In some species, but not in humans, angiotensin II also has a negative rather than a positive inotropic effect. The mechanism of these negative effects is not understood.

CHOLINERGIC RECEPTORS AND
PARASYMPATHETIC VAGAL EFFECTS

Turning now from the adrenergic system and its messengers to the parasympathetic system, there is again an extracellular first messenger (acetylcholine), a receptor system (the muscarinic receptor), and an intracellular signaling system (the G protein system). The two types of cholinergic receptors are the nicotinic receptors at the autonomic ganglia and the muscarinic receptors at the effector tissue. It is the myocardial *muscarinic receptor* (M₂) that is associated specifically with the activity of the vagal nerve endings and has as its characteristics the production of a negative inotropic response and inhibition by atropine. The *nicotinic* receptor by definition responds to nicotine and is inhibited by ganglionic-blocking agents, such as hexamethonium. This differentiation between the nicotinic ganglionic receptor sites and the tissue muscarinic sites is broadly correct, although some nicotinic receptors also have been found at the nerve endings.

The major effects of parasympathetic vagal stimulation on the heart already have been described, including bradycardia and a modest negative inotropic effect. The chief function of muscarinic cholinergic receptors is seen as the inhibitory modulation of the effects of sympathetic stimulation, known as *accentuated antagonism*, by lessening the degree of formation of cAMP in response to β-adrenergic stimulation (Figs. 7-17 and 7-18). The proposal is that muscarinic stimulation inhibits the activation of G$_s$ that results from β-receptor occupation.

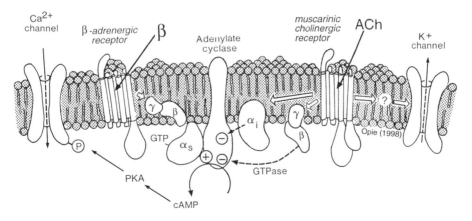

FIG. 7-17. Interaction of cholinergic and β-adrenergic receptors. The three components of the G proteins involved are the α subunit (α$_s$, stimulatory; α$_i$, inhibitory) and the β-γ unit. ACh, acetylcholine. See also Figs. 7-8 and 7-9.

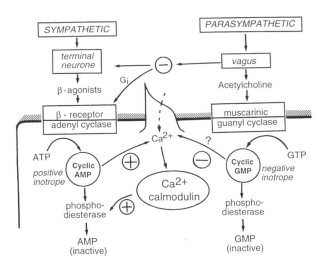

FIG. 7-18. Interaction between parasympathetic and sympathetic systems at a cellular level may involve two opposing cyclic nucleotides: cAMP and cGMP. Many effects of vagal stimulation could best be explained by the inhibitory effect on the formulation of cAMP, including formation of the inhibitory G protein G_i in response to M_2-receptor stimulation.

In more detail, stimulation of the muscarinic receptor leads to breakdown (hydrolysis) of GTP, with the end result that the binding between GTP and the α_s subunit of G_s cannot occur. The β-γ component of the G protein dissociates from the rest (α_i) to stimulate the GTPase and hence indirectly to decrease formation of cAMP (Fig. 7-9). Thus, the extent of adenylyl cyclase activation in response to a given degree of β-adrenergic stimulation is decreased. (Readers should be careful to distinguish between α_1-adrenergic receptors and the inhibitory α component of the G protein, α_i.)

In nodal tissue, opening of the G-dependent potassium channels inhibits the rate of spontaneous depolarization and slows the sinus node (see Fig. 4-19). In addition, the nitric oxide messenger system may contribute by the formation of inhibitory cGMP (next section).

In the myocardium, the ventricles are much less responsive to muscarinic agonists than are the atria, despite similar receptor densities (Lindemann and Watanabe, 1995), so that there must be postreceptor differences, probably in the degree of G-protein coupling. Nonetheless, there is a negative inotropic effect of vagal stimulation, best observed in the presence of prior β-adrenergic stimulation (Lindemann and Watanabe, 1995). The triple mechanism is: (1) heart rate slowing (negative Treppe effect, see Chapter 12); (2) inhibition of the formation of cAMP; and (3) a direct negative inotropic effect of cGMP, formed as result of activity of guanyl (guanylyl) cyclase (Fig. 7-18). According to the latter proposal, cGMP acts as a second messenger to vagal stimulation just as cAMP to β-adrenergic stimulation.

Guanylate Cyclase, cGMP, and Nitric Oxide

Besides inhibition of the formation of cAMP, increasing evidence suggests that cholinergic receptor stimulation can be linked to the enzyme complex guanylate cyclase, much as β-adrenergic stimulation is linked to adenylyl cyclase. cGMP, produced by guanylate cyclase, in general has opposite effects to those of cAMP on the myocardium. For example, calcium channel opening is promoted by cAMP but is inhibited by cGMP (Tohse and Sperelakis, 1991), which activates a cGMP-dependent kinase that induces inhibitory phosphorylation.

Nitric Oxide Signal Transduction in Cholinergic Stimulation. In *vascular smooth muscle*, guanylate cyclase responds to stimulation by nitric oxide, released by the vascular endothelium, by formation of vasodilatory cGMP. The latter reduces cytosolic calcium to act as a vasodilatory signal (see Chapter 9).

In the *sinus node*, the proposal is that cholinergic stimulation of the M_2 receptor leads to formation of nitric oxide that in turn promotes formation of cGMP (Han et al., 1995). The latter stimulates the activity of the phosphodiesterase breaking down cAMP, thereby lessening adrenergic effects on the sinus node. The result is a decreased calcium current in the sinus node, and the firing rate will diminish. Thus, cholinergic stimulation decreases the tachycardia mediated by adrenergic stimulation.

In the *myocardium*, cGMP may stimulate protein kinase G to decrease the heart rate and to have a negative inotropic effect (Lohmann et al., 1991). Such formation of cGMP could occur in response to either cholinergic stimulation or activity of the nitric oxide pathway in the cardiac myocytes (Fig. 7-19). These two mechanisms are not mutually exclusive. Cholinergic stimulation induces the activity of the myocardial (constitutive) nitric oxide synthase to increase the formation of nitric oxide (Kelly et al., 1996). Whether the myocardial nitric oxide system plays a physiologic role is still controversial.

Cross Talk Between Receptors

Thus, the picture emerges of a host of important cardiovascular receptors, with subtypes, signaling systems, and second messengers. Eventually the receptors almost all control cytosolic calcium in different ways. To avoid too many conflicting signals, the activity of the receptors needs to be integrated. There are two major ways of achieving integration. First, the process of switching on or off the adrenergic or cholinergic autonomic systems causes a coordinated series of cell changes calculated to mediate the overall adrenergic effects, in general stimulatory, or the inhibitory effects of cholinergic stimulation. Second, excess receptor stimulation can be muted by receptor downregulation or by self-regulation of internal calcium. When cytosolic calcium increases too high, for example, there may be activation of calmodulin and of the phosphodiesterase breaking down cAMP (see Chapter 6). Third and most novel is the concept of

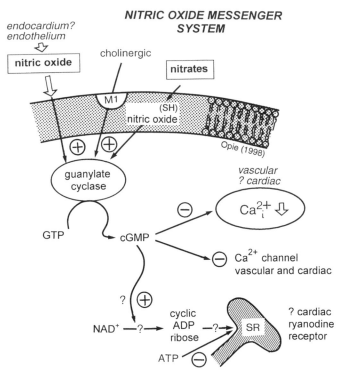

FIG. 7-19. Nitric oxide messenger system. Proposed role in stimulating guanylate cyclase and cGMP to cause vasodilation and possibly a negative inotropic effect. The physiologic significance of the cyclic adenosine diphosphate (ADP) ribose path is still speculative. RR, ryanodine receptor.

cross-talk whereby receptors can send interactive regulatory messages to each other (Port and Malbon, 1993). For example, enhanced cholinergic M_2 stimulation leads to an increase in the inhibitory G_i protein, as well as to increased formation of cGMP, thereby limiting the effects of β-adrenergic stimulation. The full implications of cross-talk are still being explored.

SIGNALS AND RECEPTORS IN DISEASE STATES

Hypertrophy and Stretch Receptors.   Both myocardial and vascular cells can respond to stretch by activation of a group of poorly described mechanoreceptors. Because the usual stimulus is stretch, they are also called stretch receptors (see Chapter 4). One concept is that the act of stretch initiates a series of conformational changes in an ion channel to allow increased entry of a specific ion. Vascular endothelial cells are also endowed with stretch receptors. In response to shear forces, the cytosolic calcium increases, which activates the synthesis of vasodilatory nitric oxide. When mechanoreceptors are chronically stretched, they appear to participate in the activation of the growth process. Thus, a sustained increase of pressure on the walls of the ventricles or the blood vessels promotes the process of myocardial or vascular hypertrophy.

Myocardial Ischemia. There is a brisk activation of the β-adrenergic–cAMP system in the first 15 to 30 minutes of severe ischemia, which may be linked to an increased propensity to ventricular tachycardia and fibrillation at the onset of a heart attack (Lubbe et al., 1992). At this stage there is the combination of intense release of norepinephrine from the nerve endings in the ischemic area and an increased density of β_1-adrenergic receptor, the latter change being a response to the rapid upregulation of the mRNA levels for this receptor (Ihl-Vahl et al., 1995). Thereafter, despite continued adrenergic stimulation and persistence of the increased receptor density, the activity of adenylyl cyclase decreases (Ungerer et al., 1996). The proposed explanation is that the β-adrenergic receptor kinase (β-ARK) is activated in response to intense adrenergic stimulation to downregulate the receptor (Fig. 7-6).

Prolonged Excess Catecholamine Stimulation. In experimental overexpression of the G_s protein, prolonged excess catecholamine stimulation can lead to a calcium-overload type of myocardial damage with cell necrosis and replacement fibrosis (Iwase et al., 1996). The human counterpart is the cardiomyopathy of pheochromocytoma.

Severe Heart Failure. The β-adrenergic–cAMP system is downregulated severe heart failure. Excess circulating catecholamines (see Chapter 16) are thought to be detrimental, and one hypothesis is that a variety of mechanisms come into play to desensitize the myocardium, thereby protecting it from excess β-adrenergic stimulation. The major changes are (1) defective functioning of adenylyl cyclase, (2) β_1-receptor downgrading, and (3) relative upgrading of the β_2-receptors, which may nonetheless be associated with an impaired contractile response (del Monte et al., 1993). In one type of heart failure caused by ischemic cardiomyopathy, the α_1-adrenergic system undergoes several changes, including increased receptor density and downstream changes that limit the ultimate inotropic response (Hwang et al., 1996). In combination, these changes may explain the poorly developed and low-amplitude calcium transients in human tissue from severe heart failure subjects (Gwathmey et al., 1987). Of the β-receptor subtypes in the human heart, 80% are normally β_1 and 20% β_2 (del Monte et al., 1993). However, in the failing left ventricle, the β_1:β_2 ratio is 60:40, a change that appears to be a true downregulation, not just an internalization. The signal for the downregulation is not clear. The excess levels of circulating catecholamines found in severe congestive heart failure would be expected to downregulate the β_2- rather than β_1-receptors (Muntz et al., 1994). In addition to loss of receptor density, there may be loss of function because levels of the inhibitory kinase, β-ARK, are much increased (Koch et al., 1996).

In the myocardium harvested at cardiac transplantation, studies on the G protein system have shown that G_i is increased (Böhm et al., 1994), which may lead to inhibition of adenylyl cyclase and, consequently, poor formation of cAMP. The G protein concerned is the α_i subunit, which may be increased as a result of increased transcription of its gene in response to excess circulating norepinephrine (Böhm et al., 1994). The same or a very similar G protein probably is the site of action of the diphtheria toxin (pertussis toxin) which causes increased activity of adenylyl cyclase. Speculatively, this sequence could explain why the disease diphtheria may be accompanied by myocardial failure (*diphtheritic myocarditis*), possibly caused by calcium overload.

Excess Nitric Oxide in Dilated Cardiomyopathy and Septic Shock. Excess nitric oxide is made in the myocardium in dilated cardiomyopathy when the inducible form of nitric oxide synthase (iNOS) is stimulated (Habib et al., 1996). The negative inotropic effect of the nitric oxide contributes to the severity of the heart failure. The hypothesis is that the inflammatory response associated with the cardiomyopathy sets off the production of cytokines, such as *tumor necrosis factor*, that induce iNOS (Schulz et al., 1995). This hypothesis can be extended to other types of heart failure, including septic shock, in which there is increased formation of tumor necrosis factor and other cytokines.

Exercise in Cardiac Transplant Patients. An interesting clinical problem has been how to understand the mechanism whereby the transplanted denervated heart still continues to respond to exercise with a tachycardia. The answer is that cardiac β_2-receptors respond to circulating catecholamines, even in the absence of neuronally released norepinephrine (Leenen et al., 1995).

SUMMARY

1. *General model.* Neurotransmitters and regulatory peptides activate intracellular processes by initial occupation of a receptor, followed by coupling via one of the G-protein family to an effector molecule, which produces an intracellular second messenger. This messenger activates protein kinases which, in turn, regulate cytosolic calcium levels by altering the activity of crucial organelles such as channels or the sarcoplasmic reticulum. When cytosolic calcium increases, cell processes are in general switched on, including the sinus node discharge rate and the force of cardiac contraction.

2. *β-adrenergic stimulation.* Occupancy of the β-receptor stimulates the reaction between the stimulatory G_s protein and GTP to increase adenylyl cyclase activity. Adenylyl cyclase converts ATP to cAMP, the second messenger that activates protein kinase A. This kinase phosphorylates a subunit of the calcium channel to admit more calcium ions. cAMP also phosphory-

lates phospholamban on the sarcoplasmic reticulum to enhance uptake of calcium by the sarcoplasmic reticulum. Thus, both the rate of contraction and the relaxation are enhanced, to explain the positive inotropic and lusitropic effects.

3. *Vagal stimulation.* Activity of the parasympathetic nervous system releases the messenger acetylcholine. The latter decreases the heart rate and force of contraction by several mechanisms, including (1) a decreased rate of release of norepinephrine from the terminal neurons by the process of neuromodulation and (2) activation of the inhibitory G protein, G_i. In addition, cGMP may be the direct second messenger of acetylcholine, and it inhibits the calcium channel. All of these changes decrease the heart rate and thereby the force of contraction (negative Treppe effect).

4. *α_1-adrenergic stimulation.* In general, the α-adrenergic system acts chiefly on vascular smooth muscle and has a relatively minor role in the control of the contractile activity of the myocardium. Its receptor is linked by another G protein (G_q) to its effector, phospholipase C, with hydrolysis of phosphatidyl inositol. Two changes result. First, the intracellular messenger, inositol trisphosphate (IP$_3$), is formed, which stimulates the release of calcium from the sarcoplasmic reticulum, leading to vasoconstriction. Second, protein kinase C is activated by its translocation from the resting cytosolic state to the active membrane-located state. Activated protein kinase C may regulate the activity of ion channels, for example, allowing an enhanced influx of calcium ions to sustain the vascular contraction initiated by IP$_3$. This kinase is also important in the growth response.

5. *Nitric oxide–cGMP system.* In blood vessels, nitric oxide formed in the vascular endothelium permeates to the vascular smooth muscle. There it stimulates guanylate cyclase to produce cGMP, which decreases cytosolic calcium and thereby causes vasodilation. A similar system may exist in the myocardium, where nitric oxide is synthesized by an inducible nitric oxide synthase. cGMP, thus formed in cardiac myocytes, may have a negative inotropic effect.

STUDENT QUESTIONS

1. What is the full messenger system involved in translating β-receptor stimulation into a positive inotropic contractile effect?
2. What is receptor desensitization?
3. How does vagal stimulation decrease the heart rate?
4. How does α_1-adrenergic stimulation cause vasoconstriction?
5. Describe the role of the G-protein family in signal transduction with special reference to the interaction between the β-adrenergic system and the cholinergic system.

CARDIOLOGIST-IN-TRAINING QUESTIONS

1. How do the two major subtypes of cardiac β-adrenergic receptors differ in their function? How are these receptors subtypes changed in severe heart failure?

2. A patient with severe acute heart failure is given the positively inotropic drug, dobutamine. An initial improvement in cardiac function rapidly tails off unless the dose is increased. Why? Describe the possible molecular mechanisms.

3. There are ten steps that follow initial β-adrenergic catecholamine stimulation, leading to a positive inotropic effect. How many can you itemize?

4. Describe the α-adrenergic signal system. Why is it of greater importance in the control of vascular than of myocardial contraction?

5. Recently the nitric oxide messenger system has attracted much attention. What is its messenger system? In which physiological responses does this system appear to be involved?

REFERENCES

1. Ahlquist RP. A study of the adrenotropic receptors. *Am J Physiol* 1948;153:586–600.
2. Allen IS, Neri M, Cohen RS, et al. Angiotensin-II increases spontaneous contractile frequency and stimulates calcium current in cultured neonatal rat heart myocytes: insights into the underlying biochemical mechanisms. *Circ Res* 1988;62:524–534.
3. Altschuld RA, Starling RC, Hamlin RL, et al. Response of failing canine and human heart cells to β$_2$-adrenergic stimulation. *Circulation* 1995;92:1612–1618.
4. Berridge MJ. Inositol trisphosphate and calcium signalling. *Nature* 1993;361:315–325.
5. Böhm M, Eschenhagen T, Gierschik P, et al. Radioimmunochemical quantification of Giα in right and left ventricles from patients with ischaemic and dilated cardiomyopathy and predominant left ventricular failure. *J Mol Cell Cardiol* 1994;26:133–149.
6. Bourne HR. Team blue sees red. *Nature* 1995;376:727–729.
7. Capogrossi MC, Kachadorian WA, Gambassi G, et al. Ca^{2+} dependence of α-adrenergic effects on the contractile properties and Ca^{2+} homeostasis of cardiac myocytes. *Circ Res* 1991;69:540–550.
8. Deckmyn H, VanGeet C, Vermylen J. Dual regulation of phospholipase C activity by G-proteins. *NIPS* 1993;8:61–63.
9. del Monte F, Kaumann AJ, Poole-Wilson PA, et al. Coexistence of functioning β$_1$- and β$_2$-adrenoreceptors in single myocytes from human ventricle. *Circulation* 1993;88:854–863.
10. Graham RM, Perez DM, Hwa J, Piascik MT. α-Adrenergic receptor subtypes. Molecular structure, function and signalling. *Circ Res* 1996;78:737–749.
11. Gwathmey JK, Copelas L, MacKinnon R, et al. Abnormal intracellular calcium handling in myocardium from patients with end-stage heart failure. *Circ Res* 1987;61:70–76.
12. Habib FM, Springall DR, Davies GJ, et al. Tumour necrosis and inducible nitric oxide synthase in dilated cardiomyopathy. *Lancet* 1996;347:1151–1155.
13. Han X, Shimoni Y, Giles WR. A cellular mechanism for nitric oxide-mediated cholinergic control of mammalian heart rate. *J Gen Physiol* 1995;106:45–65.
14. Hohl CM, Li Q. Compartmentation of cAMP in adult canine ventricular myocytes. Relation to single cell free Ca^{2+} transients. *Circ Res* 1991;69:1369–1379.
15. Hwang K-C, Gray CD, Sweet WE, Moravec CS. α$_1$-Adrenergic receptor coupling with G$_h$ in the failing human heart. *Circulation* 1996;94:718–726.
16. Ihl-Vahl R, Marquetant R, Bremerich MJ, Strasser RH. Regulation of β-adrenergic receptors in acute myocardial ischemia: subtype-selective increase of mRNA specific for β$_1$-adrenergic receptors. *J Mol Cell Cardiol* 1995;27:437–452.
17. Iwase M, Bishop SP, Uechi M, et al. Adverse effects of chronic endogenous sympathetic drive induced by cardiac G$_{s\alpha}$ overexpression. *Circ Res* 1996;78:517–524.

18. Kahn CR. Membrane receptors for hormones and neurotransmitters. *J Cell Biol* 1976;70:261–286.
19. Katz AM. Role of the basic sciences in the practice of cardiology. *J Mol Cell Cardiol* 1987;19:3–17.
20. Kelly RA, Balligand J-L, Smith TW. Nitric oxide and cardiac function. *Circ Res* 1996;79:363–380.
21. Kim D, Lewis DL, Graziadei L, et al. G-protein beta-gamma subunits activate the cardiac muscarinic K+-channel via phospholipase A2. *Nature* 1989;337:557–560.
22. Kobilka B. Molecular and cellular biology of adrenergic receptors. *Trends Cardiovasc Med* 1991;1: 189–194.
23. Koch WJ, Milano CA, Lefkowitz RJ. Transgenic manipulation of myocardial G-protein-coupled receptors and receptor kinases. *Circ Res* 1996;78:511–516.
24. Lands AM, Arnold A, McAuliff JP, et al. Differentiation of receptor systems activated by sympathomiametic amines. *Nature* 1967;214:597–598.
25. Leenen FHH, Davies RA, Fourney A. Role of cardiac β-receptors in cardiac responses to exercise in cardiac transplant patients. *Circulation* 1995;91:685–690.
26. Lefkowitz RJ. Clinical implications of basic research. G proteins in medicine. *N Engl J Med* 1995; 332:186–187.
27. Lindemann JP, Watanabe AM. Mechanisms of adrenergic and cholinergic regulation of myocardial contractility. In: Sperelakis N (ed). *Physiology and Pathophysiology of the Heart.* 3rd ed. Boston: Kluwer Academic, 1995;467–494.
28. Lohmann SM, Fischmeister R, Walter U. Signal transduction by cGMP in heart. *Basic Res Cardiol* 1991;86:503–514.
29. Lubbe WH, Podzuweit T, Opie LH. Potential arrhythmogenic role of cyclic adenosine monophosphate (AMP) and cytosolic calcium overload: implications for prophylactic effects of beta-blockers in myocardial infarction and proarrhythmic effects of phospodiesterase inhibitors. *J Am Coll Cardiol* 1992;19:1622–1633.
30. Muntz KH, Zhao M, Miller JC. Downregulation of myocardial β-adrenergic receptors. Receptor subtype selectivity. *Circ Res* 1994;74:369–376.
31. Otani H, Otani H, Das DK. α1-adrenoceptor-mediated phosphoinositide breakdown and inotropic response in rat left ventricular papillary muscles. *Circ Res* 1988;62:8–17.
32. Port JD, Malbon CC. Integration of transmembrane signalling. Cross-talk among G-protein-linked receptors and other signal transduction pathways. *Trends Cardiovasc Med* 1993;3:85–92.
33. Raymond JR, Hnatowich M, Lefkowitz RJ, Caron MG. Adrenergic receptors. Models for regulation of signal transduction processes. *Hypertension* 1990;15:119–131.
34. Schofield PR, Abbott A. Molecular pharmacology and drug action: structural information casts light on ligand binding. *TIPS* 1989;10:207–212.
35. Schulz R, Panas DL, Catena R, et al. The role of nitric oxide in cardiac depression induced by interleukin-1β and tumour necrosis factor-α. *Br J Pharmacol* 1995;114:27–34.
36. Strang KT, Sweitzer NK, Greaser ML, Moss RL. β-adrenergic receptor stimulation increases unloaded shortening velocity of skinned single ventricular myocytes from rats. *Circ Res* 1994;74: 542–549.
37. Taira Y, Panagia V, Shah KR, et al. Stimulation of phospholipid N-methylation by isoproterenol in rat hearts. *Circ Res* 1990;66:28–36.
38. Tohse N, Sperelakis N. cGMP inhibits the activity of single calcium channels in embryonic chick heart cells. *Circ Res* 1991;69:325–331.
39. Ungerer M, Kessbohm K, Kronsbein K, et al. Activation of β-adrenergic receptor kinase during myocardial ischemia. *Circ Res* 1996;79:455–460.
40. Venter JC, Ross J, Kaplan NO. Lack of detectable change in cyclic AMP during the cardiac inotropic response to isoproterenol immobilized on glass beads. *Proc Natl Acad Sci USA* 1975;72:824–828.
41. Worthington M, Opie LH. Contrasting effects of cyclic AMP increase caused by β-adrenergic stimulation or by adenylate cyclase activation on ventricular fibrillation threshold of isolated rat heart. *J Cardiovasc Pharmacol* 1992;20:595–600.

8

Myocardial Contraction and Relaxation

The most important suggestion arising from the model is that release of myosin from actin is caused by the opening of the cleft . . . when the nucleotide binds in the active site pocket.

Rayment et al., 1993

The essential components of the heart's contractile machinery are those proteins concerned primarily with contraction (actin and myosin) and those whose function is regulatory (troponin and tropomyosin). By far the greater percentage of myofibrillar protein is that concerned with contraction, with about 10% concerned with its regulation and another 10% concerned with maintenance of the structure of the myofibril (Table 8-1). In living muscle, contraction will not occur unless adenosine triphosphate (ATP) and calcium are present. According to the generally accepted sliding filament model (Huxley, 1990), the thin actin fibers slide between the thicker myosin fibers as a result of repetitive movements of the myosin heads (Plate 1). The concept of the "working stroke" of the myosin head, previously not fully proven, is now established (Irving et al., 1992). The linkage between the myosin head and the actin filament is the crossbridge. The crossbridge cycle is the repetitive attachment and detachment of myosin heads to and from actin filaments. The third and newly emphasized filament is titin, noncontractile but elastic (Plate 2).

MOLECULAR EVENTS IN THE CONTRACTILE CYCLE

The transformation of chemical energy into mechanical work involves a series of reactions that center around the splitting of ATP by hydrolysis. The term "hydrolysis" describes a reaction in which a compound is split (Greek *lysis*) by

TABLE 8-1. *The proteins of skeletal myofibrils*

Function	Location	% of myofibrillar protein	Molecular weight (kDa)
Contractile			
Myosin	Thick filament	44	460
	Two heavy chains	46–50	220×2
	Four light chains	About 10	20
Actin	Thin filament	25	42
Regulatory			
Tropomyosin	Thin filament	5	67
Troponin-I	Thin filament		24
Troponin-C	Thin filament	7	18
Troponin-T	Thin filament		38
Structural			
Titin	From Z to M lines	8–10	2.7×10^3
C-protein[a]	Thick filament		140
α-actinin[b]	Z lines		400
β-actinin	Thin filament	About 8–13	400
M-line proteins	M lines		750 (about)

Data in part from Perry (*Biochem Soc Trans* 1979;7:593–617) and Swynghedauw (*Physiol Rev* 1986;66:719–771).

[a]This protein is thought to tether or limit the degree of flexion that can be achieved by the myosin neck, thereby lessening force development (Hofmann et al. *J Physiol* 1991;439:701).

[b]Anti–α-actin antibodies alter properties of the Z line (Linke et al. *Circ Res* 1993;73:724).

the addition of water (Greek *hydor*). In the case of muscle, the enzyme that is involved is an integral part of the myosin molecule. Therefore, the enzyme is known as the myosin ATPase. For this function, the important part of ATP is the terminal pyrophosphate (P-O-P) linkage. It is customary to refer to this as a high-energy bond (a concept that was introduced by Fritz Lipmann in 1941) because when the bond is split off, useful energy is released. Thus, in general terms, all the energy needed to cause muscle contraction is obtained by splitting the terminal phosphate bond in ATP, as follows:

$$\text{ATP} + \text{H}_2\text{O} \Rightarrow \text{ADP} + \text{P}_i + \text{H}^+ + \text{energy}$$

where ADP is adenosine diphosphate and P_i is inorganic phosphate. To be exact, it is MgATP^{2-}, not ATP, that is split (see Chapter 11). A little more than 30 kilojoules of energy is released for each mole (500 g) of ATP that is hydrolyzed (or split up). The heart contains about 3 mg of ATP/g fresh weight or about 5 μmol/g or 5×10^{-6} mol/g of ATP or 10 mmol ATP/L of cytosol. Together with the roughly threefold greater pool of creatine phosphate, this represents an energy reserve sufficient for only 50 to 75 beats in an adult heart. Thus, continuous production of ATP by mitochondrial metabolism is required to sustain the contractile cycle.

In the heart, the myosin ATPase actually splits ATP in the relaxation phase of the cycle (crossbridges off), and the power stroke occurs when the products of hydrolysis (first P_i and then ADP) are released. Cyclic interaction of the two contractile proteins of the crossbridges is controlled by the regulatory proteins tro-ponin-C and -I in a calcium-dependent manner, as will be described.

Microanatomy of Contraction

To explain the contraction cycle requires first a brief recapitulation of the microanatomy of the two contractile elements, which are the thin actin fibers lying between the much thicker myosin components (Plates 1–3). A third non-contractile element, titin, tethers the myosin molecule to the Z line and provides elasticity (Trombitas et al., 1995).

Actin and Troponin-C. The thin filaments of actin (about 1 μm long and only 5 to 7 nm wide) contain two helical chains, which intertwine in a helical pattern. Each actin filament is carried on a twisting backbone of the heavier *tropomyosin* molecule. Crucial to the interaction between actin and myosin are the *troponin complexes* that occur at regular intervals of 38 nm along the tropomyosin (Plate 3). Troponin-C (C for calcium) is that component that responds to the calcium ions released from the sarcoplasmic reticulum, to start the crossbridge cycle. Troponin-C, once activated by calcium ions, binds to the inhibitory molecule *troponin-I* (I for inhibitor), which otherwise restricts the interaction between actin and the myosin heads. *Troponin-T* (T for tropomyosin binding) links the whole troponin complex to tropomyosin. *Tropomodulin* is another regulatory protein that caps the free, pointed ends of the thin actin filaments to prevent their excess elongation during growth.

Myosin Filament. Each myosin thick filament (about 1.5 μm or 1,500 nm long and 10 to 15 nm wide) is composed of about 300 individual myosin molecules, each molecule being very large and ending in a myosin head that is bilobed (Plate 3). Half of these heads are orientated toward one end of the sarcomere and half to the other, leaving a bare area in the middle of the thick filament. The bilobed head of each myosin molecule is connected to the thick filament by an elongated base or neck, which merges into the remaining body of the molecule, consisting of two helical bodies twisting around each other. These are perma-nently built into the thick myosin filament by side-to-side aggregation with other helices. The pattern in which myosin heads emerge from the body of the thick filaments is still controversial, but in a commonly accepted version, the heads appear in groups of three, each group located 14.3 nm from the next (Squire, 1981). This means that about 50 such sets occur on each half of a single thick filament (Plate 1). The heads come out in a spiral fashion, so that one myosin head will reappear in the same line as another every 43 nm. Myosin is composed of two types of chains with different molecular weights (Plate 3).

Myosin Heavy Chains. These consist of two long strands twisted together, the one end of each chain embedded in the myosin filament and the other ending in the head. The two strands each terminate in two heads that are closely linked and hence described as bilobed.

The myosin molecule is sometimes described as having two functional domains, the body or filament being the light meromyosin and the heavy meromyosin representing the crossbridge inducing the head. The latter in turn can be subdivided into the S1 subfragment that contains the myosin head, and the S2 subfragment that connects the head to the body or filament. Previously it was thought that the flexion and extension of the head at the S1–S2 junction accounted for the movements of the myosin head. The C-protein is a tethering structure that lies around the S2 subfragment. Its proposed function is to stabilize the S2 subfragment as the myosin head itself flexes and extends at the level of the light chains.

Myosin Heads.   A combination of current molecular techniques has been used to define the microanatomy of the *myosin head* (Table 8-2). Attachment of ATP to its pocket (*the ATP- or nucleotide-binding pocket*) can cause a series of configurational changes in the myosin head that initiate the crossbridge cycle (Plate 4). This ATP site is physically distinct from the actin site, also situated on the myosin head (Rayment et al., 1993). Extending from the base of the nucleotide pocket to the actin-binding face is a narrow *cleft* that splits the central 50-kDa segment of the myosin head. The proposal is that binding of either ATP or its breakdown products to the nucleotide pocket causes different changes in the physical properties of the cleft in the myosin head and hence in the physical configuration of the head (Fisher et al., 1995). ATP is split by the crucial *myosin ATPase activity*, located near the ATP binding site.

Each myosin head binds to one actin molecule with a secondary binding site on the neighboring actin molecule one turn-down on the actin helix (Plate 5). There are several strengths of interaction between actin and myosin, so that both the association and dissociation of crossbridges is a progressive molecular interaction rather than "on-off" in nature. With each successive step in the acto-

TABLE 8-2. *Microanatomy of myosin head*[a]

No. of heads per molecule	Two
Shape of head	Pear-shaped
Size of head	16.5 nm (with neck) by 6.5 nm (widest point)
Molecular weight of each head	
Heavy-chain components	95 kDa
Two light-chain components	35 kDa
Total	130 kDa
Binding sites on head	Actin
	ATP (nucleotide)
Light chains	
Regulatory	Applied to base of α-helix
Essential	Applied to helix close to the neck–head junction

[a]Rayment et al. *Science* 1993;261:50. For structure, see Fig. 8-5.

myosin interaction, the area of the binding site on actin available for myosin increases as does the binding constant.

Myosin Light Chains. Aligned to the elongated base or neck of each myosin head, there are two myosin light chains, each of a different type (MLC-1 and MLC-2), making four light chains per bilobed head. The *essential myosin light chain* (MLC-1) is an integral part of the structure of the myosin head, and it appears to interact with actin in such a way that the contractile process is inhibited (Morano, 1995). The other *regulatory myosin light chain* (MLC-2) helps to enhance the contractile response to β-adrenergic stimulation.

Titin. This molecule, the largest yet described, is extraordinarily long, about 1,000 nm, or half of the sarcomere length when the latter is stretched to 2 μm (Plate 2). Cardiac titin, flexible and slender, is composed of a folded elastic segment 200 nm in length and an inelastic anchoring segment, 800 nm long (Helmes et al., 1996). Titin acts as a third filament (the other two being actin and myosin) with a dual function. First, it tethers the myosin molecule to the Z line, thereby ensuring that myosin filaments do float around aimlessly in the sarcomere, because their central portions are physically stabilized by the centrally placed disk of the M-line proteins. Second, titin contributes to the mechanical properties of the heart. As the sarcomere stretches, the elastic segment of titin expands to help explain the pattern of the stress–strain relationship of cardiac muscle (Schmied et al., 1991). The tension thus generated largely explains the *restoring force* (Helmes et al., 1996). This force is recruited when the heart contracts and then in diastole allows the myocardium to regain its original shape, thereby aiding ventricular filling.

The Basic Crossbridge Cycle

The crossbridge cycle consists of the repetitive attachment and detachment of myosin heads to and from actin filaments. At the start of systole, muscle contraction is triggered by the arrival of calcium ions from the sarcoplasmic reticulum, in response to the process of calcium-induced calcium release (Plate 4). The end result of the arrival of calcium is that the interdigitating thin actin and thick myosin filaments slide past each other in such a way that the Z lines come closer together. Crucial to this interaction is the role of the crossbridges, which extend from the myosin filament toward the actin filament. Such crossbridges are none other than the myosin heads attached to a binding site on the actin molecule. Each crossbridge cycle produces a power stroke that drives the actin filament along the myosin. This interaction between the myosin heads and actin filaments is tightly controlled by the cytosolic calcium ion concentration and its crucial interaction with troponin-C. To understand the importance of troponin-C requires a brief recapitulation of how the internal calcium concentration changes during the contractile cycle.

The overall concept is that a single contraction of a heart cell involves a brief period (about 600 msec at an average heart rate in humans) during which the cytosolic calcium concentration increases to a peak (about 200 msec) and decreases (about 400 msec). When cytosolic calcium is high, calcium ions bind increasingly to troponin-C molecules, turning on more and more of each actin filament for interaction with any adjacent myosin heads (Plate 4). Repetitive crossbridge cycling occurs, and more and more crossbridges become activated as long as the calcium concentration increases (physiologic systole). Throughout systole, there are numerous cycles of crossbridge attachment and detachment. During the detachment phase of one cycle, tension is maintained by other crossbridges attached at that time. As soon as the calcium concentration begins to decrease, however, increasing numbers of actin filaments become unavailable to waiting myosin heads, and the number of crossbridges interacting per unit time diminishes until ultimately the beat is over when the possibility of interactions has declined to near zero (physiologic diastole).

Models of Contraction

Current concepts can be traced back to the earlier *four-step model*, still often taught. According to this model there are two major crossbridge states, the *actin-attached* and *actin-detached states*. Each exists in two stages, with the whole sequence explained as follows:

1. Myosin attaches to actin to form a state that is potentially force generating and ready to go.
2. The power stroke follows and the rigor state ensues, so that the myosin head stays attached to actin unless liberated by ATP.
3. When ATP binds to the myosin head, the rigor state is terminated, and the head detaches from actin.
4. ATP is hydrolyzed by the enzymatic activity of the myosin head, and the products of this hydrolysis energize the head, which then reattaches to another actin unit, thereby regaining the first stage.

The key events underlying the crossbridge cycle can be explained by changes in the molecular configuration of the myosin head, which alternates between two major molecular configurations (Plate 4). When ATP is bound to the head, there is a *weak binding conformation*, and when inorganic phosphate (a product of ATP hydrolysis) is released, there is a *strong binding conformation*, which explains why the power stroke is initiated. The overall concept of weak and strong binding states is now incorporated into other models and has a molecular basis (Rayment et al., 1993).

What determines the *crossbridge cycling rate*? Brenner (1988) provided the following useful concept. The cycling rate is dependent on two apparent rate constants: the f constant, which controls the rate at which crossbridges enter the attached state, and the g constant, which controls the rate of crossbridge detachment (Plate 5). Assuming that one molecule of ATP is split in each crossbridge cycle, the crossbridge cycling rate will correspond to the ATP splitting rate.

In technical terms, the ATP splitting rate corresponds to the molecular turnover number of the actin-activated myosin ATPase activity, which is proportional to fg/f + g (Brenner, 1988).

The Rayment Five-Step Model

This currently favored model provides the molecular basis for the other models (Rayment and Holden, 1994; Rayment et al., 1993). The five steps are shown in Plate 5. One of the salient features is that the molecular motor that powers the crossbridge cycle acts so that extension and flexion occur at the elongated base of the head (the neck) and not as previously thought at the S1–S2 junction. Starting with the rigor state at the end of the power stroke, this state is broken (Plate 5A) by the binding of ATP to the myosin head by a two-step procedure. First, there is binding to the pocket of most of the ATP molecule, including the terminal gamma phosphate, which opens the narrow nucleotide pocket. The resultant change in molecular configuration transforms the strong binding state into the weak binding state, and myosin detaches from actin (Plate 5B). Next, the ATP binding pocket closes around its base and there is a further molecular change in the myosin head, so that the base of the head (the flexible domain or neck) extends on the body and the myosin head comes to lie opposite a new actin unit (Plate 5C), to which it binds weakly.

Thereupon, ATP undergoes hydrolysis by the myosin ATPase activity that is located close to the nucleotide pocket. The result is that ADP is now bound to the site previously occupied by ATP and inorganic phosphate is extruded (Fig. 8-1D). The resultant molecular changes partially close the nucleotide pocket, and the strong binding state ensues. During the subsequent power stroke, the head straightens at the neck and flexes on the body so that the actin molecule is moved by 5 to 10 nm (Plate 5E). Thereafter, ADP is released (Plate 5A) to expose an empty nucleotide binding pocket where ATP can rebind, thus to terminate the rigor state (Plate 5A and B).

CONTROL OF CONTRACTILE CYCLE BY CALCIUM IONS

Although the effects of calcium on the crossbridge cycle are still not fully understood, the basic facts are as follows. Once calcium is bound to troponin-C, a molecular signal is generated within the thin filament that eventually leads to an increased rate of crossbridge attachment. How and where does calcium act?

Calcium occupancy of troponin-C strengthens the binding of troponin-C with troponin-I, thereby decreasing the negative interaction of troponin-I with actin and causing a molecular change in tropomyosin, which becomes less inhibitory to the actin–myosin interaction (Ruegg, 1988). This interaction is explained as follows.

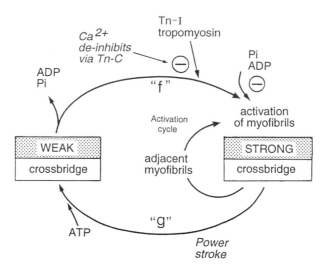

FIG. 8-1. Basic crossbridge cycle. During force generation, the molecular force generators (myosin crossbridges) cycle between weak and strong states with apparent rate constants f (forward) and g (reverse). Calcium, by activating troponin-C, increases the probability of forming strong, force-generating crossbridges. The responsiveness to calcium depends on the relative values of g and f, as well as on the calcium affinity for troponin-C. Modified from Ruegg (1990) with permission.

Troponin-C (Plate 3) has several receptor sites for calcium, of which only one is important in the case of cardiac troponin (Babu et al., 1987). When this site is occupied by calcium, it produces conformational changes in the distant regions of the troponin-C molecule.

The calcium regulatory system seems to be rather complex. When calcium levels are low, there is little interaction between troponin-I and troponin-C. The result is that troponin-I interacts with and inhibits actin. Also, when calcium is low, the tropomyosin molecule is twisted in such a way that the myosin heads cannot interact with actin. Then, when troponin-C interacts with calcium, its interaction with troponin-I is strengthened, whereas that between troponin-I and actin is lessened. As a result, the tropomyosin molecule moves to permit strong interaction between actin and myosin, allowing crossbridges to attach and to produce force. This effect is co-operative inasmuch as any attachment of crossbridges enhances the binding of calcium to troponin-C. Hence, the relationship between the free calcium concentration and force production is rather steep.

Binding Sites of Calcium on Troponin-C

Each molecule of cardiac troponin-C (TnC) has only one calcium-specific binding site. Thus, the amount of calcium-TnC formed depends on the calcium affinity and the calcium ion concentration, according to the law of mass action:

$$TnC.Ca \overset{k_{-1}}{\rightleftharpoons} TnC + Ca^{2+}$$

$$[TnC.Ca] = K[TnC][Ca^{2+}]$$

where K is the calcium affinity of troponin-C or simply the quotient of the on-rate k_{+1} and the off-rate k_{-1}. Its reciprocal value is the dissociation constant of the calcium–troponin complex (about 10^{-6} mol/L) and specifies the calcium ion concentration giving 50% calcium occupancy of troponin-C and hence half maximum activation of the contractile proteins. Interestingly, about 10^{-6} mol/L Ca^{2+} is also the calcium level reached normally during systole (see Fig. 6-2).

Mechanism of Control by Calcium. Do these effects of calcium ions control the apparent rate constants f and g for crossbridge attachment and detachment? According to Brenner (1988), it is predominantly the crossbridge attachment rate constant that is affected by calcium. Thus, any increase of the free calcium ion concentration in the myoplasm would enhance the calcium occupancy of troponin-C, which in turn would increase the probability of crossbridge attachment (Figure 8-1). The first effect of calcium ions would therefore be to increase steady-state force development. Additionally, indices of contractility, such as the rate of force increase or the rate of pressure change in the intact heart (dP/dt, where P = pressure and t = time) would also be altered by calcium acting in this manner (Ruegg, 1990).

In contrast, Hancock et al. (1993) proposed that calcium ions, interacting with troponin-C, increase the availability of the myosin binding sites on actin rather than altering the rates of transition between crossbridge states. Hancock stated that Brenner's proposals, based on data obtained from skeletal muscle fibers, may not apply to the heart.

In reality, these two apparently opposing views may not be so different, because calcium promotes binding of myosin to actin, an effect that will also change the molecular configuration of the myosin head and thereby the degree of interaction of myosin with actin. Nonetheless, Hancock does have a valid point in that models based primarily on skeletal muscle do not necessarily apply directly to the heart.

β-Adrenergic Effects and Calcium

Normally the calcium ion concentration in the cardiac cytosol during systole is such that the contractile sites are approximately half activated. Therefore, the heart has a considerable contractile reserve, which might be exploited by increasing the calcium occupancy of troponin-C. Force development would ultimately depend on the amount of calcium released from the sarcoplasmic reticulum and delivered to troponin-C, which would explain the increased force development during catecholamine stimulation (Fig. 8-2). β-adrenergic stimulation acts either indirectly through cyclic adenosine monophosphate (cAMP) or more directly to increase cytosolic calcium levels. An increased rate of crossbridge attachment increases the rate of rise of tension, dP/dt. This is the positive inotropic effect. The rate of relaxation (−dP/dt) will also be augmented. This lusitropic effect is explained by two factors. First, phosphorylation of phospholamban activates the calcium transport into the sarcoplasmic reticulum, so that the cytosolic free calcium will be lowered more rapidly in the presence of catecholamines (Katz, 1979). Second, the lowering of free calcium ion concentration causes the dissociation of the troponin-C calcium complex and hence the detachment of crossbridges and the decrease in force.

Troponin Phosphorylation

The rate constant of the dissociation of the troponin-C calcium complex is greatly enhanced when troponin-I is phosphorylated by cAMP-dependent protein kinase (Holroyde et al., 1980). The physiologic significance of this phosphorylation is likely to be that contraction can be switched off more rapidly when calcium decreases at the start of diastole, which helps contribute to an increased relaxation rate. The reduction in calcium affinity of troponin-C (Fig. 8-1) causes a rightward shift in the direction of a higher calcium ion concentration in the relationship between force and calcium ion concentration (Fig. 8-3). This negative

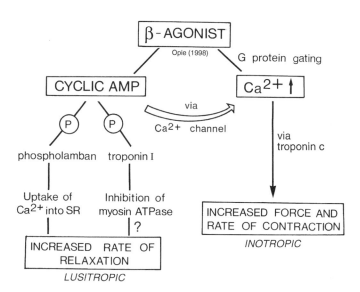

FIG. 8-2. Catecholamine regulation of contraction and relaxation. Proposed links between beta-adrenergic agonist stimulation by catecholamines and calcium-dependent changes in rates of contraction and relaxation of heart muscle. P, phosphorylation mediated by cAMP; SR, sarcoplasmic reticulum. For inotropic and lusitropic, see Fig. 7-16.

feedback may protect the heart from excessive catecholamine stimulation. Troponin-T also may undergo a similar phosphorylation in response to stimulation by protein kinase C, the latter being formed in the signaling system set in motion by α_1-adrenergic stimulation (see Fig. 7-14). Such phosphorylation of troponin-T gives inhibitory results similar to those obtained by phosphorylation of troponin-I.

Myosin Light-Chain Phosphorylation. Another factor that might also contribute to an altered calcium responsiveness during catecholamine stimulation is a change in the extent of myosin phosphorylation. Myosin is phosphorylated in the serine-13 residue of the regulatory light chains (MLC-2), which are loosely bound to the heavy myosin chains (Plate 3). This site is phosphorylated by the enzyme myosin light chain kinase, which is activated by calcium in conjunction with calmodulin, the ubiquitous calcium-binding protein (Naim and Perry, 1979). Myosin phosphorylation is increased by cAMP in response to β-adrener-

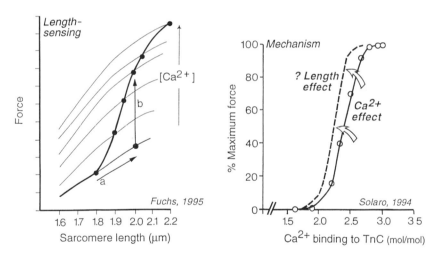

FIG. 8-3. The proposed cellular explanation for the Starling effect, whereby a greater end-diastolic fiber length develops a greater force. The left panel shows how the steep ascending limb of the cardiac force-length curve is explained by an interaction between sarcomere length and calcium ions. It is postulated that a change in end-diastolic fiber length (*left*) at any given free Ca^{2+} concentration would increase force by the Starling effect and would, in addition, cause cooperative interactions within the thin filament, the latter leading to a greater binding of Ca^{2+} to the thin filament. Hence there would be a greater force (*right*) than would be expected simply on the basis of the change in filament overlap (*left*). The right panel illustrates that the effects of Ca^{2+} and length can be explained by the properties of troponin C (TnC) and the binding of calcium to TnC. As more Ca^{2+} ions bind to troponin C in a skinned fiber preparation, more force is developed. There is a steep relationship, similar to that shown in the left panel. When the fiber is stretched and the sarcomere length increased, for any given number of Ca^{2+} ions binding to TnC, there is a greater force development, so that TnC has become sensitized to Ca^{2+}. Modified from Fuchs (1995) and Solaro et al. (1992), with permission.

gic stimulation. Such an increased phosphorylation may enhance the responsiveness of the cardiac contractile proteins to calcium (Morano et al., 1985; Resink and Gevers, 1981) or help to increase the affinity of myosin for actin (Solaro, 1992). This mechanism could explain why epinephrine increases the rate of crossbridge cycling independently of the degree of activation of the contractile proteins by calcium (Hoh et al., 1988; Saeki et al., 1990).

In vascular smooth muscle (Fig. 8-4), the regulation of contraction is again calcium dependent but by a different molecular mechanism. Calcium-calmodulin activates the myosin light chain kinase by phosphorylation of the myosin light chains. This process is essential for vascular contraction to take place.

REGULATION OF MYOSIN ATP_ASE

To recapitulate, the interaction of calcium ions with troponin-C initiates a cascade of alterations to the regulatory proteins of the thin filament (troponin-I and tropomyosin). The result is that myosin heads interact with binding sites on the actin filament in such a way that muscle shortening occurs. The greater the availability of calcium, the greater the force generated (within limits).

The multiple effects of calcium on the crossbridge cycle have already been emphasized. First, calcium initiates the contractile cycle by turning on troponin-C (Plate 4). The subsequent crossbridge attachment itself serves as a feedback mechanism to increase the calcium sensitivity of troponin-C (Fig. 8-1) (Hannon et al., 1992).

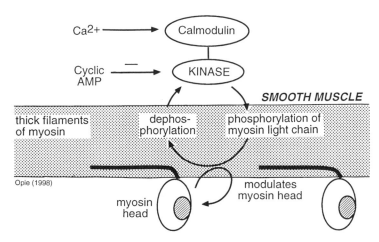

FIG. 8-4. Myosin light chain kinase plays an essential role in contraction of vascular smooth muscle. Although phosphorylation of myosin light chains also may occur in the heart, the kinase (myosin light chain kinase) is not inhibited by cAMP, an important difference from vascular smooth muscle.

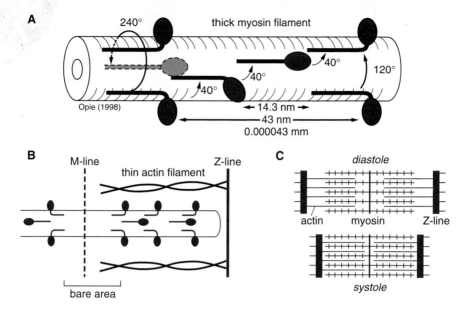

Plate 1. Sarcomere structure. (**A**) Relationship of thick myosin and thin actin filaments to sarcomere structure. The thickness of the thick filament is only relative because the length/width proportion is approximately 100:1. The heads emerge in groups of three and shift their positions by 40 degrees in succession. Thus, nine rows of about 16 heads each are placed in a line on the surface of each arm of the bipolar filament. (**B**) About 300 myosin heads come off at right angles to the body (150 heads to each side of the M line). (**C**) Compared with diastole, there is increased overlap of actin and myosin during systole, so that the Z lines move together during contraction.

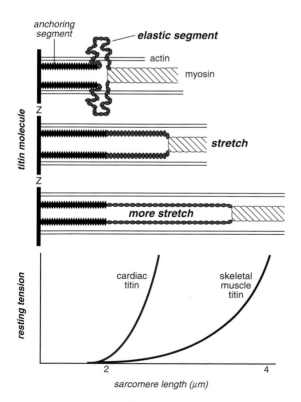

Plate 2. Titin, the elastic giant molecule. It provides structural support to actin and myosin by linking myosin to the Z line. It also has a small folded elastic segment that unfolds when stretched, which contributes to mechanical elastic properties of the sarcomere. When stretched titin relaxes, as in diastole, then restoring forces develop. Top panel modified from Helmes et al. (1996), and bottom panel, showing differences between cardiac and skeletal titin, from Trombitas et al. (1995).

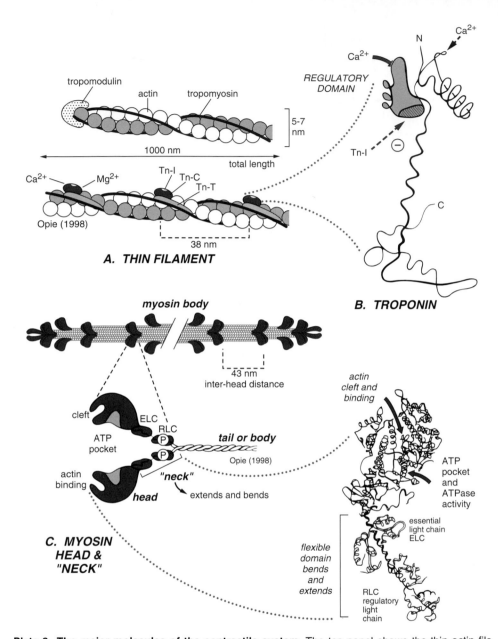

Plate 3. The major molecules of the contractile system. The top panel shows the thin actin filament, which contains troponin C (TnC). Note the Ca²⁺ binding sites in the regulatory domain of troponin-C, with another site for interaction with troponin I. When TnC is not activated by Ca²⁺, then troponin I (TnI) inhibits the actin–myosin interaction. The role of troponin T (TnT) is less well defined. The
bottom panel shows the whole myosin molecule and the myosin head. Each myosin molecule is composed of two intertwining heavy chains and four associated light chains. The myosin heads are
attached by a flexible neck to the myosin tails, also called bodies. Myosin light chains lie in apposition
to the neck of the myosin heads. The essential light chain (ELC) is part of the structure. The other regulatory light chain (RLC) influences the extent of the actin–myosin interaction. The bottom right panel
shows the myosin head molecular structure (based on Rayment et al. [1993]). The head is composed
of heavy and light chains. The heavy head chain in turn has two major domains. One interacts with
actin at the actin cleft and has an ATP-binding pocket, with a molecular weight of 70 kDa. The other
domain of 20 kDa is elongated, extends and bends, and has the two light chains attached to it.

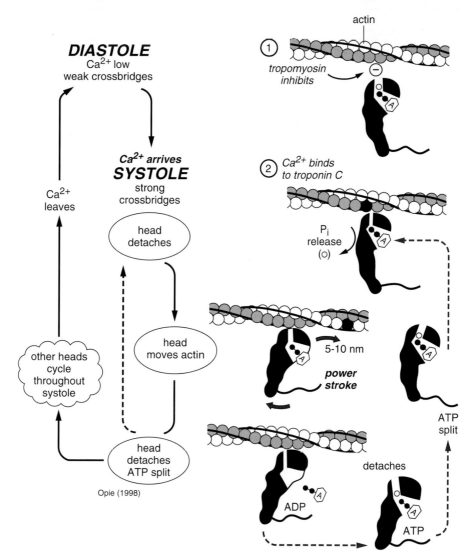

Plate 4. A simplified calcium-activated contractile cycle. The contraction phase of the cycle is initiated when the cytosolic calcium increases as calcium is released from the sarcoplasmic reticulum. The calcium interacts with a specialized component of the thin actin filament in such a way that the myosin heads are now able to interact with actin. The result is a power stroke that moves the thin actin filament 10 nm. As energy in the form of ATP reaches the myosin head, it extends again. In the meantime, the whole cycle is being repeated at other sites so that there are repetitive microcycles with flexion and extension of the myosin heads. When calcium leaves the cytosol to be sucked back into the sarcoplasmic reticulum, diastole starts.

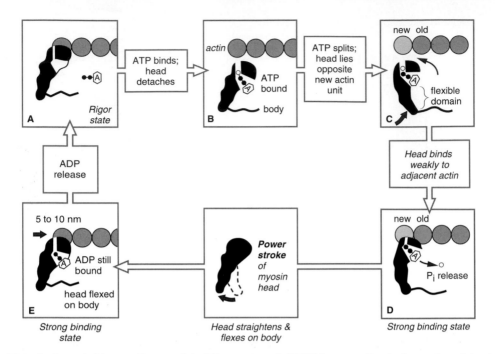

Plate 5. Crossbridge cycling model of Rayment et al. (1993) incorporating features of models of Eisenberg and Hill (*Science* 1985;227:293–309) and Lymn and Taylor (1971), with additional changes proposed by the present author. The Rayment model is based on electron density mapping of conformational changes in the myosin head. On the myosin head there is an ATP (nucleotide) binding pocket. Starting with the rigor state, binding of ATP to the binding pocket opens the cleft, and the previously strong binding state becomes a weak binding state (B). The ATP is split by the myosin ATPase and the head changes configuration (C). Next, the binding pocket closes around its base to induce further conformational changes to occur which, in turn, further closes the cleft, so that there is strong binding of myosin to actin. The result is that the affinity of myosin for Pi decreases, so that Pi is extruded, which results in a further molecular change in the myosin head to initiate the power stroke. The myosin head flexes to assume the rigor state once again. In the process, ADP is released so that the binding pocket becomes vacant. The open binding pocket is now ready to receive ATP to reinitiate the crossbridge cycle. (The increasing spatial separation between actin and myosin as contraction occurs is not shown.)

In addition, increasing the calcium concentration can enhance the myosin ATPase activity (Kuhn et al., 1990). The mechanism of this effect is still speculative, although much can be explained by the interaction of calcium with troponin-C. The latter proposal is consonant with the work of Brenner (1988). He studied an isometric model in which the sarcomere length was carefully kept constant. The kinetics of the rate of force redevelopment after an isotonic period allowed the conclusion that even at a constant number of crossbridges participating in cycling, an increased calcium level could increase myosin ATPase activity and force. A further proposal still under evaluation is that calcium can indirectly promote myosin light-chain phosphorylation and thereby convert the weakly attached crossbridges into the strongly attached force-generating state.

Isoenzymes of Myosin ATPase

The ATPase activity of cardiac muscle can vary, as is shown by the effect of thyrotoxicosis in increasing both cardiac myosin ATPase activity and the velocity of contraction. This change is caused by the re-emergence of an embryonic form of myosin (the so-called V_1 isoprotein coded by a different gene), which increases in relation to the V_3 isoprotein (Samuel et al., 1983). V_1 has an appreciably greater catalytic activity in hydrolyzing ATP than V_3, with an intermediate hybrid form, V_2 occupying an intermediate position (see Fig. 13-10). Such enzymes with similar function (breaking down ATP, myosin ATPase) but with alterations in their molecular structure are called myosin isoenzymes or myosin isoforms (Table 8-3). There are two types of molecular myosin heavy chains, the α and β. These can give rise to three types of combinations, α-α and β-β (homodimers) and α-β (heterodimer), and these correspond to V_1 (α-α), V_2 (α-β), and V_3 (β-β) isomyosins. Increased loading of the ventricles of small animals leads to a transition from dominant α to dominant β myosin heavy chains (V_1 to V_3 transition) so that contraction is slower, which is also energetically more efficient. Thus, the rat heart can change gear when loaded (Fig. 8-5). In humans, the normal isomyosin is the β type, so that the heart is already in low gear and there is little potential for gear change. An exception lies in the atria, where the myosin normally is in the α-α form even in humans, and there is a change to the β-β form (V_3 isoform) during mechanical overloading (Callens-El Amrani et al., 1989).

Myosin ATPase and Velocity of Contraction

Because the crossbridge cycling rate corresponds to the rate of splitting of ATP (Fig. 8-5), it is not surprising that the activity of myosin ATPase is often linked to the velocity (or rate) of muscle contraction. Such a link would explain the effects of changes in myosin isoenzymes in experimental models with mechanical overload. In diseased human hearts, however, the rate of contraction

TABLE 8-3. *Contractile protein isoforms with effects of mechanical overload*

	Fetus and neonate	Normal adult	Mechanical overload, heart failure
Myosin			
Ventricular heavy chain[a]	$\beta = \alpha$ ($\beta = V_3$, $\alpha = V_1$)	$\alpha > \beta$ (rat)	$\beta = \alpha$ (rat)
		$\beta > \alpha$ (humans)	Unchanged (humans)
Atrial heavy chain[b]	α	α (humans)	β (humans)
Light chain-1 in ventricles[c]	A and V forms	V form	A and V forms
Light chain-2 in ventricles[d]	No data	LC2/LC1, ratio 1:1	Ratio reduced
Troponin-I in ventricles[e]	TnIc	TnIc	TnIc
	TnIs		
Troponin-T in ventricles[f]	TnT_1	TnT_1	Increased
	TnT_{2-4}	TnT_2 (4%)	TnT_2 (12%)
Actin in ventricles[g]	Skeletal and smooth muscle α-actin	Decreased fetal form (rat)	Increased fetal form (rat)

A, atrial; V, ventricular; LC, light chain; c, cardiac; s, skeletal
[a] Mercadier et al. *Circ Res* 1983;53:52.
[b] Mercadier et al. *J Am Coll Cardiol* 1987;9:1024.
[c] Nakao et al. *Circulation* 1992;86:1727.
[d] Margossian et al. *Circulation* 1992;85:1720.
[e] Sasse et al. *Circ Res* 1993;72:932.
[f] Anderson et al. *Circ Res* 1991;69:1226.
[g] Schwartz et al. *Circ Res* 1986;59:551.

decreases but there is no change in myosin ATPase. Even artificially enhancing myosin ATPase activity by 1,000 times does not bring out any defect in the ATPase activity (Lauer et al., 1989). Hence, factors other than the myosin ATPase activity must account for the poor contractility of these human hearts.

SARCOMERE LENGTH AND CONTRACTILE ACTIVITY

Many attempts have been made to explain the pattern of the length–tension relationship of papillary muscle by changes in the sarcomere length. As the length of the latter increases, so does the tension to a certain maximum, and this pattern roughly resembles the increased performance of the whole heart as the venous return increases (Starling's law). In both cases, the contractile performance is length dependent. Thus, it may be expected that different degrees of sarcomere stretch and different extents of overlap of actin and myosin could explain both the ascending and descending limbs of the Starling curve (see Fig. 12-5). Yet neither limb can easily be explained by such factors.

Ascending Limb of the Starling Curve. The steeply ascending tension–length relationship of the myocardium cannot readily be explained by changes in the extent of actin–myosin overlap. In contrast, in skeletal muscle, pure geometric factors such as the degree of actin–myosin overlap can explain the slowly ascending limb of the force–tension line. To explain the pattern in the heart, the

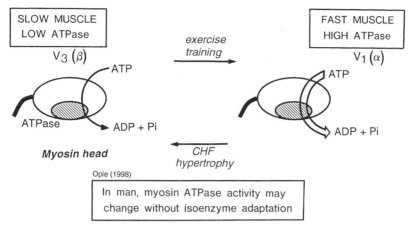

FIG. 8-5. Myosin isoenzyme hypothesis. When myosin ATPase activity is high (V1 form), there is a more rapid rate of breakdown of ATP to ADP and Pi, and cross-cycle bridging is enhanced. In rats, the transition from slow V3 to faster V1 can be achieved by vigorous exercise. Conversely, experimental congestive heart failure (CHF) or myocardial hypertrophy decreases the percentage of V1 and increases that of V3. In humans, there is no evidence for myosin isoenzyme changes in heart failure from the fast to slow form because the dominant physiologic form is already beta or V3 (slow). For further details, see Table 8-3.

currently proposed mechanism is *length-dependent activation* whereby the myofilaments become more sensitive to calcium as sarcomere length increases up to a maximum value (Fig. 8-3). In intact papillary muscles, stretching causes a large increase in force, whereas the amplitude of the intracellular free calcium transient does not increase (Fig. 8-6). Although the mechanism for this increase in calcium sensitivity in response to stretching is probably multifactorial, two favored proposals are that (1) stretch increases the calcium affinity of troponin-C by an as yet unknown mechanism (Allen and Kentish, 1988) and (2) stretch thins the sarcomere (see Fig. 12-8) to facilitate the number of interactions between actin and myosin (Hancock et al., 1993; McDonald and Moss, 1995). Technically, this hypothesis states that decreasing the lateral distance between actin and myosin lessens the interfilament lattice spacing and thereby increases the likelihood of actin–myosin interaction (McDonald and Moss, 1995). Then, it is proposed, even more crossbridges could be recruited into action by activation of near-neighbor crossbridges (Fig. 8-1). Not only do more crossbridges interact in relation to stretch, but the myosin ATPase activity also increases (Kuhn et al., 1990). Therefore, according to current concepts, length-dependent force changes and inotropic alterations of contractile activity may have ultimate similarities in the changes that they induce (Fig. 8-7).

Descending Limb of Starling Curve.   In the case of skeletal muscle, the relationship between sarcomere length and force development is more or less bell

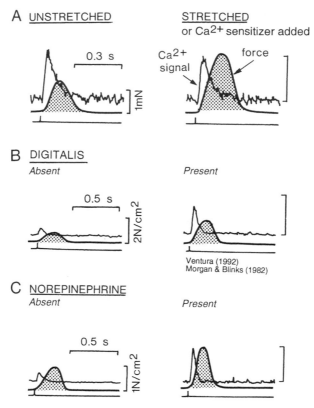

FIG. 8-6. Intracellular calcium and contraction. Contrasts between the stretch effect (**A**) and two positive inotropic interventions (**B** and **C**). Increase in force by stretching is not associated with any increase in free calcium, so that stretch is a calcium-sensitizing procedure. In (**B**) the increase in force obtained by digitalis or norepinephrine (**C**) is due to an increase in the intracellular free calcium, so that inotropic interventions increase calcium transients. A calcium sensitizing drug, like stretch, permits a greater force of contraction in the absence of any change in cytosolic calcium. Data from Ventura et al. *Circ Res* 1992;70:1081; and Morgan and Blinks. *Can J Physiol Pharmacol* 1982;60:520–528). Continuous lines, force; noisy tracings, aequorin luminescence of electrically stimulated cat papillary muscle; calibration bars, force (N) or tension (N/cm^2); Lmax, maximal luminescence signal.

shaped (Gordon et al., 1966), the optimal force being developed at a sarcomere length of about 2.2 µm (see Fig. 12-6). At greater sarcomere lengths, force declines because of the decreased overlap of actin and myosin. However, this pattern cannot explain the descending limb of the Starling curve in the failing whole heart for the following reasons. First, in the heart, the sarcomere length rarely exceeds 2.2 to 2.4 µm, even in the dilated state (Ross et al., 1971). The pericellular collagen and connecting filaments such as titin give heart muscle a high degree of resting stiffness that opposes myofibril stretching. In apparently overstretched zones, it is likely that entire fibers or myofibrils have slipped relative to each other. Rather, the explanation of the descending limb of the failing heart lies in abnormalities of the left ventricular chamber size, caused, for example, by mitral regurgitation.

CONGESTIVE HEART FAILURE AND CARDIOMYOPATHY

Isoform Changes. In general, with mechanical overload of the myocardium, a variety of isoforms of the contractile proteins revert to a more fetal type (Table 8-3). Although these changes are of great theoretical interest, at present it seems doubtful that any of them play an important role in the diminished contractile activity of the failing human heart. Rather, there appear to be a series of changes in the calcium-regulating organelles, including the sarcoplasmic reticulum (see Chapter 16).

Positive Inotropes. Agents that specifically increase the force of contraction of the heart are called positive inotropic drugs (Greek *inos,* fiber; *tropo,* active) or inotropes (Table 8-4). The oldest known inotrope is digitalis. Previously extracted from the leaf of a plant, and now synthesized in the form of digoxin,

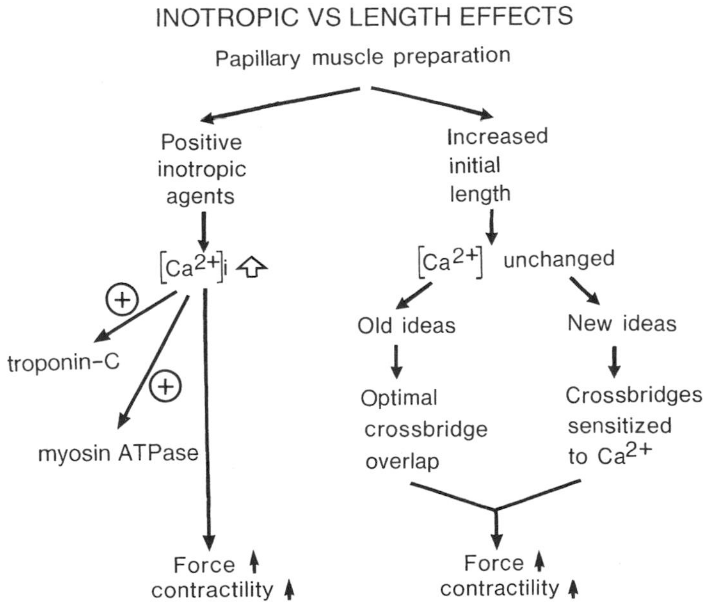

FIG. 8-7. **Length sensitivity of contractile apparatus.** This proposal means that the old ideas of "optimal" crossbridge overlap are now set aside, and it becomes clear that the crossbridge length helps to sensitize the myocardium to calcium, thus explaining the increased force and contractility in response to fiber stretching.

it is often used in the treatment of severe heart failure. It inhibits the sodium pump (see Fig. 4-27) to increase internal sodium, which promotes sodium–calcium exchange and increases internal calcium. The natural catecholamines norepinephrine and epinephrine increase contractility by increasing the formation of cAMP (see Fig. 7-16). A similar effect is found when the breakdown of cAMP is inhibited by specific drugs called the phosphodiesterase inhibitors. Such agents increasing cardiac cAMP levels may precipitate arrhythmias and increase the heart rate in patients, so these agents are being used less and less (see Fig. 20-11).

Calcium Sensitizing Drugs. Newly designed but not yet available for clinical use, these positively inotropic drugs can increase force development by increasing calcium responsiveness of the contractile proteins (Table 8-5). One such drug, levosimendan, docks to troponin-C near to its regulatory domain and may act by stabilizing troponin-C in its calcium-bound configuration (Edes et al., 1995). At high doses, such drugs may have several other effects such as increased activity of cAMP by inhibition of phosphodiesterase (Edes et al., 1995; Schmied et al., 1991). Thus, the contractile force of the heart can be regulated not only by changes in the free calcium concentration in the myoplasm, as achieved by conventional inotropic agents, but also by altering the calcium sensitivity of the myofilaments in response either to stretch or to the calcium-sensitizing drugs (Table 8-5).

Hypertrophic Cardiomyopathy. In this genetic condition, there is a single amino acid gene mutation (missense) for β-myosin heavy chains (Cuda et al., 1993). The head and head/neck areas are affected. Hypothetically, decreased myosin function of some fibers would result in hypertrophy of others, although it is at present not easy to see how these molecular changes can explain the overall hypercontractile state of the heart in this condition.

TABLE 8-4. *Agents increasing cardiac contractility (positive inotropes)*

Agent	Receptor	Effect
Digitalis (digoxin)	Na$^+$/K$^+$ ATPase (sodium pump)	Increased cytosolic Na$^+$ and hence Ca^{2+} (via Na/Ca exchange)
Catecholamines (NE + E; iso)[a]	β-adrenergic, linked to adenylate cyclase via G$_s$	Increased cyclic AMP; positive inotropic; lusitropic[b]; tachycardia; vasodilation
PDE inhibitors (milrinone, others)	None	Inhibition of breakdown of cAMP
Calcium sensitizers	None	Increased sensitivity of crossbridges to calcium

PDE, phosphodiesterase; NE, norepinephrine; E, epinephrine; iso, isoproterenol
[a]See Fig. 7-2.
[b]See Fig. 7-17.

TABLE 8-5. *Modulation of calcium sensitivity in cardiac muscle*[a]

Modulator[b]	Effect[b]
Increase in sarcomere length	+
Phosphorylation of regulatory myosin light chain	+
Phosphorylation of troponin-I or troponin-T	−
Ischemia	
Acidosis	−
Inorganic phosphate	−
New cardiotonic drugs (calcium sensitizers)	
Pimobendan and others	+

[a]See Ruegg (1992); Table 7-2.
[b]Increase (+) or decrease (−) in calcium sensitivity of cardiac myofilaments as determined in skinned cardiac muscle preparations or in vivo. Ca^{2+} sensitivity as used here is defined as the pCa (negative log of the Ca^{2+} concentration) inducing half-maximal activation of skinned fiber preparation.

ISCHEMIA AND MYOFILAMENTS

The myofilaments become desensitized to calcium when the coronary flow becomes too low, as in ischemia. There are several factors at work (see Table 17-1), yet two of the most important are the increased concentrations of hydrogen ions and inorganic phosphate (Allen and Orchard, 1987).

Rigor State and Ischemic Contracture. Hearts subjected to long periods of ischemia can become stiff and develop ischemic contracture. Under these conditions, the crossbridges are no longer inhibited at low levels of calcium, but the actomyosin ATPase activity and force-generation are potentiated (Winegrad, 1979). This change occurs because at the low ATP concentration and high cytosolic calcium levels characteristic of the ischemic state, the crossbridges are no longer occupied by ATP and become permanently attached, thereby forming so-called rigor bridges. In other words, the dominant form of the myosin head is in the strongly binding attached state, in flexion (Plate 5E). These bridges exert a cooperative effect on the thin filaments, increasing the calcium sensitivity (Guth and Potter, 1987). Thus, force development may go far beyond that caused by an increase in only the calcium ion concentration (Allen et al., 1984; Allshire et al., 1987). The high force development may then cause hypercontracture, which exerts excess tension on the sarcolemma to cause microlesions that leak so that extracellular calcium can invade the cell. However, internal calcium can increase during ischemia long before sarcolemmal rupture. For example, within minutes, lack of energy supplying the calcium uptake pump of the sarcoplasmic reticulum directly increases cytosolic calcium. The sodium–potassium pump, also energy-requiring, becomes inhibited somewhat later and causes the intracellular sodium levels to increase, after which sodium–calcium exchange brings in calcium. Also, under partially depolarized conditions, calcium channels may remain open. The term "stone heart" describes severe irreversible hypercontracture.

Creatine Kinase and Myosin ATPase.   The ATP made in the mitochondria is normally delivered to the myosin ATPase indirectly by a shuttle involving phosphocreatine (see Fig. 11-15). The enzyme creatine kinase (CK), which converts phosphocreatine back to ATP, is located in relation to the A band of the sarcomere, which contains myosin ATPase. Hence, the proposal is that this enzyme delivers ATP to the myosin ATPase. In ischemia, the CK isoenzyme concerned (A-band CK) diffuses from the A to the I band and then to outside the cell (Otsu et al., 1993), so that energy transfer within the cell is impaired. These events are associated with irreversible ischemic injury.

Release of Troponin in Myocardial Infarction.   This protein is released when the cell membranes are severely damaged, as in myocardial infarction (see Fig. 18-10). It increases rapidly in the blood and is specific for the myocardium.

SUMMARY

1. *The crossbridge cycle.* The energy that is needed to sustain the contractile activity of the heart comes from the hydrolysis of ATP by an ATPase located in the myosin head. In diastole, the force-generating interaction between actin and myosin is suppressed because of an inhibitory effect exerted by troponin-I, which forms part of the troponin complex. When calcium is supplied to troponin-C during systole, the inhibitory effect of troponin-I is overcome, and actin and myosin can then associate. The physical nature of the actin–myosin interaction involves steps in which the attached myosin heads pull the thin filaments a very small distance during the power stroke toward the center of the sarcomeres in which they are located, before detaching and reattaching further along the thin filament to repeat the crossbridge cycle. Detachment of the myosin head from the actin filament is achieved when ATP binds to a special pocket on the head. Thereafter, ATP is hydrolyzed to ADP and Pi, and the shape of this pocket changes. When Pi comes off the head, there is a further change in the molecular configuration of the myosin head, and the power stroke is initiated. During a single heart beat, tension develops by recruitment of more and more crossbridge cycles as the cytosolic calcium concentration increases to a peak, to be followed by relaxation as the crossbridge cycling activity diminishes in response to a decreasing calcium concentration. During the detachment stage of an individual crossbridge cycle, tension is maintained by other crossbridges that are attached during that time.

2. *Crossbridge interaction is enhanced by β-adrenergic receptor stimulation.* First, there is more calcium ion entry by the L channels with increased

release of more calcium from the sarcoplasmic reticulum to interact with more troponin C. In addition, the crossbridges react at a faster rate, partially the result of a direct effect of the increased quantity and rate of increase of cytosolic calcium on crossbridge kinetics, and partially an indirect effect of the associated increase of cAMP on the light chains that help to regulate myosin ATPase activity.

3. *Sarcomere length and force generation.* In the myocardium, there is no simple relationship between these factors. The previous concept of optimal or inadequate overlap of actin and myosin filaments was incorrectly based on skeletal muscle models and has now been replaced by the concept of stretch activation. It is proposed that stretch sensitizes the myofibrils to the prevailing calcium ion concentration, acting through changes in the lateral distance between actin and myosin. New positively inotropic drugs, the calcium sensitizers, also act independently of any change in the cytosolic calcium level but probably have a different molecular mode of action such as stabilizing the molecular configuration of troponin-C.

4. *Permanent rigor bonds.* During severe and prolonged ischemia, the total ATP level decreases. There is insufficient ATP to break the rigor bonds between the myosin heads and actin, with the development of the stone heart.

ACKNOWLEDGMENT

Professor J. Caspar Rüegg, Heidelberg, Germany, provided considerable advice.

STUDENT QUESTIONS

1. Describe the basic crossbridge cycle.
2. Give an outline of the properties of the major cardiac contractile proteins.
3. Why is ATP important for cardiac contraction if the power stroke can occur without any utilization of ATP?
4. Describe various mechanisms whereby calcium can increase the force of cardiac contraction.
5. What is myosin ATPase? What are its isoenzymes? What is their proposed importance?

CARDIOLOGIST-IN-TRAINING QUESTIONS

1. How does a rise of cytosolic calcium ion concentration trigger the contractile cycle? Which contractile protein is involved?
2. How is ATP split during the contractile cycle? How does the binding of ATP to the myosin head influence the molecular shape of myosin? What are the consequences for myocardial contraction and relaxation?

3. Myosin light chain phosphorylation is of crucial importance in the regulation of one type of muscle. Which and why?

4. Explain the ascending limb of the Starling curve in terms of myocardial contractile proteins.

5. How do calcium sensitizing drugs work? How could they theoretically avoid some of the adverse effects of cytosolic calcium overhead?

6. What is ischemic contracture?

REFERENCES

1. Allen DG, Eisner DA, Orchard CH. Factors influencing free intracellular calcium concentration in quiescent ferret ventricular muscle. *J Physiol (Lond)* 1984;350:615–630.

2. Allen DG, Kentish JC. Calcium concentration in the myoplasm of skinned ferret ventricular muscle following changes in muscle length. *J Physiol* 1988;407:489–503.

3. Allen DG, Orchard CH. Myocardial contractile function during ischemia and hypoxia. *Circ Res* 1987;60:153–168.

4. Allshire A, Piper M, Cuthbertson KSR, Cobbold PH. Cytosolic free Ca^{2+} in single rat heart cells during anoxia and reoxygenation. *Biochem J* 1987;244:381–385.

5. Babu A, Scordilis SP, Sonnenblick EH, Gulati J. The control of myocardial contraction with skeletal fast muscle troponin-C. *J Biol Chem* 1987;262:5815–5822.

6. Brenner B. Effect of Ca^{2+} cross-bridge turnover kinetics in skinned single rabbit psoas fibers. *Proc Natl Acad Sci USA* 1988;85:3265–3269.

7. Callens-EI Amrani F, Swynghedauw B. Transitory and permanent changes in gene expression in response to cardiac overload. Physiological and pharmacological relationships. A review. *Cardiovasc Drug Ther* 1989;3:947–958.

8. Cuda G, Fananapazir L, Zhu W-S, Epstein ND. Skeletal muscle expression and abnormal function of β-myosin in hypertrophic cardiomyopathy. *J Clin Invest* 1993;91:2861–2865.

9. Edes I, Kiss E, Kitada Y et al. Effects of levosimendan, a cardiotonic agent targeted to troponin-C, on cardiac function and on phosphorylation and Ca^{2+} sensitivity of cardiac myofibrils and sarcoplasmic reticulum in guinea pig heart. *Circ Res* 1995;77:107–113.

10. Fisher AJ, Smith CA, Thoden J. Structural studies of myosin: Nucleotide complexes: a revised model for the molecular basis of muscle contraction. *Biophys J* 1995;68(suppl):19–28.

11. Fuchs F. Mechanical modulation of the Ca^{2+} regulatory protein complex in cardiac muscle. *NIPS* 1995;10:6–12.

12. Gordon AM, Huxley AF, Julian JF. The variation in isometric tension with sarcomere length in vertebrate muscle fibres. *J Physiol (Lond)* 1966;184:170–192.

13. Guth K, Potter JD. Effect of rigor and cycling cross-bridges on the structure of troponin C and on the Ca affinity of the Ca-specific regulatory sites in skinned rabbit psoas fibers. *J Biol Chem* 1987;262:13627–13635.

14. Hancock WO, Martyn DA, Huntsman LL. Ca^{2+} and segment length dependence of isometric force kinetics in intact ferret cardiac muscle. *Circ Res* 1993;73:603–611.

15. Hannon JD, Martyn DA, Gordon AM. Effects of cycling and rigor crossbridges on the conformation of cardiac troponin C. *Circ Res* 1992;71:984–991.

16. Helmes M, Trombitas K, Granzier H. Titin develops restoring force in rat cardiac myocytes. *Circ Res* 1996;79:619–626.

17. Hoh JFY, Rossmanith GH, Kwan LJ, Hamilton AM. Adrenaline increases the rate of cycling of cross-bridges in rat cardiac muscle as measured by pseudo-random binary noise-modulated perturbation analysis. *Circ Res* 1988;62:452–461.

18. Holroyde MJ, Robertson SP, Johnson JD, et al. The calcium and magnesium binding sites on cardiac troponin and their role in the regulation of myofibrillar adenosine triphosphatase. *J Biol Chem* 1980;255:11668–11693.

19. Huxley HE. Sliding filaments and molecular motile systems. *J Biol Chem* 1990;265:8347–8350.

20. Irving M, Lombardi V, Piazzesi G, Ferenczi MA. Myosin head movements are synchronous with the elementary force-generating process in muscle. *Nature* 1992;357:156–158.

21. Katz AM. Role of the contractile proteins and sarcoplasmic reticulum in the response of the heart to catecholamine: a historical review. *Adv Cyclic Nucl Res* 1979;11:303–343.
22. Kuhn HJ, Bletz C, Ruegg JC. Stretch-induced increase in the Ca^{2+} sensitivity of myofibrillar ATPase activity in skinned fibres from pig ventricles. *Pflugers Arch* 1990;415:741–746.
23. Lauer B, Van Thiem N, Swynghedauw B. ATPase activity of the cross-linked complex between cardiac myosin subfragment 1 and actin in several models of chronic overloading. *Circ Res* 1989;64:1106–1115.
24. Lymn RW, Taylor EW. Mechanism of adenosine triphosphate hydrolysis by actomyosin. *Biochemistry* 1971;10:4617–4624.
25. McDonald KS, Moss RL. Osmotic compression of single cardiac myocytes eliminates the reduction in Ca^{2+} sensitivity of tension at short sarcomere length. *Circ Res* 1995;77:199–205.
26. Morano I, Hofmann F, Zimmer M, Ruegg JC. The influence of P-light chain phosphorylation by myosin light chain kinase on the calcium sensitivity of chemically skinned heart fibers. *FEBS Lett* 1985;189:221–224.
27. Morano I, Ritter O, Bonz A. Myosin light chain-actin interaction regulates cardiac contractility. *Circ Res* 1995;76:720–725.
28. Nairn AC, Perry SV. Calmodulin and myosin light chain kinase of rabbit fast skeletal muscle. *J Biochem (Tokyo)* 1979;179:89–97.
29. Otsu N, Yamaguchi I, Komatsu E, Miyazawa K. Changes in creatine kinase M localization in acute ischemic myocardial cells. *Circ Res* 1993;73:935–942.
30. Rayment I, Holden HM. The three-dimensional structure of a molecular motor. *TIBS* 1994;19:129–134.
31. Rayment I, Holden HM, Whittaker M. Structure of the actin-myosin complex and its implications for muscle contraction. *Science* 1993;261:58–65.
32. Resink TJ, Gevers W. Altered adenosine triphosphatase activities of natural actomyosin from rat hearts perfused with isoprenaline and ouabain. *Cell Calcium* 1981;2:105–123.
33. Ross J, Sonnenblick EH, Taylor RR, et al. Diastolic geometry and sarcomere length in the chronically dilated canine left ventricle. *Circ Res* 1971;28:49–61.
34. Ruegg JC. Towards a molecular understanding of contractility. *Cardioscience* 1990;1:163–167.
35. Ruegg JC. *Calcium in Muscle Activation. A Comparative Approach.* 2nd ed. Berlin: Springer-Verlag, 1988.
36. Saeki Y, Shiozawa K, Yanagisawa K, Shibata T. Adrenaline increases the rate of cross-bridge cycling in rat cardiac muscle. *J Mol Cell Cardiol* 1990;22:453–460.
37. Samuel J-L, Rappaport L, Mercadier J-J, et al. Distribution of myosin isoenzymes within single cardiac cells. An immunohistochemical study. *Circ Res* 1983;52:200–209.
38. Schmied R, Wang G-X, Korth M. Intracellular Na^+ activity and positive inotropic effect of sulmazole in guinea pig ventricular myocardium. Comparison with a cardioactive steroid. *Circ Res* 1991;68: 597–604.
39. Solaro RJ. Myosin and why hearts fail. *Circulation* 1992;85:1945–1947.
40. Squire JM. In: The Structural Basis of Muscular Contraction. New York: Plenum, 1981;471–521.
41. Trombitas K, Jian-Ping J, Granzier H. The mechanically active domain of titin in cardiac muscle. *Circ Res* 1995;77:856–861.
42. Winegrad S. Electromechanical coupling in heart muscle. In: Berne RM, Sperelakis N, Geiger SR (eds). *The Cardiovascular System.* Bethesda: American Physiological Society, 1979;393–428.

9

Vascular Smooth Muscle and Endothelium

*The vasculature is a complex organ capable of
sensing its environment, transducing signals to cells
within the vasculature or to the surrounding tissues,
and synthesizing local mediators that promote
functional or structural responses.*

Dzau et al., 1993

Whereas the heart is the ejecting organ, the vasculature is the receiving organ. The degree of its sustained contraction, or tone, regulates the peripheral vascular resistance and therefore is one of the main aspects of the load against which the heart must work (afterload). The interplay between the amount of blood ejected by the heart and the resistance to that ejection by the vasculature determines the blood pressure, a salient aspect of cardiovascular physiology and pathophysiology (see Fig. 2-14).

The degree of arterial tone also regulates the amount of blood reaching the tissues, and during exercise, for example, marked arterial vasodilation must occur to bring the needed oxygen and fuels to the exercising muscle. With these considerations in mind, it could be argued that the vasculature has adapted itself to its dual function by (1) devising a contractile mechanism that responds more slowly than that of the myocardium yet allows major changes in the sustained tone, and (2) responding to the metabolic needs of the tissue by reacting to metabolites formed or released during exercise. It is also clear that blood vessels should be able to close up in response to severe physical injury to avoid excess blood loss, and that this protective function should be achieved with as little risk as possible of the vessel being blocked during its normal physiologic functions (Table 9-1).

TABLE 9-1. *Functions of the peripheral vasculature*

1. Conduit function: conveys blood from the heart to the capillaries and thence back to the heart
2. Regulation of arterial tone and of peripheral vascular resistance
3. Regulation of blood flow to muscle and other tissues
4. Response to traumatic injury with vasoconstriction and hemostasis
5. Response to sustained increase in intraluminal pressure: growth and hypertrophy

To achieve these aims is an ambitious undertaking that the vasculature has apparently solved in complex ways and which we will now analyze.

VASCULAR STRUCTURE

Endothelium. Arteries consist of three basic layers: the intima, the media, and the adventitia (Fig. 9-1). The endothelium is the crucial structure in the intimal layer; it consists of a monolayer of thin cells, highly active in the control of the circulation (Fig. 9-2). It produces numerous vasoactive compounds, including (1) endothelium-derived relaxation factor (EDRF), very likely to be identical with nitric oxide; (2) endothelin, a powerful vasoconstrictor; (3) angiotensin I and possibly angiotensin II (Veltmar et al., 1991); and (4) complex cyclic compounds, the prostaglandins, such as the vasodilator prostacyclin (PGl_2) and the vasoconstrictor thromboxane A2. These and other important functions are listed

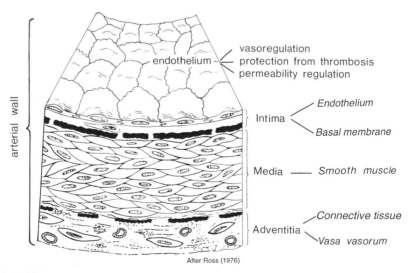

After Ross (1976)

FIG 9-1. Histologic structure of normal muscular artery, emphasizing different roles of endothelium, smooth muscle cells and fibrous tissue. Modified with permission from Ross and Glomset (1976).

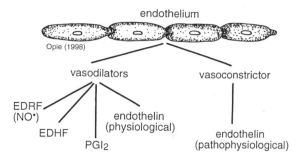

FIG. 9-2. Role of endothelium in vascular regulation. Physiologically, it produces vasorelaxing agents such as EDRF, now thought to be nitric oxide. In the presence of vascular damage, endothelin produces vasoconstriction rather than physiologic vasodilation.

in Table 9-2. The continuous secretion of nitric oxide, by a powerful antiplatelet effect, can help prevent the deposition of platelets on the intima, an event thought to occur early in the development of various types of arterial disease (see later in this chapter).

The concept is that the endothelium is a very active organ, covering an immense surface area of over 1,000 m² (Zilla et al., 1993), constantly synthesizing and releasing a variety of molecules that can all contribute to the regulation of arterial tone. "The endothelium appears to serve as a mechanoreceptor within the vasculature that senses flow or pressure and modulates vascular tone accordingly" (Gibbons and Dzau, 1990).

TABLE 9-2. *Proposed functions of vascular endothelium*

Release of vasodilatory agents
 EDRF (endothelium-derived relaxation factor) nitric oxide
 Prostacyclin
 Bradykinin
Release of vasoconstrictor agents
 Endothelin
 Angiotensin I (and possibly angiotensin II)
 Prostacyclin and thromboxane
Antiaggregatory effect
 Acts via nitric oxide and prostacyclin
Prevention of coagulation
 Thromboresistant surface
Immune function
 Supply of antigens to immunocompetent cells
 Secretion of interleukin I (a T-cell inducer)
Enzymatic activity
 Angiotensin-converting enzyme (conversion of angiotensin I to angiotension II)
Growth signal to vascular smooth muscle
 EDGF secretion (endothelium-derived growth factor)
 Heparin-like inhibitors of growth
Protection of vascular smooth muscle
 Endothelial integrity required to convert vasoconstrictory to vasodilator stimuli

Endothelial cells rest on a basement membrane, separated from smooth muscle cells by the *internal elastic lamina*, which consists of sheets of elastic fibers with openings large enough to allow the permeation of metabolites, growth factors, and mobile cells in either direction.

Tunica Media and Vascular Smooth Muscle Cells. This is the middle layer of the arterial wall (Fig. 9-1). Its two major components are (1) the smooth muscle cell that upon appropriate stimulation contracts to narrow the diameter of the arterial wall and (2) the supporting matrix that binds the muscle cells into bundles and keeps them in the correct orientation in the arterial wall. In the *small muscular arterioles* (small-bore arteries, diameter less than 1 mm), these smooth muscle cells respond to an increase of cytosolic calcium concentration by contracting and thereby decreasing the diameter of the arteriolar lumen, which increases the peripheral vascular resistance and causes the blood pressure to increase.

The *matrix* of the medial layer is that component which determines to a major extent, together with the adventitia, the mechanical properties of the artery. First, the ratio of matrix to muscle cells varies. In the large conduit arteries, like the aorta and its major branches, *elastin* is the most important component of the matrix; in the largest vessels, such as the aorta, it is the major component of the arterial wall. The elastin in the aortic wall allows the aorta to expand in systole as blood is rapidly ejected from the left ventricle, then in diastole the elastic recoil helps to propel the blood flow onward and hence to maintain the diastolic blood pressure. This is the pressure-equalizing function of the elastic layer of the aorta (see Fig. 1-8).

The *elasticity of elastin* is explained by its hydrophobic properties. When relaxed, crucial hydrophobic regions have minimal contact with the surrounding water of the extracellular space. When stretched, contact with water increases, and the hydrophobic area reacts in such a way that the fibers return to their original length. The synthesis of elastin from proelastin is triggered mechanically, whereas its breakdown by elastase is accelerated in old age.

Collagen is the other major connective tissue protein of the matrix and is closely related in structure to the collagen found in the myocardium. Collagen is an important component of the medial wall, helping it to keep its shape despite the high intraluminal pressure exerted by the blood. Hence, collagen has extremely high tensile properties, and is distributed in such a way in the medial layer that the arteries are highly resistant to the intraluminal pressure. Different types of collagen have different responses to mechanical stress. Types I and II collagen, the most common in the media, consist of fibrils about 20 to 90 nm in diameter. Type III collagen is more elastic, whereas type IV collagen is found chiefly in the intima, and type V occurs in the basement membrane of the arterial wall.

Other matrix proteins are the *glycoproteins*, including fibronectin, a biological "glue," and glycosaminoglycans (GAG), which are hydrophilic, forming aggregates that make up a gel containing both electrolytes and small molecules in passage from blood through the vessel wall to the various tissues.

Adventitia.   The adventitia, the external covering layer, is separated from the media by the external elastic lamina. The blood vessels running to the arterial wall are found here (vasa vasorum), as are lymphatics and the autonomic nerves that control arteriolar tone. Histologically, this layer contains collagen, fibroblasts, and a few muscle cells besides the blood vessels. In the large conducting arteries, the adventitia is thin and the elastic layer of the media is dominant. In the small muscular arteries, the site of the peripheral vascular resistance, the adventitia is thicker, especially its inner layer.

CONTRACTILE MECHANISMS IN VASCULAR SMOOTH MUSCLE

Many of the cellular events are similar to those already described in the cardiac contraction cycle: the entry of calcium, the calcium-induced calcium release from the sarcoplasmic reticulum, the increase in cytosolic free calcium ion concentration, the interaction of calcium with the myosin adenosine triphosphate (ATP)ase, the subsequent uptake of calcium into the sarcoplasmic reticulum, and the discharge of excess calcium via calcium exit channels. However, there are many crucial differences.

Some of the major metabolic differences between vascular smooth muscle and the myocardium are listed as follows:

1. There must be a *major difference* between the effects of cyclic adenosine monophosphate (cAMP) in the contractile cycle in the heart and peripheral smooth muscle in response to the β-receptor stimulation that causes the myocardium to contract and the peripheral vessels to dilate (Fig. 9-3).
2. Depolarization is not essential for the initiation of the contractile cycle in vascular smooth muscle, because it can be set off by the increase of calcium released from the sarcoplasmic reticulum by inositol trisphosphate (Ins 1,4,5-P_3 or Ins P_3 or IP$_3$), the second messenger of several vasoconstrictory stimuli, such as α_1-adrenergic agonism and angiotensin II.
3. Peripheral arteriolar contraction is tonic (tone-maintaining), whereas cardiac contraction is short lived and generates considerable force, so that there may be different relationships between the level of cytosolic calcium and the force generated in the two types of muscle.
4. In peripheral vascular muscle, troponin-C is absent from the actin filaments, so that calcium ions must regulate the myosin–actin interaction by a different calcium receptor. Rather, calcium ions combine with calmodulin to form calcium-calmodulin, which promotes phosphorylation of the light chains of the myosin heads (Horowitz et al., 1996).

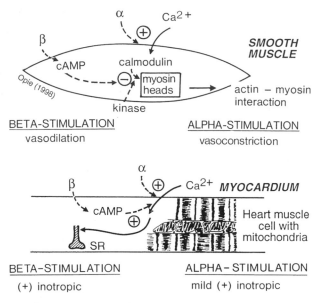

FIG. 9-3. Contrast between contractile mechanisms in vascular smooth muscle and heart. Note, in particular, that β-stimulation has a positive inotropic effect in the myocardium by an increase of cAMP, which promotes calcium ion entry and uptake into the sarcoplasmic reticulum. In contrast, β-stimulation causes vasodilation by inhibition of the myosin light chain kinase, which allows actin–myosin interaction. α-stimulation, by increasing calcium entry, activates calmodulin and actin–myosin interaction in vascular smooth muscle. A similar system responds to α-stimulation in the myocardium but is much weaker.

Calmodulin and Myosin Light-Chain Kinase

Calmodulin is a naturally occurring protein found in many cell types that binds up to four calcium ions with a high affinity and specificity. It therefore modulates the effects of calcium and plays a crucial role in the control of the tone of vascular smooth muscle (see Fig. 8-10). The binding of calcium causes conformational changes that confer biologic activity on the molecule and activate several enzymes, including that catalyzing the following reaction:

$$Ca^{2+} \cdot calmodulin + inactive \; enzyme \rightarrow Ca^{2+} \cdot calmodulin \cdot active \; enzyme.$$

The enzyme thus activated is *myosin light-chain kinase*, which exists as an inactive protein at low calcium concentrations. This kinase probably becomes active when the cytosolic calcium ion concentration increases at the start of contraction (Fig. 9-4), whereupon calcium-calmodulin forms. In this type of vascular contraction, there is a simple relationship between the cytosolic calcium concentration and force generation. For example, when a high external potassium is applied, the vascular cell depolarizes, and the voltage-dependent calcium channels open to increase the cytosolic calcium level, and both the calcium level and force generation are maintained to produce one type of tonic contraction. The

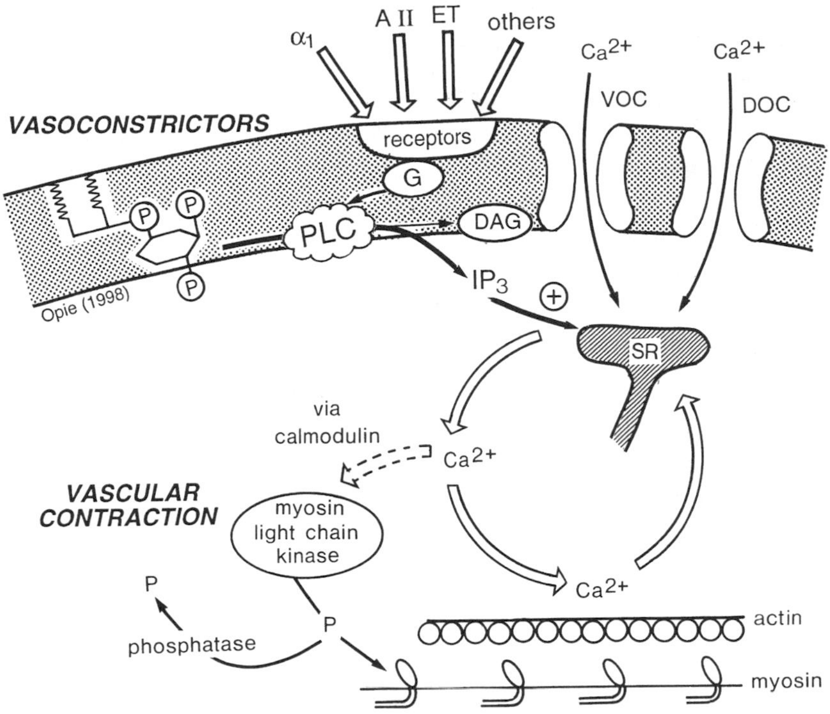

FIG. 9-4. Vasoconstrictory mechanisms. Several act by releasing calcium from the sarcoplasmic reticulum (SR). For example, stimulation of vascular receptors by endothelin (ET), angiotensin II (AII), or norepinephrine (NE) leads to increased activity of phospholipase C, which splits phosphatidyl inositol into two messengers: IP_3 (inositol trisphosphate) and 1,2-DG (1,2 diacylglycerol). IP_3 promotes the release of calcium from the SR. Membrane-bound DAG activates PKC. The latter may act by a breakdown product on the contractile apparatus to promote a sustained contractile response (Ohanian, 1993). Vasoconstriction also occurs in response to enhanced activity of the calcium channels which are either receptor-operated channels (ROC) or depolarization-operated channels (DOC).

activation of myosin light-chain kinase is reversed when the phosphate group is removed by another enzyme, *myosin light-chain phosphatase*, the control of which is not yet clarified. Because only one of the two types of light chains on myosin heads are phosphorylated, these are called the P or *regulatory light chains*, also known as the 20-kDa myosin light chains (see Fig. 8-2). In vascular smooth muscle, such phosphorylation is essential for contraction, whereas in the myocardium, the significance of the phosphorylation is still controversial.

Cyclic Nucleotides and Vascular Contraction

According to the yin–yang hypothesis, the two cyclic nucleotides, cAMP and cyclic guanosine monophosphate (cGMP), should in principle have opposing functions on any given system. That expectation is *not* met in vascular smooth muscle, where both nucleotides are vasodilators (Fig. 9-5). At least part of the mechanism for these vasodilatory effects is through interference with the regulatory myosin light-chain kinase linking calcium to contraction.

cAMP has a vasodilatory effect, the mechanism of which is by no means simple. Its major effect is probably on myosin light-chain phosphorylation, where it inhibits kinase. This process is thought to be a major vasodilatory mechanism (Bennett and Waldman, 1995). In addition, in some aortic preparations, β-stimulation decreases cytosolic calcium, possibly by enhancing the uptake of calcium into the sarcoplasmic reticulum. A possible alternate explanation is that cAMP could stimulate a pump that ejects calcium from the vascular myocyte.

cGMP has a well-established role as a vasodilatory messenger in vascular smooth muscle, in contrast to its still controversial role in the myocardium. The mechanism whereby cGMP initiates vasodilation is still under discussion. As in the case of cAMP, one proposal is that cGMP may act (via a G kinase) on myosin light-chain phosphorylation (Ishikawa et al., 1993). Alternatively, cGMP might

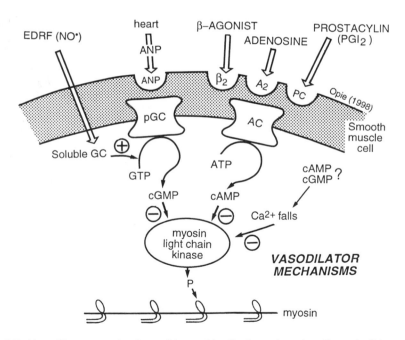

FIG. 9-5. Vasodilatory mechanisms. Most act by the formation of cyclic nucleotides, cGMP, and cAMP. These are both vasodilatory, possibly by inhibition of myosin light chain kinase. cGMP is the messenger for guanylate cyclase, which in turn is stimulated by ANP or by EDRF (i.e., nitric oxide). Vasodilatory cGMP is formed by stimulation of adenylate cyclase (AC) in response to β_2-stimulation, or by adenosine stimulation via A_2-receptors, or by the prostacyclin (PC) receptor.

stimulate the phosphatase breaking off the phosphate from the myosin light chain. An even simpler hypothesis is that cGMP inhibits voltage dependent L-type calcium channels and lessens calcium ion entry in vascular smooth muscle (Ishikawa et al., 1993).

Formation of cGMP occurs in response to several vasodilatory mechanisms (Fig. 9-5), including nitric oxide, atrial natriuretic peptide, and the nitrosovasodilators such as the nitrates and sodium nitroprusside. Previously, the term "endothelium-derived relaxation factor" (EDRF) was used more often than now. Most or all of its vasodilator activity resides in an extremely short-lived free-radical *nitric oxide* (NO), so that it is nitric oxide that is emphasized in this text, even though some workers still doubt the complete identity of EDRF and nitric oxide. A healthy endothelium is essential for formation of nitric oxide. Furchgott and Zawadzki (1980) made the fundamental discovery that acetylcholine, the messenger of the cholinergic nervous system, dilated healthy blood vessels but caused vasoconstriction when the endothelium was damaged. In atherosclerotic and other diseases, when the endothelium is damaged, release of nitric oxide is diminished and that of vasoconstrictory endothelin is enhanced.

Nitric oxide prompts vasodilation in response to both vagal stimulation and exercise. At night, the blood pressure decreases (see Fig. 1-9) as increased vagal activity releases acetylcholine, which elicits the formation of vasodilatory nitric oxide, besides inhibiting the release of vasoconstrictory norepinephrine. During exercise, as the cardiac output increases, the blood flow both to skeletal muscle and the myocardium increases. The proposed explanation is that the increased mechanical stress of the faster blood flow causes shear forces (see section on blood flow later in this chapter) to act on the endothelium, to release nitric oxide which then vasodilates. In addition, shear stress induces the activity of the nitric oxide synthase in the endothelium.

Nitrates, the widely used coronary vasodilators, act by producing nitric oxide independently of the activity of the endothelium, so that they can vasodilate even when there is endothelial damage, as occurs, for example, in coronary artery disease.

PHOSPHATIDYLINOSITOL CYCLE, INOSITOL TRISPHOSPHATE, AND VASOCONSTRICTION

Whereas the cyclic nucleotides are the messengers of the vasodilatory stimuli, such as nitric oxide and β-adrenergic activity, the vasoconstrictory messages are in contrast conveyed by the phosphatidylinositol system (compare Figs. 9-4 and 9-5).

The phosphatidylinositol cycle has two limbs: (1) the breakdown of phosphatidylinositol to inositol trisphosphate (IP$_3$) and thence to inositol, and (2) the resynthesis of phosphatidylinositol from inositol (Fig. 9-6). Phosphatidylinositol or one of its derivative compounds undergoes hydrolysis when an enzyme, a phosphodiesterase, is activated. This enzyme is often known as *phospholipase C*. Just how occupation of the vasoconstrictory receptor is coupled to phospholi-

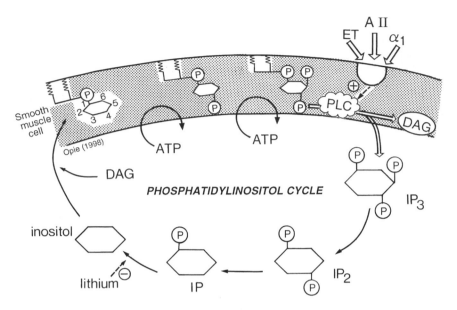

FIG. 9-6. The phosphatidylinositol cycle. In vascular tissue, the reservoir compound is phosphatidylinositol, from which phosphatidylinositol bisphosphate is formed, the substrate for the phospholipase C (PLC) which is stimulated in response to occupation of the angiotensin II receptor. The resulting formation of inositol trisphosphate, one of the intracellular messengers, precedes the formation of inositol bisphosphate and inositol monophosphate. The latter compound is converted to inositol through a reaction inhibited by the antidepressant lithium. Inositol reacts with a derivative of diacylglycerol (DAG) to reform phosphatidylinositol (top left). IP$_3$, inositol (1,4,5)-trisphosphate.

pase C activity is not fully understood, but increasing evidence involves a G-protein cycle, rather similar to that involved in linking β-receptor stimulation with formation of cAMP. Once inositol trisphosphate has formed, it can in turn undergo hydrolysis via inositol diphosphate and inositol monophosphate to inositol, from whence phosphatidylinositol is eventually reformed.

Inositol trisphosphate (IP$_3$ or Ins P$_3$) and its closely related brother inositol tetraphosphate (IP$_4$ or Ins P$_4$) act intracellularly to increase the cytosolic calcium level. IP$_3$ is thought to act on the special IP$_3$ receptor in the sarcoplasmic reticulum to liberate calcium (Berridge, 1993). The processes involved and the structure of the receptor may be similar to the release of calcium by the ryanodine receptor (see Fig. 6-7). IP$_4$ may act in a similar way or, alternatively, may increase the opening probability of the sarcolemmal calcium channel, thereby enhancing the inflow of calcium ions. The proposal is that IP$_3$, and possibly IP$_4$, act transiently to increase the cytosolic calcium level, which thereby initiates the contractile cycle in vascular smooth muscle.

Diacylglycerol (DAG) is also formed when phosphatidylinositol is split by phospholipase C. DAG stimulates the activity of protein kinase C (PKC), which is thought to induce sustained (tonic) contraction, possibly by phosphorylation of the contractile proteins calponin and caldesmon (Horowitz et al., 1996). PKC probably mediates this phosphorylation.

ROLE OF PROTEIN KINASE C

Protein kinase C is a term that refers to a family of kinases. There are four major groups and up to 11 isoforms (also called isozymes) (Horowitz et al., 1996). PKC probably plays a major role in the regulation of cell growth, both in the myocardium and in vascular smooth muscle (see Chapter 13). Situated in the cytosol when inactive, it responds to DAG by translocation to the sarcolemma and thereby becoming active. It then initiates a signal sequence that involves a complex transduction path, probably leading to the enzyme mitogen-activated protein kinase (MAP kinase), which would explain its role in growth regulation and, possibly, in sustained vascular contraction. The path concerned with contraction may eventually lead to phosphorylation of *caldesmon*. The latter is a regulatory protein that binds to both actin and calmodulin and is found in smooth but not in striated muscle. *Caldesmon* inhibits actin–myosin interaction by competing with the myosin head for a binding site on actin (Horowitz et al., 1996). This inhibition is removed by phosphorylation of caldesmon. A somewhat similar role is envisaged for *calponin*, a single low molecular weight polypeptide chain that also may be phosphorylated by a PKC to remove its inhibition of the myosin ATPase. Possibly, by such mechanisms, various PKC-linked agonists such as angiotensin II may maintain tonic contraction.

LATCH MECHANISM

The latch mechanism explains how vascular contraction is sustained for long periods in *tonic contraction* as opposed to the short-lived more regular contraction and relaxation *phasic contraction* that also occurs. The proposal is that such sustained tonic contraction requires relatively little ATP because the cross-bridges are cycling at a much reduced rate (Murphy, 1994). The contractile mechanism has no ejection work to do, as has the myocardium. Rather, contraction needs to be sustained to allow vascular smooth muscle tone to have an effect in regulating the blood pressure. Once myosin and actin are joined, they need to latch onto each other and not to relax until a further signal is given (see end of this section). Thus, the generation of initial tension (contraction) requires about double the cytosolic calcium level of that needed for maintenance of tension (Fig. 9-7). The proposed mechanism of the *latchbridge* formation is as follows. As the calcium level starts to decrease (e.g., as the effect of voltage-induced depolarization wears off), the activity of myosin kinase that phosphorylates the regulatory light chain is switched off, and myosin phosphatase removes the phosphate groups (Murphy, 1994). However, instead of returning to a simple relaxed state, the *dephosphorylated latched* bridges maintain tension. At the end

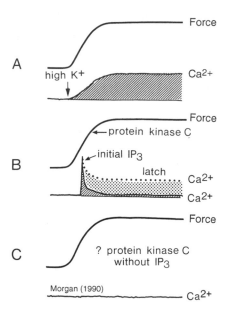

FIG. 9-7. Three types of cytosolic calcium profiles, associated with tonic contractions of vascular smooth muscle. **A:** A high external potassium concentration has caused depolarization, a sustained increase in internal cytosolic calcium, and sustained force contraction. **B:** An initial increase of cytosolic calcium is followed by a decrease either to baseline levels or to about half the previous levels, whereas there is sustained tonic contraction. Two proposed mechanisms are the latch hypothesis and an effect of PKC on the contractile mechanism. **C:** There is a sustained tonic contraction without any initial increase in calcium, and the proposal is that PKC might be formed without any associated IP$_3$. (Modified from Morgan, 1990).

of the vasoconstrictor stimulus, when the calcium channels are no longer open, the continued uptake of calcium by the sarcoplasmic reticulum of the vascular smooth muscle then relaxes the muscle by two mechanisms: first, the calcium–calmodulin complex is dissociated, and the myosin light chain is dephosphorylated by a phosphatase. Second, calcium leaves the unknown regulatory site on the latchbridges. In addition, the binding of ATP to the myosin head (as for myocardium; see Fig. 8-2) helps to unlatch. This simplified schema does not take into account the complexities of the considerable debate surrounding the latchbridge mechanism.

Calcium-Independent Contraction

Yet another pattern of vascular contraction occurs in the complete absence of any increase of internal calcium (Fig. 9-7). Possibly, phospholipase C is acting on membrane precursors other than phosphatidylinositol to release DAG without any formation of IP_3 (Horowitz et al., 1996). Of considerable interest is the proposal that mechanical stretch of vascular smooth muscle sensitizes the contractile mechanism to PKC (Osol et al., 1991).

ENDOTHELIUM AND ITS CONTROL OF VASCULAR SMOOTH MUSCLE

It might be supposed that the mechanisms thus far described for vasodilation and vasoconstriction should adequately be able to regulate vascular tone. For example, during exercise, as will be more fully discussed later in this chapter, β_2-adrenergic stimulation should achieve increased blood flow through skeletal muscle arterioles. This degree of increase of flow appears to be inadequate for the needs of the exercising muscle, and a reinforcing mechanism exists that involves the endothelium. Once blood flow has increased, the shear forces involved release nitric oxide. Thus, further vasodilation occurs.

The endothelium also releases a major vasoconstrictory substance, *endothelin*. The physiologic function of the release of endothelin probably was part of the hemostatic response to trauma in primitive circumstances. Hemostasis was of crucial importance for survival.

Endothelium-Derived Relaxation Factor (Nitric Oxide) as a Vasodilator

For practical purposes, EDRF is identical to nitric oxide (for alternate views, see Vidal et al., 1991), which travels to the vascular smooth muscle from the endothelium to stimulate guanylate cyclase in vascular smooth muscle cells to produce vasodilatory cGMP (Fig. 9-8). An important physiologic factor promoting the release of nitric oxide is enhanced blood flow acting as a shear force. When flow is increased, as during exercise, nitric oxide is formed to contribute to exercise-induced vasodilation. Local release of bradykinin may play a role in this process (Lüscher et al., 1993). Conversely, when blood flow is low, as in vascular disease, release of nitric oxide is lessened, and vasoconstrictory forces dominate. It must be stressed that nitric oxide has a very short half-life, measured in seconds or even less, so that there is almost no "downstream" activity. Nitric oxide acts locally, just at the site where it is formed.

Synthesis of Nitric Oxide. Nitric oxide is synthesized in endothelial cells from L-arginine in response to a complex messenger system involving receptors, IP_3, and calcium. The enzyme concerned is *endothelial nitric oxide synthase* (eNOS), which is calcium sensitive (de Belder and Radomski, 1994). Because nitric oxide is so labile and difficult to measure, one common way of assessing its contribution to vasodilator activity is by inhibition of its formation. This process can be achieved by L-arginine analogs, and many studies with these compounds have shown, for example, that the rate of formation of nitric

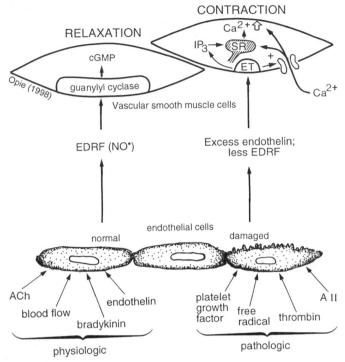

FIG. 9-8. Role of endothelial integrity in regulating vascular tone. The intact endothelium secretes vasodilatory nitric oxide (previously called EDRF), whereas in the presence of endothelial damage, endothelin is vasoconstrictory. Physiologic stimuli that cause release of nitric oxide include acetylcholine (ACh), hypoxia, increased flow, bradykinin, and (unexpectedly) endothelin. In response to certain pathologic stimuli that damage the endothelium, such as excess mechanical damage or formation of free radicals or early atheroma, release of nitric oxide is inhibited. Acetylcholine requires an intact endothelium for its vasodilatory action. When the endothelium is damaged, acetylcholine causes vasoconstriction by a direct effect on vascular smooth muscle. Vasoconstrictory endothelin is released from the damaged endothelium in response to angiotensin II, platelet-derived growth factor, free radicals, and thrombin. ER, endothelin receptor. For mode of action of IP₃, see Fig. 9-4.

oxide in some hypertensive states is diminished. Unfortunately one of these analogs (L-NAME) also inhibits muscarinic receptors and, therefore, decreases vasodilator cholinergic activity with false results (Baxton et al., 1993). Despite these technical problems, it is becoming clear that the *nitric oxide messenger system* is one of great importance, and found not only in the endothelium but probably also in the nervous system. The existence of *nitroxidergic nerves*, which release nitric oxide, is postulated to explain certain aspects of neuro-transmission in the brain and some aspects of the control of the circulation in hypertension (Toda et al., 1993).

Protective Effects of Endothelium

An intact endothelium also protects the arterioles from a number of vasoconstrictory influences, such as serotonin released from damaged platelets. A classic observation made by Furchgott and Zawadzki was that endothelial integrity was required for acetylcholine, the messenger of parasympathetic activity, to exert its physiologic vasodilatory activity. When endothelial integrity was lost, then acetylcholine became vasoconstrictory.

Thus, endothelial damage can change a physiologic vasodilatory stimulus into one that is pathologic and vasoconstrictory. Following this argument further, the endothelium can be damaged (e.g., by the mechanical stress of a raised arterial blood pressure *[hypertension]*) to change its normal vasodilatory role and to become vasoconstrictory. Speculatively, hypertensive damage to the endothelium could release vasoconstrictory endothelin that, in turn, could increase peripheral vascular resistance and exaggerate the severity of hypertension.

Endothelin

This newly discovered peptide composed of 21 amino acids is strongly vasoconstrictory in disease states, acting on vascular smooth muscle by a combination of calcium channel opening and formation of IP_3 (Yanagisawa, 1994). Physiologically, when released in small amounts, it may function as a vasodilator, probably acting on the endothelium to release nitric oxide (Fig. 9-8). The are two types of endothelin receptors: the ET_A and the ET_B. Earlier it was supposed that the former acted on smooth muscle to mediate the constrictor effects, and the latter on endothelium to promote vasodilation. Hence, it is chiefly ET_A receptors that have been developed for therapeutic testing. Currently it is agreed that the ET_B receptors mediate vasodilation but that both receptors types can cause vasoconstriction, depending on the species and the vascular bed (Yanagisawa, 1994).

Endothelin is derived from pre-pro-endothelin and pro-endothelin, from which it is formed by the action of the endothelin converting enzyme (Fig. 9-9). Of the three varieties of endothelin, it is endothelin-1 that has the greatest cardiovascular significance. The chief pathophysiologic stimulus to endothelin synthesis and hence release is angiotensin II, a mechanism counted among several others, such as enhanced release of norepinephrine and direct stimulation of vascular angiotensin II receptors, that contribute to vasoconstriction in heart failure (Kaddoura and Poole-Wilson, 1996). The biosynthesis of endothelin is also induced (1) by the thrombin that is the result of the coagulation process, (2) by the oxygen-derived free radicals that accumulate during ischemia and, particularly, reperfusion, and (3) the *platelet-derived transforming growth factor* TGF released during platelet aggregation.

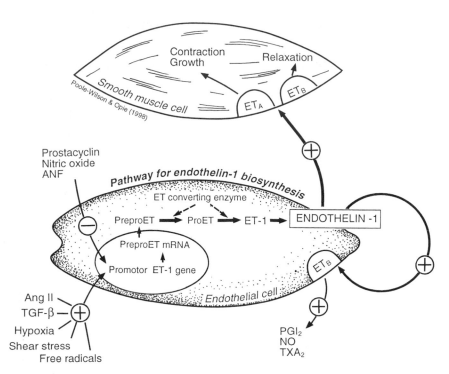

FIG. 9-9. Biosynthesis of endothelin-1. Note conflicting effects of endothelin stimulation on vascular contraction and relaxation. Modified from Kaddoura and Poole-Wilson by permission of the authors and *The Lancet.* +, stimulation; –, inhibition; ET, endothelin; ANF, atrial natriuretic factor; Ang II, angiotensin II; TGF β, transforming growth factor β; PGI₂, prostaglandin; NO, nitric oxide; TXA₂, thromboxane A₂; ET$_A$, endothelin A receptor; ET$_B$, endothelin B receptor.

The Endothelium and Platelets

The previous section argues that an intact vascular endothelium, by releasing nitric oxide, is able to prevent platelet aggregation. On the other hand, once platelet aggregation occurs, then endothelin release is promoted with vasoconstriction. Thus, the interaction between the endothelium and platelets is a crucial physiologic protective mechanism. In simplified terms, the healthy endothelium resists platelets and maintains blood flow. The damaged endothelium attracts platelets that then promote constriction.

Bradykinin. To cardiologists the term "bradykinin" may mean an agent that slows the heart (Greek *bradys,* slow, as in bradycardia; *kinein,* to move). Initially the term was given to a circulating substance that could initiate a slowly developing contraction in the gut. In reality, the major interest in bradykinin for cardiologists lies in its powerful vasodilating action. Bradykinin seems to be more of a local vasodilator, participating in local control, than a general circulating agent regulating the blood pressure. For example, when a bradykinin antagonist is experimentally injected intravenously, there is little change in the blood pressure (Maddedu et al., 1992).

Bradykinin acts on two types of endothelial receptors, the B_1 and B_2-receptors, of which the latter are more sensitive to bradykinin. B_2-receptor stimulation forms two powerful vasodilators: EDRF or nitric oxide, and prostacyclin (Mombouli et al., 1992; Schror, 1992). These bradykinin receptors must not be confused with β_1- and β_2-adrenergic receptors.

There are two major stimuli to the formation of bradykinin in vascular endothelium. The first, of greater physiologic significance, is the release of bradykinin as a result of an increased blood flow. The mechanism is thought to be that increased shear forces act on the endothelium to elicit the formation of bradykinin (Lüscher et al., 1993). Thus, local formation of bradykinin may be important in the mechanism of flow-induced dilation, and hence help to explain increased blood flow to muscles in exercise.

The second stimulus to the formation of bradykinin starts with a chain of events initiated when tissue factor XIIA is formed in response to tissue damage. Bradykinin then forms from kininogen and causes local vasodilation. Such bradykinin may promote the sensitivity to pain and may account for part of the vasodilatory component of inflammation. This sequence is probably of more pathologic than physiologic importance.

Pharmacologically, bradykinin may be an important part of the vasodilatory mechanism of drugs known as the angiotensin-converting enzyme inhibitors. Their mechanism of action is not only by inhibition of the formation of vaso-constrictory angiotensin II, but also by accumulation of bradykinin (Fig. 9-10).

PROSTAGLANDINS

Prostaglandins are compounds with a complex long-chain cyclic structure eventually derived from unsaturated fatty acids such as arachidonic acid in the endothelium and elsewhere (Fig. 9-11). The great number of different prostaglandins that exist, their wide range of biologic activity, and the major species differences make it difficult to ascribe to them an exact function. The prostaglandins with the most significance for cardiovascular function are vasodilatory prostacyclin and vasoconstrictor thromboxane A_2. Both are continuously being formed and broken down, having very short half-lives. *Prostacyclin* (PGI_2) is one of the major vasodilatory prostaglandins released from the endothelium, and it also inhibits platelet aggregation. Therefore, it has antithrombotic properties. *Thromboxane A_2*, in contrast, is a promoter of platelet aggregation and a vasoconstrictor. Thromboxane A_2 acts through vascular receptors and the IP_3 messenger system (Berridge, 1993).

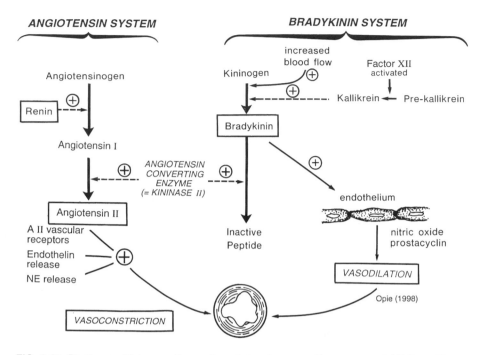

FIG. 9-10. Dual vasodilatory actions of angiotensin converting enzyme inhibitors. These agents act chiefly on the circulating and tissue renin-angiotensin systems with ancillary effects on the enzymes that inactivate bradykinin. The result of the former action is the inhibition of the vasoconstrictory systems and the result of the latter is the formation of vasodilatory nitric oxide and prostacyclin.

Leukotrienes are prostaglandin derivatives also formed from arachidonic acid. They are released from white blood cells (leukocytes) and tissue scavenger cells (macrophages) to act as powerful vasoconstrictors. The "slow-reacting substance" found in serious allergic reactions (the latter called anaphylactic shock) that mediates pulmonary vasoconstriction is now known to be a leukotriene. Certain leukotrienes, derived from leukocytes reaching the ischemic myocardium during the reperfusion period, are thought to have adverse effects by promoting the vasoconstrictory responses (Mullane and Engler, 1991).

AUTONOMIC VASCULAR CONTROL
AND NEUROMODULATION

The dominant autonomic factor governing vascular smooth muscle tone is the release of norepinephrine from the terminal neurons into the synaptic space, with stimulation of the postsynaptic vasoconstrictory α_1- and α_2-receptors (Fig. 9-12). By regulating the rate of norepinephrine release, a large number of hor-

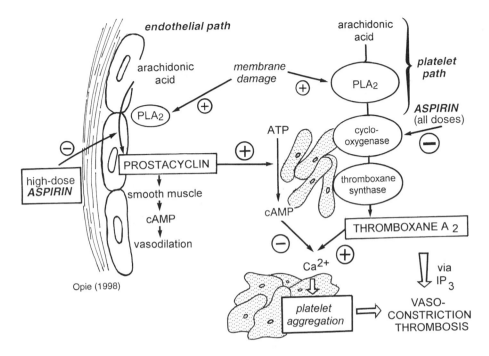

FIG. 9-11. Sources of vasodilatory prostacyclin and vasoconstrictory thromboxane A₂.
Prostacyclin formed in the vascular endothelium, inhibits vascular smooth muscle contraction, probably by formation of cAMP (see Fig. 9-5). Prostacyclin by stimulating the formation of cAMP in platelets decreases platelet calcium, which inhibits platelet aggregation. Another chain of events also leads from arachidonic acid by membrane damage to the platelets to the formation of thromboxane A₂, a powerful platelet aggregator and a promoter of endothelium-dependent contractions (Buzzard et al., 1993). The process of platelet aggregation causes release of substances such as serotonin and platelet-derived growth factor, which cause vasoconstriction. Serotonin, although normally vasodilatory, becomes vasoconstrictory when the endothelium is damaged. PG, prostaglandins.

mones and autonomic signals can achieve indirect control of the degree of vaso-constriction. For example, the parasympathetic autonomic messenger acetyl-choline can decrease release of norepinephrine acting on the receptor on the terminal neuron (presynaptic receptor). Circulating epinephrine, by acting on a presynaptic β_2-receptor, can enhance the release of norepinephrine to override the direct vasodilatory effect of this hormone when postsynaptic β_2-receptors are stimulated. It seems as if this indirect vasoconstrictory effect of epinephrine becomes particularly important during states of sustained epinephrine release as postulated in some types of hypertension. Another important neuromodulator is angiotensin II, which besides acting directly on the angiotensin II receptor to promote vasoconstriction, also increases release of norepinephrine from the terminal neuron by its action on the presynaptic angiotensin II receptor.

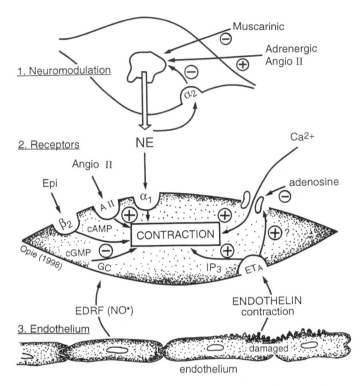

FIG. 9-12. Triple control of vascular contraction by neuromodulation, vascular receptors, and endothelium. Neuromodulation governs the rate of release of vasoconstrictory norepinephrine (NE), the rate of release of which is increased by adrenergic activation and angiotensin II (AII). The second site of control is at vascular receptors. Vasoconstrictory agonists include α_1- and α_2-adrenergic activity, angiotensin II, and endothelin (ER, endothelin receptor). Vasodilatory stimuli include β_2-adrenergic agonist activity with formation of cAMP, and also formation of nitric oxide with formation of cGMP via guanylate cyclase (GC). The endothelium may promote either relaxation via endothelium-derived relaxation factor (EDRF, nitric oxide) or when damaged vascular contraction by release of endothelin. Other endothelial factors involved include vasodilatory prostacyclin and vasoconstrictory thromboxane-A_2.

ROLE OF ION CHANNELS

Calcium Channels and Vasoconstriction. Whereas in the case of the myocardium only one type of calcium channel, operated by voltage (*voltage-operated channel* [VOC]–depolarization operated channel [DOC]) needs to be postulated, in vascular smooth muscle there are in addition *receptor-operated channels* (ROCs) (Fig. 9-13). Receptor agonists that open these channels to cause vasoconstriction include, for example, α_1-agonist activity or angiotensin II or endothelin. However, these two types of calcium channels have not been delineated by molecular biologic techniques, and it is difficult to exclude the possibil-

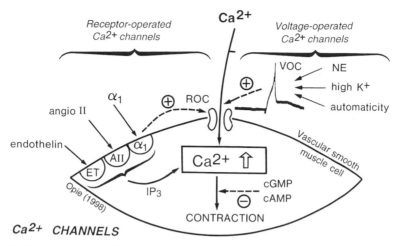

FIG. 9-13. Two types of calcium channel regulation. Receptor-operated channels (ROC) respond to α_1- or angiotensin II or endothelin receptor stimulation. Depolarization-operated channels (DOC – VOC, voltage-operated channels) operate in response to adrenergic stimulation (NE), to potassium-induced depolarization, and to spontaneous automaticity. The result is increased opening probability of the calcium channel to cause contraction of vascular smooth muscle. Note that the receptors that enhance sodium channel opening also stimulate phospholipase C with formation of vasoconstrictory IP_3. This dual mechanism of action promotes powerful vasoconstriction (see Fig. 9-4).

ity that receptor stimulation merely facilitates or inhibits the opening of the same voltage-operated channels that respond to depolarization. In general, these agonists also act on the signal system linked to formation of IP_3 so that their vasoconstrictory mechanism is rather complex: they may act on both voltage- and receptor-operated calcium channels, as well as via IP_3.

ATP-Sensitive Potassium Channel.   When this channel is open, the transferred potassium ions from within to without the cell increase the state of polarization, so that they induce hyperpolarization (the reason for this change was addressed in Chapter 4; in essence, potassium ions transferred across the sarcolemma from within to without leave behind an excess of negative charges). Such hyperpolarization closes the calcium channels because the voltage is not suitable for their operation; cytosolic calcium decreases and vascular tone decreases (Fig. 9-14).

These ATP-sensitive potassium channels can be opened either by receptor stimulation (e.g., by adenosine) or by metabolic factors, such as a decrease in ATP. The latter situation might result during hypoxia or when glycolytic flux is inhibited in severe ischemia.

The same ATP-sensitive potassium channels can be opened by a variety of vasodilator drugs, including two powerful antihypertensive agents, which are seldom used today, namely diazoxide and minoxidil. On the other hand, gliben-

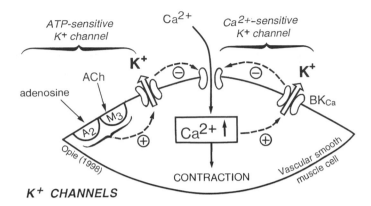

FIG. 9-14. Vasodilatory role of potassium channel activity. There are two main potassium channels. The first is the ATP-sensitive channel activated by vasodilatory adenosine and acetylcholine (ACh). As a result of the outward movement of potassium ions, the potassium ion concentration on the outer side of the cell membrane increases, there is depolarization, and the calcium channel closes. The second potassium channel that vasodilates through a similar mechanism is sensitive to internal calcium. This is the big channel, BK_{Ca} (Ch 4). When internal calcium increases, this channel opens to act as a feedback mechanism. This channel BK_{Ca} also promotes coronary vasodilation in response to estrogens (White et al., 1995).

clamide, an oral agent used in the treatment of diabetes, inhibits the potassium channel, an action that in the pancreas leads to release of insulin whereas in the heart it may limit release of potassium from the ischemic myocardium.

Calcium-Activated Potassium Channel. The existence of this channel can no longer be challenged. It provides feedback from an excess cytosolic calcium to vascular tone as follows. When the internal calcium is high, then this potassium channel opens, and there is hyperpolarization and vasodilation. This channel is therefore part of the protective feedback mechanism whereby an excessive increase of cytosolic calcium will not cause excess vasoconstriction. In addition, this channel responds to nitric oxide by opening (Bolotina et al., 1994), thereby probably playing a role in exercise-induced vasodilation.

ORGAN-DERIVED CIRCULATING PEPTIDES

There are two organs concerned with formation of peptides that send regulatory signals to the peripheral circulation. When the circulating blood volume is too high, then the left atrial pressure increases and the stretch stimulus releases atrial natriuretic peptide (ANP). ANP, besides having a diuretic function, causes arterial relaxation. The vasodilatory signal is conveyed from an ANP vascular receptor to guanylate cyclase, so that cGMP inhibits contraction (Fig. 9-5).

Conversely, when the circulating blood volume is too low, the kidney responds by release of renin, which acts on angiotensinogen to form angiotensin I. The latter is converted to vasoconstrictory angiotensin II, which stimulates the angiotensin II vascular receptors and activates the IP_3 signaling system. In addition, as already mentioned, angiotensin II acts at the level of neuromodulation on receptors on the terminal neurones to enhance the release of vasoconstrictory norepinephrine (Fig. 9-12).

Thus, the heart responding to an excess blood volume, as well as the kidney responding to a decreased blood volume, initiate two opposing peptide systems that respectively respond by vasodilation or by vasoconstriction.

OPPOSING VASODILATORY AND VASOCONSTRICTORY MECHANISMS

It is evident that there are several different powerful vasodilatory and vasoconstrictory forces at work in the control of the tone of vascular smooth muscle. There are at least seven levels at which these opposing and balancing influences are at work (Table 9-3).

First, at the level of autonomic nervous system activity, the release of acetylcholine from the cholinergic neurons is vasodilatory, whereas the release of norepinephrine is vasoconstrictory. Circulating epinephrine, largely derived from the adrenal medulla in response to acute stress such as exercise, has a predominant vasodilatory role.

TABLE 9-3. *Vasodilatory and vasoconstrictory mechanisms in vascular smooth muscle*

	Vasodilation	Vasoconstriction
Autonomic nervous system	Cholinergic, adrenergic (E)	Adrenergic (NE)
Terminal neurones	ACh inhibits NE release via neuromodulation	Adrenergic release of NE, facilitated by AII
Vascular receptors	β_2, adenosine, prostacyclin	α (α_1 and α_2 postsynaptic), AII, endothelin
Messenger systems	Receptors → G-proteins → adenylate cyclase → cAMP → PKC → myosin light chain kinase	Receptors → G-proteins → phospholipase C → IP_3 and PKC → contractile proteins
Endothelium	EDRF (nitric oxide) → vascular guanylate cyclase → cGMP → dilation (EDRF released by ACh or shear stress)	Endothelin → vascular endothelin receptors → phospholipase C → IP_3 and PKC; endothelin also releases ANP
Organ-derived peptides	Atrial natriuretic peptide from heart → ANP vascular receptors → cGMP	Renin from kidney → AII → vascular receptors → phospholipase C
Ion channels	ATP-dependent potassium channel (opens in response to adenosine, hypoxia)	Calcium channel (opens in response to depolarization or receptors)

E, epinephrine; NE, norepinephrine; ACh, acetylcholine; AII, angiotensin II; IP_3, inositol trisphosphate.

Second, activity of the terminal neurones are basically vasoconstrictory by release of norepinephrine (Fig. 9-12). The many modulating factors (neuromodulation) include acetylcholine, which inhibits norepinephrine release.

Third, there are both vasodilatory and vasoconstrictory vascular receptors. The former are those responding to β_2-adrenergic stimulation, adenosine, and prostacyclin (Fig. 9-5). Prostacyclin (PGI$_2$) is the vasodilatory prostaglandin released from the endothelium in response to circulating bradykinin. On the other hand, vasoconstrictory vascular receptors respond to α-adrenergic stimulation (α_1 and α_2 postsynaptic receptors), angiotensin II, and endothelin (Fig. 9-4).

Fourth, the opposing messenger systems involved in the vasodilatory and vasoconstrictory receptors are as follows. The vasodilatory messenger chain links the vasodilatory receptors via G proteins to adenylate cyclase, which forms cAMP, stimulates protein kinase A, and thereby inhibits myosin light-chain kinase. The vasoconstrictory messenger system leads from the vasoconstrictory receptors via G proteins to activation of phospholipase C, formation of IP$_3$, and release of calcium from the sarcoplasmic reticulum.

Fifth, the endothelium also sends out opposing signals. Vasodilatory EDRF (nitric oxide), released in response to acetylcholine or to shear stress, acts on vascular guanylate cyclase to stimulate formation of vasodilatory cGMP. Vasodilatory prostacyclin stimulates the formation of vasodilatory cAMP. The endothelium can also release (e.g., in response to injury) vasoconstrictory endothelin, which acts on vascular endothelin receptors to enhance cytosolic calcium levels.

Sixth, organ-derived peptides also give opposing signals. Atrial natriuretic peptide released from the heart is vasodilatory, acting on ANP vascular receptors that stimulate the formation of cGMP. Renin released from the kidney leads ultimately to formation of angiotensin II and has multiple vasoconstrictory signals, including an effect on vascular angiotensin II receptors and phospholipase C to stimulate the formation of IP$_3$.

Seventh, vasoconstrictory calcium channels are opposed by vasodilatory potassium channels. Chief among the vasodilatory potassium channels are the ATP-sensitive variety, which respond to adenosine or hypoxia by opening, whereupon the cell becomes hyperpolarized. The result is that the calcium channel opens less readily. In contrast, the calcium channel itself is vasoconstrictory. It opens in response to depolarization or to receptor stimulation (e.g., by α_2-adrenergic stimulation) or in response to angiotensin II or endothelin.

These multiple opposing mechanisms suggest that fine tuning of the degree of vasodilation or vasoconstriction is a physiologic necessity.

BLOOD FLOW AND SHEAR STRESS

An excellent example of the fine line between vasodilation and vasoconstriction lies in the vascular response to an increased blood flow. Endothelial cells are indispensable in the response of the vascular bed to shear stress (Morita et al., 1994). As the blood flow increases and shear forces form between the blood stream and the endothelium, endothelial cells become elongated and aligned in the direction of the blood flow. A complex response, probably mediated by a mechanoreceptor, includes not only synthesis and release of nitric oxide and opening of a potassium channel, but release of vasodilatory prostacyclin. In apparent contradiction, increased endothelial cell calcium activates PKC, which in turn switches on the gene for endothelin (Morita et al., 1994). The latter sequence is controversial and only makes sense if the physiologic role of endothelin were vasodilatory rather than vasoconstrictory, which, unexpectedly perhaps, recent data suggest is indeed the case (Masaki, 1995). This hypothesis states that it is only when endothelin is overproduced in pathologic conditions such as heart failure that it changes from being a vasodilator to a vasconstrictor and a signal to the hypertrophy of vascular smooth muscle.

PHYSIOLOGIC CONTROL BY INTEGRATION OF REGULATORY SIGNALS

It is instructive to trace out the mechanisms involved, in one physiologic vasodilatory response, namely that to exercise, and in one physiologic vasoconstrictory response, namely the catecholamine surge upon awakening.

At the *start of exercise*, central adrenergic outflow is much enhanced. The consequences are threefold. First, release of epinephrine from the adrenal gland leads to an increased circulating epinephrine level and to β-mediated (β$_2$) vasodilation (Fig. 9-15). Second, an increased β-stimulation (chiefly β$_1$) of the myocardium and the sinus node leads to an increased cardiac output that, in turn, will increase the blood pressure. As a result, baroreceptors are stimulated with a reflex decrease in peripheral vasoconstriction. Baroreflex activity also increases cholinergic activity relative to that of adrenergic activity. Cholinergic activity vasodilates through release of EDRF (nitric oxide) from the endothelium. At the same time, the increased blood pressure drives more blood through the arterioles to induce release of more nitric oxide by shear forces. At the site of skeletal muscular activity, ATP is broken down to adenosine. The latter opens the ATP-dependent potassium channel to hyperpolarize the vascular myocytes and to close the calcium channel, thereby indirectly promoting vasodilation. Tissue hypoxia also may contribute by decreasing the ATP available to inhibit the potassium channel. There are also other vasodilatory metabolites formed by exercising muscle such as increased carbon dioxide. Some workers propose that there is a direct vasodilatory effect of a low tissue oxygen tension on vascular myocytes. Possibly the mechanism to explain the effect of tissue hypoxia could be opening of the potassium channel as the ATP level decreases.

All the above mechanisms will increase blood flow to exercising muscle, thereby providing a much greater delivery of oxygen and nutrients.

The *response to awakening* includes the physiologic vasoconstrictory response caused by the catecholamine surge. Central excitation leads to adrenergic norepinephrine-mediated α-vasoconstriction. Stimulation of postsynaptic

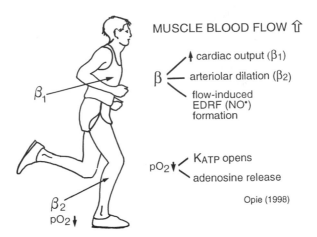

MUSCLE BLOOD FLOW ⇧

β 〈 cardiac output (β_1)
arteriolar dilation (β_2)
flow-induced
EDRF (NO·)
formation

β_1

pO_2↓ 〈 K_{ATP} opens
adenosine release

Opie (1998)

β_2
pO_2↓

FIG. 9-15. Exercise-induced peripheral arteriolar dilation. As a result of adrenergic activation during exercise, β_1-adrenergic stimulation increases the cardiac output, which increases flow to the muscles and thereby induces release of vasodilatory nitric oxide (EDRF). β_2-adrenergic stimulation directly causes vascular dilation (see Fig. 9-5). Another vasodilatory mechanism is that a decreased tissue oxygen tension opens the ATP-sensitive potassium channel (see Fig. 9-14). The mechanism involved is probably twofold, including a decrease of vascular tissue ATP (which directly opens the channel) and an increase of adenosine, resulting from breakdown of ATP, which acts via the adenosine receptor. Other vasodilatory responses to exercise are also likely to be involved.

α_1-receptors leads via G proteins to increased activity of phospholipase C, the latter resulting in formation of IP_3 and DAG, the former initiating and the latter maintaining arterial tone. Postsynaptic α_2-adrenoceptor activity leads, via G proteins, to increased opening of receptor-operated calcium channels. The net result is increased vasoconstriction with an increase in blood pressure even in the absence of any major tachycardia. Nonetheless, the associated β-adrenergic stimulation of the myocardium would also increase heart rate and cardiac output, and therefore further increase blood pressure. Vasodilatory counterregulation, in response to increased blood flow as during exercise, is overridden by the powerful norepinephrine-mediated vasoconstriction.

VASCULAR RESPONSE
IN PATHOPHYSIOLOGICAL STATES

The possible role of the endothelium in disease states is currently under intense scientific scrutiny. There are a number of states characterized by poor vasodilatory responses to acetylcholine suggesting a role for endothelial damage. These states include systemic hypertension, coronary artery disease, and vein graft rejection (Ishii et al., 1993). The endothelium, via its potent vasodilatory and antiaggregatory platelet effects, may have an important role in developing the progress of these different types of arterial disease. The protective role of the endothelium draws attention to the number of vasoconstrictory states in which excess vasoconstriction predominates to exert potentially harmful effects on the heart and circulation. Such states include hypertension (Veltmar et al, 1991), congestive heart failure, and ischemic reperfusion.

In *congestive heart failure*, there is an important regulatory disturbance whereby in compensation for the low blood pressure as a result of the myocardial contractile failure, there is activation of the adrenergic nervous system with increased α-mediated peripheral vasoconstriction and β-mediated release of renin from the kidneys with angiotensin II formation and subsequent additional vasoconstriction. Increasingly, endothelin is seen as an important vasoconstrictor that exaggerates the load against which the failing heart must work, and endothelin receptor antagonists are seen as potential therapy (Love and McMurray, 1996). Thus, in severe congestive heart failure, treatment by a variety of vasodilators plays an important therapeutic role.

In *ischemia*, when blood flow is restored either experimentally or in response to therapeutic measures, there may be the development of excess vasoconstriction, which is known as the no-reflow phenomenon. The origin of this adverse change is complex but may be mediated at least in part by endothelin release, which can be evoked by the generation of oxygen free radicals at the time of reperfusion.

In *septic shock*, the current hypothesis is that circulating compounds such as *cytokines* and endotoxins stimulate that form of nitric oxide that is inducible (iNOS) and calcium independent (de Belder and Radomski, 1994). The proposal is that intense arteriolar vasodilation leads to an unphysiologically low peripheral vascular resistance, with "warm shock."

HEMOSTATIC RESPONSE TO TRAUMA

Interactions between the vascular endothelium and the formed elements of the blood, namely the platelets, are crucial in the hemostatic process. When there is severe arterial injury, the danger is that of major hemorrhage, blood loss, and cardiovascular collapse leading to death. Therefore, adequate hemostasis is crucial. The endothelium has a crucial dual role in the hemostatic process (Fig. 9-16). First, upon injury, the endothelium releases endothelin, thereby promoting vascular contraction. Furthermore, the basal release of vasodilatory prostacyclin and nitric oxide is lost, leading to increased vasoconstriction. Second, platelets are now able to adhere to the damaged endothelium. The binding between platelets is promoted because injury activates platelet receptors, thereby facilitating the "coming together" of platelets in the process of platelet aggregation. The vascular endothelium is important in the thrombotic process (Zilla et al., 1993). Damaged platelets release serotonin, which, in the presence of endothelial damage, causes vasoconstriction. The platelets also release active thrombin, which initiates coagulation by convert-

ENDOTHELIAL DAMAGE

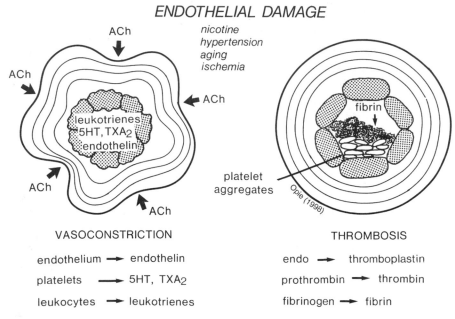

VASOCONSTRICTION

endothelium ➞ endothelin

platelets ➞ 5HT, TXA$_2$

leukocytes ➞ leukotrienes

THROMBOSIS

endo ➞ thromboplastin

prothrombin ➞ thrombin

fibrinogen ➞ fibrin

FIG. 9-16. Role of endothelial damage in promoting vasoconstriction and thrombosis. Vasoconstriction is a complex process occurring in the presence of endothelial damage through at least four mechanisms. First, the damaged endothelium directly liberates endothelin. Second, platelets liberate serotonin (5HT) and thromboxane A$_2$ (TxA$_2$). Third, leukocytes liberate leukotrienes. Fourth, activity of the parasympathetic autonomic nervous system liberates acetylcholine (ACh). Acetylcholine, normally vasodilatory, becomes vasoconstrictory in the presence of endothelial damage. Endothelial damage also initiates the process of thrombosis by release of thromboplastin, which sets in chain a sequence ending in the formation of fibrin. Platelet aggregates participate in the thrombotic process.

ing fibrinogen to fibrin. Furthermore, active thrombin binds to endothelial cells and stimulates the expression of the tissue factor thromboplastin. Thromboplastin converts prothrombin to thrombin, thereby accelerating the coagulation process.

Intense vasoconstriction is coupled to activation of the coagulation process as soon as the endothelium is injured. Such responses are entirely beneficial and desirable when there is major external trauma to the blood vessel. However, when the endothelium is pathologically damaged (e.g., by hypertension or by nicotine), then somewhat similar processes can occur chronically, ultimately to result in atheroma formation with cholesterol deposition. Therefore, maintenance of endothelial integrity is an important long-term aim in the prevention of atheroma and subsequent development of coronary artery disease, a major cause of death in Western communities.

SUMMARY

1. *The contractile mechanism* in vascular smooth muscle differs in several fundamental ways from that of the myocardium. A different signal links an increase in cytosolic calcium to muscular contraction, namely, the activation of myosin light-chain kinase by calcium-calmodulin. cAMP formed in response to β-agonist stimulation inhibits vascular contraction, in contrast to the stimulation achieved in the myocardium. cGMP plays a prominent vasodilatory role in vascular myocytes, whereas it seems to have little function in the myocardium. Vasodilatory cGMP forms in response to nitric oxide (EDRF) and atrial natriuretic peptide. The mechanism of action of cGMP is not clear but may involve inhibition of a crucial enzyme, myosin light-chain kinase.

2. *Latchbridges.* To allow for slowly sustained contractions that underlie the vascular tone of the peripheral arterioles, smooth muscle can form latchbridges. Vascular tone governs the peripheral vascular resistance, thereby indirectly controlling the blood pressure. The favored mechanism for latchbridge formation is an actin–myosin interaction that is triggered by myosin light-chain kinase in the presence of calcium, but then the actin and myosin continue to interact even after these stimuli are removed.

3. *Nitric oxide* is released from the endothelium in response to increased blood flow, thereby providing a mechanism for peripheral vasodilation during exercise. This mechanism acts in addition to the more accepted roles of adenosine and other vasodilatory metabolites produced by muscular exercise. The endothelium releases vasoconstrictory endothelin in response to trauma.

4. *Vasoconstrictory vascular receptors* include those responding to norepinephrine, released from the terminal neurons. The rate of release of norepinephrine is subject to inhibition by acetylcholine, and other regulatory substances such as angiotensin II, through a process known as neuromodulation. Norepinephrine, angiotensin II, and endothelin are all vasoconstrictors that at least in part act through the stimulation of phospholipase C. The latter, in turn, acts on the phosphatidylinositol system to form inositol trisphosphate (IP₃) and diacylglycerol. IP₃ releases calcium from the sarcoplasmic reticulum to initiate contraction. Diacylglycerol, through stimulation of the activity of PKC, is thought to lead to sustained tonic contraction. In addition, all these vasoconstrictory stimuli also promote opening of the calcium channel. They thus have a dual mode of vasoconstrictory action.

5. *Calcium channels* of the L type are the major mode of entry of calcium into vascular smooth muscle. There are two populations according to the mechanism involved: the voltage-operated and the receptor-operated channels. The cytosolic calcium level can be dissociated from the level of contraction during sustained tonic contraction. The two most favored theories to explain this phenomenon are the formation of latch crossbridges in which interaction is sustained even in the absence of calcium and a sustained actin–

myosin interaction in response to formation of protein kinase C, the latter the result of activity of the phosphatidylinositol pathway.

6. *Potassium channels* also control vascular tone. Thus, adenosine, formed from ATP during skeletal muscle exercise, is thought to open the ATP-sensitive potassium channel. The resulting hyperpolarization of the vascular smooth muscle cell moves the calcium channel away from its voltage of operation, so that the calcium channel tends to stay in the closed state.

7. *Excess peripheral vasoconstriction* occurs in a number of diseased states, especially in advanced congestive heart failure. The integrity of the endothelium and constant release of nitric oxide is thought to be important in preventing aggregation of platelets on the endothelium. Once endothelial damage occurs, vasoconstrictory mechanisms are set in motion and excess vasoconstriction will occur. Furthermore, endothelial damage may lead to intimal deposition of platelets, an early step in the formation of atheroma.

STUDENT QUESTIONS

1. List ways in which the contractile mechanism in vascular smooth muscle differs from that of the myocardium.
2. Why does β-adrenergic stimulation cause the myocardium to contract and vascular smooth muscle to relax?
3. What is the signaling system involved in vasoconstriction in vascular smooth muscle?
4. How does the vascular endothelium regulate smooth muscle tone?
5. What is EDRF? How does it cause vasodilation?
6. What are the consequences for regulation of vascular tone when the endothelium is damaged?
7. Describe how exercise causes arteriolar dilation.

CARDIOLOGIST-IN-TRAINING QUESTIONS

1. How does angiotensin II cause vascular contraction? Describe the signaling system in detail.
2. How is vascular tone maintained? Why is tone important for regulation of the blood pressure?
3. How does the vascular endothelium help regulate arteriolar tone? What are the consequences of endothelial damage? Which are the disease states in which such damage may occur?
4. What is endothelin? In which disease may it play an important role and how could it do so? If this role is confirmed, what therapeutic steps could be taken to lessen the proposed adverse effects of endothelin?
5. Describe the major ion channels that regulate vascular tone. Which of these are susceptible to drug action?
6. Describe the mechanisms whereby muscle blood flow increases during exercise.

REFERENCES

1. Bennett BM, Waldman SA. Cyclic nucleotides and protein phosphorylation in vascular smooth muscle relaxation. In: Sperelakis N, ed. *Physiology and Pathophysiology of the Heart.* 3rd ed. Boston: Kluwer Academic, 1995;975–998.
2. Berridge MJ. Inositol trisphosphate and calcium signaling. *Nature* 1993;361:315–325.
3. Bolotina VM, Najibi S, Palacino JJ, et al. Nitric oxide directly activates calcium-dependent potassium channels in vascular smooth muscle. *Nature* 1994;368:850.
4. Buxton ILO, Cheek DJ, Eckman D. N^G-nitrol-L-arginine methyl ester and other alkyl esters of arginine are muscarinic receptor antagonists. *Circ Res* 1993;72:387–395.
5. Buzzard CJ, Pfister SL, Campbell WB. Endothelium-dependent contractions in rabbit pulmonary artery are mediated by thromboxane A_2. *Circ Res* 1993;72:1023–1034.
6. de Belder AJ, Radomski MW. Nitric oxide in the clinical arena [Editorial]. *J Hypertens* 1994;12:617–624.
7. Dzau VJ, Gibbons GH, Cooke JP, Omoigui N. Vascular biology and medicine in the 1990s: scope, concepts, potentials and perspectives. *Circulation* 1993;87:705–719.
8. Furchgott R, Zawadzki JV. The obligatory role of endothelial cells in the relaxation of arterial smooth muscle by acetylcholine. *Nature* 1980;288:373–376.
9. Gibbons GH, Dzau VJ. Angiotensin converting enzyme inhibition and vascular hypertrophy in hypertension. *Cardiovasc Drug Ther* 1990;4:237–242.
10. Horowitz A, Menice CB, Laporte R, Morgan KG. Mechanisms of smooth muscle contraction. *Physiol Rev* 1996;76:967–1003.
11. Ishii T, Okadome K, Komari K, et al. Natural course of endothelium-dependent and independent responses in autogenous femoral veins grafted into the arterial circulation of the dog. *Circ Res* 1993;72:1004–1010.
12. Ishikawa T, Hume JR, Keef KD. Regulation of Ca^{2+} channels by cAMP and cGMP in vascular smooth muscle cells. *Circ Res* 1993;73:1128–1137.
13. Kaddoura S, Poole-Wilson PA. Endothelin-1 in heart failure: a new therapeutic target? *Lancet* 1996;348:418–419.
14. Love MP, McMurray JJV. Endothelin in chronic heart failure: current position and future prospects. *Cardiovasc Res* 1996;31:665–674.
15. Lüscher TF, Boulanger CM, Yang Z. Interactions between endothelium-derived relaxing and contracting factors in health and cardiovascular diseases. *Circulation* 1993;87(suppl V):V36–V44.
16. Maddedu P, Anania V, Parpaglia PP, et al. Effects of HOE 140, a bradykinin B_2-receptor antagonist, on renal function in conscious normotensive rats. *Br J Pharmacol* 1992;106:380–386.
17. Masaki T. Possible role of endothelin in endothelial regulation of vascular tone [Abstract]. *Annu Rev Pharmacol Toxicol* 1995;35:235–255.
18. Mombouli JV, Illiano S, Nagao T, et al. Potentiation of endothelium-dependent relaxations to bradykinin by angiotensin-I converting enzyme inhibitors in canine coronary artery involves both endothelium-derived relaxing and hyperpolarizing factors. *Circ Res* 1992;71:137–144.
19. Morgan KG. The role of calcium in the control of vascular tone as assessed by the Ca2+ indicator aequorin. *Cardiovasc Drug Ther* 1990;4:1355–1362.
20. Morita T, Kurihara H, Maemura K, et al. Role of Ca^{2+} and protein kinase C in shear stress-induced actin depolymerization and endothelin 1 gene expression. *Circ Res* 1994;75:630–636.
21. Mullane K, Engler R. Proclivity of activated neutrophils to cause postischemic cardiac dysfunction: participation in stunning? *Cardiovasc Drug Ther* 1991;5:915–924.
22. Murphy RA. What is special about smooth muscle? The significance of covalent crossbridge regulation. *FASEB J* 1994;8:311–318.
23. Ohanian J, Izzard A, Littlewood M, et al. Regulation of diaccylglycerol metabolism in vasoconstrictor hormones in intact small arteries. *Circ Res* 1993;72:1163–1171.
24. Osol G, Laher I, Cipolla M. Protein kinase C modulates basal myogenic tone in resistance arteries from the cerebral circulation. *Circ Res* 1991;68:359–367.
25. Ross R, Glomset J. The pathogeneis of atherosclerosis. *N Engl J Med* 1976;295:369–377.
26. Schror K. Role of prostaglandins in the cardiovascular effects of bradykinin and angiotensin-converting enzyme inhibitors. *J Cardiovasc Pharmacol* 1992;20(suppl 9):68–73.
27. Smiesko V, Johnson PC. The arterial lumen is controlled by flow-related shear stress. *News Physiol Sci* 1993;8:34–38.
28. Toda N, Kitamura Y, Okamura T. Neural mechanism of hypertension by nitric oxide synthase inhibitor in dogs. *Hypertension* 1993;21:3–8.
29. Veltmar A, Gohlke P, Unger T. From tissue angiotensin converting enzyme inhibition to antihypertensive effect. *Am J Hypertens* 1991;4:263S–269S.

30. Vidal M, Vanhoutte PM, Miller VM. Dissociation between endothelium-dependent relaxations and increases in cGMP in systemic veins. *Am J Physiol* 1991;29:H1531–H1537.
31. White RE, Darkow DJ, Lang JLF. Estrogen relaxes coronary arteries by opening BK$_{ca}$ channels through a cGMP-dependent mechanism. *Circ Res* 1995;77:936–942.
32. Yanagisawa M. The endothelin system. A new target for therapeutic intervention. *Circulation* 1994; 89:1320–1322.
33. Zilla P, Oppel Uv, Deutsch M. The endothelium: A key to the future. *J Cardiovasc Surg* 1993; 8:32–60.

PART IV

The Heart

10

Oxygen Supply: Coronary Flow

*No single mechanism predominates in control of
coronary vascular tone: neural, humoral, and local
metabolic control mechanisms all participate.*
J.M. Muller et al., 1996

Because the work production and the energy requirement of the heart vary so
much from rest to exercise, there must be some system of variable oxygen delivery to the myocardium. Blood reaches the cardiac myocytes from the coronary
circulation (Fig. 10-1). Changes in the coronary flow rate control the delivery of
oxygen (Fig. 10-2). Blood leaving the heart in the coronary sinus is markedly
deoxygenated and black in color, and in response to myocardial hypoxia, little
further extraction of oxygen is possible. When the heart needs more oxygen (as
during exercise), it is the coronary flow that must increase. Berne has proposed
that the myocardium communicates its oxygen requirements to the coronary
arteries by the rate of production of adenosine. According to his hypothesis,
when the heart lacks oxygen (as during ischemia), the breakdown of only a small
quantity of high-energy phosphate compounds, such as adenosine triphosphate
(ATP), produces enough adenosine for powerful coronary vasodilation. This
theory fails to explain events during exercise, so that there must be other
vasodilators, such as nitric oxide. The neurogenic theory for control of the coronary circulation stresses that activity of the autonomic nervous system plays an
important ancillary role, and that neurogenic stimuli may restrain the extent of
coronary vasodilation.

CORONARY CIRCULATION

The two major coronary arteries run from the base of the aorta to the left and
right ventricles, respectively, before giving off branches that run down the surface of the heart toward the apex. It is the left coronary artery that usually sup-

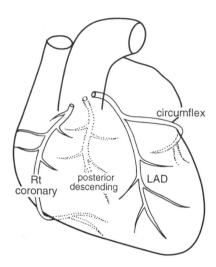

FIG. 10-1. Anatomy of major coronary arteries.

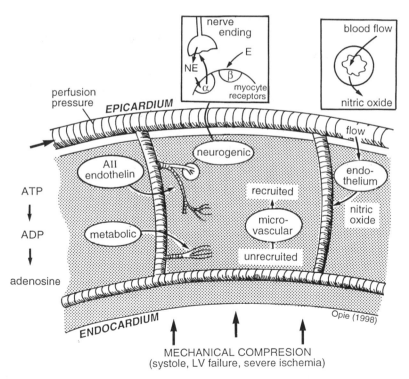

FIG. 10-2. Metabolic versus neurogenic control of the coronary circulation. Metabolic control is the basic mechanism, whereas neurogenic control is ancillary. EPI, epicardial; ENDO, endocardial.

plies the left ventricular wall. Its major branch is the left anterior descending coronary artery (anterior interventricular artery), which supplies part of the septum. This pattern is variable from species to species, as well as from individual to individual. In humans, the coronary arteries have attracted popular attention because when partially or completely occluded by coronary atherosclerosis (coronary artery disease), the myocardial oxygen supply becomes inadequate. As already emphasized, *myocardial ischemia* results from an imbalance between the oxygen supply and demand, whereby demand exceeds the supply and the myocardium starts to suffer from the effects of lack of oxygen.

Resistance Versus Conductance Arterial Vessels

From the point of view of regulation of coronary flow, there are two major types of arterial vessels. First, the small *resistance arterioles*, because they are narrow and because the resistance increases by a power of four as the radius decreases (Poiseuille's law), constitute the major resistance to flow. Second, the large conductance arteries govern the quantity of blood arriving at the resistance vessels. The coronary flow is proportional to the driving pressure across the coronary bed (coronary arterial pressure or blood pressure) divided by the resistance.

Anatomically, the major coronary vascular resistance lies in the small coronary arterioles less than 450 µm in diameter (Camici et al., 1996; Chilian et al., 1989). Going down in size, almost half of the total coronary resistance lies in vessels 100 to 450 µm in diameter, and the rest in the smaller arterioles, less than 100 µm in diameter, also called the autoregulatory vessels (see section on Coronary Autoregulation).

Capillary Microcirculation

The control of the myocardial oxygen supply lies in the *coronary arterioles*, which keep on branching until the very small, thin-walled capillaries are formed. The microcirculation is that part of the coronary circulation concerned with the regulation of the terminal arterioles and capillaries, directly responsible for the transfer of oxygen from the oxygenated arterial blood to the myocardial tissues. These aspects of the coronary circulation are remarkably similar to the peripheral circulation. Capillary flow is governed not by the properties of the capillary itself, but by tone of the feeder arteriole (see Fig. 2-17).

In the normal heart, there are over 2,000 capillaries per cubic millimeter, of which normally only 60% to 80% are open and functioning. There is about one capillary per myofiber (Table 10-1). The number of functioning capillaries increases by recruitment if the arterial oxygen tension decreases (Tables 10-1 and 10-2). Each capillary is extremely narrow so that the myocardium accommodates this astonishing abundance of open capillaries. With a mean capillary diameter of about 3 to 4µm, less than 5% of tissue volume is occupied. The nor-

TABLE 10-1. *Microanatomy of oxygen supply of myocardial cell[a]*

Capillaries per mm^2 left ventricle	About 2,500
Muscle fibers (myocytes) per mm^2	About 2,500
Muscle fiber diameter	17–18 µm
Fiber-capillary ratio	1.0
Mean capillary diameter	3–4 µm
Intercapillary distance	17 µm
Diffusion distance (half of intercapillary)	8.5 µm

[a]For data sources, see Opie, *The Heart*. Orlando: Grune and Stratton, 1984.

mal intercapillary distance is about 17 µm (Table 10-1). *During arterial hypoxia,* the precapillary sphincters relax, more capillaries are recruited, and the intercapillary distance shrinks to 14.5 µm (Table 10-2). Prolonged anoxia reduces the distance further, to 11 µm. These findings support Krogh's early idea of the regulation of capillary density by the metabolic demands of the tissue. In exercise, the coronary blood flow might double, but unless there is recruitment of capillaries with a reduction of intercapillary distance, the oxygen demands of the tissue cannot be met. Even reducing the intercapillary distance from 17 to 14 microns allows the oxygen to diffuse to an additional 1.5 µm, which is an important adjustment to avoid tissue anoxia. Only after such microvascular changes have occurred and oxygen deprivation is still severe are the reserves of oxygen dissolved in the tissue and in myoglobin used up.

Tissue Myoglobin

Myoglobin is an oxygen-binding hemoglobinlike compound found in small amounts in the heart, about 0.25 mmol/L or 0.4 g/100 g. Even the low concentrations of oxygen associated with myoglobin (as oxymyoglobin) may be important in intracellular oxygen transport because the partial pressure of oxygen required for half maximal saturation of myoglobin is very low (2.4 mm Hg) (Tamura et al., 1978). In the normal heart, oxygen bound to myoglobin or to tissue hemoglobin, or dissolved in tissue water can maintain the heart for about 8 seconds or eight contractions in the absence of any coronary blood flow. It is still

TABLE 10-2. *Recruitment of capillaries[a]*

	Intercapillary distance (µm)	Diffusion distance (µm)
Normal	17	8.5
Exercise, estimated	14	7.0
Hypoxia	14.5	7.3
Prolonged anoxia	11	5.5
Maximal recruitment	6.5	3.3

[a]For data sources, see Opie, 1984.

unclear whether myoglobin is only a reservoir for small amounts of oxygen or also facilitates the transport of oxygen.

Tissue Oxygen Tension

The cytochrome oxidase system, where oxygen acts in the mitochondria, requires a remarkably low oxygen tension of below 0.05 mm Hg (O_2 concentration, 10^{-7} mol/L). This is the minimal effective tissue oxygen tension for oxidative phosphorylation (Chance, 1976). The oxygen tension required for mitochondrial function is about 2,000 times less than that in arterial blood (say 100 mm Hg). The average myocardial tissue pO_2 (oxygen tension) should lie between these values. To measure tissue oxygen tension with a needle microelectrode requires intracellular penetration and trauma, which can be circumvented by measuring pO_2 on the surface of the beating heart or calculated from the hemoglobin oxygen saturation measured in frozen myocardium. The same message emerges irrespective of the technique: there is a marked variation both in the oxygen content of the capillary hemoglobin and in the oxygen tension of myocardial tissue, with some values apparently approaching zero. Because of the wide variety of tissue pO_2 values, any given state of oxygenation is best described by a scatter diagram. As the pO_2 decreases, so does the scatter diagram change until the majority of tissue oxygen tensions are less than 5 mm Hg. In addition, measurements of the state of oxygenation of various intracellular respiratory pigments show the probable existence of an intracellular gradient of oxygen tension from the cytosol to the mitochondria. The phasic patency of precapillary sphincters suggests that at any given overall level of capillary recruitment, some of the capillaries are opening and others closing all the time.

REGULATION OF CORONARY VASCULAR TONE

The metabolic needs of the myocardium are provided by the control of the coronary blood flow, which is tightly coupled to the energy status of the cell. During increased heart work or ischemia, myocardial metabolism, sensitive to the workload and the prevailing oxygen tension of the medium, self-regulates energy metabolism partly by release of adenosine. The latter acts largely on the small coronary resistance arterioles not on the large conductance arteries. Such metabolic vasodilation is restricted by about 30% by adrenergic vasoconstriction, mediated by α-adrenergic receptors (Table 10-3).

Vasoconstrictors Versus Vasodilators

Several neurogenic vasoconstrictor influences oppose metabolic vasodilation (Fig. 10-3), chiefly adrenergic activation of α-receptors, involving two types of postsynaptic receptors, the α_1- and the α_2-subtypes. Both of these promote vasoconstriction, acting at least in part through the IP_3 messenger system (see Fig.

TABLE 10-3. *Coronary neurogenic control*

Innervation	Messenger	Receptor	Site and function
Adrenergic sympathetic	NE	Alpha	Vasoconstrictive
		α_1	Larger conductance vessels
		D/a_2	Smaller resistance vessels
	NE, E	Beta	Vasodilatory
		β/D_1	Larger vessels
		β_2	Resistance vessels
Cholinergic parasympathetic	ACh	Muscarinic	Vasodilation via NO (vasoconstriction when endothelium damaged)
Nonadrenergic noncholinergic nerves	CGRP[a]	CGRP receptors	Modest vasodilation by opening K_{ATP} channels[b]

NO, nitric oxide; NE, norepinephrine; E, epinephrine; ACh, acetylcholine.
[a] Yaoita et al. *Circ Res* 1994;75:780.
[b] Nelson and Braydin. *Cardiovasc Drug Ther* 1993;7:605

7-14). The net result of these vasoconstrictor stimuli is an increase in free cytosolic calcium in the vascular smooth cells with formation of calcium-calmodulin (see Chapter 9) and activation of myosin light-chain kinase. Such vasoconstrictory adrenergic influences are opposed by two vasodilatory autonomic influences: first, the vasodilatory β-adrenergic receptors, and second, the vasodilatory parasympathetic cholinergic receptors. In addition, there are several platelet-derived substances, such as serotonin, that are vasodilatory only when the vascular endothelium is intact, to become vasoconstrictory when the endothelium is damaged. Cholinergic stimulation, normally vasodilatory because it releases nitric oxide (previously called the endothelium-derived relaxation factor [EDRF]), also becomes vasoconstrictory when the endothelium is damaged. Thus, there are at least three essential regulators of coronary tone: (1) the metabolic vasodilatory system, (2) the neurogenic control system, both vasoconstrictory and vasodilatory, and (3) the vascular endothelium, which can be either vasodilatory by releasing nitric oxide or vasoconstrictory by releasing endothelin (see Chapter 9). Another vasoconstrictor is angiotensin II (AII) which probably couples to the same IP_3 vasoconstrictor signal system, as does endothelin and α-receptor activity (see Chapter 9). Such AII-mediated vasoconstriction is probably of major significance only in diseased states. Of these complex control mechanisms, there is a major role for metabolic vasodilation in response to situations requiring an increased coronary blood flow, such as augmented heart work or ischemia.

Metabolic Control and Adenosine

Local metabolic control appears to be the most important mechanism that matches increases in the oxygen consumption and metabolic demand of the heart to the required increase in coronary blood flow. The precise mediators remain to

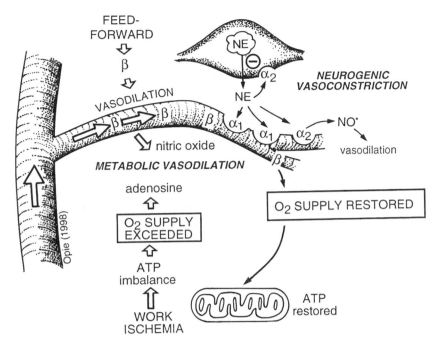

FIG. 10-3. Metabolic vasodilators. The role of vasodilators, including adenosine and nitric oxide, in local metabolic control of the coronary circulation. As a result of heart work or ischemia, the rate at which the oxygen supply to the mitochondria can synthesize ATP is temporarily exceeded so that ATP breaks down to form adenosine. Nitric oxide is released from the healthy endothelium. Neurogenic factors are both vasodilatory (β-adrenergic) and vasoconstrictory (α-adrenergic).

be identified (Muller et al., 1996). According to the hypothesis of Berne (1964), adenosine plays a critical but probably not solitary role in the local metabolic regulation of changes in the coronary circulation (Fig. 10-3). It does not help maintain coronary vascular tone in basal conditions. Adenosine is formed within the myocardial cells when, as a result of hypoxia, ischemia, or vigorous heart work, high-energy phosphate compounds are broken down. Because the molar ratio of ATP to adenosine is very high, perhaps about 1,000 to one, only a small decrease of ATP can activate the pathways producing adenosine, acting particularly at the level of the 5'-nucleotidase (Fig. 10-4). This enzyme converts adenosine monophosphate (AMP) to adenosine at the inner border of the sarcolemma. Most of the adenosine leaves the cell to reach the extracellular space, where it acts on the arteriolar vessel wall as a vasodilator. Adenosine does not have to penetrate the vascular cell to vasodilate. It can dilate even when firmly attached to molecules that prevent penetration. However, it is presumed that adenosine usually penetrates into the vascular muscle cell, where it acts to vasodilate. When adenosine reaches the circulation, it is broken down by *adenosine deami-*

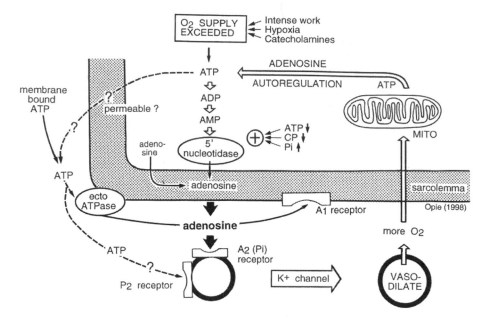

FIG. 10-4. Adenosine as vasodilator. Adenosine formed from ATP in conditions of increased myocardial work or hypoxia is thought to interact with a vascular A_2 receptor (see Table 7-1) to cause vasodilation. ATP may act as an additional dilator. CP, creatine phosphate; Pi, inorganic phosphate.

nase (Fig. 10-5), present both in red cells and in the vessel wall. Agents such as dipyridamole inhibit adenosine deaminase, allow adenosine to accumulate, and increase coronary vasodilation. Because it is chiefly the small and intermediate *resistance arterioles* (less than 100 μm in diameter) that are dilated by adenosine, the enhanced coronary flow in normal zones may steal much needed blood flow from the ischemic myocardium so that these agents, which act by increasing adenosine formation, have limited antianginal potential. Somewhat surprisingly, the methylxanthines, including the bronchodilator theophylline, compete with adenosine for the vascular sites, thereby inhibiting the vasodilation caused by adenosine.

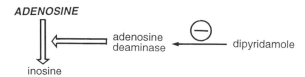

FIG. 10-5. Coronary vascular reserve is measured by the principle of maximum vasodilation achieved, for example, by the inhibition of adenosine deaminase activity by the drug dipyridamole.

Because adenosine is a purine compound, it acts on *purinergic receptors*. These are further subdivided into the P_1-receptors sensitive to adenosine and the P_2-receptors sensitive to ATP. The P_1-receptors can be further subdivided into the *A_1-myocardial receptors* and *A_2-vascular receptors* (see Table 7-1). The myocardial receptors inhibit the formation of cyclic AMP (cAMP), acting on the inhibitory G protein, G_i, and hyperpolarize nodal cells (see Fig. 5-10), so that adenosine in high doses arrests the heart by two mechanisms. The vascular A_2-receptors situated on the vascular smooth muscle cells stimulate the formation of cAMP, thereby giving a second mechanism for coronary artery dilation. The adenosine hypothesis is widely accepted as explaining part of the coronary vasodilation resulting during hypoxia or ischemia. During physiologic exercise, the evidence that adenosine plays a role is not strong (Bache et al., 1988), and endothelial-dependent factors such as formation of nitric oxide or other metabolic vasodilators are probably at work.

Nonetheless, the adenosine hypothesis has been recast in a new mode by the discovery of the ATP-sensitive potassium channel, which when open causes hyperpolarization of the vascular smooth muscle cells and coronary vasodilation (see Fig. 9-14). These channels are normally inhibited by ATP, even in low concentrations, but adenosine is one of the factors relieving this inhibition. Thus, when adenosine formation is increased as in severe heart work or ischemia (Chapter 11), then there is preliminary evidence that this mechanism may operate (Muller et al., 1996).

Other Metabolic Vasodilators

Oxygen and carbon dioxide.   A decreasing tissue oxygen and increasing carbon dioxide tension (pCO_2) may account for about 40% of the changes in coronary flow during pacing (Broten et al., 1991). Hypoxia may act as a vasodilator by opening the ATP-sensitive potassium channels (Nelson and Brayden, 1993). An increasing pCO_2 may act similarly to intracellular acidosis.

Protons produced by anaerobic metabolism have a direct effect in causing coronary vasodilation and also sensitize the coronary arteries to the effects of added adenosine.

ATP is normally found within the cell and does not cross the sarcolemma. There is an unexpected controversial proposal that small amounts of superficial ATP (Fig. 10-4) liberated by hypoxic or working heart muscle into the circulation can have a vasodilatory effect. Measurements of ATP and adenosine in the effluent from the hypoxic heart argue against a direct vasodilatory role of ATP (Vial et al., 1987).

Potassium in a modestly increased concentration is also vasodilatory, whereas very high values vasoconstrict. The mechanisms involved are complex and include effects on neurotransmitters and adrenergic receptors, as well as release of nitric oxide by potassium (Rubanyi and Vanhoutte, 1988). When extracellular potassium is sufficiently high, it depolarizes the cell membrane to

increase the opening probability of the calcium channel, leading to vasoconstriction.

Atrial natriuretic peptide (ANP) is released from the atria in response to
stretch. ANP promotes diuresis and renal loss of sodium. In addition, ANP is an
arterial vasodilator, acting on guanylate cyclase.

Prostaglandins can be released into coronary venous blood when angina is
provoked by rapid pacing of the heart. Therefore, it is not surprising that
prostaglandins have been regarded as physiologic vasodilators. These early
observations have been supported by the isolation of *prostacyclin (PGI₂)*, which
is made by the endothelium, powerfully relaxing coronary arteries and inhibiting
platelet aggregation. The real role, if any, for prostaglandins in the control of the
coronary circulation is still controversial.

Endothelial-Dependent Dilation and Nitric Oxide

The crucial role of an intact vascular endothelium in determining vascular
smooth muscle tone has already been discussed (see Chapter 9). In response to
well-defined stimuli, healthy endothelial cells liberate a short-lived vasodilatory
factor, now known to be nitric oxide or a very similar compound, previously
called EDRF. Nitric oxide vasodilates because it stimulates guanylate cyclase in
the vascular smooth muscle to form cyclic guanosine monophosphate (cGMP)
and inhibits platelet aggregation by increasing the platelet level of cGMP to
decrease cytosolic calcium, i.e., to promote vasorelaxation. Therefore, the risk of

A. **NORMAL VESSEL**

FLOW ➡ Nitric oxide release (⇧)

⌈ dilation
⌊ antiaggregation (o=platelet)

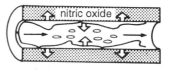

B. **FLOW LIMITING STENOSIS**

⬇FLOW   : ⬇ Nitric oxide

⌈ loss of dilation
⌊ loss of antiaggregation

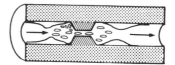

C. **DILATION OF STENOSIS**

⬆FLOW   ⬆ Nitric oxide

– release from
   adjacent endothelium

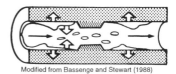

Modified from Bassenge and Stewart (1988)

FIG. 10-6. Flow-dependent coronary dilation is diminished in severe coronary stenosis. In
response to dilation of coronary stenosis, for example by angioplasty, increased release of nitric
oxide causes dilation of the artery downstream from the site of stenosis. Antiaggregation, inhibition of platelet aggregation by nitric oxide. (Modified from Bassenge and Stewart. *Cardiovasc
Drugs Ther* 1988;2:27–34.)

occlusion of small arterioles in response to physiologically induced platelet aggregation is lessened. Nitric oxide is released by vascular shear forces associated with increased coronary flow (Fig. 10-6). In addition, when platelets aggregate, as tends to occur in response to catecholamine stimulation as part of the stress reaction, they release serotonin and adenosine diphosphate, both of which stimulate nitric oxide release from the healthy endothelium. When the coronary perfusion pressure increases, as in exercise, the flow also tends to follow suit. The increased flow releases more nitric oxide from the endothelium. Such *flow-induced vasodilation* may occur in exercise independently of the formation of adenosine (Bache et al., 1988).

When the endothelium is damaged, as in coronary artery disease, the release of nitric oxide is diminished and the release of vasoconstrictory endothelin is increased. In the presence of coronary artery disease and endothelial damage, platelet aggregation occurs and is likely to release vasoconstrictory factors from the endothelium, which may precipitate myocardial ischemia. In such conditions, the vasoconstrictory stimuli overcome metabolic vasodilation. Some clinical workers believe that such a sequence is at the basis of *unstable angina*, when severe repetitive ischemic chest pain heralds the more serious event of myocardial infarction.

AUTONOMIC CONTROL

Sympathetic stimulation activates vasoconstricting α-adrenergic receptors in the coronary arteries (Fig. 10-7). Whether such α-mediated vasoconstriction

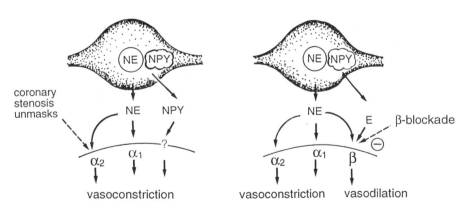

FIG. 10-7. Neurogenic vasodilation. Physiologically, the catecholamines norepinephrine (NE) and epinephrine (E) both mediate coronary vasodilation. The positive inotropic effect also indirectly promotes vasodilation. In coronary disease, norepinephrine released from the terminal neurons may cause vasoconstriction. Increasing coronary stenosis may unmask α₂-mediated vasoconstriction. β-adrenergic blockade by propranolol may promote unopposed vasoconstriction. NPY, neuropeptide Y, a vasoconstrictor coreleased with NE (Warner and Levy, 1990) and hypothetically playing a role in coronary spasm.

serves any physiologic function still remains to be shown (Baumgart et al., 1993). One view is as follows (Muller et al., 1996). Supposing that during exercise, as part of sympathetic stimulation, there is increased α-adrenergic receptor activation with constriction of arterioles greater than 100 μm in diameter, then the lowered pressure in the downstream arterioles could induce myogenic vasodilation.

Adrenergic Receptor Subtypes. α_1-Receptor-mediated coronary vasoconstriction acts chiefly on the larger coronary arteries, whereas both α_1- and α_2-receptor activity are involved in regulating the degree of vasoconstriction of the smaller resistance vessels (Heusch, 1990). Enhanced sympathetic tone may increase flow through small arterioles when the circulation is healthy. When there is a decrease in coronary perfusion pressure, then vasoconstriction mediated by both receptor subtypes occurs throughout the coronary microcirculation (Muller et al., 1996). Thus, in the presence of coronary disease, adrenergic stimuli such as emotional stress or cold exposure or smoking could lead to a relative preponderance of α-adrenergic vasoconstrictive mechanisms, with increased risk of myocardial ischemia. α_2-postjunctional adrenergic receptors could have greater functional significance when adrenergic activity is enhanced, as in heart failure (Parker et al., 1995). Experimentally, coronary stenosis unmasks α_2-adrenergic activity (Fig. 10-7), perhaps because endothelial damage removes the vasodilatory effects of nitric oxide.

Neuropeptide Y is co-stored and co-released with norepinephrine from adrenergic terminal neurons, and the ratio of its release to that of norepinephrine increases with sympathetic stimulation (Fig. 10-7). Neuropeptide Y is concentrated around the coronary arteries and is a potent vasoconstrictor. It may, hypothetically, contribute to coronary vasoconstriction at high levels of sympathetic activation.

Vasodilatory Coronary Vascular β-Adrenergic Receptors. In addition to vasoconstrictory α-adrenergic receptors, there are coronary β-adrenergic receptors that, when stimulated, should lead to vasodilation. On first principles, it might be expected that coronary vascular β-receptors should be of the noncardiac β_2 subtype, yet the contrary may be the case (Amenta et al., 1991; Murphree and Saffitz, 1988). Different β-receptor subtypes may regulate coronary resistance in the small vessels (β_2-receptors) than in the larger vessels (chiefly β_1). In large human coronary arteries, β_1-receptors dominate and are localized to the muscular medial layer (Amenta et al., 1991). According to the *feed-forward* hypothesis, β-stimulation by norepinephrine causes vasodilation of healthy coronary arteries, independently of any increase in heart rate or contractility (Miyashiro and Feigl, 1993). In the presence of a diseased endothelium, however, norepinephrine is likely to have predominantly coronary vasoconstrictive effects.

Cholinergic Coronary Vasodilation. Acetylcholine, the cholinergic messenger, is a powerful coronary vasodilator when given by the intracoronary route in the presence of an intact endothelium, acting by release of nitric oxide. Yet with vagal stimulation, the dilator response is transient and weak.

To summarize these extremely complex control mechanisms, the major effect of sympathetic α-adrenergic stimulation is vasoconstriction to increase the tone of both large and small coronary arteries, and this is overridden by metabolic vasodilation and feed-forward β-adrenergic vasodilation. The net effect is coronary vasodilation during exercise when the coronary arteries are healthy, but when they are diseased and the endothelium does not secrete nitric oxide, then overall vasoconstriction is more likely.

CORONARY FLOW VARIATIONS

Reactive hyperemia is a phenomenon somewhat better explained by the metabolic than by the neurogenic theories of coronary control. When the coronary arteries are transiently occluded and then reperfused, there is a period of apparent overperfusion as the blood flow increases substantially for a short period. Such reactive hyperemia can be found in patients in whom the coronary artery is briefly occluded by a balloon during percutaneous transluminal angioplasty, a procedure used increasingly to relieve certain types of coronary artery disease. Adenosine appears to be involved because when adenosine receptors are blocked by theophylline, reactive hyperemia is reduced by 40% to 100% (Warner and Levy, 1990). Also, in response to intracoronary adenosine, there is marked coronary hyperemia similar to that caused by papaverine (Wilson et al., 1990). Additionally, flow-induced vasodilation may be operative (Muller et al., 1996).

The complex mechanisms, chiefly metabolic, whereby coronary blood flow can increase severalfold to meet the increased demands placed on the circulation during exercise emphasize the capacity for coronary vasodilation.

Phasic Coronary Flow

The changing intraventricular pressures during the cardiac cycle will alter coronary flow. During systole, subendocardial but not subepicardial arteries are compressed (Fig. 10-8). An important hypothesis is that systolic blood flow in the subendocardium decreases and even stops as the left ventricular pressure increases to compress the arteriolar flow, whereas conversely, subendocardial blood flow increases in diastole. Of the total coronary flow, most occurs in diastole. The remaining component occurs in systole but chiefly in the epicardial zone. Early diastolic flow, which is the peak flow rate, can be impaired when the rate of myocardial relaxation in early diastole decreases, as in ischemia and reperfusion (Domalik-Wawrzynski et al., 1987). When the coronary perfusion pressure is increased experimentally (Fig. 10-9), then both systolic and diastolic components of epicardial flow increase, with diastolic flow dominating (Recchia et al., 1996).

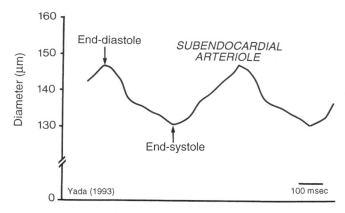

FIG. 10-8. Epicardial arteriolar diameter in systole and diastole. Adapted from Yada et al. (1993), with permission of American Heart Association.

When the normal phasic coronary flow is impaired, there is greater risk of periodic platelet aggregation, especially in the presence of endothelial damage, which can worsen the reduction in the cyclical flow.

Coronary Autoregulation

The process whereby coronary flow is regulated by the myocardial oxygen demand independently of the arterial perfusion pressure is called *autoregulation*,

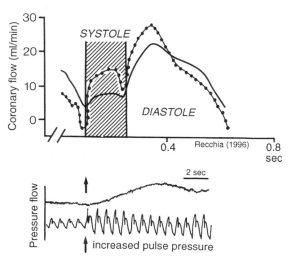

FIG. 10-9. Phasic coronary flow: effect of systole (S) and diastole on phasic coronary flow in dogs. The dotted lines indicate increased pulse pressure (see bottom panel) as may occur during exercise. Adapted from Recchia et al. (1996), with permission of the American Heart Association.

which basically means that coronary blood flow stays relatively constant within wide limits of blood pressure changes (Fig. 10-10). This mechanism helps to protect the myocardium against sudden changes in blood pressure. Most of the autoregulation takes place in coronary arterioles larger than 150 μm in diameter, but smaller arterioles may be recruited as the perfusion pressure progressively decreases (Chilian and Layne, 1990). There are definite limits to autoregulation above which an increased perfusion will augment coronary flow and below which myocardial ischemia will result. In the presence of severe coronary stenosis, when the coronary perfusion pressure decreases below 50 mm Hg, coronary autoregulation is progressively lost. The signal systems involved in autoregulation are not fully understood; at the lower end of the range both formation of nitric oxide (Smith and Canty, 1993) and opening of the vascular ATP-sensitive potassium channel may play a role (Narishige et al., 1993). In addition, myogenic regulation may be involved (Chilian and Layne, 1990).

Myogenic Control.   Such control originates in the intrinsic properties of the vascular smooth muscle (hence the name "myogenic"). Vascular smooth muscle responds to increased force by contracting, so that an alternate name is "stretch-induced contraction." That is, as the distending pressure across the vessel wall increases, so does the inherent vascular tone, and vice versa. The inherent tendency of an increased intravascular pressure to distend the vessel is opposed, so that myogenic control could contribute to coronary autoregula-

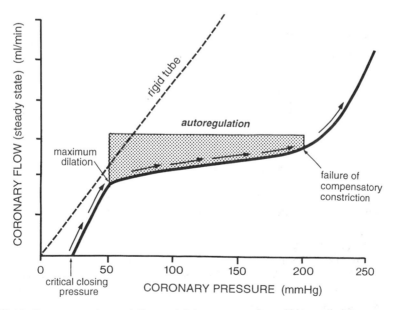

FIG. 10-10. Coronary autoregulation maintains coronary flow within a rather narrow range.

tion, particularly in coronary arterioles less than 100 μm in diameter (Muller et al., 1996). The mechanism of myogenic tone is not understood, but stretch-activated channels could be important.

Exercise

Coronary blood flow can almost double during acute exercise in conscious dogs (Vogel et al., 1982), and during heavy exercise in humans, the flow may increase three times (see second edition of this book). The explanation includes the increased mean arterial pressure of exercise (see Chapter 15), with a greater coronary perfusion pressure and a greater pulse pressure (Fig. 10-9). Factors improving systolic flow may include β-adrenergic–induced vasodilation and flow-induced formation of nitric oxide. When nitric oxide synthesis is inhibited, then the coronary vasodilation of exercise is much less (Wang et al., 1993). Such formation of nitric oxide is probably induced by the effect of mechanical shear stress on the endothelium (Fig. 10-6). Nitric oxide may have an additional metabolic effect by decreasing the myocardial oxygen uptake for a given workload (Bernstein et al., 1996), rendering the heart more efficient and decreasing the oxygen requirement.

Garden Hose and Erectile Effects

To recapitulate, the accepted view is that the coronary arteries dilate in response to an increased myocardial oxygen demand. Although the evidence for this supposition is good (Schulz et al., 1991), there is also some evidence for an opposite sequence of events (Opie, 1965), as originally found by Gregg (1963). The proposed explanation may be that the greater coronary flow may stiffen the ventricle, thereby increasing the oxygen demand (Iwamoto et al., 1994; Vogel et al., 1982). Colorful names such as the "garden hose" or "erectile" effect have perhaps given this phenomenon more prominence than it deserves. Nonetheless, it is logical that as coronary flow decreases during coronary occlusion, there will be a reversed erectile effect as the arteries empty, so that the ischemic segments will have less work to do.

EFFECT OF ISCHEMIA ON CORONARY FLOW

Before considering the complex and highly variable effects of coronary disease on coronary flow, the consequences of ischemia by itself need evaluation. Experimental ischemia will vasodilate by two mechanisms. First, there will be breakdown of ATP to adenosine (Fig. 10-4). Second, lack of ATP will activate the *ATP-sensitive potassium channel*, K_{ATP}. Opening of this channel may contribute to early potassium loss from the ischemic myocardium and to the associated electrocardiographic (ECG) changes (see Chapter 17). Even during exercise, such ischemia-induced vasodilation is not maximal, possibly owing to the influence of neurogenic vasoconstriction induced by α-adrenergic receptor stimulation or due to the commonly associated endothelial dysfunction. Hypothetically, drugs closing this channel, such as the oral antidiabetic agent glibenclamide, may prevent ischemia-mediated vasodilation. Therefore, in diabetic patients with acute myocardial infarction, it may be preferable to avoid such agents and to change antidiabetic therapy to insulin (Hofmann and Opie, 1993).

CORONARY DISEASE

The effects of coronary artery disease on the coronary arteries are highly variable, from diffuse damage to a localized narrowing or stenosis. Ischemia has many different consequences. First, the direct hemodynamic effect of coronary stenosis is to decrease the coronary perfusion pressure in the distal segment of the diseased artery. Second, the indirect effect of tissue ischemia causes contractile failure, thereby increasing the left ventricular end-diastolic pressure, which, in turn, compresses subendocardial tissue and reduces coronary perfusion further to increase ischemia (Fig. 10-2). Third, as discussed in the preceding section, ischemia has direct vasodilatory effects on the coronary circulation, acting by formation of adenosine and opening of the ATP-sensitive vascular potassium channel. Fourth, because the vascular endothelium is damaged in coronary artery disease, such vasodilatory stimuli are usually overcome by endothelium-mediated vasoconstrictory force.

To reduce coronary flow by stenosis requires a large reduction in arterial lumen. The most important factor is the severity of the stenosis and the consequent increase in resistance to blood flow across the stenosis (Klocke, 1983). The resistance increases by a power of 4 as the radius decreases (Poiseuille's law), and reducing the internal diameter from 80% to 90% dramatically elevates the resistance (Fig. 10-11). Resting flow is not affected until the stenosis is very severe, and one estimate is that a 70% reduction of internal diameter with a 90% to 95% decrease in luminal area is required for basal coronary flow to decrease. When the internal diameter is reduced beyond 30%, maximal vasodilation flow starts to be impaired (Klocke, 1983).

For a given severity of stenosis, the longer the stenotic segment, the more marked the effects of any given degree of occlusion. For any given degree of *fixed coronary stenosis*, there are complex additional factors, such as the degree of turbulence across the stenosis and added vascular spasm, which may further decrease the flow (*dynamic stenosis*).

As the coronary perfusion pressure decreases below the limits of autoregulation (Fig. 10-10), the extraction of oxygen from the arterial blood increases. Nonetheless, because extraction is normally nearly complete (Parsons et al., 1993), this mechanism cannot fully compensate so that tissue oxygen stores of hemoglobin and myoglobin decrease, and the respiratory chain cytochromes become less oxidized. When the myocardial blood flow decreases below 50% of control, tissue oxygen stores decrease to a minimum (Fig. 10-12) and any further flow reduction

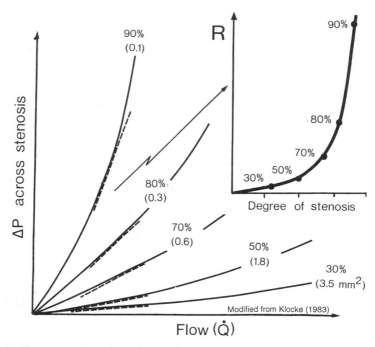

FIG. 10-11. Coronary stenosis and vascular resistance. The effect of the severity of coronary stenosis (internal diameter) on vascular resistance (R) (Klocke, 1983). %, percentage reduction of internal diameter.

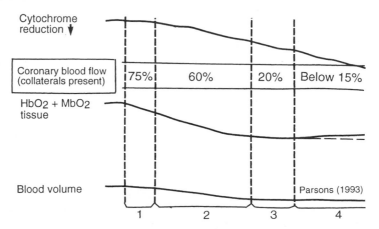

FIG. 10-12. Progressive flow reduction in left anterior descending coronary artery in dog. Note initial protective role of tissue oxygen stores (myoglobin and hemoglobin) with progressive reduction of respiratory chain cytochrome enzymes. Modified from Parsons et al. (1993), with permission of American Heart Association.

means that the respiratory chain becomes even less oxidized (Fig. 10-12). The result is the development of anaerobic metabolism (see Chapter 11).

Coronary Vascular Resistance in Coronary Stenosis

Just as the peripheral vascular resistance can be calculated from the aortic pressure divided by the cardiac output (see Chapter 14), so the coronary vascular resistance (CVR) is calculated from the following formula.

$$CVR = \frac{\text{aortic pressure}}{\text{coronary flow}}$$

The CVR of a stenosed coronary artery is called the *stenosis resistance*. It must not be supposed that the stenosis resistance is necessarily fixed. The influence of dynamic stenosis has already been described. Hemodynamic factors also are important. In severe stenosis, the poststenotic pressure can decrease below a certain critical value of about 50 mm Hg required for normal vasodilation and autoregulation (Klocke, 1983). The failure of compensatory vasodilation further robs the already ischemic myocardium of blood flow. In the presence of severe subendocardial or transmural ischemia, there is left ventricular failure, which increases the intracavity pressure and further decreases the actual perfusion (driving) pressure across the stenosis. Other mechanical and flow factors also can determine the stenosis resistance. For example, peripheral vasodilation with a decrease in the perfusion pressure available to the coronary stenosis may passively narrow the stenotic segment, or platelet aggregation may further impair flow. Such variable stenosis resistance may account for the variable oxygen demand at which effort angina occurs.

If the coronary perfusion pressure decreases low enough, below a certain value (about 20 to 40 mm Hg), the capillaries clam up and shut—*the critical closing pressure* (Fig. 10-10). The mechanism is controversial. During reperfusion after ischemia, restoration of blood flow may be impaired because of persistent critical closing, because of endothelial damage and swelling, and because of release of endothelin.

Poststenotic Coronary Flow

Distal to a flow-limiting coronary stenosis, several factors help to vasodilate. Nitric oxide production decreases as the flow rate decreases, yet hypoxia compensates to some extent by increasing the production of nitric oxide (Duncker and Bache, 1994). As already discussed, adenosine production from ATP breakdown will dilate small resistance vessels. The vascular ATP-sensitive K^+ channel is also likely to open, thereby promoting metabolic vasodilation (Gollasch et al., 1996).

Anatomic Site of the Occluded Artery: Collateral Flow

The severity of ischemia is greater when a main left coronary artery rather than a branch is restricted, probably because collateral flow is better maintained with smaller ischemic lesions resulting from branch occlusions. Once subendocardial ischemia has occurred, left ventricular failure compresses the coronary arteries further, and an advancing wave-front phenomenon occurs and the epicardial zones are eventually involved (Fig. 10-13). With occlusion of smaller coronary arteries, subendocardial flow first decreases, with metabolic changes developing at about 60% and contractility and ECG changes at 75% flow reduction (Gregg and Bedynek, 1978). With major artery occlusions, such events occur with lesser flow reductions.

The *collateral flow* is the coronary blood flow reaching the ischemic zone by means of alternate arteries that have developed and supply the zone that was formerly reached by the occluded artery (*collateral*, coming in from the side). In some species, such as the guinea pig, collateral flow is so extensive that even complete coronary artery occlusion by ligation results in no detectable ischemia. In other species, such as the rat, the flow is so low that severe ischemia results—as Schaper has so eloquently stated, "guinea pigs win the rat race" (1984). In humans, it is thought that gradual coronary occlusion provokes a variable growth

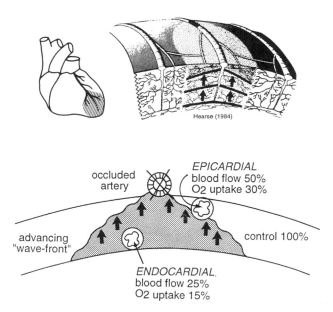

FIG. 10-13. Complete coronary occlusion damages subendocardial tissue first. A wavefront phenomenon then involves the epicardial zones, according to the model of Reimer et al. (*Circulation* 1977;56:786–794). The mechanism is probably by a progressive increase in subendocardial pressure as the left ventricle fails. (Upper right panel is reproduced with permission of Professor David Hearse).

TABLE 10-4. *Metabolic vasodilation*

Agent	Site of action	Signal system
Adenosine	Resistance arterioles <100 μm	A_2 receptor, promotes formation of vasodilatory cAMP
Nitric oxide	Resistance arterioles >200 μm	Guanylate cyclase, cGMP
ATP	ATP-sensitive K^+ channel	Decreased ATP and increased adenosine remove inhibition by ATP on channel opening

of collateral arteries, and the results of complete arterial occlusion vary significantly from patient to patient. Never is the collateral flow high enough in humans to align them to guinea pigs.

Subendocardial Ischemia

A traditional point of view has been that the subendocardial zone of the heart has a lower oxygen tension and a more anaerobic type of metabolism. The lower oxygen tension could cause a lower oxygen uptake. When the coronary flow is reduced, the endocardial zone suffers from even lower values of oxygen tension (Fig. 10-13), and there is greater depletion of creatine phosphate and more accumulation of lactate.

Subendocardial layers, being subject to greater mechanical stress, require an increased oxygen uptake, which accounts for the lower tissue oxygen tension and higher rates of oxidative metabolism (Table 10-4). A higher rather than lower capillary density in the endocardial zones also supports the idea of a higher rate of oxidative metabolism in the subendocardium. These metabolic factors, in addition to blood flow factors, may account for the increased vulnerability of the subendocardium to ischemic damage with increased risk of necrosis.

CORONARY ARTERY VASOCONSTRICTION AND SPASM

Besides anatomic stenosis resulting from coronary artery disease, a second mechanism of coronary artery narrowing is by vasoconstriction (Fig. 10-14). Sometimes, especially in the large epicardial arteries, the vasoconstriction is focal and called *coronary spasm*. When the narrowing caused by such spasm is added to organic coronary artery disease, the term is *dynamic stenosis*, which can be relieved by drugs inducing coronary vasodilation, such as the nitrates or calcium antagonists. Clinically, the degree of vasoconstriction or coronary spasm is thought to be variable, with the critical finding being the induction of myocardial ischemia at rest and not by effort as in the case of classic angina. The result can vary from minor degrees of vasoconstriction shown only by certain changes on the ECG (asymptomatic ST-segment deviations, thought to result from different degrees of ischemic loss of potassium) to transmural ischemia

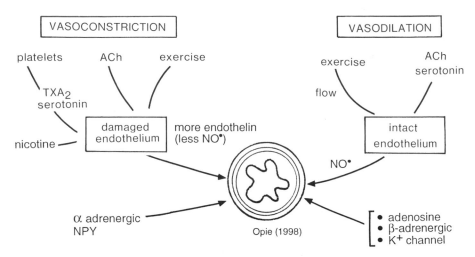

FIG. 10-14. Endothelium and coronary diameter. The endothelium plays an important role in determining the degree of coronary vasoconstriction or coronary vasodilation in response to certain stimuli such as acetylcholine (ACh), exercise, and serotonin released from damaged platelets. When the endothelium is intact, exercise, acetylcholine, and serotonin are all vasodilatory, acting by release of nitric oxide. Exercise may act by release of adenosine, by β-adrenergic stimulation, and by flow-mediated release of nitric oxide (see Fig. 10-6). In the presence of a damaged endothelium, these factors promote vasoconstriction, possibly by the release of endothelin. In addition, β-adrenergic stimuli become vasoconstrictive instead of vasodilatory. Besides releasing serotonin, platelets also release thromboxane-A_2 (TXA$_2$). Vasoconstrictory stimuli enhance the risk of coronary vasoconstrictive spasm. NPY, neuropeptide Y; see Fig. 10-7.

with severe chest pain at rest and the typical ST-segment elevation of what is called *Prinzmetal's angina.*

There are two explanations for the association of spasm and organic stenosis. First, platelet thrombi may form at the stenotic site to liberate agents, such as *serotonin* and *thromboxane* A_2, which are vasoconstrictive in the presence of endothelial damage. White cells (leukocytes) may liberate other vasoconstrictive substances called *leukotrienes.* Second, coronary atheroma damages the vascular endothelium with lessened production of several vasodilating substances, including nitric oxide and the vasodilatory prostaglandin (PGI$_2$), and enhanced production of vasoconstrictory endothelin. Endothelial damage may remove some physiologic vasodilatory influences to allow the arteries to become sensitized to vasoconstrictive stimuli. Cigarette smoking promotes coronary spasm (Sugiishi and Takatsu, 1993), hypothetically by causing endothelial damage. Nonetheless, the exact vasoconstrictory mechanism in coronary artery spasm in humans still has not been identified despite intensive studies.

Abnormal Coronary Vasomotion. The normal coronary response to exercise is vasodilation, whereas in coronary disease there is vasoconstriction, also called abnormal vasomotion (Kaufmann et al., 1995). Likewise in hypertensives there is impaired coronary vasodilation on exercise, even when there is no visible angiographic evidence of coronary artery disease (Frielingsdorf et al., 1996). The most probable explanation is that both coronary disease and hypertension cause endothelial dysfunction.

CORONARY FLOW RESERVE

The *coronary vascular reserve* (or coronary vasodilatory reserve or coronary flow reserve) is measured by the ratios of the coronary flow found during the period of reactive hyperemia and basal coronary flow. Methods of achieving maximal flow include (1) intracoronary administration of the drug dipyridamole, which inhibits the breakdown of adenosine (Fig. 10-5), and (2) the evocation of maximal hyperemic flow after the transient ischemia caused by injection of the radio-opaque contrast material used for coronary angiography. Coronary vascular reserve is reduced in ischemic heart disease, by chronic smoking, and in the hypertrophied myocardium of chronic hypertension or aortic stenosis. Mechanisms whereby coronary vascular reserve is reduced in the hypertrophied myocardium, even in the absence of any apparent coronary artery disease, may relate either to small vessel damage (microvascular disease) or to endothelial damage evoked by the shear forces associated with a sustained blood pressure increase.

MYOCARDIAL BLOOD FLOW MEASUREMENTS

Although coronary blood flow can be measured experimentally by several techniques, including flow probes, the actual rate of delivery of blood to the myocardium requires different techniques. In animals, radiolabeled microspheres provide an accurate index of regional myocardial blood flow. Such microspheres are injected into the circulation and are then caught in the capillaries throughout the heart. The dissected tissue is analyzed, and the flow in that segment of tissue is proportional to the counts. Using this method, coronary blood flow can be measured even in minute areas of the myocardium. If different radionuclide traces are used, coronary blood flow before or after an intervention can be quantified precisely. Microsphere data in dogs show a normal resting myocardial blood flow of about 100 ml/100 g/min with about 70 ml/100 g/min in pigs. Such values correspond rather well with the results obtained in humans with an entirely different technique, namely the use of positron emission tomography (PET).

Positron emission tomography in humans uses ^{13}N-ammonia as an indicator of myocardial blood flow (Camici et al., 1996). The principle is that dynamic imaging monitors the uptake and retention of the tracer ^{13}N-NH$_3$. Technical refinements allow the separation of the first arrival phase, dependent on blood flow, with distinction from the later myocardial retention phase, which depends on conversion of the ammonia into the amino acid glutamine. It is assumed that the rate of conversion of ammonia to glutamine remains constant and can be compensated for mathematically. Even if uncorrected, however, this factor is only about 10%. The rate constant (K_1) for delivery of ^{13}N-NH$_3$ into the tissue incorporates a mass factor (i.e., positrons emitted per unit mass), so that the myocardial blood flow is ultimately given as, for example, 90 to 100 ml/100 g/min (Camici et al., 1996). Similar values are found if H$_2$^{15}O is used as the tracer. This technique allows more frequent repetition of flow measurements because of the shorter half-life of ^{15}O than of ^{13}N, but the image quality is better with ^{13}N (De Silva and Camici, 1994). Values for myocardial blood flow obtained by PET in humans correspond well with other techniques and with microsphere data in large animals such as dogs and pigs. PET also can image glucose extraction. Therefore, it is possible to compare the uptake of ^{18}F-deoxyglucose relative to that of ^{13}N-ammonia, the ratio being increased in reversible ischemia. The major problems with PET are its great expense, as well as its limited spatial and transmural resolution.

Thallium 201 (^{201}Tl) is an analog of potassium, and its uptake by the myocardium is impaired in ischemia. The myocardial distribution of ^{201}Tl is the result of two processes. The initial distribution reflects the distribution of the coronary blood flow to the various zones of the myocardium. The second phase of redistribution reflects actual uptake by the myocardial cells. The uptake of thallium by the myocardium is dependent on the same sodium-potassium pump (Na$^+$-K$^+$-ATPase) that transports potassium, but thallium binds 10 times more avidly at two sites as compared with the one site for potassium. In the underperfused but potentially viable myocardium, both the uptake and washout of ^{201}Tl are slow, so that in time the levels of radioactivity in the normal and ischemic zones tend to equalize. In infarcted, scarred myocardium, the tissue cannot take up ^{201}Tl, and no equalization can occur. These differences can be useful in distinguishing the potential viability of poorly contracting myocardial segments. Nonetheless, thallium studies do not give absolute blood flow measurements.

SUMMARY

1. *Capillaries.* The myocardium has a rich supply of capillaries, with about one capillary for each myofiber. Normally, not all the capillaries are open. Recruitment, or opening up of capillaries, occurs when the myocardial oxygen demand increases during exercise or ischemia, so that the available oxygen has a shorter distance to diffuse to the mitochondria where it is required.
2. *Regulation of the caliber of the coronary arterial tree.* There are four major systems. First, metabolic mechanisms respond to exercise or ischemia. A small fraction of the ATP broken down is converted ultimately to the vasodilator adenosine, a mechanism less important than previously thought. Second, the healthy vascular endothelium produces the important vasodilator nitric oxide, previously called EDRF. Third, neural stimulation also regulates the extent of vasodilation. Adrenergic stimulation causes both

vasodilatory β-adrenergic stimuli and vasoconstrictory α-adrenergic stimuli. Fourth, myogenic control is still poorly understood but important.

3. *During exercise, coronary flow increases substantially.* Flow-mediated release of nitric oxide from the endothelium is important, but all the exact signals are not yet known.

4. *Ischemia* promotes vasodilation, acting both by formation of adenosine and by opening of the ATP-sensitive potassium channels.

5. *In coronary artery disease,* the vascular endothelium is damaged, with lessened release of nitric oxide and increased activity of vasoconstrictory endothelin. Thus, normal vasodilatory stimuli, including serotonin released from platelets during their aggregation, can become vasoconstrictory. Thus the normal vasodilatory effect of ischemia per se is overcome by the effects of associated endothelial dysfunction, which results in endothelial-mediated coronary vasoconstriction or even spasm.

6. *Positron emission tomography* measures coronary blood flow in humans by monitoring the uptake of ^{13}N-NH$_3$. It becomes a powerful tool when combined with the uptake of glucose to estimate the viability of tissue in coronary artery disease.

STUDENT QUESTIONS

1. Nitric oxide. What is it? Where and how is it formed? What are its physiologic effects?
2. What is the coronary vascular resistance? Why is it important?
3. Describe the autonomic control of the coronary arteries?
4. What is coronary autoregulation? Propose a mechanism for this effect.
5. How does metabolic vasodilation take place?

CARDIOLOGIST-IN-TRAINING QUESTIONS

1. Why does the coronary blood flow increase during exercise?
2. What role does the vascular endothelium play in the physiological regulation of coronary blood flow?
3. What is endothelial dysfunction and what role may it play in altering the response to ischemia?
4. How may coronary disease alter normal physiologic coronary vascular responses?
5. Describe the principles of measurement of myocardial blood flow in humans.

REFERENCES

1. Amenta F, Coppola L, Gallo P, et al. Autoradiographic localization of β-adrenergic receptors in human large coronary arteries. *Circ Res* 1991;68:1591–1599.

2. Bache RJ, Dai XZ, Schwartz JS, Homans DC. Role of adenosine in coronary vasodilation during exercise. *Circ Res* 1988;62:846–853.
3. Baumgart D, Ehring T, Kowallik P, et al. Impact of α-adrenergic coronary vasoconstriction on the transmural myocardial blood flow distribution during humoral and neuronal adrenergic activation. *Circ Res* 1993;73:869–886.
4. Berne RM. Regulation of coronary blood flow. *Physiol Rev* 1964;44:1–29.
5. Bernstein RD, Ochoa FY, Xu X, et al. Function and production of nitric oxide in coronary circulation of the conscious dog during exercise. *Circ Res* 1996;79:840–848.
6. Broten TP, Romson JL, Fullerton DA, et al. Synergistic action of myocardial oxygen and carbon dioxide in controlling coronary blood flow. *Circ Res* 1991;68:531–542.
7. Camici PG, Groplert RJ, Jones T, et al. The impact of myocardial blood flow quantitation with PET on the understanding of cardiac diseases. *Eur Heart J* 1996;17:25–34.
8. Chance B. Pyridine nucleotide as an indicator of the oxygen requirements for energy-linked functions of mitochondria. *Circ Res* 1976;38(suppl I):I31–I38.
9. Chilian WM, Layne SM. Coronary microvascular responses to reductions in perfusion pressure. Evidence for persistent arteriolar vasomotor tone during coronary hypoperfusion. *Circ Res* 1990;66:1227–1238.
10. Chilian WM, Layne SM, Klausner EC, et al. Redistribution of coronary microvascular resistance produced by dipyridamole. *Am J Physiol* 1989;256:H383–H390.
11. De Silva R, Camici PG. Role of positron emission tomography in the investigation of human coronary circulatory function. *Cardiovasc Res* 1994;28:1595–1612.
12. Domalik-Wawrzynski LJ, Powell J Jr, Guerrero L, Palacios I. Effect of changes in ventricular relaxation on early diastolic coronary blood flow in canine hearts. *Circ Res* 1987;61:747–756.
13. Duncker DJ, Bache RJ. Inhibition of nitric oxide production aggravates myocardial hypoperfusion during exercise in the presence of a coronary artery stenosis. *Circ Res* 1994;74:629–640.
14. Frielingsdorf J, Seiler C, Kaufmann P, et al. Normalisation of abnormal coronary vasomotion by calcium antagonists in patients with hypertension. *Circulation* 1996;93:1380–1387.
15. Gollasch M, Ried C, Bychkov R, et al. K⁺ currents in human coronary artery vascular smooth muscle cells. *Circ Res* 1996;78:676–688.
16. Gregg DE. Effect of coronary perfusion pressure or coronary flow on oxygen usage of the myocardium. *Circ Res* 1963;13:497–500.
17. Gregg DE, Bedynek JL. Compensatory changes in the heart during progressive coronary artery stenosis. In: Maseri A, Klassen GA, Lesch M (eds). *Primary and Secondary Angina Pectoris.* Orlando, FL: Grune & Stratton, 1978;3–11.
18. Heusch G. Alpha-adrenergic mechanisms in myocardial ischemia. *Circulation* 1990:81:1–13.
19. Hofmann D, Opie LH. Potassium channel blockade and acute myocardial infarction: implications for management of the non-insulin requiring diabetic patient. *Eur Heart J* 1993;14:1585–1589.
20. Iwamoto T, Bai X-J, Downey HF. Coronary perfusion related changes in myocardial contractile force and systolic ventricular stiffness. *Cardiovasc Res* 1994;28:1331–1336.
21. Kaufmann P, Vassalli G, Utzinger U, Hess OM. Coronary vasomotion during dynamic exercise: influence of intravenous and intracoronary nicardipine. *J Am Coll Cardiol* 1995;26:624–631.
22. Klocke FJ. Measurements of coronary blood flow and degree of stenosis: current clinical implications and continuing uncertainties. *J Am Coll Cardiol* 1983;1:31–41.
23. Miyashiro JK, Feigl EO. Feedforward control of coronary blood flow via coronary β-receptor stimulation. *Circ Res* 1993;73:252–263.
24. Muller JM, Davis MJ, Chilian WM. Integrated regulation of pressure and flow in the coronary microcirculation. *Cardiovasc Res* 1996;32:668–678.
25. Murphree SS, Saffitz JE. Delineation of the distribution of beta-adrenergic receptor subtypes in canine myocardium. *Circ Res* 1988;63:117–125.
26. Narishige T, Egashira K, Akatsuka Y, et al. Glibenclamide, a putative ATP-sensitive K⁺ channel blocker, inhibits coronary autoregulation in anesthetized dogs. *Circ Res* 1993;73:771–776.
27. Nelson MT, Brayden JE. Regulation of arterial tone by calcium-dependent K⁺ channels. *Cardiovasc Drug Ther* 1993;7:605–610.
28. Opie LH. Coronary flow rate and perfusion pressure as determinants of mechanical function and oxidative metabolism of isolated perfused rat heart. *J Physiol* 1965;180:529–541.
29. Parker JD, Newton GE, Landzberg JS, et al. Functional significance of presynaptic α-adrenergic receptors in failing and nonfailing human left ventricle. *Circulation* 1995;92:1793–1800.

30. Parsons WJ, Rembert JC, Bauman RP, et al. Myocardial oxygenation in dogs during partial and complete coronary artery occlusion. *Circ Res* 1993;73:458–464.
31. Recchia FA, Senzaki H, Saeki A, et al. Pulse pressure-related changes in coronary flow in vivo are modulated by nitric oxide and adenosine. *Circ Res* 1996;79:849–856.
32. Rubanyi GM, Vanhoutte PM. Potassium-induced release of endothelium-derived relaxing factor from canine femoral arteries. *Circ Res* 1988;62:1098–1103.
33. Schaper W. Experimental infarcts and the microcirculation. In: Hearse DJ, Yellon DM (eds). *Therapeutic Approaches to Myocardial Infarct Size Limitation.* New York: Raven, 1984;79–90.
34. Schulz R, Guth BD, Heusch G. No effect of coronary perfusion on regional myocardial function within the autoregulatory range in pigs. Evidence against the Gregg phenomenon. *Circulation* 1991; 83:1390–1403.
35. Smith TP, Canty JM Jr. Modulation of coronary autoregulatory responses by nitric oxide. Evidence for flow-dependent resistance adjustments in conscious dogs. *Circ Res* 1993;73:232–240.
36. Sugiishi M, Takatsu F. Cigarette smoking is a major risk factor for coronary spasm. *Circulation* 1993;87:76–79.
37. Tamura M, Oshino N, Chance B, Silver I. Optical measurements of intracellular oxygen concentration of rat heart in vitro. *Arch Biochem Biophys* 1978;191:8–22.
38. Vial C, Owen P, Opie LH, Posel D. Significance of release of adenosine triphosphate and adenosine induced by hypoxia or adrenaline in perfused rat heart. *J Mol Cell Cardiol* 1987;19:187–197.
39. Vogel WM, Apstein CS, Briggs LL, et al. Acute alterations in left ventricular diastolic chamber stiffness. Role of the "erectile" effect of coronary arterial pressure and flow in normal and damaged hearts. *Circ Res* 1982;51:465–478.
40. Wang J, Wolin MS, Hintze TH. Chronic exercise enhances endothelium-mediated dilation of epicardial coronary artery in conscious dogs. *Circ Res* 1993;73:829–838.
41. Warner MR, Levy MN. Sinus and atrioventricular nodal distribution of sympathetic fibers that contain neuropeptide gamma. *Circ Res* 1990;67:713–721.
42. Wilson RF, Wyche K, Christensen BV, et al. Effects of adenosine on human coronary arterial circulation. *Circulation* 1990;82:1595–1606.
43. Yada T, Hiramatsu O, Kimura A, et al. In vivo observation of subendocardial microvessels of the beating porcine heart using a needle-probe videomicroscope with a CCD camera. *Circ Res* 1993;72: 939–946.

11

Fuels: Aerobic and Anaerobic Metabolism

Every day the human heart must synthesize about 35 kg of adenosine triphosphate (ATP) to keep pumping (Taegtmeyer, 1994). For this process, it needs a continuous supply of oxygen, delivered by a coronary circulation that is sufficiently flexible to meet increases in energy needs, as during exercise. The heart also requires a constant supply of fuels, largely derived from the coronary circulation but with cardiac glycogen acting as a reserve to support sudden increases in heart work. These fuels are broken down by the processes of intermediary metabolism to acetyl CoA, the two-carbon fragment that can enter the citrate cycle in the mitochondria (Fig. 11-1).

The uptake of fuels by the heart is partly dependent on their arterial concentrations and partly dependent on energy demand. In every case, normal coronary arteries are required to respond to any increase in the energy demand. If ischemia (poor blood flow) results from coronary disease, then oxidative patterns of metabolism are replaced by the breakdown of glucose or glycogen to lactate with the production of anaerobic energy, to play an essential role in the survival of the myocardium.

When the oxygen supply of the heart is normal, the rate of glycolysis is inhibited by high levels of citrate and ATP formed by oxidative metabolism in the citrate cycle (Randle and Morgan, 1962). When there is anoxia or severe hypoxia, oxidative metabolism ceases, citrate and ATP levels decrease, and glycolysis is stimulated (Fig. 11-2). Glycolysis can provide limited amounts of energy even in the absence of oxygen (anaerobic ATP). When there is not only extreme hypoxia but severe ischemia, the delivery of both oxygen and glucose decreases, and glycolysis may decrease. Thus, severe ischemia limits the capacity of the tissue to survive.

Another way of dealing with hypoxia or ischemia is to downgrade the ATP requirements of the myocytes to a new *hypometabolic state* (Hochachka et al., 1996), which could be one explanation for the adaptive processes that underlie the hibernating myocardium (see Chapter 19).

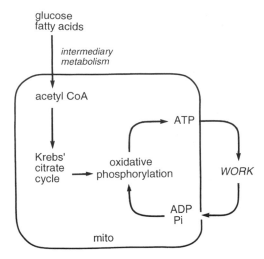

FIG. 11-1. Intermediary metabolism is the process whereby the fuels (glucose and fatty acids) are prepared for energy production in the mitochondria. Figure designed by L.H. Opie.

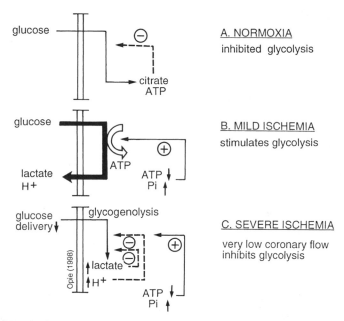

FIG. 11-2. Glycolysis. A: In the normally oxygenated heart, tissue citrate and ATP are high and inhibit glycolysis. **B:** When coronary flow is mildly decreased (mild ischemia), glycolysis is stimulated. **C:** In severe ischemia (severe deprivation of both oxygen and coronary flow), the decreased delivery of glucose and glycogen depletion, as well as the accumulation of lactate and protons, inhibits glycolysis despite any tendency toward acceleration by a low cardiac content of ATP.

FUELS OF THE HUMAN HEART

The heart see-saws between carbohydrate in the fed state and fatty acids in the fasted state as the major sources of energy, as suggested by Bing in the early 1950s (Table 11-1). In the fasted state, the level of blood free fatty acids (FFAs) is high. The high rates of uptake of fatty acids are preferentially used for oxidative metabolism (Fig. 11-3) so that fatty acids become the major source of energy (Neely and Morgan, 1974; Opie, 1968). When fatty acids are oxidized, glucose oxidation is inhibited and the glucose taken up is increasingly converted to glycogen: the glucose sparing effect of fatty acid oxidation (Randle et al., 1963). Conversely, in the carbohydrate-fed state (Fig. 11-4), when the levels of circulating glucose and insulin are high, then circulating fatty acid levels are suppressed. The uptake of fatty acids by the heart decreases, the inhibition of glycolysis by fatty acids is removed, and glucose oxidation increases. Furthermore, glucose metabolism also directly suppresses the oxidation of fatty acids.

In patients who have just consumed a high-fat meal of cream and cheese, there is a marked increase in blood triglycerides during postprandial lipemia. Triglyceride is converted by the enzyme lipoprotein lipase to FFAs, which then enter the pathways of fatty acid oxidation. In these exceptional circumstances, circulating triglyceride becomes the major myocardial fuel. During acute exercise, the blood lactate increases, and lactate becomes the major fuel. Lactate inhibits the oxidation of glucose and the uptake of FFAs, each of which now contributes only 15% to 20% of the energy needs of the heart during exercise. Ketone bodies contribute significantly to the energy metabolism of the heart only in starvation or severe diabetic ketosis, because like fatty acids or lactate, their uptake is concentration dependent. In ischemia, the pattern of substrate uptake changes from a predominant reliance on lipids to a predominant carbohydrate pattern.

The above balance studies depend on two assumptions: that there is a steady state and that the fuel concerned is fully oxidized. Nonetheless, it may be that there are substantial nonoxidative fates or that there is a considerable delay between the uptake of a molecule and its ultimate oxidation. In the case of glucose, this delay may result from its prior conversion to glycogen (Taegtmeyer, 1994).

Glucose–Fatty Acid Cycle. The marked variation in the relative roles of glucose and fatty acid as major fuel between the fed and fasted states is impressive (Figs. 11-3 and 11-4) and forms the basis of the glucose–fatty acid cycle first described by Randle et al. (1963). It is the cyclical switching on and off of production of FFA by adipose tissue that is the basic event in the cycle. During fasting, adipose tissue is broken down to release FFA, which inhibits the metabolism of glucose by the heart. In the fed state, glucose and insulin inhibit such release of fatty acid, and glucose becomes the major fuel. The contribution of any given fuel to the oxidative metabolism of the heart varies throughout the day according to the circulating levels, and probably even from minute to minute in relation to the effects of food or exercise.

TABLE 11-1. *Effect of nutritional state or exercise on fuel for oxidative metabolism of the human heart: Ratio of oxygen uptake accounted for by extraction of various substrates if fully oxidized*

Conditions	Glucose (OER %)	Pyruvate (OER %)	Lactate (OER %)	Total CHO (OER %)	FFA (OER %)	TG (OER %)	Ketones (OER %)	Amino acids (OER %)	Respiratory quotient
Insulin (glucose 5 mmol/L)[a]	6	44	51	101	3	—	—	—	Approaches 1.0
Feeding	—	—	—	92	5	—	—	—	Approaches 1.0
Postprandial, CHO meal[b]	68	4	28	100	—	—	—	—	0.94
Postprandial, lipid meal	10	—	10	20	30	50	—	—	—
Fasting, few hours[c]	31	2	28	61	34	—	5	0	—
Same during exercise	16	0	61	77	21	—	2	0	—
Same with recovery	21	2	36	59	36	—	3	0	—
Fasting overnight, resting	27	1	11	38	62	14	7	—	0.74
Fasting overnight, corrected[d]	5	1	11	17	62	14	7	—	0.74

OER, oxygen extraction ratio; CHO, carbohydrate; TG, triglyceride; —, absence of data.

[a]Ferrannini. *Am J Physiol* 1993;26:E308.
[b]Subjects studied 2–3 hours after a light low-fat breakfast.
[c]Subjects studied in the early afternoon after a light breakfast.
[d]Corrected for actual glucose oxidation rates. See Wisneski et al. *J Clin Invest* 1985;76:1819.
For other references, see Opie (1989).

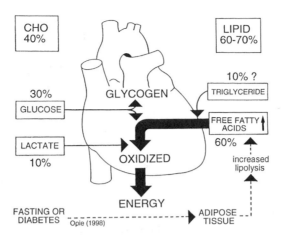

FIG. 11-3. Substrate metabolism: fasted state. Patterns of substrate metabolism when blood levels of FFAs are high, as in the fasted state or poorly controlled diabetes mellitus. High levels of blood FFAs are oxidized by the heart in preference to glucose and lactate. Use of lipid accounts for 60% to 70% of the oxygen uptake of the heart, whereas use of carbohydrate accounts for less than 40%. Potential errors in the indirect methods used mean that the sum of the oxidation extraction ratios (see Table 11-1) will not equal exactly 100%. CHO, carbohydrate.

Oxidative Metabolism of Glucose. The uptake of glucose from the blood stream across the sarcolemma and into the cells of the heart is controlled by the glucose transporters *GLUT 4 and GLUT 1,* which are stereospecific and prefer glucose to other circulating sugars (Lopaschuk and Stanley, 1997; Pessin and Bell, 1992). No energy is required for such glucose transport because the glucose concentration in the extracellular space is so much higher than in the cytosol. The uptake of glucose increases whenever the glucose transporter is

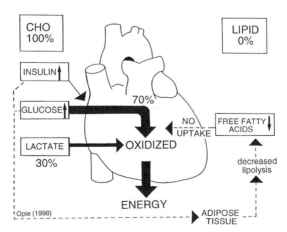

FIG. 11-4. Substrate metabolism: fed state. After a high-carbohydrate meal or glucose feeding, blood glucose and insulin are high, and blood FFAs are low. Glucose becomes the major fuel of the heart, and carbohydrate can account for 100% of the oxygen uptake. CHO, carbohydrate.

stimulated, as during increased heart work, in the fed state, or during hypoxia or ischemia. All these conditions also enhance glycolysis. Conversely, the uptake of glucose is reduced by those factors inhibiting glycolysis: a low workload, the fasted state, or severe diabetes mellitus. The factor common to the latter two conditions is the high blood fatty acid level, which in turn inhibits the glucose transporters in muscle (Roden et al., 1996).

Insulin, a circulating hormone, the level of which rises in the fed state, increases the number of glucose carriers in the sarcolemma (Fig. 11-5). Insulin translocates the glucose carriers GLUT 4 and GLUT 1 from internal unavailable sites to external sarcolemmal sites (Russell et al., 1996; Young et al., 1997). Thus, insulin stimulates the rates at which the carriers are recycled between internal and external sites. Insulin binds to specific insulin receptors, consisting of an external α-subunit and an internal β-subunit. When insulin occupies the external subunit, there is a rapid self-phosphorylation of the β-subunit (White and Kahn, 1994). This *autophosphorylation* greatly amplifies the effect of insulin and in turn activates peptide kinases to phosphorylate tyrosine. Thereafter, the downstream events are not yet finalized (White and Kahn, 1994). A brief summary of one current view is as follows. Tyrosine phosphorylation

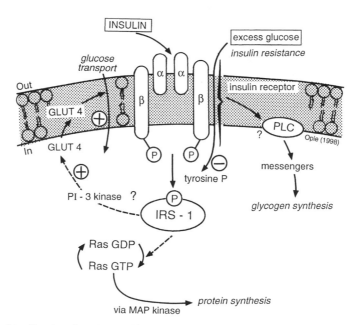

FIG. 11-5. Insulin signal systems. Note crucial role of tyrosine phosphorylation and its proposed inhibition by hyperglycemia, which could contribute to insulin resistance. GLUT 4, glucose transporter 4; α and β, alpha and beta subunits of insulin receptor; P, phosphorylation; IRS, insulin receptor substrate; MAPK, mitogen-activated protein kinase; PI, phosphotidyl inositol; PLC, phospholipase C.

increases the activity of the insulin receptor substrate-1 (IRS-1), which in turn passes on the message to several different signal systems to increase by phosphorylation the activity of diverse crucial enzymes, including glycogen synthase and pyruvate dehydrogenase. In addition, through an entirely different signal system that involves mitogen-activated protein kinase (MAPK), IRS-1 promotes growth pathways (Fig. 11-5). It is not clear how the glucose carriers are activated. Thus, insulin achieves its multiple actions through diverse mechanisms that are not fully understood.

Insulin resistance refers to the impaired glucose transport found in response to apparently normal or even elevated levels of insulin in diverse diseases such as maturity-onset diabetes, congestive heart failure, and some types of hypertension (see section on Clinical Applications in this chapter).

PATHWAYS OF GLYCOLYSIS

Glycolysis is the metabolic pathway converting glucose to pyruvate. During normal oxidative metabolism, glycolysis yields pyruvate, which is then oxidized in the citrate cycle. Thus, ATP is produced from glycolysis not only during anaerobic conditions, although it is chiefly during anaerobiosis that the relatively small amounts of glycolytic ATP are of importance in preserving membrane function.

The pathway of glycolysis can be divided into two stages (for details, see Table 10-5 of the 2nd edition of this book). Very little free glucose is found in the cytosol, so that any glucose taken up in cardiac myocytes is trapped and rapidly converted by the unidirectional enzyme *hexokinase* to glucose 6-phosphate. The latter compound is then directed either to glycogen synthesis or to glycolysis. Glycolysis converts glucose 6-phosphate into a compound containing two phosphate groups, fructose 1,6-diphosphate (fructose 1,6-bisphosphate) under the influence of the enzyme phosphofructokinase (PFK). Of the many enzymes participating in the reactions of the glycolytic pathway, PFK is one of the few that actually regulate flux. When its activity increases, as in hypoxia, glucose 6-phosphate is converted at an increased rate via fructose 6-phosphate to fructose 1,6-bisphosphate:

$$\text{Glucose} + \text{ATP} \rightarrow \text{glucose 6-phosphate} + \text{adenosine diphosphate (ADP)}$$

$$\text{Glucose 6-phosphate} \rightarrow \text{fructose 6-phosphate}$$

$$\text{Fructose 6-phosphate} + \text{ATP} \overset{\text{PFK}}{\rightarrow} \text{fructose 1,6 bisphosphate} + \text{ADP}$$

Thereafter, glycolysis converts each six-carbon hexose phosphate into two three-carbon triose phosphates. During the next stages of glycolysis that form two molecules of pyruvate, four molecules of ATP are made independently of oxygen:

$$\text{Fructose 1,6 bisphosphate} + 2Pi + 4\,\text{ADP} \rightarrow 2 \times \text{pyruvate} + 4\,\text{ATP}$$

There is a coordinated intracellular control of glycolysis such that glucose uptake, glucose phosphorylation, the activity of PFK, and that of pyruvate dehydrogenase can all speed up or slow down simultaneously in response to increased heart work and other stimuli (Table 11-2).

Fructose 2,6-bisphosphate is an additional product of glycolysis, not an intermediate, with the capacity for potent stimulation of PFK that overrides the inhibitory effects of ATP and citrate. It is produced from fructose 6-phosphate by an enzyme (PFK-2) whose activity increases when glycolytic flow is increased in response to insulin or increased heart work (Depré et al., 1993).

Pyruvate and Lactate

Pyruvate stands at the crossroads of glycolysis and oxidative metabolism in the citrate cycle. It is formed both from lactate taken up by the heart and from glycolysis. In the anaerobic heart, pyruvate forms lactate. In the aerobic heart, the major fate of pyruvate is oxidative decarboxylation and entry into the citrate cycle, which requires the activity of pyruvate dehydrogenase (Fig. 11-6). Before pyruvate can be oxidized fully in the Krebs citrate cycle, it must undergo oxidative decarboxylation through the action of the enzyme complex pyruvate dehydrogenase, which is found in the inner mitochondrial membrane. The products of the multistage reaction include acetyl CoA, which is ready to enter the citrate cycle, and $NADH_2$, which will eventually form ATP by oxidative phosphorylation. Pyruvate dehydrogenase can exist in either active or inactive forms. Normally, this enzyme is largely inactive but is activated by increased heart work (McCormack et al., 1982), by catecholamines, or by the high glycolytic rates of the fed state (Table 11-2). Conversely, the enzyme is inhibited by $NADH_2$ formed by ischemia or hypoxia or by fatty acid oxidation. Inhibition of pyruvate dehydrogenase is a key factor in the inhibition of glycolysis during oxidation of fatty acids (Weiss et al., 1989).

Lactate is taken up by the aerobic heart and produced during anaerobiosis, so that in its release into coronary sinus blood it is sometimes used as a sign of myocardial ischemia (Gertz et al., 1980). The contribution of lactate to the energy needs of the well-oxygenated myocardium increases by up to 60% when the circulating lactate levels are high (e.g., during and soon after exercise) and by up to

TABLE 11-2. *Major factors controlling glycolysis and sites of action*

Conditions	Glucose uptake	Glycogen content	Activity of PFK	Activity of pyruvate dehydrogenase
Increased heart work	+	↓	+	+
Inotropic agents	+	↓	+	+
Fed state, insulin	+	↑	+	+
Starvation, high blood fatty acids or ketones	–	↑	–	–
Hypoxia, mild ischemia	+	↓	+	–
Severe ischemia	–	↓	–	–

+, stimulation; –, inhibition; ↓, decreased content; ↑, increased content.

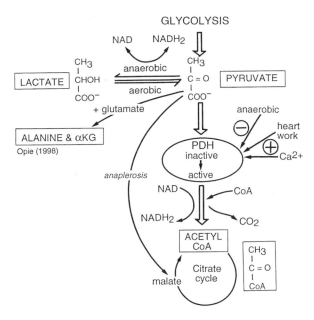

FIG. 11-6. The major fates of pyruvate. In the normal aerobic heart, lactate is taken up and converted to pyruvate, the major part of which enters the citrate cycle. Transamination is a pathway of minor significance. In the anaerobic heart, lactate is produced from pyruvate derived from glycolysis. There is also formation of alanine and the possibility of ATP production via GTP as succinate is ultimately formed. During postischemic reperfusion, pyruvate can be converted to malate to help replenish the citrate cycle intermediates by anaplerosis. αKG, α-ketoglutarate; PDH, pyruvate dehydrogenase.

90% during a lactate infusion. Lactate is a much less important fuel when its level is low or when FFA levels are high. The uptake of lactate by the heart depends on a specific transport system (sensitive to inhibition by cinnamate) because the sarcolemma is not freely permeable to lactate. Once taken up, intracellular lactate is converted into pyruvate by *lactate dehydrogenase* (LDH) and thus joins the pool of pyruvate in the cytosol. The reaction catalyzed by LDH is freely reversible.

$$\text{Lactate} + NAD^+ \leftrightarrow \text{pyruvate} + NADH + H^+$$

The myocardial activity of LDH is high enough to make it unlikely that it could be a controlling step for lactate metabolism by the heart. There are five *LDH isoenzymes,* named in order of rapidity of their electrophoretic migrations. Each isoenzyme is a tetrameric unit composed of four subunits of the H or M type. The H type, predominating in the heart muscle, is also known as LDH_1 or as α-hydroxybutyrate dehydrogenase because α-hydroxybutyrate can replace lactate as substrate. In acute myocardial infarction, an estimate of infarct size may be found by measuring the rate of appearance and disappearance in the blood of the LDH cardiac isoenzyme (LDH_1), with peak values 35 to 43 hours after the onset of symptoms (Hermens and Witteveen, 1977).

TABLE 11-3. *Comparative energy yields of various fuels per molecule fully oxidized*

Molecule	ATP yield per molecule		ATP yield per carbon atom		ATP yield per oxygen atom taken up (P/O ratio)[a]	
	Old	New	Old	New	Old	New
Glucose	38[c]	32[d]	6.3	5.2	3.17	2.58
Lactate	18	14.75	6.0	4.9	3.00	2.46
Pyruvate	15	12.25	5.0	4.1	3.00	2.50
Palmitate[b]	130	105	8.1	6.7	2.83	2.33

[a]P/O, phosphorylation/oxidation.
[b]For palmitate details, see Brand. *Biochemist* Aug–Sept 1994:20.
[c]n = 36 via mitochondria, two via glycolysis.
[d]n = 30 via mitochondria, two via glycolysis.
Old, conventional; new, revised. See Hinkle et al. *Biochemistry* 1991;30:3576.

Is There a Role for Glycolysis in the Oxygenated Myocardium?

In the normal well-oxygenated (aerobic) heart, FFA or lactate can be the major source of energy, and the function of *aerobic glycolysis* may appear obscure. Yet glucose remains an important fuel for the heart, providing up to 30% of the energy needs of the heart in the fasted state and up to 70% after a carbohydrate meal. After a high-fat meal, glucose still accounts for about 10% of the oxygen uptake. It is not known if the low remaining rates of glycolytic flux have a function beyond that of merely keeping the pathway slowly ticking over to accelerate more easily during the onset of a sudden increase of heart work. When heart work is increased by exercise, glycolysis rapidly accelerates within 5 seconds, the glucose probably being derived from glycogen. Thus, there is increased input of pyruvate and acetyl CoA into the citrate cycle, so that an extra 30 ATP units (or 36 according to the phosphorylation to oxygen uptake (P/O) ratios previously thought to be correct) are generated by the citrate cycle (Table 11-3).

A further role for glycolysis is to provide energy for the maintenance of normal ATP-requiring membrane functions such as the sodium pump. This role was first proposed in the context of ischemia but now established for normoxia, at least in the case of the ATP-sensitive potassium channels (Weiss and Lamp, 1987; Coetzee, 1992). Key glycolytic enzymes, situated near the sarcolemma, may be involved in the production of such membrane-related glycolysis.

More controversial functions of glycolysis are to sustain maximal heart work and to promote diastolic relaxation especially during ischemia.

GLYCOGEN

Glycogen is a polysaccharide (i.e., a combination of many molecules of glucose) that forms large granules in the cytoplasm of the heart. Although frequently thought of as a storage carbohydrate, glycogen molecules are in a constant state of turnover as a result of variable rates of synthesis and degradation.

The pathways of *glycogen synthesis* function separately from those of glycogen breakdown because two different enzyme systems are involved. Glycogen synthesis (Fig. 11-7) proceeds at a high rate in the fed state under the influence of insulin, which both increases glucose uptake and stimulates the synthase (through a complex and controversial mechanism). Glycogen synthesis also appears to take place after intense heart work or after ischemia has depleted glycogen (Camici et al., 1989a, 1989b; Henning et al., 1996). This proposal is in accord with animal data, suggesting that low glycogen levels promote glycogen synthesis. In the fasted state, despite the lack of insulin, glycogen synthesis can still proceed, albeit at a lower rate, because glycogen synthase is stimulated by the high myocardial levels of glucose 6-phosphate that result from blocked glycolysis. The energy required for glycogen synthesis is derived from a special high-energy phosphate, uridine triphosphate (UTP), which is formed from ATP.

The two major mechanisms underlying glycogen breakdown are (1) activation of phosphorylase by cyclic adenosine monophosphate (cAMP) or (2) in ischemia, by a decrease in high-energy phosphate levels (Fig. 11-6). An increase

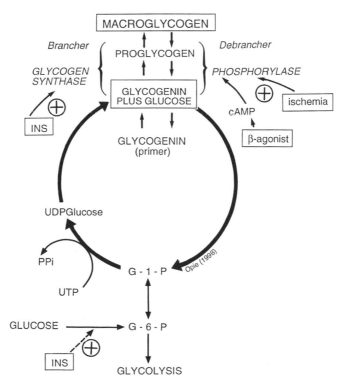

FIG. 11-7. Glycogen synthesis and breakdown. Note different pathways for synthesis, which is controlled by glycogen synthase (synthetase), when compared with glycogen breakdown, which is controlled by glycogen phosphorylase.

in cAMP promotes the cascade of events that eventually converts the inactive enzyme phosphorylase *b* to the highly active phosphorylase *a*:

Catecholamine stimulus → β-receptor → adenylate cyclase → cAMP activation of protein kinase → activation of phosphorylase *b* kinase → change of phosphorylase *b* to *a* → breakdown of glycogen.

An unexpected finding is that calmodulin, the intracellular calcium-binding receptor protein, is one of the subunits of phosphorylase *b* kinase, which explains why calcium ions are required for the formation of phosphorylase *a* (Werth et al., 1982). Phosphorylase is the enzyme controlling the initial burst of glycogenolysis during hypoxia or ischemia, and thereafter the activity of the *debranching enzyme* becomes significant.

Function of Cardiac Glycogen.   Cardiac glycogen is a potential source of myocardial energy, producing three ATP units during glycolysis and the standard amount of ATP through the citrate cycle in aerobic conditions. It has an established role as energy source during myocardial hypoxia or ischemia (Cross et al., 1996).

Apart from these short-lived conditions, glycogen turnover may contribute substantially to aerobic glycolysis in the normal working heart and may be oxidized in preference to external glucose, especially soon after the onset of enhanced β-adrenergic stimulation (Goodwin et al., 1996). The glycogen thus oxidized is not only that most recently synthesized, so the "last on, first off" hypothesis receives only partial support (Goodwin et al., 1995; Henning et al., 1996). Some workers speculate that exogenous glucose, after uptake and conversion to glucose 6-phosphate, passes through glycogen on the way to glycolytic breakdown (Taegtmeyer, 1994). These proposals provide a physiologic role for glycogen (Achs et al., 1982). Because glycogen is situated in proximity to the sarcoplasmic reticulum, its turnover might provide on-site ATP for the calcium uptake pump.

Glycogenin and Proglycogen

Glycogenin is a primer or backbone for glycogen synthesis, well described in the liver and presumably also present in the heart. It is autocatalytic in that it glucosylates itself before glucosylation to glycogen synthesis (Alonso et al., 1995). Proglycogen is an abundant stable glycogen precursor molecule, found in the heart. Hypothetically, glycogen may oscillate between proglycogen and the higher molecular weight storage glycogen called *macroglycogen,* depending on energy supply and demand (Alonso et al., 1995).

Glycogen Storage Disease of the Heart.   In the lysosomes of the heart, the breakdown of some of the glycogen is mediated by a different pathway dependent on α-1,4 glucosidase (acid maltase). The congenital absence of this enzyme has drastic consequences because the heart cells become stuffed with glycogen,

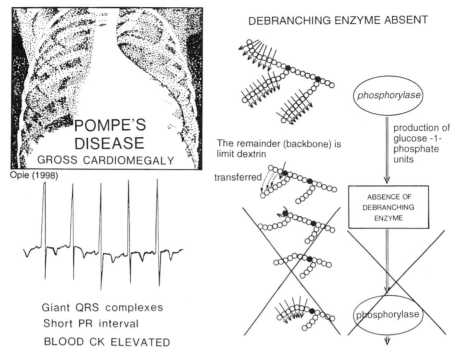

FIG. 11-8. Glycogen storage disease of Pompe. Clinical features are shown.

and the fatal condition of cardiomegalic glycogenolysis or Pompe's disease results (Fig. 11-8). Cytoplasmic glycogenolysis, dependent on phosphorylase and the debrancher enzyme, proceeds normally in these cases. Because of distention of the lysosomes by glycogen, the lysosomal membranes rupture with risk of destruction of heart muscle.

FREE FATTY ACIDS DURING AEROBIC METABOLISM

Although long-chain FFAs are the major myocardial fuel during fasting, their oxidation in the mitochondria can only take place after complex but essential transformational steps. In ischemia, when mitochondrial metabolism is inhibited, accumulated long-chain metabolites exert adverse influences on the myocardial cell membranes (Fig. 11-9). Myocardial metabolism of FFA starts with the blood level, because the higher the FFA level and the greater the FFA/albumin molar ratio, the greater the uptake of FFA by the myocardium. FFA molecules traversing the sarcolemma appear to link up with an intracellular *fatty acid binding protein* (Vyska et al., 1991) before further metabolism. Eventually, if sufficient FFA is taken up, accumulated intracellular intermediates will limit the fatty acid activation (Fig. 11-10).

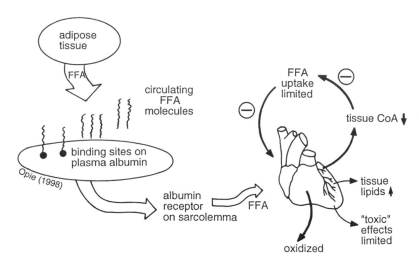

FIG. 11-9. Uptake of FFAs at high circulating levels, exceeding the tight binding sites on plasma albumin (the two black circles), is uncontrolled and may give rise to toxic effects. For details of tissue CoA and acyl CoA, see Fig. 11-10.

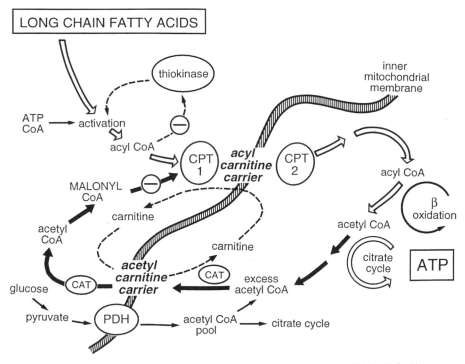

FIG. 11-10. The carnitine carrier functions to transfer activated fatty acid (acyl CoA) into the mitochondrial space for oxidation in the fatty acid oxidation space. For detail, see p. 309. Acyl CoA, long-chain acyl CoA compounds; acyl carnitine, long-chain acyl carnitine compounds.

After uptake into the myocardial cell, a series of intricate steps changes the long-chain fatty acid into acetyl CoA, which can enter the citrate cycle and which in turn will yield ATP. The details of this complex sequence have been well reviewed (Lopaschuk et al., 1994). The first step is the activation of the intracellular fatty acid by CoA (coenzyme A) to form fatty acyl CoA derivatives. The mitochondrial membrane is not permeable to these acyl CoA molecules, which need transformation and transfer from the cytosol to within the mitochondria by a staged transfer system that requires carnitine and formation of acyl carnitine, as well as transport into the mitochondrial space. Thereafter, the long-chain acyl CoA molecules are progressively broken into two-carbon units of acetyl CoA by β-oxidation, and finally acetyl CoA is oxidized in the citrate cycle. Any activated intracellular fatty acid not oxidized can be stored as triglycerides or can be transformed to structural lipids by lengthening and alterations in the degree of saturation. Tissue triglyceride (also called triacylglycerol) may be a reserve source of fatty acids when the circulating levels are low (Lopaschuk et al., 1997). Complex intracellular controls exist to prevent any undue accumulation of lipid intermediates that may have toxic effects.

The overall steps can be summarized as follows. Palmitate is the standard example, although in human the chief fatty acid taken up is oleic acid (Table 11-4).

1. Extramitochondrial acyl CoA (example, palmityl CoA) forms from fatty acid (Fig. 11-10):

$$\text{Palmitate} + \text{CoA} + \text{ATP} \rightarrow \text{palmityl CoA} + \text{AMP} + \text{PPi}$$

2. Extramitochondrial acyl carnitine forms from extramitochondrial acyl CoA, catalyzed by the enzyme carnitine palmityl transferase 1 (CPT 1).

TABLE 11-4. *Myocardial uptake of plasma free fatty acids in fasting human*

Fatty acid	Structure	Site of unsaturated bonds	Percentage of total plasma FFA[a,b]	Percentage of uptake of FFA by human heart
Palmitic	C16:0	—	About 25	16
Palmitoleic	C16:1	9	2	2
Stearic	C18:0	—	14	7
Oleic	C18:1	9	30–45	53
Linoleic	C18:2	9,12	10–14	7
Linolenic	C18:3	6,12,15	8 in guinea pig	No data
Arachidonic	C20:4	5,8,11,14	5	No data in humans, no uptake in dog heart[c]
Erucic	C22:1	13	Normally low	No data but may increase with rapeseed ingestion

[a]Spector. *Prog Biochem Pharm* 1971;6:130.
[b]Calculated from data of Rothlin and Bing. *J Clin Invest* 1961;40:1380.
[c]Van der Vusse et al. *Circ Res* 1982;50:538.

3. The enzyme carnitine acyl translocase transfers extramitochondrial acyl carnitine to within the mitochondrial space.
4. Mitochondrial carnitine acyl transferase 2 allows intramitochondrial acyl carnitine to react with CoA to liberate intramitochondrial acyl CoA and carnitine; the carnitine is exported outward to the cytosol as in step 3.
5. Intramitochondrial acyl CoA enters the fatty acid oxidation spiral to form acetyl CoA, which enters the citrate cycle.
6. During high rates of FFA uptake and subsequent metabolism by the above steps, more acetyl CoA may form than can enter the citrate cycle. Such acetyl CoA also can react with intramitochondrial carnitine to form acetyl carnitine that is transported outward from the mitochondria by the enzyme carnitine-acetyl translocase (CAT), and in the process cytoplasmic acetyl CoA is formed. This can then undergo transformation into malonyl CoA, which provides feedback inhibition.

Malonyl CoA is produced whenever high cytosolic levels of acetyl CoA are produced by rapid rates of either fatty acid metabolism (as above) or high rates of glucose oxidation. Malonyl CoA potently inhibits step 2 (Fig. 11-10), to provide a mechanism whereby high rates of aerobic glycolysis could switch off FFA metabolism. The enzyme that synthesizes malonyl CoA, acetyl CoA carboxylase, is inhibited during early postischemic reperfusion, so that the rates of fatty acid oxidation are enhanced with postulated harmful effects (Kudo et al., 1995).

β-Oxidation

β-Oxidation converts intramitochondrial long-chain acyl CoA to the two-carbon fragment acetyl CoA. The fatty acid oxidation spiral continuously removes acetyl CoA from the carboxyl (–COOH) end of the chain. The enzymes of β-oxidation are loosely organized into a multienzyme complex in which the intermediates never leave the complex except for entering and departing. The products of each reaction are simply displaced by the arrival of fresh substrates for that reaction, to move on in the spiral. The net ATP production per palmitate molecule may be only 105, although classically still regarded as 130, depending on the phosphorylation/oxidation ratio used (Table 11-3).

During *increased heart work,* the mitochrondria become more oxidized. Intramitochondrial levels of $NADH_2$ and $FADH_2$ decrease, and there is an increased turnover of the whole fatty acid oxidation spiral. A series of signals tells the cytosol that the mitochondria need a higher rate of production of acetyl CoA derived from fatty acid oxidation during increased heart work. Such cytosolic acetyl CoA then enters the mitochondria after transformation to acetyl carnitine. Thereby, free cytosolic CoA forms, and the rate of fatty acid activation is enhanced.

Conversely, during anaerobiosis, intramitochondrial $NADH_2$ increases, as does $FADH_2$, as a result of impaired β-oxidation due to decreased electron transport. Intermediates of fatty acid metabolism accumulate, including β-hydroxy-fatty acids, acyl carnitine, and acyl CoA.

Oxygen Wastage

When the heart is exposed to high circulating levels of catecholamines or FFA, the oxygen uptake may increase much more than expected from the change in respiratory quotient in switching from carbohydrate to fatty acids as fuel. This phenomenon, also found in humans (Simonsen and Kjekshus, 1978), may be mediated in part by increased turnover of intracellular *futile cycles,* thereby wasting ATP. Alternatively, pathways of respiration producing not ATP but free oxygen radicals may be enhanced, with the potential for myocardial damage. Similar mechanisms may underlie the development of *lipid peroxides,* which together with formation of phospholipids, free radicals, and lipid intermediates may all contribute to ischemic reperfusion damage (see Chapter 19). Thus, when catecholamine activity is high in acute myocardial infarction, part of the benefit of β-adrenergic blockade may be by reduction of blood FFA levels (Oliver and Opie, 1994).

Structural Lipids of the Heart

Phospholipids, the major structural lipids of the heart, form an important part of the various cell membranes, including the sarcolemma. The outer phospholipid layer binds calcium ions, which in some way appear to be involved in excitation–contraction coupling (Langer, 1985). In prolonged ischemia, all membranes are damaged, and products of phospholipid breakdown are formed (Corr et al., 1982). One view is that ischemic injury becomes irreversible when the molecular structure of the cell membranes is damaged beyond repair. In phospholipid molecules, both the free base group (choline or ethanolamine) and the phosphate are charged, providing a polar head in contrast to the nonpolar tail. It is this polarity of the molecule that allows the formation of the lipid bilayer of the cell membranes. The polar heads point outward, and the nonpolar tails point inward. Into the lipid bilayer are inserted various complex proteins, including enzyme systems that may require specific phospholipids for optimal activity. Such lipid–enzyme complexes include adenylate cyclase and the sarcolemmal sodium–potassium pump.

Plasmalogens are phospholipids with an ether band and an unknown function, possibly stabilizing the membranes. They constitute more than 50% of the phospholipids of the sarcolemma and the sarcoplasmic reticulum in the heart (Davies et al., 1992).

ATP SYNTHESIS AND EXPORT

The breakdown of ATP is the only immediate source of energy for contraction, the maintenance of ion gradients, and other vital functions. The complex metabolic pathways already described transform the major fuels (glucose, FFAs, and lactate) to acetyl CoA, which enters the citrate cycle to produce $NADH_2$ (NADH + H^+). $NADH_2$ is the reduced form of the cofactor nicotinamide adenine dinucleotide. The two H, in turn, yield the protons that are pumped across the mitochondrial membrane, as well as the electrons that flow along the cytochrome chain, the end result being the conversion of ADP into ATP by oxidative phosphorylation. Once produced in the mitochondria, ATP must be transported outward to the cytosol by the ATP/ADP transport system for use in the cytoplasm, chiefly in contraction. As cytosolic ATP is used, it is replenished by synthesis from ADP in the mitochondria. The rates of synthesis and breakdown of ATP are therefore closely linked.

The rate at which the citrate cycle of Krebs (Fig. 11-11) operates is a major factor controlling the rate of production of ATP by the heart. The standard dogma is that each turn of the cycle produces 12 molecules of ATP, but reality (allowing for technical factors often ignored) may be closer to 10 (Table 11-5). An increased rate of the Krebs cycle occurs with increased heart work. Conversely,

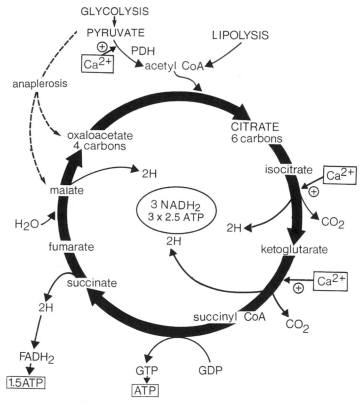

FIG. 11-11. **The citrate cycle of Krebs.** In reality, the following reactions are readily reversible: citrate → isocitrate; succinate → oxaloacetate via the intervening reactions. The most important potential sites of control are citrate synthase, isocitrate dehydrogenase, α-ketoglutarate dehydrogenase, and malate dehydrogenase (by regulating the supply of oxaloacetate). Of these, isocitrate dehydrogenase and α-ketoglutarate dehydrogenase are calcium sensitive, as is pyruvate dehydrogenase (PDH). These dehydrogenases respond to increased cytosolic calcium (as in inotropic stimulation) by increased activity.

TABLE 11-5. *Sites of production of 2H, CO_2 and high-energy phosphates in citrate cycle*

Product	Sites of production	Fate
4 × 2H in total	Isocitrate dehydrogenase	Formation of NADH plus H⁺ (NADH₂) and electron transport to produce 2.5 ATP
	α-Ketoglutarate dehydrogenase	As above
	Succinate dehydrogenase	FADH₂ formation and electron transport via CoQ to produce 1.5 ATP
	Malate dehydrogenase	2.5 ATP as above
GTP	Succinate dehydrogenase by substrate level phosphorylation	1 ATP ultimately
One turn of citrate cycle	Various dehydrogenase reactions as above	10 ATP[a]

[a]For conventional data with phosphorylation/oxidation ratio of 3.0, see Table 11-3; likewise there would be 12 ATP per turn of cycle.

decreased rates of operation of the cycle occur during states of oxygen deprivation, such as hypoxia or ischemia or during cardioplegic arrest.

Increased Heart Work and Citrate Cycle

How can the activity of the citrate cycle be matched to the varying energy requirements of the heart (Fig. 11-12)? Hypothetically, as the heart works harder, more ATP is broken down to ADP to drive oxidative phosphorylation, which in turn uses H from NADH₂, so that the ratio NAD/NADH₂ within the mitochon-

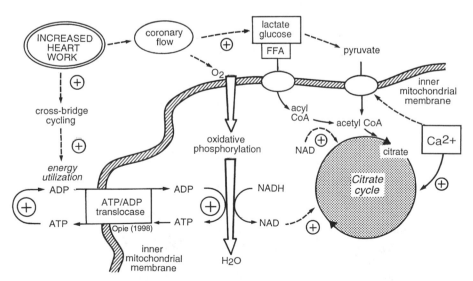

FIG. 11-12. Work and citrate cycle. The proposed effects of increased heart work in providing an increased supply of circulating substrates and in stimulating oxidative phosphorylation and citrate cycle activity.

dria increases, thereby stimulating the activity of certain key enzymes of the citrate cycle (isocitrate dehydrogenase, α-ketoglutarate dehydrogenase, malate dehydrogenase). The change in the mitochondrial $NAD/NADH_2$ ratio toward NAD also helps the formation of oxaloacetate from malate. Oxaloacetate is one of the substrates for the key enzyme citrate synthase, which regulates the formation of citrate. The other substrate for citrate synthase is acetyl CoA, the formation of which also is stimulated during increased heart work by increases in the rates of glycolysis and the fatty acid oxidation spiral. The above sequence is supported both by direct and indirect measurements of the mitochondrial ratio of NAD to $NADH_2$, which decreases at the start of increased work in the isolated heart (Opie and Owen, 1975). Nonetheless, the control mechanisms are far from clarified, and the evidence remains controversial (Heineman and Balaban, 1993).

Inotropic Stimulation and Regulation of Citrate Cycle by Calcium

Thus, for practical purposes, it may be accepted that the citrate cycle responds to the decrease in the ATP/ADP and $NAD/NADH_2$ ratios when the oxygen uptake of the heart is increased by a volume or a pressure load. When the primary stimulus to increased heart work is increased contractility associated with an increased cytosolic concentration of calcium ions, a current proposal is that the intramitochondrial calcium concentration also increases as the cytosolic level increases (Brandes and Bers, 1997). There are two dehydrogenases of the citrate cycle—isocitrate dehydrogenase and α-ketoglutarate dehydrogenase—that are both sensitive to calcium ions in the concentrations thought to be found in the cytosol. Calcium also causes the conversion of the inactive to the active form of pyruvate dehydrogenase (Fig. 11-6). In addition, because the positive inotropic effect of calcium by definition increases heart work, increased provision of ADP to the mitochondria will promote the rate of oxidative phosphorylation (Lehninger, 1975). Even when increased heart work is achieved by an increased preload, cytosolic calcium could still increase because stretch of the muscle fibers could stimulate mechanoreceptors.

Respiratory Control

"Mitochondrial respiration" refers to all those processes concerned with the uptake of oxygen and the associated production of ATP, including the activity of the citrate cycle and the respiratory chain. Besides the evident need for oxygen, there are three important regulators of the respiratory rate: (1) the supply of ADP that regulates respiration by its rate of transfer into the mitochondria, (2) the ratio of $NAD/NADH_2$ in the mitochondria, which regulates the activity of citrate cycle dehydrogenases (Fig. 11-12), and (3) the mitochondrial calcium concentration, which also regulates these dehydrogenases (Brown, 1992). With the exception of the regulatory role of calcium, these key factors can be deduced from the overall equation for phosphorylation of ADP to ATP:

$$NADH + H^+ + 3\ ADP + 3\ Pi + \tfrac{1}{2}\ O_2 \rightarrow NAD^+ + H_2O + 3\ ATP$$

The response of mitochondria to oxygen is steep, needing only minute amounts of oxygen for full operation. Therefore, in conditions of oxygen lack, the mitochondria are probably fully functioning until suddenly switched off as the mitochondrial oxygen tension decreases below a critical point. Provided there is sufficient oxygen, the processes of respiration are so regulated that ATP is resynthesized as rapidly as it is used, so the level tends to stay constant.

Calcium Uptake and Release by Mitochondria

Calcium is an important controller of mitochondrial respiration. *Calcium uptake* by the mitochondria occurs by a uniporter system that is not linked to the transport of any other ion. Inward transport of calcium is increased when cytosolic calcium increases. This uptake of calcium ions by mitochondrial matrix effectively requires energy to pump the protons out to balance the charges brought in with calcium ions. The fact that mitochondria contain much less calcium than previously thought suggests that the main function of calcium transfer in and out of the mitochondria is to regulate internal matrix calcium, and thereby Krebs cycle activity (Carafoli, 1988).

Calcium release from mitochondria occurs by an antiporter system, whereby two sodium ions are taken up for each calcium ion released. This carrier system is electrically neutral. There are separate pathways and separate control mechanisms for calcium uptake and release. The flux of calcium ions can be varied in either direction so that the mitochondrial pool of calcium can act as a calcium buffer for the cytosol.

The uptake of excess calcium in conditions of cytosolic calcium overload is serious. It impairs the proton gradient across the mitochondrial membranes, thereby reducing the ability of mitochondria to synthesize ATP. Irreversible reperfusion damage may be mediated by calcium (see Chapter 19). About two calcium ions and one phosphate ion accumulate for each pair of electrons passing through each energy-conserving site of the respiratory chain. Calcium forms insoluble calcium phosphate in the mitochondrial matrix, seen as irreversible granular densities on electron microscopy.

COUPLED OXIDATIVE PHOSPHORYLATION

Oxidation is an increase in positive charges or loss of negative charges; *reduction* is the reverse. When an electron donor donates e^- it undergoes oxidation. When an electron acceptor accepts e^- it undergoes reduction. Transfer of hydrogen is regarded as an equivalent process (because the hydrogen atom equals H^+ plus e^-).

The exact mechanisms linking the oxidation of $NADH_2$ (formed from the activity of the citrate cycle or pathways of substrate breakdown) to the formation of ATP are still poorly understood, despite the obvious importance of this critical process. The basic oxidative reaction in coupled oxidative phosphorylation is the oxidation of $NADH_2$ (which is more correctly given in the ionized form as NADH and H^+).

$$NADH + H^+ + \tfrac{1}{2} O_2 \rightarrow NAD^+ + H_2O$$

This is coupled to phosphorylation of ADP:

$$3\ ADP + 3\ Pi \rightarrow 3\ ATP$$

Classically it has been taught that three molecules of ATP are formed for each atom or half molecule of oxygen taken up (*P/O ratio of 3*), yet current evidence favors a lower value of about 2.5 (Ferguson et al., 1986). Production of ATP is coupled to proton production, and four protons produce enough proton motive force for one ATP. Thus, according to these current views, and depending on the substrate oxidized, the P/O ratio may vary from 2.28 to 2.58, in contrast to the old values of 2.83 to 3.17 (Table 11-3). That means that the oxygen uptake can be changed by the nature of the substrate by a factor of just over 11%. The physiologic variations in the P/O ratio simply reflect the number of oxygen atoms in the substrate used. Thus, glucose, already containing some oxygen atoms in its structure, needs less oxygen added to produce H_2O than does fatty acid.

Electron Transport Through Respiratory Chain

Electrons derived from $NADH_2$ (NADH + H^+) flow along the respiratory transport (electron transmitter) chain as follows:

$$NADH + H^+ + \text{flavoprotein (FP)} \rightarrow FP + 2e^- + NAD^+ + 2H^+$$

$$FP + 2e^- + \text{coenzyme Q} \rightarrow \text{reduced coenzyme Q (ubiquinone)} + \text{flavoprotein}$$

$$\text{Reduced coenzyme Q} + \text{cytochromes} \rightarrow \text{reduced cytochromes} + \text{coenzyme Q}$$

$$\text{Reduced cytochromes} + 2\ H^+ + \tfrac{1}{2} O_2 \rightarrow \text{cytochromes} + H_2O$$

Electrons are transferred through the cytochromes (b, c, and a), which are electron-transferring proteins containing iron porphyrin (heme) groups. The iron atoms undergo reversible changes in valency from the ferrous to the ferric form, and vice versa. Heart mitochondria, with their high rate of respiration and extensive surface area of inner membranes, each contain 60,000 to 70,000 molecules of cytochrome in all, compared with 17,000 in each liver mitochondrion (Lehninger, 1975).

The respiratory chain may be divided into three spans, each associated with the pumping of protons and with the production of ATP (Fig. 11-13). Site 1 is the span between NADH and coenzyme Q 10, site 2 is the span between cytochrome b and cytochrome c, and site 3 is the span between cytochrome c and oxygen. Together,

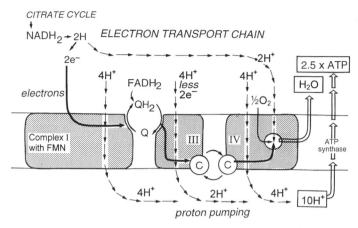

FIG. 11-13. Proton pumping and ATP synthesis. According to Mitchell's chemiosmotic hypothesis, the electron transfer components of the respiratory chain are arranged spatially and in sequence so that alternate electron and proton transfers occur. The consequence of such an arrangement is that protons are transferred from the mitochondrial matrix spaced out across the inner membrane, leaving negative charges behind. The exact mechanism of proton pumping is uncertain. The result is the establishment of an electrochemical proton gradient across the mitochondrial inner membrane (the *proton motive force*) made up of a proton concentration gradient and a charge separation or membrane potential. Coupling of the proton motive force to the synthesis of ATP from ADP and Pi occurs via a protein complex located in and on the inner mitochondrial membrane as protons re-enter the mitochondrial matrix. FMN, flavin mononucleotide; Q, coenzyme Q10; C, cytochrome C. For stoichiometry of oxidative phosphorylation, see Hinkle. *Biochemistry* 1991;30:3576.

these sites transfer 10 protons outward across the mitochondrial membrane, and each four protons produce one ATP according to the current view. The mitochondrial oxidation of three molecules of $NADH_2$ produced by the citrate cycle therefore yields two and a half molecules of ATP per atom of oxygen reduced (with a P/O ratio of 2.5). Other reactions (e.g., pyruvate dehydrogenase) forming $NADH_2$ will also have a P/O ratio of 2.5, but reactions feeding into the chain at the level of coenzyme Q will have a lower P/O ratio (succinate dehydrogenase produces $FADH_2$, which reacts with coenzyme Q so that only eight protons are transferred with the potential for the synthesis of two ATP).

Proton Pumping and ATP Synthesis

The actual mechanism for ATP manufacture is closely linked with the fate of protons rather than of electrons. Thus,

$$Hydrogen\ atom = proton + electron$$

$$H = H^+ + e^-$$

It is simple to suppose that the two H^+ link up with the two electrons and with oxygen eventually to form water. According to Mitchell's theory of oxidative phosphorylation, protons are pumped outward across the inner mitochondrial membrane to yield a gradient of H^+ across the membrane (Fig. 11-13). This H^+ gradient is the driving force for phosphorylation of ADP because protons re-enter the mitochondrial matrix through a complex of membrane proteins called the *ATP synthetase,* which is a protein ionophore. Formation of ATP from ADP is driven by proton movements caused by the transmembrane proton gradient.

To recapitulate, for oxidative phosphorylation to proceed requires a continuous supply of (1) oxygen, delivered by the coronary circulation; (2) protons and electrons, delivered by the citrate cycle; and (3) ADP. Both ADP and ATP are large, highly charged molecules that must be transported rapidly and continuously across the impermeable inner mitochondrial membrane. Such counterexchange of ADP inward and ATP outward across the inner membrane occurs by the activity of a very active transport system, the ADP–ATP carrier, or antiporter, also called the *translocase.* It is the most abundant protein in cardiac mitochondria. The carrier system is highly selective, transporting only ADP and ATP. The entry process of the translocase greatly prefers ADP to ATP, possibly by over 50 times. As the cytosolic ATP is converted to ADP during increased heart work, ADP transport to within the mitochondrial matrix is encouraged. Thus, there is an inverse relationship between the external ATP/ADP ratio and the oxygen uptake.

Free Radicals and Respiration

During normal mitochondrial respiration, small quantities of free oxygen radicals, such as the superoxide anion, are produced.

$$\text{Reduced flavin-enzyme} + O_2 \rightarrow \text{flavin-enzyme} + \cdot O_2$$

The rate of formation of superoxide is increased in ischemia when more reduced flavin-enzyme is available, and especially during reperfusion (for details see Chapter 19). Free radicals also may be produced by the xanthine oxidase reaction, which is not very active in the human heart. Such free radicals are normally removed by various enzyme systems, such as superoxide dismutase, which converts the superoxide anion into hydrogen peroxide, which is then acted on by catalase and peroxidase to yield water and molecular oxygen. *Glutathione reductase* also helps to remove spare electrons by aiding the formation of reduced glutathione. Because it is suspected that the increased formation of free radicals may contribute to ischemic and especially to reperfusion damage, *scavenger* compounds have been used experimentally. Examples include the enzymes superoxide dismutase and catalase.

HOW IS THE ENERGY USED?

How is the vast amount of ATP made every day by the heart actually used? Quite simply, most is for contraction (Fig. 11-14) and all the associated essential phenomena, such as calcium uptake by the sarcoplasmic reticulum. About 11%

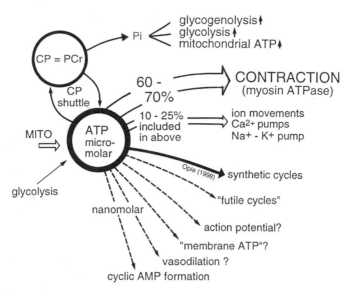

FIG. 11-14. Functions of ATP and CP. Note major use in contraction and related activities, such as ion transfer across membranes.

to 15% of ATP may be used for active transport by the sodium-potassium pump (see Table 4-7). Very little (less than 5%) is used for the actual generation of the action potential or the conduction of the cardiac impulse. Very small amounts of ATP are needed to phosphorylate the proteins in response to the formation of protein kinase or to form cAMP. An ill-defined small percentage is used for the futile cycles of glycogen and triglyceride turnover and of mitochondrial calcium uptake and release, and a further small percentage is used for protein synthesis. In pathologic states, *ATP wastage* occurs if futile cycles speed up and if abnormal nonphosphorylating pathways of oxygen uptake are stimulated by excess FFA (oxygen wastage).

In all these calculations, it must be appreciated that the actual energy liberated by ATP hydrolysis is largely converted to heat. Thus, only about 20% to 25% of the ATP used is actually converted into mechanical work. When allowance is made for the inevitable loss of heat, the heart is in fact very efficient in its ability to convert free energy into mechanical work plus heat.

Creatine Phosphate as Reserve Energy. At first sight, it would appear that creatine phosphate (CP; also called phosphocreatine, PCr) rather than ATP is the immediate source of energy for contraction. In several types of heart failure, loss of CP exceeds that of ATP. Yet the overall evidence is that it is ATP and not CP that is used directly in muscular contraction because it is ATP that causes isolated actomyosin threads to shorten. It is logical (and in agreement with the classical concepts of skeletal muscle physiology) that the ATP concentration in the myocardial cell should be maintained at the expense of CP, with the pool of CP suffering from more marked depletion than the pool of ATP. Very careful measurements show what is expected. Thus, a small early decrease of ATP precedes the large decrease in CP when all the coronary flow is abruptly stopped (global ischemia).

Energy Transfer Between ATP and CP.   The transfer of energy from CP to ATP occurs under the influence of creatine kinase (CK; also called creatine phosphokinase), which catalyses the following reaction

$$CP + ADP \rightarrow ATP + creatine$$

and the equilibrium favors formation of ATP by about 50 times. The function of CP as a reserve of energy can be seen during an acute work jump in the isolated heart when CP decreases and ATP is kept virtually constant or when skeletal muscle exercises. Why does the content of ADP increase rather than decrease as would be expected from the above equation? This is partly because the initial event is ATP hydrolysis.

$$ATP \xrightarrow{\text{myosin ATPase}} ADP + Pi + free energy$$

ATP is reformed from CP and ADP. Therefore, combining the above two equations, ATP should not decrease at all.

$$CP \rightarrow creatine + Pi + free energy$$

In reality, ATP decreases and ADP increases, showing that the rate of ATP hydrolysis during the work jump can exceed the rate at which ATP is formed from CP.

Creatine Kinase (Creatine Phosphokinase).   The heart has a high content of CK, and the loss of this enzyme in large amounts into the circulation is taken as proof of cell necrosis in acute myocardial infarction. The larger proportion of the cardiac CK exists in the cytosol as the *MB isoenzyme* (having one subunit of M muscle type and one of B brain type). The MM isoenzyme is present in small amounts in the myofibrils and possibly the microsomes. Different localization of isoenzymes within the extramitochondrial space could be one way in which local aliquots of energy are transferred from CP to ATP, so that ATP can be used at various localized sites in the cytoplasm (Fig. 11-15). This process is the *CP shuttle* (Kammermeier, 1987), which is required to shuttle energy from one site in the cytosol to another. The very low cytosolic concentration of free ADP (most is protein bound) means that ADP produced by heart work could not rapidly diffuse to the mitochondria.

   A mitochondrial CK isoenzyme is situated on the outside of the inner mitochondrial membrane, where it is thought to be in close juxtaposition to the adenine nucleotide translocase. The kinetic properties of the enzyme support the role of

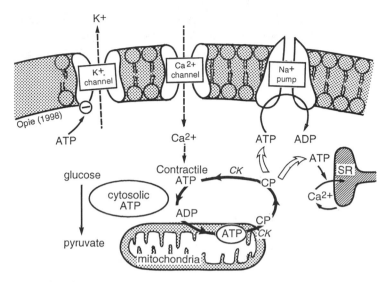

FIG. 11-15. ATP pools and compartments. The major ATP compartments are mitochondrial and cytosolic. Minor localized pools are associated with the potassium channel, where ATP acts as a regulatory ligand, and external surface ATP, which may function as a vasodilator. ATP is used in many noncontractile processes, such as sodium pumping and uptake of calcium by the sarcoplasmic reticulum (SR). CK has an important role in the functional compartmentalization of ATP. The mitochondrial CK isoenzyme is situated between the inner and outer mitochondrial membranes to form CP from creatine. The outer mitochondrial membrane is freely permeable to CP, which can then reform ATP from ADP generated by cellular activity (e.g., contraction). This is the function of the cytoplasmic CK isoenzyme.

this enzyme in dealing with ATP newly synthesized and newly exported from mitochondria (Kuznetsov et al., 1989). ATP produced in the mitochondria by oxidative phosphorylation is thought to be transferred by the mitochondrial CK isoenzyme to cytoplasmic CP. Thus, the real end product of oxidative phosphorylation in the heart is CP (Jacobus, 1985). The latter compound then transfers high-energy phosphate bonds back to ATP at the site of ATP use, under the influence of a cytosolic isoenzyme of CK (Fig. 11-15). When creatine transport is inhibited by a specific inhibitor, heart failure ensues, which again supports the concept of the importance of the CP shuttle for cardiac contractile function (Kapelko et al., 1988). A corollary of this proposal is that ADP produced by the mitochondrial CK should have preferential access to the translocase, as proposed by Jacobus (1985). When the CP shuttle is obliterated in a mouse knock-out model, then the hearts maintain energy production by a higher ADP concentration (Saupe et al., 1996).

This doctrine of privileged access of mitochondrial ATP to mitochondrial CK is challenged by counterproposals that the cytoplasmic CKs are so active that they promote rapid equilibrium of the substrate throughout the cytosol (Altschuld and Brierley, 1977).

Whichever view is adopted, CK plays a vital role in the maintenance of cytosolic ATP at the expense of cytosolic CP. By transferring energy-rich bonds from ATP as it emerges from the mitochondria to cytosolic CP, and then back again to ATP, CK also controls the transport of energy in the cytosol.

During irreversible ischemia, the sarcolemma becomes permeable and various enzymes, including CK, leak into the circulation. When the blood level of CK increases above a certain arbitrary level, then the diagnosis of cardiac cell necrosis (myocardial infarction) is made.

ATP COMPARTMENTS

At the onset of ischemia, there is a surprising discrepancy between the rapid cessation of contraction and the small decrease in the level of myocardial ATP. Cellular compartmentation of ATP is one of several possible explanations. Compartmentation means that certain compounds are not distributed uniformly throughout the cell. Rather, different concentrations are found in different compartments within the cell. Compartmentation of ATP between its site of production in mitochondria and its site of use in the cytoplasm is well accepted. At least 90% of the ATP is found in the cytosol. During acute heart work, it is the ATP in the cytosol that is broken down so that the very small amount of cytosolic ADP doubles. Cytosolic ADP will therefore increase with increased work to drive mitochondrial respiration, according to the classic concept that the rate of mitochondrial respiration is set by ADP.

It is the possibility of *cytosolic subcompartments of ATP* that has provoked abundant controversy (Fig. 11-15). Evidence favoring cytoplasmic subcompartmentation is as follows. First, unequal distribution of CK isoenzymes throughout the cytoplasm could form more ATP from CP in specific cytosolic sites. Similar evidence is provided by the role of the phosphocreatine energy shuttle (Kapelko et al., 1988). Second, the existence of a small subcompartment of rapid-turnover ATP would explain those situations in which small changes in total ATP occur but appear to have large effects, such as the abrupt loss of contractile activity in ischemic hearts, while the ATP is still relatively high. Such low rates of decrease of ATP in regional ischemia, compared with the much faster declines in CP, have been shown by numerous workers. Depletion of only a small pool of ATP could cause contractile failure, but it is equally possible that other factors, such as an increase of tissue pCO_2 or Pi, could cause contractile failure. Third, ATP produced by glycolysis appears to have a special function in protecting the cell membrane, particularly the activity of the ATP-sensitive potassium channel (Weiss and Lamp, 1987) and the sodium pump (Cross et al., 1996), and in promoting relaxation of the ischemic heart. When ischemic contracture develops in underperfused hearts, it is the source of ATP and not the total ATP that is important in preventing contracture. Thus, ATP made by glycolysis is effective, whereas ATP from residual mitochondrial metabolism is not (Owen et al., 1990). Fourth, ATP injected directly into altered cells helps to prolong the action potential duration (Taniguchi, 1983), suggesting a role of cytoplasmic ATP in electrogenesis.

Evidence arguing against ATP compartments chiefly relates to doubtful correlations found between the decrease in the total ATP and the onset of irreversible ischemic injury. An additional biochemical argument is that the cytosol can be viewed as a uniform space, throughout which CP and ATP are in equilibrium (Altschuld and Brierley, 1977).

PHYSIOLOGIC BREAKDOWN OF ATP

To release energy from ATP requires its breakdown to ADP and inorganic phosphate (Pi) (Fig. 11-16), which form during each cardiac contraction cycle. It is usually forgotten that there is a proton produced and that ATP is chelated to magnesium.

Thus, the standard equation

$$ATP \rightarrow ADP + Pi + \text{free energy}$$

becomes

$$MgATP^{2-} \rightarrow MgADP^{1-} + Pi^{2-} + H^+ + \text{free energy}$$

The exact charges depend on the intracellular pH. ADP can (1) reform ATP via the CK reaction, (2) be further split to form ATP and AMP by the adenylate

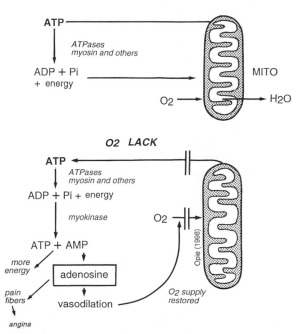

FIG. 11-16. ATP breakdown. The influence of oxygen supply on the extent of ATP breakdown. In normoxia, ATP is broken down by heart work (myosin ATPase) to ADP and Pi, which are resynthesized to ATP in the mitochondria. In hypoxia, further breakdown yields more energy and stimulates glycolysis to provide anaerobic energy and causes a compensatory vasodilation (probably via adenosine).

kinase reaction, or (3) enter the mitochondria under the influence of the adenine nucleotide translocase to stimulate respiration. The proton produced is important during anaerobic glycolysis, when it is the major source of the intracellular acidosis (Gevers, 1977).

The total content of ADP in the normal heart is about 0.5 to 1 μmol/g wet weight. However, the real concentration dissolved in cell water (as opposed to the overall level) is difficult to assess because most ADP is bound to actin, some to myosin, and only a smaller portion is freely dissolved in the cytosol. The breakdown of even small amounts of cytosolic ATP to ADP can markedly increase the concentration of free ADP in the cytosol (estimated at only 0.02 μmol/g wet weight), thereby stimulating mitochondrial metabolism.

Adenylate kinase (AMP kinase, myokinase) allows the breakdown of ADP to proceed to AMP, thereby increasing the cardiac content of AMP.

$$2 \text{ ADP} \xrightarrow{\text{myokinase}} \text{ATP} + \text{AMP}$$

This reaction is reversible and will proceed toward formation of AMP only when ADP is elevated. Thus, under the influence of myosin ATPase

$$2 \text{ ATP} \rightarrow 2 \text{ ADP} + 2 \text{ Pi} + 2 \text{ (free energy)}$$

and under the influence of myokinase

$$2 \text{ ADP} \rightarrow \text{ATP} + \text{AMP}$$

and myosin ATPase again catalyzes

$$\text{ATP} \rightarrow \text{ADP} + \text{Pi} + \text{free energy}$$

so that the overall reaction is

$$2 \text{ ATP} \rightarrow \text{ADP} + \text{AMP} + 3 \text{ Pi} + 3 \text{ (free energy)}$$

This overall equation liberates 1.5 times as much high-energy phosphate as does simple ATP hydrolysis (compare above equations). The extra energy provided by the added breakdown of ATP beyond ADP to AMP is associated with further metabolism of AMP to IMP (inosine monophosphate) and adenosine. Because the ratio of ATP to adenosine is so high, perhaps about 1,000 to 1, the breakdown of only a small amount of ATP to adenosine can markedly increase the levels of the latter.

Adenosine

In view of its multiple important functions, adenosine has been given colorful names, such as the "homeostatic metabolite" (Schrader, 1990) and the "signal of life" (Mullane and Engler, 1991), which can be harnessed for endogenous cardioprotection (Mullane and Bullough, 1995).

Adenosine interacts with two receptors, the A_1 myocardial receptors and the A_2 vascular receptors and is linked to multiple signal systems. One key function of adenosine, acting on the A_2 receptors, is to keep energy metabolism in bal-

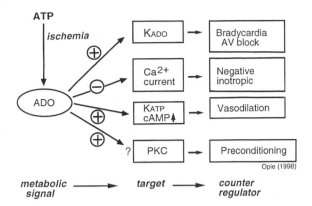

FIG. 11-17. Adenosine signaling. Proposed role of adenosine (ADO) in (1) inhibition of sino-atrial (SA) and atrioventricular (AV) nodes and of atrial muscle via potassium channel (K_{ADO}) opening and hyperpolarization, (2) inhibition of ventricular contraction by increasing calcium channel closing times, (3) opening of ATP-sensitive potassium channel (K_{ATP}), and (4) activation of protein kinase (PKC). For function of adenosine in coronary flow regulation, see Chapter 10.

ance by providing the signal to compensatory vasodilation. When acting on the A_1 receptors, there are additional and other cardioprotective roles, including potassium channel opening, catecholamine antagonism, therapeutic inhibition of the atrioventricular node in supraventricular tachycardias, and an important role in preconditioning (Fig. 11-17). These possibilities are discussed in more detail in the section on Clinical Applications.

ATP BREAKDOWN IN ISCHEMIA

When ATP is broken down acutely, as in hypoxia or ischemia, it is protected by CP. Then, release from the heart of breakdown products of ATP can be expected. During regional ischemia, the concentration of Pi in the coronary sinus increases. This phosphate is derived only in part from ATP, with a larger component coming from the breakdown of CP. Adenosine, inosine, and hypoxanthine can all cross the cell membrane, and it is therefore not surprising that the ischemic myocardium releases these compounds.

Is It the Decrease in ATP That Causes Cell Death?

A simplistic view of cell death in ischemia would be that ATP decreases to a critical level, vital functions cease, and all is over. Considering the pains to which the cell goes to maintain and replenish its ATP, it would not be surprising if there was a critical level of ATP required to keep the cell alive. For example, in *regional ischemia,* Jennings et al. (1978) have linked irreversible ultrastructural changes about 40 minutes after coronary artery occlusion to ATP levels of 2 to 3 μmol/g dry weight (0.4 to 0.6 μmol/g fresh weight). Similarly, the onset of rigor mortis could be linked to endocardial ATP values of 0.6 μmol/g fresh weight (Lowe et al., 1979).

Nonetheless, this concept is oversimplified. ATP levels below those regarded as critical are still compatible with cell survival. In *low flow ischemia* (Owen et al., 1990), the development of ischemic contracture could be dissociated from the total tissue ATP value. In the *nonischemic zone* after coronary occlusion, there was an unexpected decrease in the ATP content in some experiments (Gudbjarnason et al., 1970). Nonischemic muscle contracted normally and survived at ATP values as low as 1.5 to 2.0 μmol/g fresh weight. In *reperfusion* after ischemic arrest, Schaper et al. (1979) showed that ATP might decrease as low as 1 μmol/g wet weight and the hearts could still survive.

Such evidence shows that it is very unlikely that there is a single critical level of ATP, especially because (1) the duration of the deficit of ATP may be as important as the level reached and (2) compartmentation of ATP can selectively save membrane function. Furthermore, as cells die, a great number of events besides loss of ATP takes place, and the true cause of lethality could be the combination of ATP deficits with the accumulation of calcium and potentially toxic metabolites, such as fatty acid derivatives, lactate, protons, and CO_2. ATP depletion is harmful for ischemic cells, but low ATP levels in well-oxygenated or reperfused cells can be withstood. Measurements of ATP are no substitute for direct measurements of irreversible ischemic injury, such as ultrastructural changes or ischemic contracture.

ATP Products and Energy Status

A decrease of ATP stimulates both the primitive energy supply systems of glycogenolysis and glycolysis and also the more evolved mitochondrial oxidative systems. Stimulation of the latter is assisted by an increased coronary blood flow via adenosine formation and provides more oxygen to increase oxidative phosphorylation in the mitochondria. The detailed mechanisms whereby the decline in ATP acts on the different pathways vary (Table 11-6), yet the principle is constant. It is not the level of ATP itself that regulates the compensatory pathways but the ATP breakdown products (adenosine monophosphate, Pi, adenosine) that act as regulators. Breakdown of only a small amount of ATP potentially can markedly increase the cellular levels of the real regulators, such as AMP and adenosine.

The *phosphorylation potential* relates change in high-energy phosphates to mitochondrial metabolism (Brown, 1992).

$$\text{Phosphorylation potential} = \frac{[\text{ATP}]}{[\text{ADP}][\text{Pi}]}$$

AMP is omitted because it does not play a direct role in the regulation of mitochondrial respiration. The value of this ratio is that it is reciprocally related to the

TABLE 11-6. *Compensatory metabolic pathways sensitive to decrease of ATP and CP and increase of ADP, AMP, and Pi*

Pathway	Site of regulation	Mode of regulation
Glycogenolysis	Phosphorylase	CP inhibits; AMP and Pi stimulate phosphorylase *b*
Glycolysis	PFK (and glucose uptake)[a]	ATP and CP inhibit; increase of AMP and Pi stimulates
Adenosine formation	5'-Nucleotidase	Decrease in energy status activates
ATP synthesis	Oxidative phosphorylation	ADP and Pi stimulate mitochondrial oxidative phosphorylation

[a]Regulated by coronary flow rate and glucose transporters, GLUT 4 and GLUT 1.

rate of mitochondrial oxidative metabolism. The problem is that the cytosolic ADP concentration is required and cannot readily be measured but only calculated (Clarke and Willis, 1987).

The *free energy of hydrolysis of ATP* is not an arbitrary ratio, but gives absolute values. It is calculated from the following equation (Lawson and Veech, 1979):

$$\Delta G_{ATP} = \Delta G^{\circ}_{obs} + RT \ln \frac{[ADP][Pi]}{[ATP]}$$

where ΔG°_{obs} is the standard change in free energy, taken as -30.5 kJ/mol, R is the gas constant, and T is the absolute temperature. A high (ATP)/(ADP)(Pi) ratio is associated with a high value of $-\Delta G$ ATP. The lower the ATP and the higher the ADP and Pi, the less the value of the negative free energy of ATP hydrolysis. In general, in ischemia, the most negative values (e.g., -58 kJ/mol) are associated with the best postischemic recoveries (Cross et al., 1996). In severe ischemia, when the ΔG drops as low as -47 kJ/mol, there appears to be a thermodynamic restriction on the use of ATP for the sodium pump; that is, not only is the ATP low, but the ATP there is not yielding the energy that might be expected.

In humans, the *ratio CP/Pi* can be measured by ^{31}P nuclear magnetic resonance (NMR) techniques and therefore assessed in vivo (Schaefer et al., 1989). This ratio represents a simple approach because it is closely related to the breakdown of ATP to ADP and Pi (Chance et al., 1981). Another NMR ratio that has been used on the human heart is *CP/ATP*, the principle being that in conditions of myocardial metabolic stress, ATP is maintained at the expense of CP (Conway et al., 1991).

ANAEROBIC GLYCOLYSIS

Strictly, anaerobic means no oxygen but that does not mean no life. Anaerobic metabolism refers to any state of suboptimal oxygenation that accelerates glycolysis and increases the production of lactate (Fig. 11-18). Anaerobic glycolysis is part of the defense mechanism that allows sufficient production of oxygen-inde-

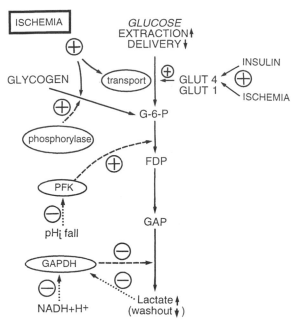

FIG. 11-18. Regulation of glycolysis in ischemia. Two major hypotheses are (1) rate-limiting steps as shown in ovals and (2) distributive control, regulated by rates of glucose delivery or glycogenolysis (King et al., 1995). G-6-P, glucose 6-phosphate; FDP, fructose 1,6 bisphosphate; GAP, glyceraldehyde 3-phosphate.

pendent energy to sustain the noncontractile ischemic myocardium. To explain how glycolysis is accelerated during hypoxia and ischemia requires an analysis of the properties of two crucial enzymes: PFK and glyceraldehyde 3-phosphate dehydrogenase. The PFK reaction is ideally suited for metabolic control of glycolysis during hypoxia because it is so sensitive to the energy status of the myocardial cells. Low molecular weight metabolites, such as ATP, AMP, ADP, and Pi interact with the enzyme at *allosteric sites* (Greek *allos,* alongside; *stereos,* configuration) that are distant from the site of interaction between substrates and enzyme. During hypoxia and mild ischemia, ATP levels decrease, and those of ADP and AMP increase, as does that of Pi. These changes enhance the activity of the enzyme (increased anaerobic glycolysis). During severe ischemia, glycolysis is inhibited by low rates of delivery of glucose, glycogen depletion, and intracellular acidosis, which all inhibit the enzyme PFK. In addition, just before the onset of irreversible damage in severe ischemia, PFK is translocated from cytosol to myocardial membranes, and thereby inactivated (Hazen et al., 1994).

A second and equally important control step is that regulating the flow through glycolysis at the level of the enzyme glyceraldehyde 3-phosphate dehydrogenase (Mochizuki and Neely, 1979), which is inhibited in severely ischemic tissue by the end products of anaerobic glycolysis, such as lactate, protons, and $NADH_2$.

Thus, to recapitulate, mild ischemia stimulates glycolysis and has potentially beneficial effects by provision of oxygen-independent ATP. Severe ischemia limits glycolysis by decreasing the delivery of glucose to the ischemic cells, by glycogen depletion, by enzyme inhibition at the levels of PFK and glyceraldehyde 3-phosphate dehydrogenase, and by translocation and inactivation of PFK. The consequent decrease in the rate of anaerobic production of ATP has potentially harmful or even lethal consequences for the ischemic myocardium.

Energy Production by Anaerobic Glycolysis

For anaerobic glycolysis to produce as much ATP as during aerobic metabolism of glucose would require an acceleration of glycolysis by nearly 20 times, in contrast to the more modest acceleration that even total anoxia produces when coronary flow is maintained artificially. The anaerobic heart therefore develops a severe deficit of energy unless arrested by potassium (Fig. 11-19) or hypothermia. When glucose is the source of glycolysis, the whole glycolytic path uses two ATP and produces four ATP, that is, the net production is two. When glycogen is the source, ATP production is three per six-carbon molecule passing through glycolysis. An important point is that glycolytic ATP will be made whenever glucose 6-phosphate is converted to pyruvate even during oxidative metabolism.

Anaerobic glycolysis changes the normal uptake of lactate by the aerobic myocardium to discharge, and the level in the coronary sinus may exceed that in

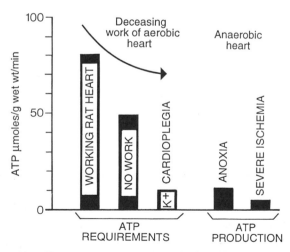

FIG. 11-19. Anaerobic ATP cannot meet energy needs of the heart unless it is arrested by cardioplegia, even when ATP is produced at maximal rates (anoxia with sustained coronary flow). During total ischemia, the rate of anaerobic glycolysis decreases so that the best way of preserving the ischemic myocardium is by reducing the ATP demand (cardioplegia-hypothermia). For details of calculations, see Opie, *Cardiology* 1971;56:2.

arterial blood during myocardial ischemia. This is not a very sensitive procedure because apparent net uptake of lactate can mask local lactate production by the ischemic zone (Ferrannini et al., 1993). The formation of protons during anaerobic glycolysis is, strictly speaking, not from glycolysis itself but from the associated breakdown of ATP. The *malate-aspartate shuttle* is crucial in transferring protons in the form of $NADH_2$ from the cytosol to the mitochondria. During anaerobic glycolysis, such protons accumulate in the cytosol, as discussed in Chapter 17.

CLINICAL APPLICATIONS OF ENERGY METABOLISM

Despite the wealth of possible metabolically based interventions that could be of clinical relevance, it is disappointing that only a few have been subject to thorough appraisal.

Cardioplegia.   This is the most successful and widely used application of metabolic principles to myocardial preservation (Fig. 11-19). A low temperature diminishes the ATP requirements by decreasing the rate of enzyme reactions and the force of contraction, and a high external potassium mechanically arrests the heart by depolarization. Provision of glucose as glucose-insulin-potassium in the preoperative period increases cardiac glycogen and gives added protection (Oldfield et al., 1986).

Insulin Resistance.   This diagnosis is of increasing clinical importance and is applied to a variety of common clinical conditions that share the inability of skeletal muscle to respond to insulin by adequately increasing the glucose uptake. These conditions include congestive heart failure, obesity, diabetes mellitus, some cases of hypertension (see Fig. 14-14), and postinfarct patients with low ejection fractions (Paternostro et al., 1996). Whether insulin resistance can occur in cardiac as well as in skeletal muscle is controversial. Studies on heart failure patients suggest that insulin resistance can be found in the heart in proportion to the severity of the failure (Swan et al., 1994). In two animal models, insulin resistance is associated with cardiac hypertrophy, allowing the speculation that insulin could be acting as a growth factor and promoting the hypertrophy (Katz et al., 1995; Paternostro et al., 1995).

Insulin resistance seems to be multifactorial in origin, including (1) glucose-induced phosphorylation of the serine/threonine components of the insulin receptor, which diminishes the capacity of this receptor to undergo the crucial phosphorylation of tyrosine in response to insulin (Pillay et al., 1996); and (2) inhibition of the glucose transporter by circulating FFAs (Roden et al., 1996). Of interest, these fatty acids may be elevated in several of the conditions associated with insulin resistance, such as obesity and maturity-onset diabetes.

For the patient, the major problem with insulin resistance is that it is potentially a self-perpetuating vicious circle, because as it progresses, the blood levels of glucose and FFAs are both likely to increase. As a result, the diabetic state could worsen or the nondiabetic patient could be edged nearer and nearer to frank diabetes. In heart failure or hypertension, these adverse trends could be exaggerated by concurrent diuretic therapy, which may promote the diabetic state. Despite these grave possibilities, there is no pharmacologic therapy specifically designed to avoid or to ameliorate insulin resistance. Hypothetically, insulin resistance could be overcome or prevented by exercise training, which increases glucose transport into muscle. There are already data supporting such a proposal in obese diabetic patients. In the obese and in diabetics, weight loss lessens insulin resistance. In heart failure, a reasonable but thus far unproven speculation is that effective treatment would lessen insulin resistance.

Hemodynamic Effects of Insulin. There are controversial proposals that insulin could decrease the peripheral vascular resistance by vasodilation or act as an inotropic agent to increase cardiac performance. Nonetheless, no such effects were found in healthy humans in a careful study with full hemodynamic and metabolic monitoring (Ferrannini et al., 1993).

Metabolic Therapies of Ischemia. Because the ATP needs of contraction are so high and the rate of anaerobic production of ATP is so low, the first principle in preserving ischemic cells is to lessen the myocardial oxygen demand (see Chapter 12). Thus, when the myocardial cells are threatened by ischemia, as in angina pectoris (see Chapter 17), the heart rate and the blood pressure should be reduced by drugs such as β-adrenergic blockers. Experimentally, provision of glycolytic ATP is crucial to the survival of ischemic cells (Apstein et al., 1983) (Fig. 11-20). Whether the increase of glucose extraction achieved by the ischemic process itself can be further enhanced by insulin is not clear. Formation of intracellular protons needs to be kept low (e.g., by the use of Na^+/H^+ exchange inhibitors, which are currently under clinical trial for unstable angina). Experimentally, accumulation of lactate, which is probably harmful in its own right apart from any associated formation of protons, may be lessened by giving inosine to divert pyruvate from lactate to alanine (Lewandowski et al., 1991).

During severe ischemia, which threatens to kill myocytes, glycolysis is limited by the low rate of delivery of glucose (King et al., 1995), so that *reperfusion by thrombolysis* is an important procedure to accelerate glycolysis. During the early phase of acute myocardial infarction, the levels of circulating catecholamines and FFAs are high, and both can have toxic effects on myocardial cells. Blood FFAs can be reduced by either β-blockade or glucose-insulin infusions. Of these, β-blockade is the best tested in acute infarction, and this procedure also increases the glucose extraction by the ischemic zone after coronary ligation in the dog. Although theoretically thrombolysis should be initiated and β-blockade given as soon as possible after the onset of symptoms, this combination has not yet been subject to strict clinical trials.

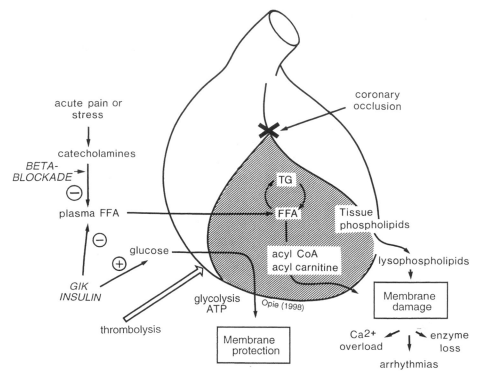

FIG. 11-20. Mechanisms of fatty acid toxicity and metabolic protection by glycolysis.
TG, triacylglyceride; CoA, coenzyme A; GIK, glucose-insulin-potassium, –, negative effect; +, positive effect.

Regarding the vexed question of GIK (glucose-insulin-potassium) infusions for acute myocardial infarction, it is not certain that insulin has an added effect on top of ischemia in enhancing the activity of the glucose transporters. It should also be considered that excess stimulation of glycolysis, greater than the capacity for washout of inhibitory protons and lactate, might have adverse effects. Therefore, thrombolytic reperfusion might be the most effective mode of increasing glucose delivery to ischemic cells. A trial of GIK in acute infarction is currently under way. In diabetic patients with acute myocardial infarction, an infusion of glucose and insulin followed by insulin therapy was more beneficial than oral antidiabetic therapy by sulfonylureas, and long-term prognosis improved (Malmberg et al., 1995). Such an infusion may work, in part, by suppression of blood FFA levels, which tend to be high in diabetic patients.

Lipid Metabolites in Ischemic Injury.   In the normal heart, the cytosolic concentration of acyl carnitine is very low, with none in the mitochondria. During ischemia, the concentrations in both cytosol and mitochondria increase to about

2,000 μmol/L. Acyl carnitines also inhibit the activity of the sodium–potassium pump at concentrations likely to be present in the ischemic tissue. The ensuing loss of potassium is also arrhythmogenic. Lysophosphoglycerides are membrane-active fatty acids that are released from the phospholipids of the sarcolemma and other membranes during ischemia. It is proposed that accumulated lysophosphatidyl choline (LPC) can depolarize the cell membrane, thereby having arrhythmogenic properties (Sato et al., 1993). No therapy is available to limit such lipid accumulation; several trials with carnitine or propionyl carnitine have not been promising. Theoretically, β-blockade may help by decreasing blood FFAs and by lessening the rate of breakdown of myocardial triglycerides.

Adenosine. Perhaps best known as a vasodilator, according to the Berne hypothesis (see Chapter 10), adenosine has further interesting cardioprotective properties. Acting through the A_1 receptor and a G protein, it links to the potassium and calcium channels and thereby inhibits nodal and muscular activity, respectively (Fig. 11-17). Adenosine is often successful in the therapy of paroxysmal supraventricular tachycardias (see Chapter 5). During ischemia, adenosine produced from the breakdown of ATP may act as a protective negative feedback signal by causing atrioventricular block, decreasing the ventricular response rate, and conserving the limited supply of oxygen available (Jenkins and Belardinelli, 1988). Adenosine also inhibits myocardial adenylate cyclase and the L-calcium current, thereby providing potential protection against excess β-adrenergic stimulation. Of considerable current interest and debate is the proposed role of adenosine in the protective phenomenon of preconditioning (see Chapter 19). One proposal is that adenosine acts via A_1 receptors and phospholipase C to activate protein kinase C, which may then help open ATP-sensitive potassium channels, which in turn confers the protection.

During effort angina, stimulation of the myocardial pain fibers by adenosine, ultimately derived from the ischemic breakdown of ATP, may hypothetically cause the chest pain.

In ischemic cardiac arrest, there is loss of total adenine nucleotides. Experimentally, the rate of resynthesis of ATP during the recovery period is stimulated by the therapeutic provision of adenosine or its precursors. In all these cases, the adenosine concentrations used probably are far higher than the very low amount of adenosine found in normal heart tissue. Such high concentrations of adenosine may not be well tolerated by humans.

Experimental Myocarditis and Cardiomyopathy. The activity of the mitochondrial ATP-ADP *translocase* is vital to life of the heart, and compounds inhibiting the carrier can literally kill the heart. One such inhibitor is bongkrekate, a deadly poison produced by bacteria growing on coconut food products in Indonesia. Another inhibitor of pharmacologic interest is *atractyloside,* which is similar in structure to the physiologic inhibitor acyl CoA. When infused into the coronary circulation, atractyloside can induce deficits of tissue high-energy phosphate compounds and an elevation of the ST segment of the epicardial electrocardiogram.

During experimental myocardial damage by virus infection (*myocarditis*), circulating antibodies to adenine nucleotide translocase form. Such antibodies can in turn penetrate the myocytes to interact with and damage the translocase system (Schulze et al., 1990). This defect in oxidative metabolism may contribute further to the myocardial damage and promote the process of cardiomyopathy (cardiac muscle disease). In patients with human dilated cardiomyopathy, studies with positron emission tomography (PET) show defects in oxidative metabolism.

Metabolic Imaging: Positron Emission Tomography.   Pathways of intracellular metabolism, previously studied only in animal tissues, can now be traced in humans by the technique of PET scanning. Radiolabeled *2-deoxyglucose* (^{18}F-deoxyglucose) can be visualized by PET (Fig. 11-21) when it is given in tracer amounts that accumulate within myocardial cells as the phosphorylated compound, without glycolysis being inhibited. In addition, the compound ^{13}NH$_3$ can be used to measure coronary blood flow (see Chapter 12). As expected, mild ischemia increases the glucose extraction, so that the metabolic severity of ischemia can be measured and used clinically to distinguish between those myocardial segments that are ischemic but viable (increased glucose extraction in relation to decreased coronary flow, mismatch pattern) in contrast to those that are nonviable (decreased glucose extraction and low coronary flow), a test that has practical potential in diagnosing hibernation (see Chapter 19) and hence in

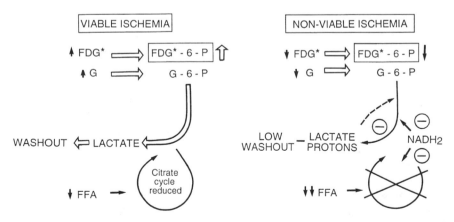

FIG. 11-21. Glucose imaging and viability. Proposed use of F18-fluorodeoxyglucose (FDG˙) in acting as a marker for glucose uptake. FDG-G-P is not metabolized. Hence, the intensity of extraction of FDG by the myocardium as detected by positron emission tomography is an index of viability. In "mismatch," glucose extraction is increased in relation to coronary blood flow, measured by NH$_3$. In very severe ischemia or infarction, glucose delivery is decreased, glycolysis is inhibited, and extraction of FDG decreases.

selecting patients for coronary artery surgery. It is not clear whether accurate additional information is given by calculation of the absolute glucose uptake from the rate of arrival of ^{18}F-deoxyglucose in the human heart. Those using this technique argue that valuable information is achieved. For example, the very low basal rate of glucose uptake in the fasted state is increased about four times in unstable angina (Camici et al., 1989b), or insulin resistance of the human heart can be defined (Paternostro et al., 1996). The problem is that a number of fundamental limitations are involved in the calculations of the glucose uptake (Hariharan et al., 1995).

The uptake of *^{11}C-acetate* is related directly to the rate of acetate oxidation, which, in turn, is closely related to the myocardial oxygen uptake because acetate enters the citrate cycle without requiring preparation by complex metabolic pathways, as in the case of glucose or fatty acid fuels. Thus, the use of ^{11}C-acetate may allow noninvasive determination of the oxygen uptake of the intact heart (Armbrecht et al., 1990).

Measurement of High-Energy Phosphates by Nuclear Magnetic Resonance. Nuclear magnetic resonance techniques (^{31}P NMR) allow repetitive measurements of ATP and CP in the animal heart in situ. This powerful technique is now being applied to the human heart in situ and may have application in assessing the viability of a donor heart before transplantation. It should be noted that ^{31}P NMR cannot directly measure the low cytosolic levels of ADP, a crucial regulator of mitochondrial activity. The decline of contractile activity during oxygen lack can be linked not so much to decreased high-energy phosphate levels but rather to decreased rates of production of ATP and CP (Bittl et al., 1987). In heart failure, the ratio of CP to ATP decreases in relation to the severity of failure (Conway et al., 1991; Neubauer et al., 1992).

Novel Therapies. *Taurine* is an amino acid of unknown function that lessens sodium accumulation during ischemia by promotion of Na-taurine efflux (Chapman et al., 1993). Thus, the potentially lethal increase of internal sodium may be lessened. This benefit of intracellular taurine is not achieved by taurine infusions because the very high intracellular level of taurine limits uptake from the blood.

Glutamate, by interacting with pyruvate, can form alanine and α-ketoglutarate, the latter then giving increased succinyl CoA, which can then undergo substrate level phosphorylation with production of a high-energy compound, guanosine triphosphate (GTP). All of this could theoretically happen independently of oxygen and thereby benefit the ischemic myocardium, as suggested in some clinical trials (Thomassen et al., 1991).

Postreperfusion abnormalities are multiple. Experimentally, provision of glucose and pyruvate is protective. A rundown of citrate cycle intermediates can be remedied by conversion of pyruvate to malate (Fig. 11-9). This topping-up process is called anaplerosis (Taegtmeyer, 1995). Excessive cytosolic calcium in the reperfused myocardium can be normalized by promotion of glycolysis (Jeremy et al., 1993), which provides the cytosolic ATP required for the uptake of calcium by the sarcoplasmic reticulum and for extrusion of sodium by the sodium pump. Promotion of glycolysis is not enough, because a high glycolytic rate can be uncoupled from low rates of glucose oxidation and poor cardiac performance (Kudo et al., 1995). Levels of malonyl CoA can be very low, the proposed result of an accumulation of AMP, which in turn inhibits the synthesis of malonyl CoA to lessen the inhibition of fatty acid oxidation (Kudo et al., 1995). Increased fatty acid oxidation and reduced glucose oxidation appear to be adverse in the context of reperfusion and may have to be countered. Increased glucose oxidation and cardiac function may be achieved by activation of pyruvate dehyrogenase (e.g., by dichloroacetate), as well as by provision of pyruvate. None of these measures have been subject to clinical trials during thrombolysis.

SUMMARY

1. *Myocardial fuels.* The heart is omnivorous in its requirements for fuels that it can convert to energy required chiefly for contractile purposes. Glucose is the major myocardial fuel only after a high-carbohydrate meal. Glucose is transported into heart cells by the insulin-sensitive transporter GLUT 4 to undergo phosphorylation to glucose 6-phosphate. Glycogen is a reserve fuel that can be broken down to glucose 6-phophate in emergency situations, such as the sudden onset of increased heart work or of ischemia. Glycolysis is the process common to glucose uptake and glycogen breakdown that converts glucose 6-phosphate to two molecules of pyruvate. In anaerobic conditions (lack of oxygen), pyruvate is converted to lactate, whereas aerobically it forms the two-carbon compound acetyl CoA, which enters the citrate cycle.

2. *Energy yield.* During glycolysis (glucose 6-phosphate to pyruvate), there is a net yield of two ATP, as well as two H_2 (the latter from dehydrogenation step). The two H_2 cannot immediately form water but must first interact with an important carrier molecule, NAD, to form $NADH_2$ which enters the mitochondrial space by a shuttle mechanism to yield aerobic energy. The additional energy yield of the oxidative metabolism of glucose is about 30 ATP molecules per glucose molecule, with a total yield of 32 ATP (these are lower than values previously given).

3. *Role of free fatty acids.* Long-chain free fatty acids (FFAs), usually the major myocardial fuel, readily pass through the sarcolemmal membrane before irreversible activation to acyl CoA, which cannot penetrate the mitochondrial barrier without a carnitine carrier system. Acyl CoA is carried within the mitochondria as acyl carnitine, there to enter the pathways of β-oxidation that sequentially chop off two carbon fractions to form acetyl CoA, which in turn enters the citrate cycle. That part of the FFA uptake that is not oxidized can form triglyceride and myocardial structural lipids, the latter by changes in the degree of saturation and chain length.

4. *Citrate cycle.* The citrate cycle functions within the mitochondrial matrix to produce both CO_2 and hydrogen atoms and, ultimately, ATP by oxidative phosphorylation. The last process takes place as hydrogen atoms are transferred outward across the mitochondrial membrane by the process of proton pumping, which is coupled with the generation of high-energy phosphate compounds. Normally one ATP molecule is made for every four protons transferred, with a phosphorylation-to-oxidation ratio of 2.5, not 3 as previously held. An important mechanism regulating the activity of the citrate cycle is the mitochondrial ratio of $NAD/NADH_2$ (the redox state), which decreases during increased heart work when more cytosolic ATP is also broken down to ADP per unit time. The increased supply of cytosolic ADP is transferred to within the mitochondria by the ADP-ATP translocase, and this stimulates mitochondrial oxidative phosphorylation, using up both reducing equivalents and oxygen to form ATP and H_2O.

5. *Ischemia.* In ischemia, when oxidative metabolism is impaired, the use of ATP decreases dramatically. The ATP content of the myocardium also decreases, but less rapidly, because ischemic arrest of contractility decreases use of ATP and because of replenishment from creatine phosphate. As ATP decreases, the level of breakdown products such as ADP, AMP, adenosine, inosine, and hypoxanthine all increase to stimulate various pathways and restorative processes. In the phase of recovery from ischemic arrest (reperfusion), ATP can be reformed either by salvage pathways or by de novo synthesis. It seems unlikely that there is a fixed critical ATP level below which the cell dies, although ATP is always low in dying cells.

6. *Adenosine.* Adenosine is probably the most important breakdown product of ATP. It has multiple protective functions, including compensatory coronary vasodilation. It also slows the heat rate (by the current K_{ADO}), inhibits the calcium current, and probably plays an important role in preconditioning by activation of protein kinase C.

7. *Anaerobic glycolysis.* During anaerobiosis, metabolism shifts from predominant dependence on oxygen-requiring fatty acids to glycolysis. Lactate is produced instead of being taken up by the myocardium. Pyruvate is converted to lactate because $NADH_2$ formed cannot enter the anaerobic mitochondria. Formation of ATP by glycolysis may be important for the survival of ischemic cells. Hypothetically, glycolytic ATP can protect the membrane by providing energy for the membrane-related pumps, such as the sodium pump and the calcium uptake pump of the sarcoplasmic reticulum. Further harm results from accumulation of the membrane-active intermediates of lipid metabolism, such as intracellular FFA, acyl CoA, and acyl carnitine.

8. *Insulin resistance.* This is a clinically common condition occurring in such diverse situations as obesity, type 2 diabetes, hypertension, and recently found also in severe heart failure. The mechanism is not well understood, but the resulting impairment of glucose transport into muscle could precipitate or exaggerate the diabetic state.

9. *Positron emission tomography.* This technique allows noninvasive monitoring of myocardial metabolic pathways. For example, 18-fluorodeoxyglucose is extracted more by the mildly ischemic than by the normal myocardium, and this increase relative to the coronary blood flow is called mismatch. In severely injured tissue, the extraction is decreased. Thus, myocardial viability may be defined by mismatch, which helps to select patients for coronary artery surgery.

STUDENT QUESTIONS

1. Which are the major fuels of the heart in (a) fasting and (b) the fed state? Explain why these differences exist.
2. Outline the pathways of glycolysis and the major rate-controlling steps. In which conditions are these pathways (a) increased and (b) decreased?
3. In which conditions is fatty acid oxidation (a) increased and (b) decreased?
4. How is ATP produced in mitochondria? Discuss phosphorylation/oxidation ratios.
5. What is the effect of oxygen deprivation (anaerobiosis) on myocardial use of fuels? How well are the energy needs of the myocardium covered during anaerobiosis?

CARDIOLOGIST-IN-TRAINING QUESTIONS

1. During increased heart work in a patient with coronary artery disease, the blood supply is limited and ischemia develops. What changes in the patterns of myocardial energy utilization can be expected?
2. Glycolytic flux is important during ischemia. Critically consider procedures to increase the flux.
3. Insulin resistance is found in a number of clinically diverse conditions. List these conditions. Does insulin resistance matter to the patient? If so, what are the therapeutic implications?
4. Adenosine can be harnessed for endogenous cardioprotection—do you agree? Give reasons for your opinion.
5. What is the scientific basis for the concept of mismatch whereby certain changes in myocardial metabolism, detectable by positron emission tomography (PET), can indicate myocardial viability or otherwise?

REFERENCES

1. Achs MJ, Garfinkel D, Opie LH. Computer simulation of metabolism of glucose perfused rat heart in a work-jump. *Am J Physiol* 1982;243:R389–R399.
2. Alonso MD, Lomako J, Lomako WM, Whelan WJ. A new look at the biogenesis of glycogen. *FASEB J* 1995;9:1126–1137.
3. Altschuld RA, Brierley GP. Interaction between the creatine kinase of heart mitochondria and oxidative phosphorylation. *J Mol Cell Cardiol* 1977;9:875–896.

4. Apstein CS, Gravino FN, Haudenschild CC. Determinants of a protective effect of glucose and insulin on the ischemic myocardium. Effects of contractile function, diastolic compliance, metabolism, and ultrastructure during ischemia and reperfusion. *Circ Res* 1983;52:515–526.
5. Armbrecht JJ, Buxton DB, Schelbert HR. Validation of [1–11C] acetate as a tracer for noninvasive assessment of oxidative metabolism with positron emission tomography in normal, ischemic postischemic and hyperemic canine myocardium. *Circulation* 1990;81:1594–1605.
6. Bittl JA, Balschi JA, Ingwall JS. Contractile failure and high energy phosphate turnover during hypoxia: 31-P NMR surface coil studies in living rat. *Circ Res* 1987;60:871–878.
7. Brandes R, Bers DM. Intracellular Ca^{2+} increases the mitochondrial NADH concentration during elevated work in intact cardiac muscle. *Circ Res* 1997;80:82–87.
8. Brown GC. Control of respiration and ATP synthesis in mammalian mitochondria and cells. *Biochem J* 1992;284:1–13.
9. Camici P, Ferrannini E, Opie LH. Myocardial metabolism in ischemic heart disease: basic principles and application to imaging by positron emission tomography. *Prog Cardiovasc Dis* 1989;32:217–238.
10. Camici P, Marraccinni P, Marzilli M, et al. Coronary hemodynamics and myocardial metabolism during and after pacing stress in normal humans. *Am J Physiol* 1989;257:E309–E317.
11. Carafoli E. Intracellular calcium regulation, with special attention to the role of plasma membrane calcium pump. *J Cardiovasc Pharmacol* 1988;12(suppl 3):77–84.
12. Chance B, Eleff S, Leigh JS Jr, et al. Mitochondrial regulation of phosphocreatine/inorganic phosphate ratios in exercising human muscle: a gated 31P NMR study. *Proc Natl Acad Sci USA* 1981;78:6714–6718.
13. Chapman RA, Suleiman M-S, Earm YE. Taurine and the heart. *Cardiovasc Res* 1993;27:358–363.
14. Clarke K, Willis RJ. Energy metabolism and contractile function in rat heart during graded, isovolumic perfusion using 31-P nuclear magnetic resonance spectroscopy. *J Mol Cell Cardiol* 1987;19:1153–1160.
15. Coetzee WA. ATP sensitive potassium channels and myocardial ischemia: why do they open. *Cardiovasc Drugs Ther* 1992;6:201–208.
16. Conway MA, Allis J, Ouwerkerk R, et al. Detection of low phosphocreatinine to ATP ratio in failing hypertrophied human myocardium by ^{31}P magnetic resonance spectroscopy. *Lancet* 1991;338:973–976.
17. Corr PB, Gross RW, Sobel BE. Arrhythmogenic amphiphilic lipids and the myocardial cell membrane [Editorial]. *J Mol Cell Cardiol* 1982;14:619–626.
18. Cross HR, Opie LH, Radda GK, Clarke K. Is a high glycogen content beneficial or detrimental to the ischemic rat heart? *Circ Res* 1996;78:482–491.
19. Davies NJ, Lonlin RE, Lopaschuk GD. Effect of exogenous fatty acids on reperfusion arrhythmias in isolated working perfused hearts. *Am J Physiol* 1992;262:H1796–H1801.
20. Depré C, Rider MH, Veitch K, Hue L. Role of fructose 2,6-bisphosphate in the control of glycolysis. *J Biol Chem* 1993;268:13274–13279.
21. Ferguson TB, Smith PK, Lofland GK, et al. The effects of cardioplegic potassium concentration and myocardial temperature on electrical activity in the heart during elective cardioplegic arrest. *J Thorac Cardiovasc Surg* 1986;92:755–765.
22. Ferrannini E, Santoro D, Bonadonna R, et al. Metabolic and hemodynamic effects of insulin on human hearts. *Am J Physiol* 1993;264:E308–E315.
23. Gertz EW, Wisneski JA, Neese R, et al. Myocardial lactate extraction: multi-determined metabolic function. *Circulation* 1980;61:256–261.
24. Gevers W. Generation of protons by metabolic processes in heart cells. *J Mol Cell Cardiol* 1977;9:867–874.
25. Goodwin GW, Ahmad F, Taegtmeyer H. Preferential oxidation of glycogen in isolated working rat heart. *J Clin Invest* 1996;97:1409–1416.
26. Goodwin GW, Arteaga JR, Taegtmeyer H. Glycogen turnover in the isolated working rat heart. *J Biol Chem* 1995;270:9234–9240.
27. Gudbjarnason S, Mathes P, Ravens KG. Functional compartmentation of ATP and creatine phosphate in heart muscle. *J Mol Cell Cardiol* 1970;1:325–339.
28. Hariharan R, Bray M, Ganim RT, et al. Fundamental limitations of [18F]2-deoxy-2-fluoro-D-glucose for assessing myocardial glucose uptake. *Circulation* 1995;91:2435–2444.
29. Hazen SL, Wolf MJ, Ford DA, Gross RW. The rapid and reversible association of phosphofructokinase with myocardial membranes during myocardial ischemia. *FEBS* 1994;339:213–216.
30. Heineman FW, Balaban RS. Effects of afterload and heart rate on NAD(P)H redox state in the isolated rabbit heart. *Am J Physiol* 1993;264:H433–H440.

31. Henning SL, Wambolt RB, Schönekess BO, et al. Contribution of glycogen to aerobic myocardial glucose utilization. *Circulation* 1996;93:1549–1555.
32. Hermens WT. Witteveen SAGJ. Problems in estimation of enzymatic infarct size. *J Mol Med* 1977;2: 233–239.
33. Hochachka PW, Buck LT, Doll CJ, Land SC. Unifying theory of hypoxia tolerance: molecular/metabolic defense and rescue mechanisms for surviving oxygen lack. *Proc Natl Acad Sci USA* 1996;93: 9493–9498.
34. Jacobus WE. Respiratory control and the integration of heart high energy phosphate metabolism by mitochondrial creatine kinase. *Ann Rev Physiol* 1985;47:707–725.
35. Jenkins JR, Belardinelli L. Atrioventricular nodal accommodation in isolated guinea pig hearts: physiological significance and role of adenosine. *Circ Res* 1988;63:97–116.
36. Jennings RB, Hawkins HK, Lowe JE, et al. Relation between high energy phosphate and lethal injury in myocardial ischemia in the dog. *Am J Pathol* 1978;92:187–214.
37. Jeremy RW, Ambrosio G, Pike MM, et al. The functional recovery of post-ischaemic myocardium requires glycolysis during early reperfusion. *J Mol Cell Cardiol* 1993;25:261–276.
38. Kammermeier H. Why do cells need phosphocreatine and a phosphocreatine shuttle? *J Mol Cell Cardiol* 1987;19:115–118.
39. Kapelko VI, Kupriyanov VV, Novikova NA, et al. The cardiac contractile failure induced by chronic creatine and phosphocreatine deficiency. *J Mol Cell Cardiol* 1988;20:465–479.
40. Katz EB, Stenbit AE, Hatton K, et al. Cardiac and adipose tissue abnormalities but not diabetes in mice deficient in GLUT4 [Letter]. *Nature* 1995;377:151–155.
41. King LM, Boucher F, Opie LH. Coronary flow and glucose delivery as determinants of contracture in the ischemic myocardium. *J Mol Cell Cardiol* 1995;27:701–702.
42. Kudo N, Barr AJ, Barr RL, et al. High rates of fatty acid oxidation during reperfusion of ischemic hearts are associated with a decrease in malonyl-CoA levels due to an increase in 5′-AMP-activated protein kinase inhibition of acetyl-CoA carboxylase. *J Biol Chem* 1995;270:17513–17520.
43. Kuznetsov AV, Khuchua ZA, Vassilèva EV, et al. Heart mitochondrial creatine kinase revisited: the outer mitochondrial membrane is not important for coupling of phosphocreatine production to oxidative phosphorylation. *Arch Biochem Biophys* 1989;268:176–190.
44. Langer GA. The effect of pH on cellular and membrane calcium binding and contraction of myocardium. A possible role for sarcolemmal phospholipid in EC coupling. *Circ Res* 1985;57: 374–382.
45. Lawson JWR, Veech RL. Effects of pH and free Mg on the Keq of the creatine kinase reaction and other phosphate hydrolyses and phosphate transfer reactions. *J Biol Chem* 1979;254:6528–6537.
46. Lehninger AL. *Biochemistry.* New York: Worth, 1975;513.
47. Lewandowski ED, Johnston DL, Roberts R. Effects of inosine on glycolysis and contracture during myocardial ischemia. *Circ Res* 1991;68:578–587.
48. Lopaschuk GD, Belke DD, Gamble J, et al. Regulation of fatty acid oxidation in the mammalian heart in health and disease. *Biochem Biophys Acta* 1994;1213:263–276.
49. Lopaschuk GD, Stanley WC. Glucose metabolism in the ischemic heart. *Circulation* 1997;95: 313–315.
50. Lowe JE, Jennings RB, Reimer KA. Cardiac rigor mortis in dogs. *J Mol Cell Cardiol* 1979;11: 1017–1031.
51. Malmberg K, Ryden L, Efendic S, et al. Randomized trial of insulin-glucose infusion followed by subcutaneous insulin treatment in diabetic patients with acute myocardial infarction (DIGAMI Study): effects on mortality at one year. *J Am Coll Cardiol* 1995;26:57–65.
52. McCormack JG, Edgell NJ, Denton RM. Regulation of rat heart pyruvate dehydrogenase activity. *Biochem J* 1982;202:419–427.
53. Mochizuki S, Neely JR. Control of glyceraldehyde-3-phosphate dehydrogenase in cardiac muscle. *J Mol Cell Cardiol* 1979;11:221–236.
54. Mullane K, Bullough D. Harnessing an endogenous cardioprotective mechanism: cellular sources and sites of action of adenosine. *J Mol Cell Cardiol* 1995;27:1041–1054.
55. Mullane K, Engler R. Proclivity of activated neutrophils to cause postischemic cardiac dysfunction: participation in stunning? *Cardiovasc Drug Ther* 1991;5:915–924.
56. Neely JR, Morgan HE. Relationship between carbohydrate and lipid metabolism and the energy balance of heart muscle. *Ann Rev Physiol* 1974;36:413–459.
57. Neubauer S, Krahe T, Schindler R, et al. ^{31}P magnetic resonance spectroscopy in dilated cardiomyopathy and coronary artery disease. Altered cardiac high-energy phosphate metabolism in heart failure. *Circulation* 1992;86:1810–1818.

58. Oldfield GS, Commerford PJ, Opie LH. Effects of preoperative glucose-insulin-potassium on myocardial glycogen levels and on complications of mitral valve replacement. *J Thorac Cardiovasc Surg* 1986;91:874–878.

59. Oliver MF, Opie LH. Effects of glucose and fatty acids on myocardial ischaemia and arrhythmias. *Lancet* 1994;343:155–158.

60. Opie LH. Metabolism of the heart in health and disease. Part I. *Am Heart J* 1968;76:685–698.

61. Opie LH. Substrate and energy metabolism of the heart. In: Sperelakis N (ed). *Physiology and Pathophysiology of the Heart.* Boston: Kluwer Academic, 1989;327–359.

62. Opie LH, Owen P. Assessment of mitochondrial free NAD+/NADH ratios and oxaloacetate concentrations during increased mechanical work in isolated perfused rat heart during production or uptake of ketone bodies. *Biochem J* 1975;148:403–415.

63. Owen P, Dennis S, Opie LH. Glucose flux rate regulates onset of ischemic contracture in globally underperfused rat hearts. *Circ Res* 1990;66:344–354.

64. Paternostro G, Camici PG, Lammerstma AA, et al. Cardiac and skeletal muscle insulin resistance in patients with coronary heart disease. *J Clin Invest* 1996;98:2094–2099.

65. Paternostro G, Clarke K, Heath J, et al. Decreased GLUT-4 mRNA content and insulin-sensitive deoxyglucose uptake show insulin resistance in the hypertensive rat heart. *Cardiovasc Res* 1995;30:205–211.

66. Pessin JE, Bell GI. Mammalian facilitative glucose transporter family: structure and molecular regulation. *Ann Rev Physiol* 1992;54:911–930.

67. Pillay TS, Xiao S, Olefsky JM. Glucose-induced phosphorylation of the insulin receptor. *J Clin Invest* 1996;97:613–620.

68. Randle PJ, Garland PB, Hales CN, Newsholme EA. The glucose-fatty acid cycle. Its role in insulin sensitivity and the metabolic disturbances of diabetes mellitus. *Lancet* 1963;1:785–789.

69. Randle PJ, Morgan HE. Regulation of glucose uptake by muscle. *Vitamins Horm* 1962;20:199–249.

70. Roden M, Price TB, Perseghin G, et al. Mechanism of free fatty acid-induced insulin resistance in humans. *J Clin Invest* 1996;97:2859–2865.

71. Russell RR, Yin R, Xiaoyue H, et al. Insulin stimulates translocation of both GLUT 4 and GLUT 1 in the heart [Abstract]. *Circulation* 1996;94(suppl 1):1–308.

72. Sato T, Arita M, Kiyosue T. Differential mechanism of block of palmitoyl lysophosphatidylcholine and of palmitoylcarnitine on inward rectifier K$^+$ channels of guinea-pig ventricular myocytes. *Cardiovasc Drug Ther* 1993;7:575–584.

73. Saupe KW, Spindler M, Ingwall JS. Altered energetics but not contractile-function in mouse hearts with deleted M-CK and mitochondrial-CK genes. *Circulation* 1996;94(suppl 1):1–308.

74. Schaefer S, Camacho A, Gober J, et al. Response of myocardial metabolites to graded regional ischaemia: 31-P NMR spectroscopy of porcine myocardium in vivo. *Circ Res* 1989;64:968–976.

75. Schaefer S, Grober JR, Schwartz GG, et al. In vivo phosphorus-31 spectroscopic imaging in patients with global myocardial disease. *Am J Cardiol* 1990;65:1154–1161.

76. Schaper J, Mulch J, Winkler B, Schaper W. Ultrastructural, functional, and biochemical criteria for estimation of reversibility of ischaemic injury: a study on the effects of global ischaemia on the isolated dog heart. *J Mol Cell Cardiol* 1979;11:521–541.

77. Schrader J. Adenosine. A homeostatic metabolite in cardiac energy metabolism. *Circulation* 1990;81:389–391.

78. Schulze K, Becker BF, Schauer R, Schultheiss HP. Antibodies to ADP-ATP carrier—an autoantigen in myocarditis and dilated cardiomyopathy—impair cardiac function. *Circulation* 1990;81:959–969.

79. Simonsen S, Kjekshus JK. The effect of free fatty acids on myocardial oxygen consumption during arterial pacing and catecholamine infusion in man. *Circulation* 1978;58:484–491.

80. Swan JW, Walton C, Godsland IF, Clark AL, Coats AJ, Oliver MF. Relationship of insulin resistance to the severity and etiology of chronic heart failure. *Circulation* 1994;90:1–174.

81. Taegtmeyer H. Energy metabolism of the heart: from basic concepts to clinical applications. *Curr Prob Cardiol* 1994;19:59–113.

82. Taegtmeyer H. Metabolic support for the postischaemic heart. *Lancet* 1995;345:1552–1555.

83. Taniguchi J, Noma A, Irisawa H. Modification of the cardiac action potential by intracellular injection of adenosine triphosphate and related substances in guinea pig single ventricular cells. *Circ Res* 1983;53:131–139.

84. Thomassen A, Nielsen TT, Bagger JP, et al. Antiischemic and metabolic effects of glutamate during pacing in patients with stable angina pectoris secondary to either coronary artery disease or syndrome X. *Am J Cardiol* 1991;68:291–295.

85. Vyska K, Meyer W, Stremmel W, et al. Fatty acid uptake in normal human myocardium. *Circ Res* 1991;69:857–870.
86. Weiss JN, Lamp ST. Glycolysis preferentially inhibits ATP-sensitive K+ channels in isolated guinea pig cardiac myocytes. *Science* 1987;238:67–70.
87. Weiss RG, Chacko VP, Gerstenblith G. Fatty acid regulation of glucose metabolism in the intact beating rat heart assessed by carbon-13 NMR spectroscopy: the critical role of pyruvate dehydrogenase. *J Mol Cell Cardiol* 1989;21:469–478.
88. Werth DK, Hathaway DR, Watanabe AM. Regulation of phosphorylase kinase in rat ventricular myocardium. Role of calmodulin. *Circ Res* 1982;51:448–456.
89. White MF, Kahn CR. The insulin signalling system. *J Biol Chem* 1994;269:1–4.
90. Young LH, Renfu Y, Russell R, et al. Low-flow ischemia leads to translocation of canine heart GLUT-4 and GLUT-1 glucose transporters to the sarcolemma in vivo. *Circulation* 1997;95:415–422.

12

Ventricular Function

THE CARDIAC CYCLE

Wiggers' (1915) diagram is one of the most frequently reproduced and modified figures in cardiology (Fig. 12-1). Although conceived by Wiggers, the earliest complete diagram showing the phases of the cardiac cycle and the pressures in aorta, ventricles, atria, and veins, as well as the relationship to the electrocardiogram (ECG) and heart sounds was by Lewis in 1920. The message of this cycle is so important that it must be committed to memory by every student of cardiology. The basic events are (a) left ventricular (LV) contraction, (b) LV relaxation, and (c) LV filling (Table 12-1). These events generate the pressure to propel blood received from the lungs to the body via the aorta. Similarly, right ventricular contraction, undergoing a similar sequence of events, propels blood to the lungs and thence to the left heart. For simplicity, we focus on events in the left side of the heart, where the pressure changes are greater and the ventricle is correspondingly thicker. This increased wall thickness of the left ventricle is a natural adaptation to the higher pressures in aorta and left ventricle than in pulmonary artery and right ventricle.

The Ventricle Contracts: Systole

LV pressure increases when the arrival of calcium ions at the contractile protein starts to trigger actin-myosin interaction. On the electrocardiogram, the arrival of the wave of depolarization that opens the L-calcium channels is indicated by the peak of the R wave (Fig. 12-1). Soon the LV pressure builds up to exceed that in the left atrium (normally 10 to 15 mmHg), followed about 30 msec later by the mitral component of the first sound, M_1. The exact relationship of M_1 to mitral valve closure is still open to dispute (Laniado et al., 1973; Parisi and Milton, 1973). Mitral valve closure, often thought to coincide with the crossover point at which the LV pressure initially exceeds the left atrial pressure, is in reality delayed because the valve is kept open by the inertia of

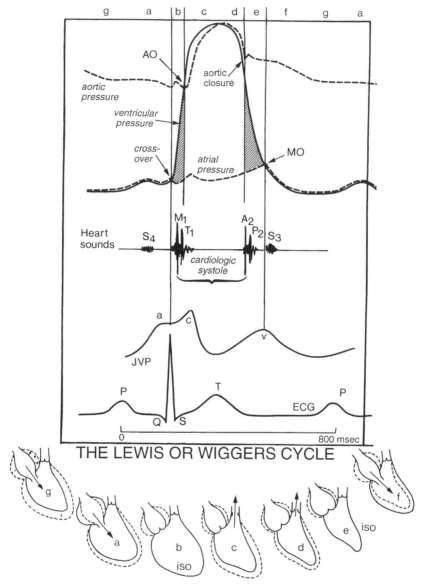

FIG. 12-1. The cardiac cycle, first assembled by Lewis in 1920 although conceived by Wiggers (1915). Note that mitral valve closure occurs after the crossover point of atrial and ventricular pressures at the start of systole. The "a" and "c" waves of jugular venous pressure (JVP) coincide with "a" and "c" in the bottom panel. (Visual phases of the ventricular cycle are modified from Shepherd and Vanhoutte. *The Human Cardiovascular System*. New York: Raven, 1979;68.) For explanation of phases a to g, see Table 12-1. M_1, mitral component of the first sound at time of mitral valve closure; T_1, tricuspid valve closure, second component of first heart sound; AO, aortic valve opening, normally inaudible; A_2, aortic valve closure, aortic component of second sound; P_2, pulmonary component of second sound, pulmonary valve closure; MO, mitral valve opening, sometimes audible in mitral stenosis as the opening snap; S_3, third heart sound; S_4, fourth heart sound; a, wave produced by right atrial contraction; c, carotid wave artefact during rapid LV ejection phase; v, venous return wave that causes pressure to increase while tricuspid valve is closed. Cycle length of 800 msec for 75 beats per minute.

TABLE 12-1. *The cardiac cycle*

LV contraction
Isovolumic contraction (b)
Maximal ejection (c)
LV relaxation
Start of relaxation and reduced ejection (d)
Isovolumic relaxation (e)
Rapid LV filling and LV suction (f)
Slow LV filling (diastasis) (g)
Atrial booster (a)

The letters a through g refer to the phases of the cardiac cycle shown in the Wiggers' diagram (Fig. 12-1).

the blood flow (Hirschfeld et al., 1976). The second component of the first heart sound, T_1, occurs shortly thereafter, as pressure increases in the right ventricle, similarly to that in the left ventricle, although lesser in magnitude. The result is that the tricuspid valve closes, thereby creating the second component of the first heart sound. These two components cannot be distinguished clinically under normal circumstances.

Isovolumic contraction occurs between the times of mitral closure and aortic valve opening. The LV volume is fixed because both these valves are shut, and pressure development proceeds as the interaction of actin and myosin increases. Thereafter, the aortic valve opens when the pressure in the left ventricle exceeds that in the aorta. Opening of the aortic valve is followed by *rapid ejection.* The speed of ejection of blood is determined both by the pressure gradient across the aortic valve and by the elastic properties of the aorta and the arterial tree. Particularly the aorta undergoes systolic expansion (see Fig. 14-10).

Pattern of Contraction of the Whole Heart. There is a complex wringing motion, with the apex swinging up to the chest wall and the base rotating in the opposite direction, around a relatively fixed equatorial mid-zone (Maier et al., 1992).

Ventricular Relaxation

After the LV pressure increases to a peak, it then starts to decrease. As the cytosolic calcium is taken up into the sarcoplasmic reticulum under the influence of phosphorylated phospholamban, more and more myofibers enter the state of relaxation. As a result, the rate of ejection of blood from the aorta decreases (*phase of reduced ejection*). Although the LV pressure is decreasing, blood flow is maintained by aortic distensibility: the Windkessel effect (Belz, 1995). Next, the aortic valve closes as the pressure in the aorta exceeds the decreasing pressure in the LV. The first component of the second sound, A_2, results from aortic valve closure, and the second component, P_2, results from closure of the pulmonary valve as pressure in the RV decreases below that in the pulmonary artery. In contrast to S_1, the two components of S_2 are clinically distinguishable. Thereafter, the ventricle relaxes without changing its volume (*isovolumic relaxation*) because it is sealed off as both aortic and mitral valves are closed. Next, the mitral valve opens as the LV pressure decreases to below that in the left atrium. The filling phase of the cardiac cycle starts (Fig. 12-1). Mitral valve opening, normally silent, may be audible as an opening snap in mitral stenosis.

Ventricular Filling

Just after mitral valve opening, as the LV pressure decreases below that in the left atrium, the *phase of rapid or early filling* accounts for most of ventricular filling. Active diastolic relaxation of the ventricle (*ventricular suction*) also may contribute to early filling, particularly during exercise. A *physiologic third heart sound* (S_3) may result from rapid filling during exercise or with sinus tachycardia. LV filling *temporarily* stops as pressures in the atrium and ventricle equalize, called the phase of diastasis, which means separation. *Atrial systole* or the *left atrial booster* increases the pressure gradient from the atrium to the ventricle to renew filling. When LV fails to relax normally as in LV hypertrophy, then increased atrial contraction can enhance late filling (Ohno et al., 1994). The *fourth heart sound* may accompany atrial systole in the diseased heart (Table 12-2). Unlike S_3, S_4 is not audible physiologically.

Definitions of Systole and Diastole

Systole is the contraction phase and diastole the relaxation phase. *Systole* means contraction in Greek and *diastole* is derived from two Greek words to *send* and *apart*. For the physiologist, systole starts with isovolumic contraction when LV pressure crosses the atrial pressure (Fig. 12-1). Physiologic diastole commences as the LV pressure starts to decrease (Table 12-3). For the cardiologist, systole is demarcated by the heart sounds, lasting from the first heart sound (M_1) to the closure of the aortic valve (A_2). The remainder of the cardiac cycle is cardiologic diastole. Mitral valve closure (M_1) actually occurs about 20 milliseconds after the onset of physiologic systole at the crossover point of

TABLE 12-2. *Origins of the heart sounds*

Sound	Origin
1. Mitral component (M1)	Mitral valve closure
Tricuspid component (T1)	Tricuspid valve closure
2. Aortic component (A2)	Aortic valve closure
Pulmonary component (P2)	Pulmonary valve closure
3. Physiologic	Rapid LV filling
Pathologic	Ventricular wall vibrations
4. Pathologic	Enhanced atrial systole

TABLE 12-3. *Physiologic versus cardiologic systole and diastole*

Physiologic systole	Cardiologic systole
1. Isovolumic contraction 2. Maximal ejection	1. From M_1–A_2 2. Only part of isovolumic contraction* (includes maximal and reduced ejection phases)
Physiologic diastole	Cardiologic diastole
1. Reduced ejection 2. Isovolumic relaxation 3. Filling phases	1. A_2–M_1 interval (filling phases included)

*Note that M_1 occurs with a definite delay after the start of LV contraction.

pressures. Thus, cardiologic systole starts and ends later than physiologic systole. *Protodiastolic* (early diastole) for the physiologist refers to the early part of the relaxation phase from the time when aortic flow begins to decline until the mitral valve shuts. For the cardiologist, protodiastole is the early phase of rapid filling, when the *third heart sound* (S₃) may be heard. This sound probably reflects ventricular wall vibrations during rapid filling. A *pathologic S₃* (protodiastolic gallop) results from an increase in LV diastolic pressure, as in heart failure, or increased wall stiffness and is distinguished from a *physiologic S₃* (normal LV, increased rate of filling due to exercise, pregnancy, or youth).

PRELOAD AND AFTERLOAD

To understand how an increased venous return, as during exercise, enhances ventricular function, a simple circuit diagram can be proposed (Fig. 12-2). The *preload* is the load present before contraction has started and is provided by the venous return that fills the atrium and empties into the left ventricle during diastole. During systole, the left ventricle contracts against the *afterload* (load after the ventricle starts to contract). When the preload increases (Fig. 12-3), the left ventricle distends and the stroke volume increases. Because the heart rate also increases (for mechanism, see Chapter 15), cardiac output increases. A similar mechanism explains at least in part the increased cardiac output of exercise or of volume expansion (infusion of intravenous fluids).

Starling's Law of the Heart

Starling law may be stated in many forms, one of which is that the energy of contraction is a function of the length of the muscle fiber. "Within physiological limits, the larger the volume of the heart, the greater the energy of its contraction and the amount of chemical change at each contraction" (Starling, 1918) (Fig. 12-4).

Put differently, an increased venous pressure stretches the fibers more at the end of diastole, and systolic contraction is more vigorous with an increased

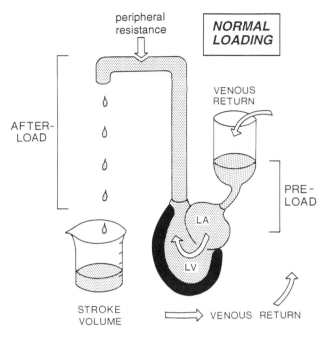

FIG. 12-2. Simplified model of circulation under normal loading conditions. The venous return provides the preload, and the afterload is regulated by the peripheral (systemic) vascular resistance. LA, left atrium; LV, left ventricle.

stroke volume. To obtain the end-diastolic fiber length and the stroke volume, Starling measured the heart volume and the stroke volume and cardiac output. Because the heart volume is difficult to determine even with modern echocardiographic (echo) techniques, the LV diastolic *filling pressure* (the difference between the left atrial pressure and the LV diastolic pressure) is often taken as a surrogate for heart volume. As the filling pressure increases, so does the preload on the myocardium and the ventricular performance (Fig. 12-5). An invasive procedure using the Swan-Ganz catheter measures both the LV filling pressure and the cardiac output, the latter by a temperature-sensitive device at the tip of the catheter in the pulmonary capillary bed. Nonetheless, LV pressure and volume are not linearly related because the myocardium cannot continue to stretch indefinitely. Rather, as the LV end-diastolic pressure increases, so does the cardiac output reach a plateau.

Although LV volume can be measured with two-dimensional echocardiography, the value found depends on a number of simplifying assumptions such as a spherical LV shape and neglects the confounding influence of the complex anatomy of the left ventricle (Schiller and Foster, 1996). Nevertheless, a portable nuclear vest can show the Starling relationship between heart volume and contractile performance in humans (Legault et al., 1995).

Force–Length Relationship and Starling's Law

In the past, "optimal sarcomere length" was linked to Starling's law. Supposedly, ventricular stretch gives rise to such optimal overlap of actin and myosin with an increased force of contraction. Whereas the overlap theory holds for skeletal muscle, in the heart the situation is different (Fig. 12-6). In the case of skeletal muscle, Fuchs pointed out that each actin filament projects about 1 μm from each side of the Z disk, so that the active force would decline when the sarcomere length was less than the sum of the lengths of the individual actin filaments, i.e., less than 2.0 to 2.2 μm. In cardiac muscle, however, only 10% or less of the maximal force is developed, even at 80% of the optimal length (Fig.

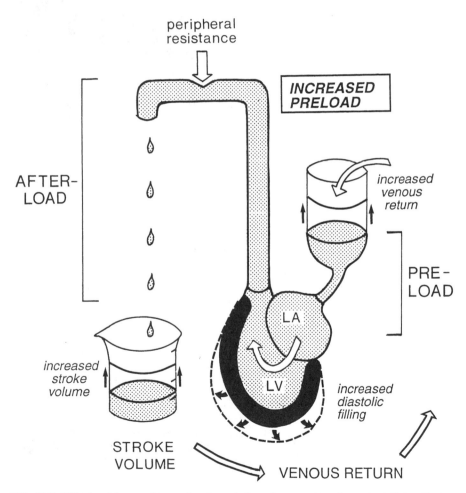

FIG. 12-3. Effects of increasing preload on stroke volume and cardiac output. Note effect on LV volume. For Starling's actual observations, see Fig. 12-4.

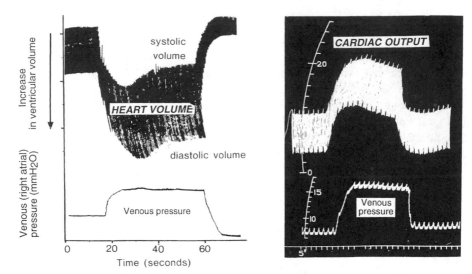

FIG. 12-4. Starling's law of the heart as applied to the preload (venous filling pressure). As the preload increases (bottom in both figures), the heart volume increases (left top), as does the cardiac output (right top). On present evidence, both SV and HR would have increased. Starling's explanation was: *"The output of the heart is a function of its filling; the energy of contraction depends on the state of dilatation of the heart's cavities."* VP, venous pressure in the right atrium. (Left figure adapted from Patterson et al. *J Physiol* 1914;48:465. Right figure adapted from Halliburton and McDowall. *Handbook of Physiology and Biochemistry.* London: John Murray, 1942.)

12-6). Thus, cardiac sarcomeres must function near the upper limit of their maximal length (L_{MAX}), which is 2.2 μm (Rodriguez et al., 1992). The change in sarcomere length from approximately 85% of L_{MAX} to L_{MAX} itself is able to affect physiologic LV volume changes (Fig. 12-7).

The favored explanation for this steep length–tension relationship of cardiac muscle (Fig. 12-8) is *length-dependent activation* (see Chapter 8). Direct evidence for this point of view is that the calcium transient does not increase as the sarcomere length is extended (Backx and ter Keurs, 1993). In contrast, when forces increase by a true inotropic intervention such as β-adrenergic stimulation, there is also an increase in the calcium transient.

Frank and Isovolumic Contraction

Whereas Starling emphasized the role of increasing the initial length of the muscle fiber by increasing the heart volume, it was his German predecessor, Frank, who in 1895 established another important principle. When an isolated heart was filled to several increasing volumes, each of which was fixed throughout the cardiac cycle through an ingenious perfusion system, the isovolumically (Greek *iso,* equal) contracting heart could generate an increasing

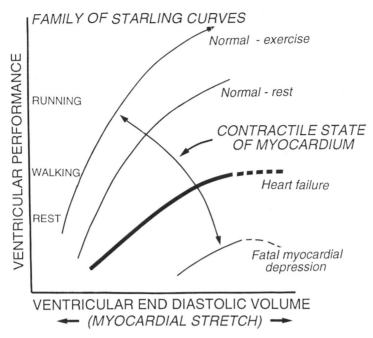

FIG. 12-5. Family of Starling curves. According to Starling's law, increased stretch of myocardial fibers, which increases the ventricular end-diastolic volume, results in greater ventricular performance. Modified with permission from Braunwald et al. (1968). The line for heart failure is based on that shown in Figs. 1 and 2 of Holubarsch et al. (1996).

and decreasing pressure trace (Fig. 12-9). The greater the initial volume, the more rapid the rate of increase, the greater the peak pressure reached, the faster the rate of relaxation. Frank therefore was able to show that an increasing diastolic heart volume stimulated the ventricle to contract more rapidly and more forcefully, which is a positive *inotropic effect* (Greek *ino,* fiber; *tropus,* move). Thus, the observation of Frank explained the contractile behavior of the heart during the operation of Starling's law. These findings of Frank and Starling are so complementary that they often are referred to as the *Frank-Starling law.* Of interest, the cellular mechanism of this law is still not well understood (see Chapter 8); stretch may act by a reduction of the lateral distance between the filaments.

Measurement of Afterload

Starling and his colleagues gave a simple picture of how afterload could influence an isolated muscle: "The extent to which it will contract depends on . . . the amount of the weight which it has to overcome" and "the tension aroused in it" (Starling, 1918).

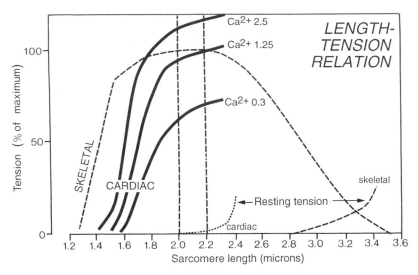

FIG. 12-6. Effect of sarcomere length on tension. The relationship between sarcomere lengths and tension for cardiac muscle in comparison with skeletal muscle. Note (i) the effect of increasing calcium ion concentration and (ii) the absence of any decrease of tension at maximal sarcomere lengths, so that there is no basis for the descending limb of the Starling curve. Recent sophisticated laser-diffraction techniques invalidate previous curves based on apparent sarcomere length–tension relationships of imperfect papillary muscle preparations. For data on failing human heart, see Holubarsch et al. (1996).

Hypothetically, the increased afterload stimulates sarcolemma stretch receptors to allow cytosolic calcium levels to increase. Generally, in clinical practice, the arterial blood pressure can be taken as one important measure of the afterload, provided there is no significant aortic stenosis. Increased afterload by itself will increase the intraventricular pressure that has to be generated to open the aortic valve and also the pressure against which the myocardium contracts during the ejection phase (Fig. 12-10). These increases will translate themselves to an increased wall stress, which can be measured either as an average value throughout systole or at a given phase of systole. A second important component of the afterload lies in the *aortic compliance*: the extent to which the aorta can "yield" during systole. *Aortic impedance* is an index of the afterload and is the aortic pressure divided by the aortic flow of that incidence, so that the afterload varies during each phase of the contraction cycle. Factors reducing aortic flow, such as high arterial blood pressure or aortic valve narrowing (stenosis), will increase impedance and hence the afterload (see Fig. 14-10).

Preload and Afterload Are Interlinked

The preceding approach presumes that preload and afterload are two separate unconnected entities. Nonetheless, supposing that the LV end-diastolic pressure

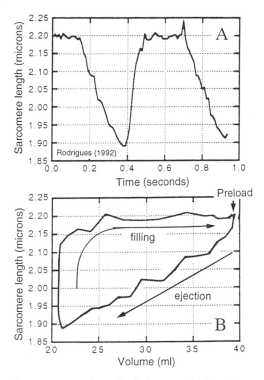

FIG. 12-7. Changes in sarcomere length during a typical cardiac contraction–relaxation cycle in the intact dog heart. Top panel shows that during diastole the sarcomere length is 2.2 μm, reducing to 1.90 μm during systole. Bottom right panel relates sarcomere length to LV volume. Starting at the top right, the preload is the maximum sarcomere length just before the onset of contraction. Then ejection decreases the LV volume, in this case by about half. Sarcomere length decreases from 2.20 to 1.90 μm. Then, during the rapid phase of filling (see Fig. 12-22), the sarcomere length increases from 1.90 to 2.15 μm, to be followed by the phase of constant sarcomere length (diastasis). Modified from Rodriguez et al. (1992).

increases, as during exercise, the preload increases by definition. When the left ventricle then starts to contract, the tension in the LV wall will be higher because of greater distention of the left ventricle by the greater pressure. The load during systole also will increase, and the afterload will increase. Another example is heart failure, when there is a depressed contractile state. One of the compensations is an increase in the peripheral (systemic) vascular resistance, initiated chiefly by an increased sympathetic drive. In that situation, the poorly functioning myocardium cannot cope with the afterload, the degree of myocardial failure becomes more severe, the relative amount of blood ejected with each contraction becomes less, more blood is retained in the left ventricle, and the preload increases. Therapy aimed at reduction of the afterload (arterial vasodilator therapy) will improve myocardial performance, allow the left ventricle to empty better, and reduce the end-diastolic volume and preload. Once

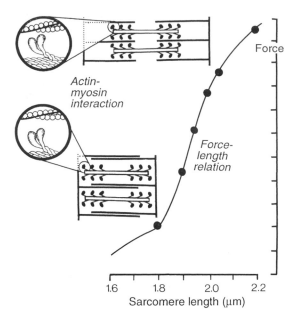

FIG. 12-8. The force length relationship of the cardiac sarcomere. This is explained in part by sensitization of troponin C to the prevailing calcium level and, in part, by closer proximity of the myosin leads to actin. For force–length data, see Fig. 8-8. See Fuchs (1995).

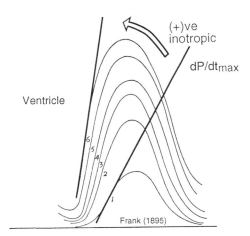

FIG. 12-9. Frank's family of isometric (isovolumic) curves. Each curve was obtained at a greater initial filling of the left ventricle by an increased left atrial filling pressure (Frank, 1895). Then valves were shut to produce isovolumic conditions. Curve 6 has a greater velocity of shortening, reflecting greater contractility. Hence, the initial fiber length (volume of ventricle) can influence contractility. This effect of initial fiber length on contractility recently has been rediscovered. One index of contractility is the maximal rate of change of the intraventricular pressure (max dP/dt) that could be obtained, indicated by the two tangential lines added to the curves of the original figure of Frank. The line on curve 6 has the much steeper slope and, therefore, indicates a greater rate of contraction or a greater contractility, in contrast to the line drawn on curve 1, which ascends more slowly and indicates a lower contractile state.

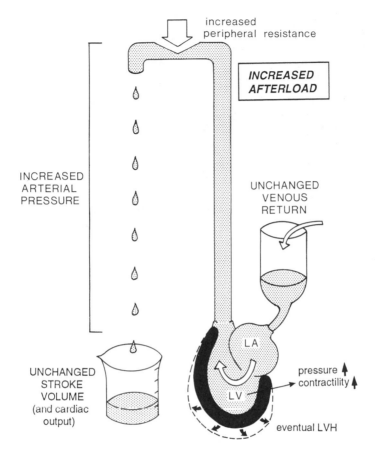

FIG. 12-10. Effect of increasing afterload by increasing the peripheral vascular resistance and the arterial blood pressure. LV pressure development is enhanced because of increased contractility. Eventually chronically increased LV pressure causes LV hypertrophy.

again, it is difficult to separate preload from afterload. Nonetheless, it is useful to emphasize that, in general, the preload is related to the degree to which the myocardial fibers are stretched at the end of diastole, and the afterload is related to the wall stress generated by those fibers during systole.

HEART RATE AND FORCE–FREQUENCY RELATIONSHIP

The heart rate is one of the three basic mechanisms that acutely regulate the contractile state, the other two being the Frank-Starling law and autonomic control by the sympathetic and parasympathetic systems (Holubarsch et al., 1996). Heart rate is also one of the two major determinants of the myocardial oxygen demand, the other being myocardial wall stress. As expected, an increased heart rate increases the myocardial oxygen demand when the stroke volume is fixed by increasing the external work of the heart. Unexpectedly, an increased heart rate also increases the oxygen demand by progressively enhancing the force of ventricular contraction (Fig. 12-11). This phenomenon is called the Bowditch staircase effect, the *treppe* (German for steps) effect, the positive inotropic effect of activation, or the force–frequency relationship. Conversely, a decreased heart rate has a negative staircase effect. To explain the *treppe* effect during rapid stimulation, the proposal is that more sodium and calcium ions enter the myocardial cells than can be handled by the sodium pump. Sodium overload leads to an increase of cytosolic calcium by the sodium–calcium exchanger, with an increased force of contraction.

Too rapid a rate of stimulation causes the force of contraction to decrease (Mulieri et al., 1993). In the whole heart, high rates decrease the duration of ventricular filling and thereby oppose the force–frequency effect. On the other hand, the longer the filling interval, the better the filling of the ventricle and the stronger the subsequent contraction by the Frank-Starling law. In other words, changes in the preload to some extent correct for the *treppe* effect.

Force–Frequency Relationship in Humans

In the failing human heart, there is a very different response to an increased frequency of stimulation (Fig. 12-12). At a fixed muscle length (*isometric contraction*) peak contractile force occurs at about 150 to 180 stimuli per minute (Mulieri et al., 1993), which is the human equivalent of the *treppe* phenomenon.

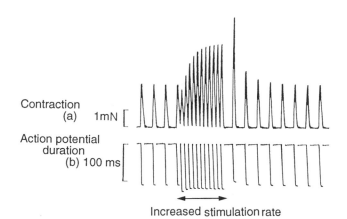

FIG. 12-11. The Bowditch or *treppe* phenomenon, whereby a faster stimulation rate (bottom panel) increases the force of contraction (top panel). The stimulus rate is shown as the action potential duration of an analog analyzer (ms, milliseconds). The tension developed by papillary muscle contraction is shown in milliNewtons (mN) in the top panel. On cessation of rapid stimulation, the contraction force gradually declines. Hypothetically, the explanation for the increased contraction during the increased stimulation is repetitive Ca^{2+} entry with each depolarization and, hence, an accumulation of cystolic calcium. (From Noble MIM. Excitation-contraction coupling. In: Drake-Holland AJ, Noble MIM (eds). *Cardiac Metabolism.* Chichester, England: John Wiley, 1983;49–71.)

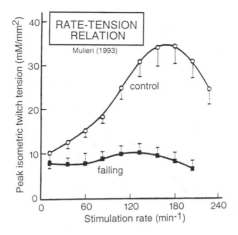

FIG. 12-12. Heart rate–tension relationship. Plot of average steady-state isometric twitch tension versus stimulation frequency. Each point represents the mean ± SEM of eight nonfailing control preparations (NF) and eight failing mitral regurgitation preparations (MR). Temperature 37°C. Data from Mulieri et al. (1993). By permission of authors and American Heart Association.

In patients with mitral stenosis complicated by atrial fibrillation, the variable filling interval influences contraction, with longer filling intervals and greater diastolic stretch causing stronger contractions (Schneider et al., 1983). In contrast, there is hardly any response to an increased frequency of stimulation in patients with severe mitral regurgitation.

In the human heart in situ, pacing rates of up to 150 beats per minute can be tolerated, whereas higher rates cause AV block. During exercise, however, a maximal heart rate of 170 beats per minute can be tolerated, presumably because of the enhanced rate of conduction through the AV node associated with adrenergic stimulation. A concept currently under test is that incessant or chronic tachycardias can cause or contribute to LV failure.

CONTRACTILITY OR THE INOTROPIC STATE

Although difficult to define with exactness, increased contractility results in a greater velocity of contraction, which reaches a greater peak tension or pressure when other factors influencing the myocardial oxygen uptake, such as the heart rate, the preload, and the afterload, are kept constant. An alternate name for contractility is the *inotropic state*. Contractility is an important regulator of the myocardial oxygen uptake. Factors that increase contractility include adrenergic stimulation, digitalis, and other inotropic agents. At a molecular level, *an increased inotropic state is an enhanced load-independent interaction between calcium ions and the contractile proteins.* Such an interaction could result from either increased calcium transients or from sensitization of the contractile proteins to a given level of cytosolic calcium, as during the action of certain drugs acting through this mechanism. With conventional inotropes, as internal calcium increases within physiologic limits, so does the myosin ATPase activity and the maximum tension development.

Problems with the Contractility Concept*

The concept of contractility has at least two serious defects, including (1) the absence of any potential index that can be measured in situ and is free of significant criticism and, in particular, the absence of any acceptable noninvasive index; and (2) the impossibility of separating the cellular mechanisms of contractility changes from those of load or heart rate. Thus, an increased heart rate through the sodium pump lag mechanism gives rise to an increased cytosolic calcium, which is thought to explain the *treppe* phenomenon. An increased preload involves increased fiber stretch, which in turn causes length activation, explicable by sensitization of the contractile proteins to the prevailing cytosolic calcium concentration. An increased afterload may increase cytosolic calcium through stretch-sensitive channels. Thus, there is a clear overlap between contractility which should be independent of load or heart rate and the effects of load and heart rate on the cellular mechanisms. Hence, the traditional separation of inotropic state from load/heart rate effects as two independent regulators of cardiac muscle performance is no longer simple now that the underlying cellular mechanisms have been uncovered. In clinical terms, it nonetheless remains important to separate the effects of a primary increase of load or heart rate from a primary increase in contractility. This distinction is especially relevant when attempting to dissect the multiple abnormalities found in congestive heart failure, where a decreased contractility could indirectly or directly result in increased afterload, preload, and heart rate, all of which factors then predispose to a further decrease in myocardial performance. Thus, decreased contractility is eventually self-augmenting. Because muscle length can influence contractility, the traditional separation of length and inotropic state into two independent regulators of cardiac muscle performance is no longer true if the end result is considered. In clinical terms, however, it still remains useful to separate the effects of a primary increase of load from a primary change in contractility. Thus it remains true that β-adrenergic stimulation has a calcium-dependent positive inotropic effect independent of loading conditions (Fig. 12-13).

Force–Velocity Relationship and Idealized Contractility in Muscle Models

If the concept of contractility is truly independent of the load and the heart rate, then unloaded heart muscle stimulated at a fixed rate should have a max-

---

*Section taken with permission from Opie LH. Mechanisms of cardiac contraction and relaxation. In: Braunwald E (ed). *Heart Disease.* 5th ed. Philadelphia: Saunders, 1997;360–393.

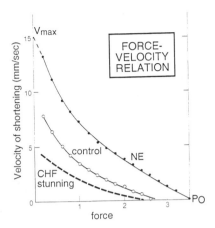

FIG. 12-13. Force–velocity relationship. Effects of the addition of norepinephrine (NE) on the force–velocity relationship of the cat papillary muscle. NE induces an increase in the velocity of shortening at any load, in the maximum force and isometric contraction (P_0), and in the maximum velocity of zero-load shortening (V_{max}). The dashed line adds hypothetical data from congestive heart failure (CHF). (Modified from Braunwald E et al. Normal and abnormal circulatory function. In: Braunwald E (ed). *Heart Disease: A Textbook of Cardiovascular Medicine.* 4th ed. Philadelphia: Saunders, 1992;351–392.) For original data on stunning, see McDonald et al. (1995).

imum value of contractility for any given magnitude of the cytosolic calcium transient. This value, the V_{MAX} of muscle contraction, is defined as the *maximal velocity of contraction* when the isolated muscle is not loaded at all (Fig. 12-13). β-adrenergic stimulation increases V_{MAX}, and converse changes are found in the failing myocardium. V_{MAX} is also termed V_0 (the maximum velocity at zero load). The problem with this relatively simple concept is that V_{MAX} cannot be measured directly but is extrapolated from the peak rates of force development in unloaded muscle obtained from the intercept on the velocity axis. In another extreme condition, there is no muscle shortening at all (zero shortening), and all the energy goes into development of pressure (P_0) or force (F_0). This situation is an example of *isometric shortening* (Greek *iso,* the same; *metric,* length). Because the peak velocity is obtained at zero load when there is no external force development, the relationship is usually termed the *"force–velocity relationship."*

The concept of V_{MAX} has been subject to much debate over many years, chiefly because of the technical difficulties in obtaining truly unloaded conditions. Braunwald et al. used cat papillary muscle to define a hyperbolic force velocity curve, with V_{MAX} relatively independent of the initial muscle length but increased by the addition of norepinephrine (Fig. 12-13).

Another preparation used to examine force–velocity relationships uses single cardiac myocytes isolated by enzymatic digestion of the rat myocardium and then permeabilized with a staphylococcal toxin. Again, the force–velocity relationship is hyperbolic, suggesting the existence of intracellular *passive elastic elements* that contribute to the load on the isolated myocyte (Schweitzer and Moss, 1993). In fact, the more hyperbolic and increased curvilinear nature of the force–velocity relationship in isolated myocytes than in the papillary muscle suggests that internal passive forces such as those generated by titin are greater than expected in the isolated myocytes. In the intact heart, the noncontractile components contribute relatively little to overall mechanical behavior, at least in physiologic circumstances (Campbell et al., 1994).

Mechanism of β-Adrenergic Effects on Force–Velocity Relationship

The data on papillary muscles showing that norepinephrine can increase V_{MAX} could be explained by either an effect of β-adrenergic stimulation on enhancing calcium ion entry or a direct effect on the contractile proteins, or both (see Fig. 7-16). Either isoproterenol (β-stimulant) or protein kinase A (intracellular messenger) can increase V_{MAX} by about 40% concurrently with phosphorylation of troponin-I and C protein in an isolated ventricular myocyte preparation (Strang et al., 1994). Hypothetically, such phosphorylations increase the rate of cross-bridge cycling (Schweitzer and Moss, 1993).

Drugs given therapeutically that act by increasing cyclic adenosine monophosphate (cAMP) levels and having a similar signaling chain to that shown in Fig. 7-16 include the β-adrenergic stimulant dobutamine and the phosphodiesterase inhibitor milrinone.

Isometric Versus Isotonic Contraction

Despite the similarities in the force–velocity patterns between the data obtained on papillary muscle and isolated myocytes, it should be considered that a number of different types of muscular contraction may be involved. For example, data for P_0 are obtained under isometric conditions (length unchanged). When muscle is allowed to shorten against a steady load, the conditions are *isotonic* (Greek *iso,* the same; *tonic,* contractile force). Yet measurements of V_{MAX} have to be under totally unloaded conditions, both in the papillary muscles and in permeabilized myocytes (Schlant and Sonnenblick, 1994). Thus, the force–velocity curve may be a combination of initial isometric conditions followed by isotonic contraction and then may follow abrupt and total unloading to measure V_{MAX}. Although isometric conditions can be found in the whole heart as an approximation during isovolumic contraction, isotonic conditions cannot prevail because the load is constantly changing during the ejection period, and complete unloading is impossible. Therefore, the application of force–velocity relationships to the heart in vivo is limited.

WALL STRESS

Myocardial wall stress or wall tension increases when the myofilaments slide over each other during cardiac contraction as they are squeezing blood out of the

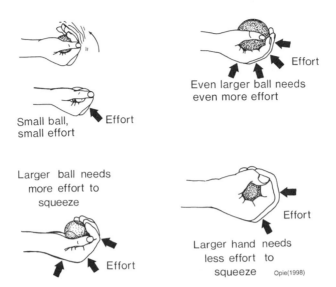

FIG. 12-14. Model of wall stress. The effort required to squeeze a ball in the hand has some analogies to the development of wall stress in the heart. When the volume of blood in the ventricle is increased, the wall stress increases, and more effort is required for contraction. When the heart hypertrophies, the wall tension decreases, and a larger volume of blood in the ventricle can be ejected more easily. The analogy is that a bigger hand needs less effort to squeeze the big ball than does a smaller hand.

ventricles into the circulation. An analogy is the human effort required to squeeze a ball in the palm of the hand (Fig. 12-14). A small rubber ball can be compressed easily. A larger rubber ball (tennis ball in size) is compressed less readily, and two large rubber balls (or one really large ball) could be compressed only with the greatest difficulty. As the size of the object in the hand increases, so does the force required to compress it. Intuitively, the stress on the hand increases as the ball increases in diameter. However, what is wall stress?

At this point it is appropriate to deviate briefly into a description of force, tension, and wall stress. *Force* is a term frequently used in studies of muscle mechanics. Strictly,

$$Force = mass \times acceleration$$

Thus, when a load is suspended from one end of a muscle as the muscle contracts, it is exerting force against the mass of that load. In many cases, it is not possible to define force with such exactitude, but generally force has the following properties. First, force is always applied by one object (such as muscle) on another object (such as a load). Second, force is characterized both by the direction in which it acts and its magnitude. Hence, it is a vector, and the effect of a combination of forces can be established by the principle of vectors. Third, each object exerts a force on the other, so that force and counterforce are equal and opposite (Newton's third law of motion).

Tension exists when the two forces are applied to an object so that the forces tend to pull the object apart. When a spring is pulled by a force, tension is exerted; when more force is applied, the spring stretches, and the tension increases.

Stress develops when tension is applied to a cross-sectional area, and the units are force per unit area. According to the *Laplace law* (Fig. 12-15),

$$\text{Wall stress} = \frac{\text{pressure} \times \text{radius}}{2 \times \text{wall thickness}}$$

The increased wall thickness due to hypertrophy balances the increased pressure, and the wall stress remains unchanged during the phase of compensatory hypertrophy (see Chapter 16). In congestive heart failure, the heart dilates to increase the radius factor, thereby elevating wall stress. Furthermore, because ejection of blood is inadequate, the radius stays too large throughout the contractile cycle, and both end-diastolic and end-systolic tensions are higher.

Wall Stress, Preload, and Afterload

Wall stress is a useful concept in the understanding of preload and afterload in the human heart. *Preload* can be defined as the wall stress at the end of diastole and therefore at the maximal resting length of the sarcomere (Figs. 12-6 and 12-7). Measurement of wall stress in vivo is difficult because the radius of the left ventricle (see preceding sections) neglects the confounding influence of the complex anatomy of the left ventricle (Borow, 1988). Surrogate measurement of the indices of preload include LV end-diastolic pressure or dimensions

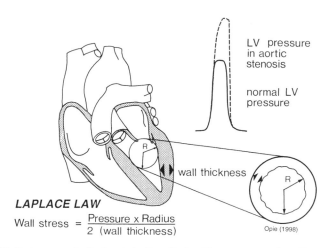

LV pressure in aortic stenosis

normal LV pressure

wall thickness

LAPLACE LAW

Wall stress $= \dfrac{\text{Pressure} \times \text{Radius}}{2 \ (\text{wall thickness})}$

Opie (1998)

FIG. 12-15. Wall stress and afterload. As the afterload increases, so does the wall stress. The formula is derived from the Laplace law. The increased LV pressure in aortic stenosis is compensated for by LV wall hypertrophy, which decreases the denominator on the right side of the equation, thereby maintaining wall stress at control levels.

(the latter being the major and minor axes of the heart in a two-dimensional echocardiographic view). The *afterload,* being the load on the contracting myocardium, is the wall stress during LV ejection. Increased afterload means that an increased intraventricular pressure has to be generated first to open the aortic valve and then during the ejection phase. These increases translate themselves into an increased myocardial wall stress, which can be measured either as an average value or a given phase of systole, such as end-systole. Systolic wall stress reflects the two major components of the afterload, namely the arterial blood pressure and the arterial compliance. Decreased arterial compliance and increased afterload can be anticipated when there is aortic dilation as in severe systemic hypertension or in the elderly. Generally, in clinical practice, it is a sufficient approximation to take the arterial blood pressure as a measure of the afterload, provided that there is no significant aortic stenosis nor change in arterial compliance.

Wall Stress and Myocardial Oxygen Demand

At a fixed heart rate, the myocardial wall stress is the major determinant of the myocardial oxygen uptake. Because myocardial oxygen uptake ultimately reflects the rate of mitochondrial metabolism and adenosine triphosphate (ATP) production, any increase of ATP requirement will be reflected in an increased oxygen uptake. It is not only external work that determines the requirement for ATP. Rather, tension development (increased wall stress) is oxygen requiring even without external work being done. The difference between external work and tension developed can be epitomized by the man standing and holding a heavy suitcase, doing no external work yet becoming very tired, compared with the man lifting a much lighter suitcase, doing external work yet not getting tired. The greater the LV chamber size, the greater the radius, the greater the wall stress (Fig. 12-15). Hence, ejection of the same stroke volume from a large left ventricle against the same blood pressure will produce as much external work as ejection of the same stroke volume by a normal sized left ventricle, yet with a much greater wall stress in the case of the larger ventricle. Therefore, more oxygen will be required. In clinical terms, heart size is an important determinant of myocardial oxygen demand, and in a patient with angina in a large left ventricle, the appropriate therapy to reduce LV size will also reduce the myocardial oxygen demand.

The overall concept of wall stress includes afterload because an increased afterload generates an increased systolic wall stress. Wall stress also includes preload, which generates diastolic wall stress. Wall stress increases in proportion to the pressure generated and to the radius of the LV cavity (Fig. 12-15), factors which are responsive to increases in afterload and preload respectively. Wall stress allows for energy required for generation of muscular contraction that does not result in external work. Furthermore, in states of enhanced contractility, wall stress is increased. Thus, thinking in terms of wall stress provides a comprehensive approach to the problem of myocardial oxygen demand. Apart from a metabolic component, usually small but which may be prominent in certain special circumstances, such as when circulating free fatty acids are abnormally high, *changes in heart rate and wall stress account for most of the clinically relevant changes in myocardial oxygen uptake.*

OXYGEN COST OF HEART WORK

To what extent is external work a determinant of the myocardial oxygen uptake? That index is the heart work. External work is done, for example, when a mass is lifted a certain distance. In terms of the heart, the cardiac output is the mass moved, and the resistance against which it is moved is the afterload, chiefly the blood pressure (for reservations, see Chapter 14). The following are clinical approximations:

Minute work = systolic or mean BP × CO

where BP is blood pressure and CO is cardiac output in liters per minute. The cardiac output reflects both heart rate and stroke volume, the stroke volume reflects preload, and the blood pressure reflects afterload.

Stroke work = mean BP × stroke volume

Stroke work index = stroke work, corrected for body surface area

where SV = end-diastolic volume − end-systolic volume. When the end-diastolic volume is increased, as in the enlarged heart of heart failure, and the stroke volume remains the same, external work is unchanged, but internal work increases (because of the need to overcome greater wall stress). This deleterious change is important because it means that the enlarged failing heart has a greatly increased internal workload and, hence, increased oxygen demand, in attempting to maintain a normal cardiac output.

Kinetic Versus Pressure Work

In strict terms, the work performed (*power production*) needs to take into account not only pressure but kinetic components. Thus far, it is pressure work that has been discussed. It is the larger component, and an approximate clinical index of pressure work is the product of the cardiac output and the peak systolic pressure. The kinetic work is that component required to move the blood against the pressure of the arterial system. Kinetic work depends on the cardiac output, the density of the blood, the cross-sectional area of the major resistance site (e.g., the aortic valve), and the ejection time. Normally, kinetic work is only a fraction of the total work (Kannengiesser et al., 1979), but it increases substantially in aortic stenosis.

The formulae for work production are:

$$\text{Pressure power} = K_1 \times Ps \times CO$$

$$\text{Kinetic power} = K_2 \times \frac{(CO)^3}{A^2} \times \left(\frac{T}{Te}\right)^2$$

where Ps is peak systolic pressure in mm Hg, CO is cardiac output in ml/minute, A is area of aortic valve in cm², T is total cycle time, Te is ejection time, and the units for power are milliwatts (i.e., milliJoules per second). Instead of the peak systolic pressure, another formula uses the mean systolic pressure. Even these formulae are simplifications because in reality the pressure power is the product of the integrated sum of the instantaneous arterial pressure, which changes all the time, and the instantaneous aortic flow (also changing).

Work Diagram of Left Ventricle

Bearing in mind that the major factor in cardiac work is the product of pressure and volume, it follows that external work can be quantified by the integrated pressure–volume area that represents the product of the systolic pressure and the stroke volume (Fig. 12-16). As contractile force develops in the LV wall in systole, so does the pressure buildup in the cavity (a → b in Fig. 12-16) until the moment when the aortic valve opens to eject the blood, and the isovolumic phase of LV contraction is over. When the aortic valves open, the flow of blood

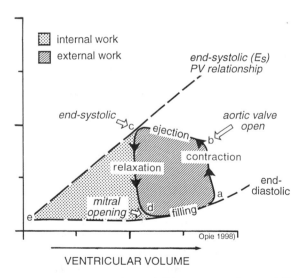

VENTRICULAR VOLUME

FIG. 12-16. Pressure–volume loops. Normal LV pressure–volume relationship. The aortic valve opens at b and closes at c. The mitral valve opens at d and closes at a. External work is defined by a, b, c, and d, and internal work by e, d, and c. The pressure–volume area is the sum of external and internal work.

commences, the ventricular pressure still increases because the pressure in the aorta must be overcome, and the LV volume decreases (b → c). The intraventricular pressure is highest at the peak of ejection (point c). As the heart relaxes in early diastole, the pressure decreases nearly to zero (c → d), and the ventricle is nearly empty. Then, as the mitral valve opens and the left ventricle fills, the volume increases as the pressure stays low (d → a). When systole starts, the cycle is repeated. This sequence should be studied in conjunction with the Wiggers diagram (Fig. 12-1). To relate work to the oxygen consumption, account must be taken of both the external work (a, b, c, d) and internal work, which is the volume–pressure triangle joining the end-systolic volume–pressure point to the origin (c, d, e). In addition, a small portion of the work of moving the blood can be accounted for by factors external to the left ventricle, such as atrial contraction and venous return.

Pressure Versus Volume Work.   In analyzing the difference between oxygen cost of pressure work and volume work, an established clinical observation is that the myocardium can tolerate a chronic pressure load less well than a volume load. Suga et al. (1982) made the following proposals. If, starting at the same end-diastolic volume the amount of external stroke work is artificially kept the same during a volume and pressure load, there will be large differences in the total oxygen uptake (Fig. 12-17). To keep the stroke work the same, the area within the loop has to be the same, so that the stroke volume during a pressure load is initially less (to compensate for the higher pressure). However, the remaining area between the pressure–volume loop and the end-systolic PV relationship line (c, d, e in Fig. 12-16) is greater for the same amount of work done under the increased pressure. Thus, when cardiac work is increased by increasing the afterload, as during severe hypertension or narrowing of the aortic valve by aortic stenosis, the peak systolic pressure in the left ventricle must increase, and pressure power increases. However, because of the complex way in which the muscle fibers of the myocardium run, a greater proportion of the work is against the internal resistance. The result is that the efficiency decreases. An extreme example of the loss of efficiency during pressure work would be if the aorta were completely occluded, so that none of the work would be external and all would be internal. Internal work is done against the noncontractile elements of the myocardium and is not useful work in terms of calculating efficiency.

When the heart is subject to a volume load (e.g., in mitral regurgitation when the mitral valve leaks and part of the stroke volume is ejected into the left atrium, thereafter returning to the left ventricle), the increased work that the heart must perform is met by an increased end-diastolic volume. The myofibers stretch, and the phenomenon of length-dependent activation occurs (Fig. 12-8). The primary adaptation to increased heart volume is an increased fiber length and not increased pressure development, so the amount of external work done is more,

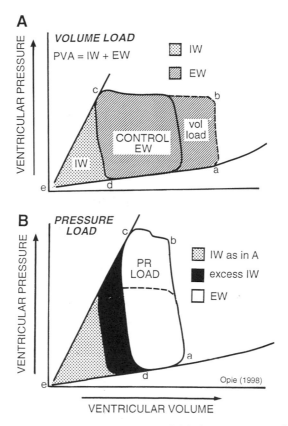

FIG. 12-17. Pressure versus volume work. In artificial circumstances, and using an isovolumic preparation, it is possible to compare equal amounts of stroke work performed by volume loading (top panel) and pressure loading (bottom panel), which have different consequences for the oxygen uptake (Schwinger et al., 1994). Both external work (a, b, c, d) and internal work (c, d, e) require oxygen. The slashed area in the upper panel indicates the control conditions including a triangle (c, d, e) to the left of the PV loop, which is the requirement for internal work (IW). The stippled area in both panels indicates extra stroke work, the same for the volume-loaded as for the pressure-loaded heart because total stroke work is designed to be the same in this experiment. The black area during the pressure load indicates the extra internal work and hence the extra oxygen requirement of the pressure-loaded heart when compared with the volume-loaded heart at equal levels of external work (EW).

but the work against the internal resistance is unchanged; therefore, the efficiency increases. A secondary adaptation is fiber slippage so that the ventricular wall thins and becomes more compliant. During β-adrenergic stimulation, the slope of the pressure–volume diagram (E_s, Fig. 12-18), an index of the positive inotropic effect, increases. Concurrently, the lusitropic effect pushes down the filling curve. External work increases substantially, with a relatively lesser increase in internal work.

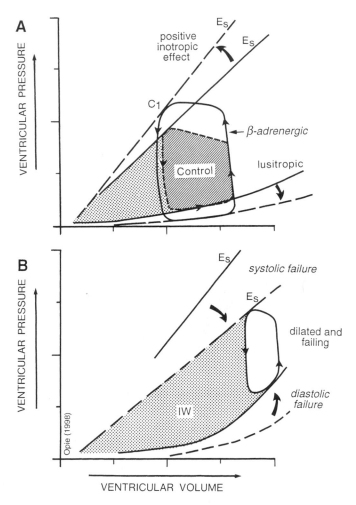

FIG. 12-18. PV loops: β-adrenergic effects versus heart failure. A: Effects of β-adrenergic stimulation, with both positive inotropic and increased lusitropic (relaxant) effects. Compare position of C1 with C in Fig. 12-16, and note changes in E_s. Also compare with effects of dynamic exercise (see Fig. 15-6). **B:** Pressure–volume relationship in severe left ventricular failure (LVF) with both systolic and diastolic failure. Decreased compliance moves the end-diastolic pressure–volume curve upward and to the left. A decreased inotropic effect moves the pressure–volume slope to the right. A decreased stroke volume is indicated by the smaller volume changes. Note greatly increased internal work (IW), with much less external work (area within the loop).

Efficiency of Work

The efficiency of work relates the amount of work performed to the myocardial oxygen uptake. An ideal definition of efficiency of work would be:

$$\text{Efficiency} = \frac{\text{work performed}}{\text{maximum work possible}}$$

The denominator of this equation cannot be measured. A simpler measure of the efficiency of the work is to relate the external measured work to the oxygen uptake.

$$\text{Efficiency} = \frac{\text{work performed}}{\text{oxygen uptake}}$$

To improve the efficiency of work requires an analysis of whether it requires more oxygen to increase pressure or volume work. To conserve the myocardial oxygen balance, it would be desirable to achieve more work for the same oxygen uptake (improved efficiency). In practice, this means less pressure and more volume work, an aim that can be achieved therapeutically by arterial vasodilation. Conversely, increasing internal work (e.g., by allowing aortic stenosis to progress) promotes inefficient pressure work, which is one reason why aortic stenosis is so deleterious to patients with coronary artery disease.

Heat Production and the Efficiency of Work. The assessment of heat production is of most use when trying to marry the analyses of skeletal muscle mechanics by A.V. Hill and colleagues to the much more complex mechanics of cardiac muscle (Gibbs, 1974). From the metabolic view, however, all heat production is nothing other than the use of ATP, partially for contraction and relaxation but also for ionic movements. However, the production of heat is the major product of ATP hydrolysis. A major requirement of all tissue, including the heart, is to be at the optimum temperature (37°C) for enzyme activity so that the generation of heat by ATP hydrolysis is teleologically desirable. Furthermore, the percentage of ATP converted to heat cannot be substantially changed except by breaking ATP down further than ADP. Taking these facts into account, it is not surprising that the efficiency of external work of the heart is only 12% to 20%.

Efficiency of Work in Heart Failure. The failing myocardium is unable to generate enough pressure to keep the arterial blood pressure high enough without compensatory support mechanisms such as increased peripheral arteriolar vasoconstriction (see Chapter 16). In the pressure–volume loop, external work is much decreased, whereas internal work is considerably more (Fig. 12-18). Thus, the failing myocardium is called to work much more. The failing myocardium is in an energetically unfavorable situation, and the efficiency of work declines. This harmful situation can be partially countered by therapeutically reducing the afterload (Asanoi et al., 1996).

CLINICAL INDICES OF CONTRACTILITY

Whereas it is relatively easy for the clinician to reach approximations of the preload or the afterload of the heart by measuring the LV filling pressure or the blood pressure and to relate these to the stroke volume, it is very difficult to assess the inotropic state (or the contractile state) of the myocardium. It is also not easy to link the parameters of myocardial mechanical function to the pro-

TABLE 12-4. *Proposed mechanisms for some parameters of mechanical cardiac function*

Parameter of function	Definition	Proposed explanation
End-diastolic fiber length	Acts by Starling's law	Increased fiber sensitivity to Ca^{2+}
Peak force (peak tension increment); developed pressure	Difference between maximum systolic tension and minimum diastolic tension	Total number of crossbridges attached since beginning of systole, a function of (1) initial fiber length; (2) systolic Ca^{2+} increase; (3) calcium responsiveness of filaments; (4) myosin light chain phosphorylation; (5) loading
V_{max} of isolated papillary muscle	Maximal rate of shortening at zero load (see Fig. 12-4)	Proportional to (1) myosin ATPase activity, (2) rate-limiting steps in crossbridge cycle, (3) cytosolic Ca^{2+}: rate of increase and peak level
P_0	Maximal tension at zero shortening rate	Related to number of attached crossbridges and to peak Ca^{2+} level
Indices of contractility	See Table 12-5	As for V_{max} but variously influenced by preload and afterload

posed subcellular mechanisms (Table 12-4). By definition, the types of studies undertaken on papillary muscle to obtain V_{MAX} are virtually impossible in humans, and a variety of indices are used (Table 12-5).

Left Ventricular Function Curves

Ventricular function curves can be obtained by varying the end-diastolic volume with repetitive measurements during a volume load (intravenous infusion). These curves are based on the Starling relationship indirectly assessed by Swan-Ganz catheterization using not the heart volume nor the end-diastolic fiber length, but the end-diastolic LV filling pressure as a surrogate (Fig. 12-5). The extrapolation from the one to the other usually is reasonable but can be substantially altered by changes in the LV compliance (see section on Compliance). Furthermore, to produce an LV function curve by altering the preload over a wide range in humans is not easy. Yet another problem is the wide overlap among the different patterns of LV function curves, so that it is not a simple matter to decide whether a given function curve decreases into the normal category, into impaired LV function without clinical heart failure, or into clinical heart failure. Nonetheless, by comparing the LV end-diastolic pressure with the stroke volume and relating this point to the normal range (Fig. 12-5), an approximation of cardiac function can be obtained.

Maximal Rate of Left Ventricular Pressure Generation

In relation to the cardiac contraction–relaxation cycle, it is easiest to consider LV function during the early period of isovolumic contraction (Fig. 12-19).

TABLE 12-5. *Some applicable clinical indices of myocardial contractile (inotropic) state*

Index	Advantage	Comment
Isovolumic indices		
dP/dt$_{max}$	Classic invasive index	Requires LV catheterization; preload sensitive
Noninvasive +dP/dt	Can be determined by echocardiogram and phonocardiogram	dt measured from M$_1$ (phono) to AO (echo); dP from aortic diastolic pr and assuming LVEDP
Load-sensitive indices		
Ejection fraction (EF)	Noninvasive radionuclide scan or from echo-cardiographic volumes	Volume ejected during systole compared with initial ventricular volume; index of LV systolic function; load-dependent; normal >55%
Percentage fractional shortening (FS)	Simple noninvasive echocardiographic technique	(EDD-ESD)/(EDD); like ejection fraction; load-dependent
Long to minor axis shortening	Echocardiographic index claimed to be sensitive	Compares well with fractional shortening
Velocity of circum-ferential fiber shortening (V$_{cf}$)	Noninvasive echocar-diographic technique	Calculated from end-systolic and end-diastolic diameters and ejection time; consider end-systolic wall stress
End-systolic indices		
End-systolic volume	Echocardiographic	Normal mean 34 ml in males, 29 in females; limit 55 ml (Carabello, 1996; Schiller and Foster, 1996)
End-systolic volume/pressure relation-ship	Echocardiographic or radionuclide determination; measured noninvasively	A small end-systolic volume reflects high contractility but is also afterload dependent
End-systolic wall stress/V$_{cf}$	Corresponds approximately to force-velocity relationship of isolated papillary muscle	Needs complex echocardiographic analyses
End-systolic stress/end-systolic volume	Corresponds approximately to one end-point of PV loop	Wall stress difficult to measure
Pressure-volume loop	Part of loop can be monitored noninvasively as end-systolic volume-pressure relationship	Increased slope indicates increased contractility

EDP, end-diastolic pressure; EDD, end-diastolic dimension; ESD, end-systolic dimension; LV, left ventricle; pr, pressure; echo, echocardiography; phono, phonocardiography. For dP/dt$_{max}$, see Fig. 12-5.

During this period of isovolumic contraction, the preload and afterload are constant, and the maximal rate of pressure generation should be an index of the inotropic state:

$$Inotropic\ index = max\ dP/dt$$

where P is LV pressure, t is time, and d indicates rate of change. This index has stood the test of years and gives some absolute values. Unfortunately, this index is not fully independent of the preload, which when increased will enhance the contractile state by length–activation.

The measurements required for dP/dt can be obtained only by LV catheterization, except in mitral regurgitation when Doppler echocardiography can measure changes in the LV–atrial pressure gradient (Chen et al., 1991). Bearing in

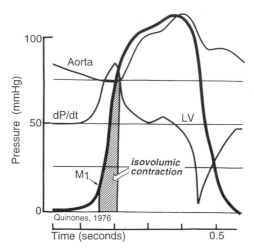

FIG. 12-19. Isovolumic contraction phase and its characteristics. Based on original data of Quinones et al. (1976). For dP/dt$_{max}$, see Table 12-5.

mind that LV pressure is changing during the period of isovolumic contraction, some workers prefer to make a correction for the change in pressure by dividing dP/dt by a fixed developed pressure, e.g., dP/dt(dP$_{40}$), or by the pressure at the instant of the maximal rate of pressure development, (dP/dt)/P. Such corrections add little except complexity.

Ejection Phase Indices of Contractile State

During the ejection phase, the left ventricle contracts against the afterload. Hence, all indices of function in this period are afterload dependent (Table 12-5), a problem that is especially serious in the case of the failing myocardium, which is adversely affected by afterload increases (Vahl et al., 1994). The initial fiber length helps to determine contractility, which in turn influences the afterload, because a greater contractile state in the presence of a fixed peripheral (systemic) vascular resistance will increase the blood pressure and the afterload.

The *ejection fraction* of the left ventricle, measured via radionuclide or echocardiographic techniques, is one of the most frequently used indices and one of the least sensitive. The ejection fraction relates stroke volume to end-diastolic volume and is therefore an index of the extent of LV fiber shortening. Nonetheless, this index is easy to obtain and particularly useful in evaluating the course of chronic heart disease. Because the ejection fraction measures the contractile behavior of the heart during systole, it is by definition afterload sensitive. Another defect is that the ejection fraction relates the systolic emptying to the diastolic volume without measuring that volume, and the left ventricle could theoretically be markedly enlarged yet have reasonable systolic function by this measure. Thus, the correlation between the degree of clinical heart failure and the ejection fraction is often only imperfect.

Echocardiographic Indices of Contractile State

The major advantages of echocardiographic indices is that the techniques are widely available and relatively rapid. The *fractional shortening* uses the percentage of change of the minor axis (defined in the next paragraph) of the LV chamber during systole. An approximation often used by clinicians is to estimate the ejection fraction from *fractional shortening*. Despite obvious defects, this easily defined index is pragmatically useful in the management of heart failure. More accurately, ejection fraction can be determined from volume measurements.

The *end-systolic volume* reflects contractile state because the normal left ventricle ejects most of the blood present at the end of diastole (ejection fraction exceeds 55%). Impaired contractility, shown by an abnormally increased end-systolic volume, is a powerful predictor of adverse prognosis after myocardial infarction (Schiller and Foster, 1996). The *end-diastolic volume* is a less powerful predictor but essential for the accurate measurement of the ejection fraction.

Much more sophisticated measurements of the pumping function of the heart can be obtained via echocardiography. In particular, the velocity at which the circumference of the heart in its minor axis changes during systole is a useful index of myocardial contractility (Table 12-5). The *minor axis* of the heart is the distance from the left side of the septum to the posterior endocardial wall. The *major axis* lies in the direction of the septum, which introduces an additional factor, septal contraction, so that major axis changes cannot be used to assess contractile activity. The mean *velocity of circumferential fiber shortening* (mean V_{cf}) can be determined from echocardiographic measurements of the end-diastolic and end-systolic sizes and the rate of change. The difference between the calculated circumferences is divided by the duration of shortening, which is the ejection time. The *mean V_{cf}* compares favorably with more sophisticated invasive measurements of the contractile state.

Contractility Indices Based on Pressure–Volume Loops

There are two fundamental aspects of the Frank-Starling relationship that can be seen readily in a pressure–volume loop (Fig. 12-16). First, as the preload increases, the volume increases. On the other hand, for any given preload (initial volume of contraction), a positive inotropic agent increases the amount of blood ejected, and for the same final end-systolic pressure, there is a smaller end-systolic volume. Thus, the slope of the end-systolic pressure–volume relationship is increased. It follows that relating pressure to volume is one way of assessing both the Starling effect and the contractility of the left ventricle.

Accordingly, measurements of pressure–volume loops are among the best of the current approaches to the assessment of the contractile behavior of the intact heart, and hence the key to one of the major determinants of the myocardial oxygen demand. The end-systolic pressure–volume relationship can be estimated noninvasively from the arterial systolic pressure and the end-systolic echocardiographic dimension. Invasive measurements of the LV pressure are required for the full loop, which is an indirect measure of the Starling relationship between the force (as measured by the pressure) and the muscle length (measured indirectly by the volume). It is proposed that conditions associated with a higher contractile activity (increased inotropic state) will have higher end-systolic pressures at any for a given end-systolic volume (point c1) (Fig. 12-18), have a steeper slope Es, and have correspondingly higher oxygen uptakes. Although useful, like all systolic phase indices, it is still afterload dependent and thus not totally load independent.

DIASTOLE AND DIASTOLIC FUNCTION

Among the many complex cellular factors influencing ventricular relaxation, four are of chief interest. First, the cytosolic calcium level must decrease to cause the relaxation phase, a process requiring ATP and phosphorylation of phospholamban for uptake of calcium into the sarcoplasmic reticulum (Fig. 12-20). Second, the inherent viscoelastic properties of the myocardium are of importance. In the hypertrophied heart, relaxation occurs more slowly. Third, increased phosphorylation of troponin-I enhances the rate of relaxation (Zhang et al., 1995). Fourth, relaxation is influenced by the systolic load. The history of

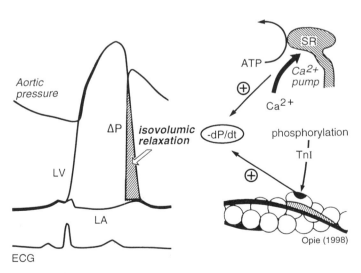

FIG. 12-20. Isovolumic relaxation. This phase of the cardiac cycle is shaded in. It extends from the aortic second sound (A_2) to the crossover point between the left ventricular and left atrial pressures (Fig. 12-1). The rate of relaxation is given by –dP/dt.

contraction affects crossbridge relaxation (Hori et al., 1991; Leite-Moreira and Gillebert, 1994). Within limits, the greater the systolic load, the faster the rate of relaxation. This complex relationship has been explored in detail by Brutsaert (1993), but could perhaps be simplified as follows. When the workload is high, peak cytosolic calcium is also thought to be high. A high end-systolic cytosolic calcium level means that the rate of decrease of calcium also can be greater, provided that the uptake mechanisms are functioning effectively. In this way a systolic pressure load and the rate of diastolic relaxation can be related. Furthermore, a greater muscle length (when the workload is high) at the end of systole should produce a more rapid rate of relaxation by the opposite of length-dependent sensitization, so that there is a more marked response to the rate of decline of calcium in early diastole. Yet, when the systolic load exceeds a certain limit, then the rate of relaxation is delayed (Leite-Moreira and Gillebert, 1994), perhaps because of too great a mechanical stress on the individual crossbridges. Thus, in congestive heart failure caused by an excess systolic load, relaxation becomes increasingly afterload dependent, so that therapeutic reduction of the systolic load should improve LV relaxation (Eichhorn et al., 1992).

The *isovolumic relaxation* phase of the cardiac cycle is energy dependent, requiring ATP for the uptake of calcium ions by the sarcoplasmic reticulum (Fig. 12-20), which is an active, not a passive process. Impaired relaxation is an early event in angina pectoris. A proposed metabolic explanation is that there is impaired generation of energy, which diminishes the supply of ATP required for the early diastolic uptake of calcium by the sarcoplasmic reticulum. The result is that the cytosolic calcium level, at a peak in systole, delays its return to normal in the early diastolic period. In other conditions, too, there is a relationship between the rate of diastolic decay of the calcium transient and diastolic relaxation, with a relation to impaired function of the sarcoplasmic reticulum (Corey et al., 1994). When the rate of relaxation is prolonged by hypothyroidism, the rate of return of the systolic calcium elevation is likewise delayed, whereas opposite changes occur in hyperthyroidism (Morgan and Morgan, 1989). In congestive heart failure, diastolic relaxation also is delayed and irregular, as is the rate of decay of the cytosolic calcium elevation. Most patients with coronary artery disease have a variety of abnormalities of diastolic filling, probably related to those also found in angina pectoris. Theoretically, such abnormalities of relaxation are potentially reversible because they depend on changes in patterns of calcium ion movement. Indices of the isovolumic phase and other indices of diastolic function are shown in Table 12-6. Of interest is the echocardiographic determination in patients with regurgitant valve disease of $-dP/dt_{max}$ (Yamamoto et al., 1995) and of *tau,* the time constant of relaxation (Chen et al., 1992).

Phases of Diastole

Hemodynamically, diastole can be divided into four phases (Fig. 12-21), using the clinical definitions of diastole according to which diastole extends

TABLE 12-6. *Some indices of diastolic function*

1. *Isovolumic relaxation*
   $(-)dP/dt_{max}$
   Aortic closing, mitral opening interval
   Peak rate of LV wall thinning
   Time constant of relaxation, tau[a]
2. *Early diastolic filling*
   Relaxation kinetics on ERNA (rate of volume increase)
   Early filling phase (E phase) on Doppler transmitral velocity trace
3. *Diastasis*
   Pressure–volume relationship indicates compliance
4. *Atrial contraction*
   Invasive measurement of atrial and ventricular pressures
   Doppler transmitral pattern (late or A phase)
5. *E/A ratios*
   Normally E > A unless A increased by age or disease; decreased LV compliance increases E to A (Yamamoto et al., 1996)

[a]For noninvasive measurements by continuous wave Doppler velocity profile in mitral regurgitation, see Chen et al. (1992). ERNA, equilibrated radionuclide angiography.

from aortic valve closure to the start of the first heart sound. The first phase of diastole (see preceding section) is the isovolumic phase, which, by definition, does not contribute to ventricular filling. The second phase of rapid filling provides most of the ventricular filling. The third phase of slow filling or diastasis accounts for only 5% of the total filling. The final atrial booster phase accounts for the remaining 15%.

Does the Left Ventricle "Suck" During Early Filling? Whether the LV suction by active relaxation could increase the pressure gradient from the left atrium to the left ventricle during the early filling phase remains controversial although well supported by data. An LV suction effect can be found by carefully comparing LV and left atrial pressures, and it occurs especially in the early diastolic phase of rapid filling (Fig. 12-22). The sucking effect may be of most importance in mitral stenosis, when the mitral valve does not open as it otherwise should in response to diastolic suction. During catecholamine stimulation, the rate of relaxation may increase to enhance the sucking effect and to prolong the period of filling. The proposed mechanism of sucking is as follows. When the end-systolic volume is less than the equilibrium volume, the shortened muscle fibers and collagen matrix may act as a compressed spring, to generate recoil forces in diastole.

Atrial Function. The left atrium, besides its well-known function as a blood-receiving chamber, also acts as follows. First, by presystolic contraction and its booster function, it helps to complete LV filling (Hoit et al., 1994). Second, it is the volume sensor of the heart, releasing atrial natriuretic peptide (ANP) in response to intermittent stretch. Third, the atrium contains receptors for the affer-

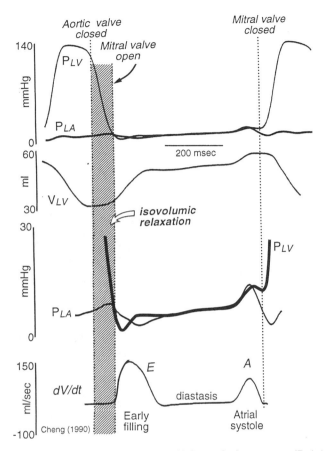

FIG. 12-21. Diastolic filling phases. Recording of left ventricular pressure (P$_{LV}$), left atrial pressure (P$_{LA}$), left ventricular volume (dV/dt), which indicates the rate of LV filling. LV filling occurs early in diastole and during atrial systole in response to pressure gradient from the left atrium to the left ventricle. The early diastolic pressure gradient is generated as LV pressure decreases below left atrial pressure, and the late diastolic gradient is generated as atrial contraction increases left atrial pressure above LV pressure. (Data from Cheng et al. Effect of loading conditions, contractile state and heart rate on early diastolic left ventricular filling in conscious dogs. *Circ Res* 1990;66:814; Copyright 1990 American Heart Association.)

ent arms of various reflexes, including mechanoreceptors that increase sinus discharge rate, thereby contributing to the tachycardia of exercise as the venous return increases (*Bainbridge reflex*).

The atria have a number of differences in structure and function from the ventricles (Table 12-7), having smaller myocytes with a shorter action potential duration as well as a more fetal type of myosin (both in heavy and light chains). Furthermore, the atria are more reliant on the phosphatidylinositol signal transduction pathway, which may explain the relatively greater positive inotropic

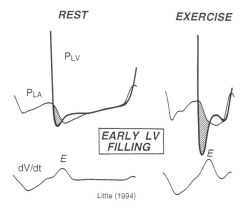

FIG. 12-22. Apparent LV sucking effect. Recording of P_{LV}, P_{LA}, and dV/dt at rest and during exercise. During exercise, minimal P_{LV} decreases without any increase in P_{LA}. This leads to an increase in the peak mitral valve gradient and produces a larger peak filling rate (E). From Little and Cheng. Modulation of drastic dysfunction in the intact heart. In: Lorell BH, Grossman W (eds). *Diastolic Relaxation of the Heart.* Boston: Kluwer Academic, 1994:167–176, with permission.

effect in the atria than in the ventricles in response to angiotensin II (Holubarsch et al., 1993). The more rapid atrial repolarization is thought to be due to increased outward potassium currents, such as I_{to} and I_{kACh} (Koumi et al., 1994). In addition, some atrial cells have the capacity for spontaneous depolarization. In general, these histologic and physiologic changes can be related to the decreased need for the atria to generate high intrachamber pressures, while retaining enough contractile action to help with LV filling and to respond to inotropic stimuli (Hoit et al., 1994).

TABLE 12-7. *Major differences between atria and left ventricle*

Parameter	Atria	Left ventricle
Hemodynamic function	Receives venous blood and transmits it to ventricles	Ejects blood into aorta to maintain BP and CO
Blood volume control	Volume sensor	Volume ejector
Wall dimension	Thin	Thick
Myocyte size	20×5 μm	$75 \times (10\text{–}25)$ μm
Pressure generated	Low, 15–30 mmHg	High, over 100 mmHg
Myosin phenotype, heavy	Fetal (α-α)	Adult (β-β)
Myosin phenotype, light	Fetal (A-LC1)	Adult (V-LC1)
ANP synthesis	Physiologic	Pathologic (also BNP)
Action potential	Prominent phase 1; short plateau; triangular	Small phase 1; long plateau; square

BP, blood pressure; CO, cardiac output; A-LC1, atrial type myosin light chain 1; V-LC1, ventricular type myosin light chain 1; ANP, atrial natriuretic peptide; BNP, brain natriuretic peptide. Also see Table 8-3.

DIASTOLIC LEFT VENTRICULAR DYSFUNCTION: DIASTOLOGY

Diastolic dysfunction is now increasingly emphasized as a cause of cardiac disability (Table 12-8). Although abnormalities of the filling phases are usually prominent, the first phase of isovolumic relaxation also must be considered. The rate of such relaxation can be measured by negative dP/dt_{max} at invasive catheterization (Fig. 12-20). *Tau,* the time constant of relaxation, describes the rate of decrease of LV pressure during isovolumic relaxation and also requires invasive techniques for precise determination (Chen et al., 1992). Tau is increased as the systolic LV pressure increases (Leite-Moreira and Gillebert, 1994). In mitral regurgitation, the Doppler velocity profile can be used to calculate *tau* (Chen et al., 1992). Another index of relaxation can be obtained echocardiographically from the peak *rate of wall thinning* (Douglas et al., 1989). The *isovolumic relaxation time,* because it lies between aortic valve closure and mitral valve opening, can be measured by signals of valve movements at Doppler echocardiography (Fig. 12-21). In each case, precise measurement is difficult, and the range of normality is large.

Diastolic Dysfunction in Hypertrophy and Failure

In *hypertrophic hearts,* as in chronic hypertension or severe aortic stenosis (Villari et al., 1995), abnormalities of diastole are common and may precede systolic failure, from which there are a number of important differences. The mechanism is not clear, although it is thought to be related to the fibrosis that accompanies ventricular hypertrophy or indirectly to a stiff left atrium (Mehta et al., 1991). Conceptually, impaired relaxation must be distinguished from prolonged systolic contraction with delayed onset of normal relaxation (Brutsaert et al., 1993). Experimentally, there are several defects in early hypertensive hypertrophy, including decreased rates of contraction and relaxation, as well as

TABLE 12-8. *Systolic and diastolic dysfunction of the myocardium*

	Systolic	Diastolic
Exertional dyspnea	Yes	Yes
Ejection fraction	Low	Normal (or increased in myocardial hypertrophy)
Mechanical parameter on pressure-volume loop	Impaired inotropic state	Impaired lusitropic state
PV[a] relationship	End-systolic PV altered	End-diastolic PV altered
Relaxation indices	Abnormal	Abnormal
$(-)dP/dt_{max}$	Abnormal	Abnormal
Rapid filling phase	Abnormal	Abnormal
Atrial booster function	Responds to the associated diastolic failure	Increased early in course of development of failure; A-to-E ratio increased[b]

[a]PV, pressure-volume (Fig. 12-15).
[b]A-to-E ratio (Fig. 12-23).

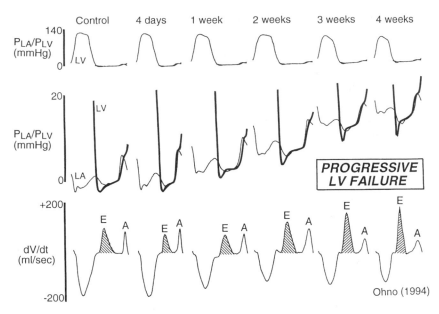

FIG. 12-23. Diastolic filling during progressive heart failure. Analog record of P_{LA} and P_{LV} and the time derivative of left ventricular volume (dV/dt) indicate the filling pattern. Peak filling rate occurring early in diastole is indicated (E) and during late diastole after atrial contraction (A). Time for early filling deceleration (t_{dec}) is also indicated. For A wave, see Fig. 12-1. Modified from Ohno et al. (1994) with permission of authors and American Heart Association.

decreased peak force development (Corey et al., 1994). Loss of the load-sensitive component of relaxation may be due to impaired activity of the sarcoplasmic reticulum. Impaired relaxation is associated with an increase of the late (atrial) filling phase, so that the E/A ratio on the mitral Doppler pattern declines (Fig. 12-23). In time, with both increased hypertrophy and the development of fibrosis, LV chamber compliance decreases and the E wave again becomes more prominent. Thus, it becomes difficult to separate truly normal from *pseudonormal patterns of mitral inflow.*

In *myocardial failure,* multiple abnormalities can be detected in the transmitral flow pattern, including an early change in the E/A ratio (Fig. 12-23). It must be stressed that the E/A ratio changes considerably as the LV failure progressively becomes more severe with late-phase pseudonormalization (Fig. 12-23). Currently, much emphasis is placed on new Doppler echocardiography methods to assess diastolic dysfunction more accurately (Yamamoto et al., 1996).

COMPLIANCE

The diastolic volume of the heart is influenced not only by the loading conditions but by the elastic properties of the myocardium. *Elasticity* means that the myocardium recovers its normal shape after removal of the systolic stress. Compliance is strictly defined as the relationship between the change in stress and the resultant *strain* (percentage change in dimension or size). In clinical practice, it is taken as the ratio of dP/dV, that is, the rate of pressure change divided by the rate of volume change. The relationship is curvilinear, and the initial slope of the change is gentle. As the pressure increases, the volume increases less and less so that there is a considerable increase of pressure for only a small increase of volume (Fig. 12-24).

The term *diastolic distensibility* has been used in preference to the more traditional compliance because distensibility refers not to the slope of the pressure–volume relationship but to the diastolic pressure required to fill the ventricle to the same volume. Thus, when compliance decreases, the distensibility is less (Wyman et al., 1989), as in the failing human heart (Fig. 12-25).

Whereas resting skeletal muscle is truly in a state of relaxation (so that the resting tension is close to zero), the heart has a very high resting tension. Resting *stiffness* may be attributed in part to the unique myocardial collagen network, thought to counter the high systolic pressure normally developed in the ventricles. Pathologic loss of compliance is usually due to abnormalities of the myocardium. For example, in *myocardial hypertrophy,* a greater pressure increase is required to achieve any given volume increase (the thicker the wall, the more intraluminal pressure is needed to make it stretch). When corrected for the increased mass, however, the muscular compliance in myocardial hypertrophy is close to normal. One approach to the problem of measuring true compli-

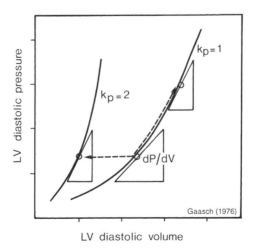

LV diastolic volume

FIG. 12-24. Left ventricular compliance. The compliance reflects the relationship between the increase in heart volume for a given increase in pressure (dP/dV). On the left, the compliance is decreased because the modulus of chamber stiffness (K_p) is increased. Such a true increase of stiffness can occur in acute myocardial infarction. (From Gaasch et al. *Am J Cardiol* 1976;38: 645, with permission.)

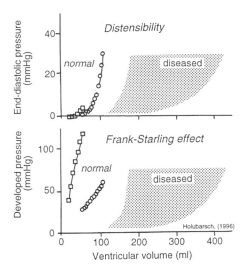

FIG. 12-25. Failing human heart. Poor response to increased ventricular volume in both (1) end-diastolic pressure and (2) developed pressure (systolic-diastolic pressure). Therefore, there is both decreased distensibility and a decreased Frank-Starling response. For original data see Holubarsch et al. (1996). Modified with permission of authors and American Heart Association.

ance in hypertrophy is to plot LV stress against volume so that there is a built-in compensation for the increased wall thickness.

A true loss of muscular compliance occurs from a variety of causes: acute ischemia as in angina, fibrosis as after myocardial infarction, and infiltrations causing a restrictive cardiomyopathy. In angina, the increased temporary stiffness probably is caused by a combination of an increase of intracellular calcium and of altered myocardial properties. In myocardial infarction, the connective tissue undergoes changes after 40 minutes of occlusion. Eventually, healing and fibrosis permanently increase stiffness. When muscle stiffness increases, so does *chamber stiffness* (the chamber referred to is the ventricle). When the functioning of the chambers is indirectly impaired by constrictive pericarditis, a hemodynamic situation similar to restrictive cardiomyopathy may arise. Because the basic problem is extracardiac, the decrease of compliance is more apparent than real. Nonetheless, extracardiac mechanical factors, such as those exerted by the pericardium and the lungs on the heart, also help determine the diastolic pressure–volume relationship (Gilbert and Glantz, 1989).

The compliance of the heart influences both the Starling curve and the pressure–volume loop, as well as the early diastolic filling rate of the heart. A stiffer heart will be on a lower Starling curve, and the baseline of the pressure–volume loop will increase upward more steeply, so that a higher left atrial pressure will be required for early diastolic filling. For these reasons, compliance is a fundamental mechanical property of the heart.

VENTRICULAR INTERACTION

Thus far, LV function has been discussed as if the left ventricle were working in isolation. In reality, its function is intimately linked to that of the right ventricle, both functionally and anatomically. The cardiac output of the left ventricle must equal that of the right ventricle unless there is a state of imbalance, as in conditions of acute LV failure when blood may accumulate in the lungs to cause pulmonary edema. In general, the right ventricle is working against a low resistance circuit, and afterload is not a major problem in physiologic conditions. What the right ventricle receives by means of its filling pressure in the venous system, it will empty in response to the Starling effect. The amount of pressure work generated by the right ventricle is relatively low, which explains the thinner right ventricular wall and the dominance of LV function in calculations of pressure work or of myocardial oxygen uptake.

Anatomically, the two ventricles are interlinked. They share a common septum. That septum constitutes part of the load against which each ventricle must work. In LV hypertrophy, which includes the septum, the right ventricle must therefore work harder and tends to become hypertrophied. This is *systolic ventricular interaction.* One type of diastolic ventricular interaction is the *Bernheim effect,* whereby a large left ventricle can compress the right ventricle, the volume on the left side being so great that the right side is unable to fill properly. A converse ventricular interaction can occur in severe heart failure, when the dilated right ventricle may impinge on the left. When the right ventricle is unloaded by the venodilator agent nitroglycerin, it can decrease in size and allow the LV function to improve.

When there is a physical impairment of the mechanical function of one ventricle on the other as a result of volume overloading with blood, the result is *diastolic ventricular interference.*

PERICARDIUM AND ENDOCARDIUM

The normal *pericardium* has an important restraining effect on the diastolic properties of the ventricles, especially the right ventricle. Without the pericardium, the right ventricle would dilate by about 40% and the right atrium by about 70%. Therefore, the physical properties of the pericardium help to determine ventricular pressure–volume relationships and, indirectly, the compliance. Normally LV diastolic pressure is greater than that in the other chambers by the amount of its transmural pressure (5 to 10 mmHg), the low pericardial pressure being equally applied to all chambers. During pericardial disease with cardiac tamponade, the pressure within the pericardial cavity increases as the volume increases, especially with a volume above 200 ml, so that the intrapericardial pressure equals or exceeds the normal diastolic filling pressure. When this happens, diastole is severely impaired.

Regarding the *endocardium,* the vascular and endocardial endothelium constitute "one continuous sheet of tissue" (Li et al., 1993). A current proposal is that there is intracavity autoregulation by endocardial endothelial cells. It has been proposed that release of an endothelinlike agent, endocardin, from the stretched endocardium could increase the duration of contraction (Brutsaert and Andries, 1992). Thereby, the dilated failing left ventricle could generate an autoregulating inotropic stimulus. Yet there is thought to be a defect in the endocardial endothelium in heart failure, causing, for example, a decreased response to α_1-adrenergic inotropic stimulation (Li et al., 1993). What is thus far not explained is how, if the properties of endocardin resemble those of endothelin, a preferential positive inotropic effect rather than vasoconstriction could be achieved. Presumably endocardin preferentially stimulates the adjacent papillary muscle cells of the endocardium.

CONTRACTILE PROPERTIES IN HUMAN HEART DISEASE

The *failing human myocardium* has impaired contractile properties so that even when the venous filling pressure is adequate, the stroke volume is reduced when compared with normal, and the blood pressure tends to decrease. An increased heart rate provides some compensation to help maintain the cardiac output and, thereby, the blood pressure. Nonetheless, the *treppe* effect is lost (Fig. 12-12), and internal work is increased relative to external work (Fig. 12-18). Homeostatic mechanisms that come into play sustain the blood pressure (see Chapter 16), but the severely failing myocardium does this at the cost of decreased efficiency of work (Asanoi et al., 1996). Other defects include an impaired response to an increased preload (Fig. 12-25), defective generation of cAMP in response to β-adrenergic stimulation, and numerous defects of the patterns of handling of intracellular calcium (see Chapter 16). In response to an increased afterload, the intracellular calcium transient of trabecular myocardium from the severely failing human heart shows an abnormally prolonged and exaggerated pattern of increase, despite poor generation of force (Vahl et al., 1994). It is controversial whether there is truly a defective Frank-Starling response, as claimed by Schwinger et al. (1994) or whether apparent defects can be explained by the decreased distensibility, as claimed by Holubarsch et al. (1996). According to the latter point of view, there still is a Starling response, so that the LV filling pressure of patients with severe heart failure could be therapeutically set to be high enough to achieve an optimal Starling effect without being too high and causing pulmonary edema. For other methods of enhancing cardiac performance, see Table 12-9.

In *aortic valve disease,* the increased volume load of aortic regurgitation contrasts with the pressure load of aortic stenosis. In aortic stenosis, kinetic work increases sharply as the cross-sectional area narrows, whereas pressure work increases as the gradient across the aortic valve increases. Therefore, the myocardial oxygen demand is increased by both types of work in aortic stenosis. In aortic regurgitation, heart work and oxygen demand is increased by the

TABLE 12-9. *Stimuli to enhanced cardiac performance*

Stimulus	Physiologic mechanism
1. *Rate-dependent effects*	
Treppe phenomenon	Sodium pump lag; calcium entry exceeds rate of exit
2. *Load-dependency*	
Preload increase	Length-dependent sensitization of contractile proteins to calcium
Afterload reduction	Failing myocardium is afterload dependent
3. *Receptor stimulation*	
β-adrenergic (or similar drugs)	Positive inotropic and lusitropic effects; increased calcium entry; increased calcium-induced calcium release; increased uptake of calcium into SR
α-adrenergic	Inconsistent effects on contraction
Angiotensin II	Variable positive inotropic
Endothelin	Positive inotropic (marked vascular effects)
4. *Sodium pump inhibition*	
Digoxin	Increased sodium-calcium exchange
5. *Calcium sensitizers*	
Levosimendan, others	Increased calcium sensitivity of troponin-C?

increased wall stress resulting from the greater ventricular volume (see Chapter 16) and by an increased afterload. The latter results from (1) associated systolic hypertension after the ejection of an increased stroke volume into the arterial tree, and (2) increased wall stress from the volume load.

SUMMARY

1. *The cardiac cycle.* Left ventricular (LV) contraction shuts the mitral valve so that the blood inside the LV cavity is trapped for the duration of the isovolumic contraction phase, until the aortic valve is forced open, so that blood shoots out during the phase of maximal ejection. LV relaxation follows. It results first in the phase of reduced ejection and then, after the aortic valve has closed, in isovolumic relaxation, until the pressure in the left ventricle decreases below that in the left atrium, which opens the mitral valve. Rapid LV diastolic filling is followed by a slow phase (diastasis) before the atrial booster contraction, whereupon the heart is ready to re-enter a new cycle.

2. *Preload and afterload.* The preload is the load on the ventricle before contraction starts, at the end of diastole. The afterload is that against which the left ventricle contracts.

3. *Effect of load on myocardial performance.* When either preload or afterload increases acutely, so does ventricular performance. There are two major mechanisms. First, an increased preload increases ventricular filling and the end-diastolic fiber length to enhance performance (Starling's law) by the process of length-dependent activation. If the afterload is increased, the proposed mechanism may be by activation of stretch receptors.

4. *Contractility or inotropic state.* This concept relates to changes in performance independently of the load, either because the cytosolic calcium level

has increased (e.g., during β-adrenergic stimulation), or the myofibrils have become sensitized to calcium (e.g., in response to a calcium-sensitizing drug). In clinical practice, it is not easy to measure the inotropic state. Inaccurate but practical load-dependent indices include the fractional shortening and the ejection fraction measured echocardiographically. Load-independent indices include end-systolic wall stress, much more difficult to measure, and invasive measurement of pressure–volume loops.

5. *Pressure–volume loops.* The inotropic state (contractility) is reflected in the end-systolic pressure–volume relationship, which moves leftward and upward during inotropic stimulation. On the other hand, the end-diastolic volume–pressure relationship is an index of the compliance of the myocardium, which decreases in chronic congestive heart failure.

6. *Diastolic dysfunction.* Whereas decreased contractility is a classic feature of myocardial systolic failure, changes in the lusitropic state (ability to relax) are at least equally important and often occur in LV hypertrophy before systolic abnormalities.

STUDENT QUESTIONS

1. Starling's law relates an increased diastolic fiber length to an increased force of contraction. How is this observation explained at a cellular level?
2. What role do calcium ions play in the regulation of cardiac contractility (inotropic state)?
3. Describe in detail the complete signal systems involved in the positive inotropic effect of β-adrenergic stimulation.
4. Distinguish between preload and afterload. Describe the effects of each on left ventricular performance.
5. Give the major factors that increase myocardial oxygen demand, and provide an example of how each operates.

CARDIOLOGIST-IN-TRAINING QUESTIONS

1. What is myocardial wall stress? Can it explain preload and afterload? How does it influence the myocardial oxygen demand?
2. Diastolic filling of the ventricles: describe the phases and diastolic dysfunction.
3. Is it really possible to distinguish between the effects of load independently from changes in contractility? List reasons for your answer.
4. Which classes of drugs increase myocardial cAMP levels, and what are the expected effects on myocardial performance? What is the role of calcium in these responses?
5. What is a positive lusitropic effect? Give the cellular mechanism and signal systems involved when this effect is obtained by adrenergic stimulation.

6. Heart failure. Describe the contractile abnormalities (both at the cellular and at the organ level) in early and in advanced heart failure.

REFERENCES

1. Asanoi H, Kameyama T, Ishizaka S, et al. Energetically optimal left ventricular pressure for the failing human heart. *Circulation* 1996;93:67–73.
2. Backx PH, ter Keurs HE. Fluorescent properties of rat cardiac trabeculae microinjected with fura-2 salt. *Am J Physiol* 1993;264:H1098–H1110.
3. Belz GG. Elastic properties and Windkessel function of the human aorta. *Cardiovasc Drug Ther* 1995;9:73–83.
4. Borow KM. Clinical assessment of contractility in the symmetrically contracting left ventricle: Part 1. *Modern Concepts Cardiovasc Dis* 1988;57:29–34.
5. Braunwald E, Ross Jr J, Sonnenblick EH. In: *Mechanisms of Contraction in the Normal and Failing Heart.* Boston: Little, Brown & Co, 1968.
6. Brutsaert DL, Andries LJ. The endocardial endothelium. *Am J Physiol* 1992;263:H985–H1002.
7. Brutsaert DL, Sys SU, Sillebert TC. Diastolic failure: Pathophysiology and therapeutic implications. *J Am Coll Cardiol* 1993;22:318–325.
8. Campbell KB, Kirkpatrick RD, Tobias AH. Series coupled non-contractile elements are functionally unimportant in the isolated heart. *Cardiovasc Res* 1994;28:242–251.
9. Carabello BA. Aortic regurgitation in women. Does the measuring stick need a change. *Circulation* 1996;94:2355–2357.
10. Chen C, Rodiguez L, Levine RA. Non-invasive measurement of the time constant of left ventricular relaxation using the continuous-wave Doppler velocity profile of mitral regurgitation. *Circulation* 1992;86:272–278.
11. Chen C, Rodriguez MD, Guerrero JL, et al. Noninvasive estimation of the instantaneous first derivative of left ventricular pressure using continuous-wave Doppler echocardiography. *Circulation* 1991;83:2101–2110.
12. Cory CR, Grange RW, Houston ME. Role of sarcoplasmic reticulum in loss of load-sensitive relaxation in pressure overload cardiac hypertrophy. *Am J Physiol* 1994;266:H68–H78.
13. Douglas PA, Berko B, Lesh M, Reichek N. Alterations in diastolic function in response to progressive left ventricular hypertrophy. *J Am Coll Cardiol* 1989;13:461–467.
14. Eichhorn EJ, Willard JE, Alvarez L. Are contraction and relaxation coupled in patients with and without congestive heart failure. *Circulation* 1992;85:2132–2139.
15. Frank O. Zur dynamik des Herzmuskels. *Z Biol* 1895;32:370–447.
16. Fuchs F. Mechanical modulation of the Ca^{2+} regulatory protein complex in cardiac muscle. *NIPS* 1995;10:6–12.
17. Gibbs CL. Cardiac energetics. In: Langer GA, Brady AJ (eds). *The Mammalian Myocardium.* New York: Wiley, 1974;105–133.
18. Gilbert JC, Glantz SA. Determinants of left ventricular filling and of the diastolic pressure-volume relation. *Circ Res* 1989;64:827–852.
19. Hirschfeld S, Meyer R, Korfhagen J. The isovolumic contraction time of the left ventricle. An echographic study. *Circulation* 1976;54:751–756.
20. Hoit BD, Shao Y, Gabel M, Walsh RA. In vivo assessment of left atrial contractile performance in normal and pathological conditions using a time-varying elastance model. *Circulation* 1994;89: 1829–1838.
21. Holubarsch C, Hasenfuss G, Schmidt-Schweda S, et al. Angiotensin I and II exert inotropic effects in atrial but not in ventricular human myocardium. An in vitro study under physiological experimental conditions. *Circulation* 1993;88:1228–1237.
22. Holubarsch C, Ruf T, Goldstein DJ, et al. Existence of the Frank-Starling mechanism in the failing human heart. Investigations on the organ, tissue and sarcomere levels. *Circulation* 1996;94:683–689.
23. Hori M, Kitakaze M, Ishida Y, et al. Delayed and ejection increases isovolumic ventricular relaxation rate in isolated perfused canine hearts. *Circ Res* 1991;68:300–308.
24. Kannengiesser GJ, Opie LH, Van der Werff T. Impaired cardiac work and oxygen uptake after reperfusion of regionally ischemic myocardium. *J Mol Cell Cardiol* 1979;11:197–207.
25. Koumi S, Arentzen C, Backer C, Wasserstrom A. Alterations in muscarinic K^+ channel response to

acetylcholine and to G protein-mediated activation in atrial myocytes isolated from failing human hearts. *Circulation* 1994;90:2213–2224.

26. Laniado S, Yellin EL, Miller H, Frater RW. Temporal relation of the first heart sound to closure of the mitral valve. *Circulation* 1973;47:1006–1014.

27. Legault SE, Freeman MR, Langer A, Armstrong PW. Pathophysiology and time course of silent myocardial ischaemia during mental stress: clinical, anatomical and physiological correlates. *Br Heart J* 1995;73:242–249.

28. Leite-Moreira AF, Gillebert TC. Non-uniform course of left ventricular pressure fall and its regulation by load and contractile state. *Circulation* 1994;90:2481–2491.

29. Li K, Rouleau JL, Calderone A, et al. Endocardial function in pacing-induced heart failure in the dog. *J Mol Cell Cardiol* 1993;25:529–540.

30. Maier SE, Fischer SE, McKinnon GC, et al. Evaluation of left ventricular segmental wall motion in hypertrophic cardiomyopathy with myocardial tagging. *Circulation* 1992;86:1919–1928.

31. McDonald KS, Mammen PPA, Strang KT, et al. Isometric and dynamic contractile properties of porcine skinned cardiac myocytes after stunning. *Circ Res* 1995;77:964–972.

32. Mehta S, Charbonneau F, Fitchett DH. The clinical consequences of a stiff left atrium. *Am Heart J* 1991;122:1184–1191.

33. Morgan JP, Morgan KG. Intracellular calcium and cardiovascular function in heart failure: effects of pharmacologic agents. *Cardiovasc Drug Ther* 1989;3:959–970.

34. Mulieri LA, Leavitt BJ, Martin BJ, et al. Myocardial force-frequency defect in mitral regurgitation heart failure is reversed by forskolin. *Circulation* 1993;88:2700–2704.

35. Ohno M, Cheng CP, Little WC. Mechanism of altered patterns of left ventricular filling during the development of congestive heart failure. *Circulation* 1994;89:2241–2250.

36. Parisi AF, Milton BG. Relation of mitral valve closure to the first heart sound in man. Echocardiographic and phonocardiographic assessment. *Am J Cardiol* 1973;32:779–782.

37. Quinones MA, Gaasch WH, Alexander KJ. Influence of acute changes in preload, afterload, contractile state and heart rate on ejection and isovolumic indices of myocardial contractility in man. *Circulation* 1976;53:293–302.

38. Rodriguez EK, Hunter WC, Royce MJ, et al. A method to reconstruct myocardial sarcomere lengths and orientations at transmural sites in beating canine hearts. *Am J Physiol* 1992;263:H293–H306.

39. Schiller NB, Foster E. Analysis of left ventricular systolic function. *Heart* 1996;75(suppl 2):17–26.

40. Schlant RC, Sonnenblick EH. Normal physiology of the cardiovascular system. In: Schlant RC, Alexander RW (eds). *The Heart.* New York: McGraw-Hill, 1994;113–151.

41. Schneider J, Berger HJ, Sands MJ, et al. Beat-to-beat ventricular performance in atrial fibrillation: radionuclide assessment with the computerized nuclear probe. *Am J Cardiol* 1983;51:1189–1195.

42. Schwinger R, Bohm M, Koch A, et al. The failing human heart is unable to use the Frank-Starling mechanism. *Circ Res* 1994;74:959–969.

43. Sweitzer NK, Moss RL. Determinants of loaded shortening velocity in single cardiac myocytes permeabilized with α-hemolysin. *Circ Res* 1993;73:1150–1162.

44. Starling EH. In: *The Linacre Lecture on the Law of the Heart.* London: Longmans, Green and Co, 1918.

45. Strang KT, Sweitzer NK, Greaser ML, Moss RL. β-adrenergic receptor stimulation increases unloaded shortening velocity of skinned single ventricular myocytes from rats. *Circ Res* 1994;74:542–549.

46. Suga H, Hisano R, Hirata S, et al. Mechanism of higher oxygen consumption rate: pressure-loaded vs volume-loaded heart. *Am J Physiol* 1982;242:H942–H948.

47. Udelson JE, Bacharach SL, Canon RO, Bonow RO. Minimum left ventricular pressure during beta-adrenergic stimulation in human subjects. *Circulation* 1990;82:1174–1182.

48. Vahl CF, Bonz A, Timek T, Hagl S. Intracellular calcium transient of working human myocardium of seven patients transplanted for congestive heart failure. *Circ Res* 1994;74:952–958.

49. Villari B, Vassalli G, Monrad ES, et al. Normalization of diastolic dysfunction in aortic stenosis late after valve replacement. *Circulation* 1995;91:2353–2358.

50. Wiggers CJ. In: *Modern Aspects of Circulation in Health and Disease.* Philadelphia: Lea & Febiger, 1915.

51. Wyman RM, Farhi ER, Bing OHL, et al. Comparative effect of hypoxia and ischemia in the isolated, blood-perfused dog heart: evaluation of left ventricular diastolic chamber distensibility and wall thickness. *Circ Res* 1989;64:121–128.

52. Yamamoto K, Masuyama T, Doi Y, et al. Non-invasive assessment of left ventricular relaxation using

continuous wave Doppler aortic regurgitant velocity curve. Its comparative value to the mitral regurgitation method. *Circulation* 1995;91:192–200.

53. Yamamoto K, Redfield M, Nishimura R. Analysis of left ventricular diastolic function. *Heart* 1996;75(suppl 2):27–35.

54. Zhang R, Zhao J, Mandveno A, Potter JD. Cardiac troponin I phosphorylation increases the rate of cardiac muscle relaxation. *Circ Res* 1995;76:1028–1035.

13

Overload Hypertrophy and Its Molecular Biology

When an excessive workload on the heart is sustained, ventricular myocytes grow in response to a complex series of events. A mechanical event, the hemodynamic load, must be translated into the biochemical signal for growth. Hypertrophy is the process whereby each cell becomes larger (Fig. 13-1) as opposed to what happens when there are more cells (hyperplasia). Once hypertrophied, the initially excessive mechanical stress on the myocardium is corrected toward normal by operation of the Laplace law, whereby an increased wall thickness decreases wall stress (see Chapter 16). Nonetheless, the overall properties of the hypertrophied myocardium are by no means normal and, in particular, diastolic function seems impaired as a relatively early event. When the increased mechanical load is prolonged or exceeds a certain limit, it seems that the myocardial cells also can undergo hyperplasia. In contrast, nonmyocardial cells of the heart, such as those of the coronary vascular tree and interstitial space, undergo both hypertrophy and hyperplasia even as an early response to overload (Fig. 13-1).

Hypertrophy also sets in motion a complex reprogramming of cardiac gene expression, with the emergence of a more fetal phenotype.

PHASES OF PRESSURE-INDUCED HYPERTROPHY

The adjustment of cardiac mass to hemodynamic load is a fundamental characteristic of the heart. Any sustained increase in the hemodynamic function due either to physiologic activity or to pathologic alterations in the cardiovascular system eventually leads to changes in the heart/body weight ratio.

A pressure load causes the myocyte to become greater chiefly in volume but not in length. The mitochondria increase in number but decrease in relation to the overall cell volume, and the capillary network may be inadequate. A volume load, in contrast, causes the myocyte to elongate (Fig. 13-2) but retains the same ratio of mitochondrial volume to the cell. Why pressure and volume load should

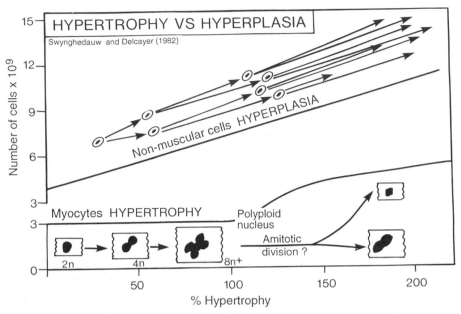

FIG. 13-1. Cell growth in cardiac overload in humans. As hypertrophy occurs, polypoid nuclei become more common and may undergo amitotic division. Evidence for an increased number of myocytes in the human heart at a certain critical level is based on the results of Astorri et al. (1977) and Linzbach (1952). Note that nonmuscular cells undergo mitotic division over the whole range of growth. (From Swynghedauw and Delcayre. *Pathobiol Ann* 1982; 12:137–183).

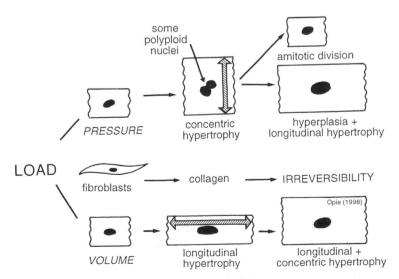

FIG. 13-2. Pressure versus volume load. Note initial differences in response to pressure and volume load. However, end results are similar due to compensatory mechanisms.

have different effects on the cell shape is not known. Teleologically, however, during pressure overload, an increased cell thickness is required to decrease the wall stress (see Chapter 16). During a volume load, longitudinal hypertrophy combines with slippage between myocytes to thin the walls to allow a greater cavity size, thereby increasing the compliance and decreasing the wall stress (see Chapter 16).

Meerson (1983) divided the development of hypertrophy into three stages:

Phase I: *Developing hypertrophy,* a period when the workload exceeds the work output that is normal for the initial mass of the heart.

Phase II: *Compensatory hypertrophy,* a period when the work-induced growth of the heart compensates for the increased workload/cardiac mass ratio. Although gross mechanical function is often apparently normal, more subtle tests show a decreased rate of shortening velocity, delayed relaxation, and a diminished coronary vascular reserve.

Phase III: *Heart failure,* a period when the work output per unit of cardiac mass decreases again due to the progressively decreasing ability of the heart to fill normally and to generate force.

The duration of these three stages, as well as the progression from one to the next, depends on several variables, of which magnitude and type of overload are the most important. Generally, acute pressure overload results in the earliest onset and the fastest rate of compensatory growth and molecular adaptation to the new hemodynamic situation.

Left Ventricular Hypertrophy

Left ventricular hypertrophy (LVH) needs to be distinguished from an increase in LV wall thickness (Fig. 13-3). LVH means an increase in the LV mass related to the body surface area, which is the LV mass index, with an arbitrary upper limit of 125 g/m^2. If the LV wall thickens without any increase in the LV mass index, then there is *concentric remodeling,* a process not well understood but possibly the result of adaptation to a mild pressure load. When both thickness and mass increase, there is *concentric hypertrophy,* the result of a sustained pressure load. When LV volume increases without an increase in wall thickness, there is eccentric hypertrophy, the result of a sustained volume load. In chronic hypertension, there may be mixed features. For example, *eccentric hypertrophy* may be accompanied by a thicker wall, presumably the result of both a pressure and volume load, as in hypertensive heart failure.

MOLECULAR BASIS OF CARDIAC HYPERTROPHY

Hyperplasia is the increase in the number of cells by means of nuclear division and is the principal feature of cardiac growth during the fetal and neonatal periods and also occurs in vascular cells (Fig. 13-1). As development progresses,

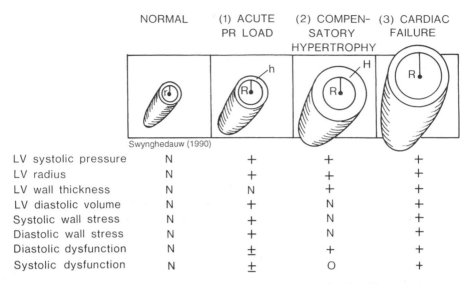

	NORMAL	(1) ACUTE PR LOAD	(2) COMPEN-SATORY HYPERTROPHY	(3) CARDIAC FAILURE
LV systolic pressure	N	+	+	+
LV radius	N	+	+	+
LV wall thickness	N	N	+	+
LV diastolic volume	N	+	N	+
Systolic wall stress	N	+	N	+
Diastolic wall stress	N	+	N	+
Diastolic dysfunction	N	±	+	+
Systolic dysfunction	N	±	O	+

FIG. 13-3. Meerson's three stages, as modified for clinical application. The acute hemodynamic load (stage 1) calls forth protein synthesis and compensated hypertrophy (stage II) before failure develops (stage III). This figure shows Laplace's law (see Fig. 13-15) and wall stress as factors determining modifications of genomic expression. The modifications induced on wall stress by an acute pressure overload are corrected by the development of hypertrophy. N, normal; +, increased. Adapted from Swynghedauw et al. (1990).

particularly during the late gestation period, the number of dividing cells rapidly decreases, and an increase in size of existing myocytes becomes the mode of cardiac enlargement. During the first 3 to 4 weeks of life, the number of cardiac myocytes in the heart doubles. Thereafter, the normal growth of the heart is accomplished solely by the enlargement of existing cells, so that the diameter of myocytes increases from about 5 μm at birth to 12 to 17 μm in the adult heart. Interestingly, ventricular myocytes of various mammals appear to have the same diameter irrespective of animal size. The number of muscle cells thus varies directly with the size of the heart. A blue whale has about 10^6 more cells than a rat heart. Cell death, previously thought to be rare in the healthy heart, occurs increasingly with age, although it remains true that most myocytes have the same life span as the entire organism.

Outline of Protein Synthesis

The response of the protein synthetic machinery to a change in the myocardial workload is dramatic (Weber et al., 1987). Within 2 hours or even earlier, there is an increase in RNA and overall protein synthesis in the isolated heart, with a similar increase within 24 hours in the intact heart, which peaks at 2 days. To understand this response to a workload requires the application of molecular biology. During the development of hypertrophy, hemodynamic stimuli are thought to evoke growth signals that can promote protein synthesis at several different levels, including the formation of growth factors, the stimulation of the activity of growth factor receptors, increased activity of intracellular effectors, such as protein kinases, and enhanced activity of transcription factors. Proto-oncogenes, to be discussed later, promote several steps of these processes.

Only a brief review of the overall process of protein synthesis is given here (Fig. 13-4). The two major nucleic acids are DNA (deoxyribonucleic acid) and RNA (ribonucleic acid). DNA molecules with their double-helical structure are the master file of genetic information. RNA is newly synthesized on part of the DNA molecule by the process of *transcription.* The molecular structure of the corresponding part of DNA is copied or transcribed onto premessenger RNA. These premessenger RNAs contain both sequences that correspond to the DNA

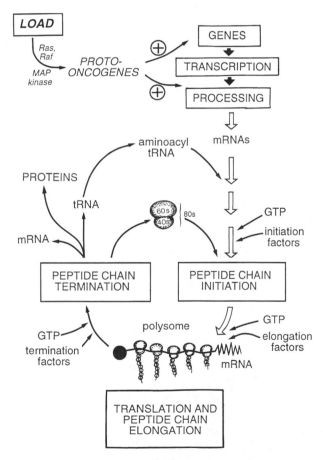

FIG. 13-4. Protein synthesis. Proposed sites of action of mechanical overload. Adapted from Morgan et al. (1979). +, stimulatory sites; −, inhibitory sites.

code (exons) and noncoding stretches of varying lengths (including introns) that will be lost at the stage of formation of messenger RNA (mRNA) processing. The enzymes catalyzing the synthesis of RNA from DNA are called *RNA polymerases* and initiate gene expression by binding to the promoter region of each gene. This binding can be regulated by various factors, including some hormone receptors, which interrelate with the *enhancer* part of the gene. Molecules of mRNA carry the genetic signals to *ribosomes,* which are particles composed of many different molecules of proteins, including some enzymes. Groups of ribosomes are known as *polysomes* (Fig. 13-4). The mRNA merely instructs the ribosome how to make the peptide bonds required for protein synthesis, the peptides having been transported to the ribosomes by transfer RNA (*tRNA*). To get the process of protein synthesis on the go in the ribosomes requires *initiation factors,* themselves proteins. *Elongation factors* help the chain to grow. At the ribosome, the mRNA translates the genetic message to the growing peptide chains. *Posttranslational events* include the assembly and storage of the newly made proteins. Thus, the hemodynamic load, a physical stimulus, has undergone *transduction* to a biochemical signal that has enhanced the rate of gene expression and protein synthesis, resulting in hypertrophy.

DNA and Cardiac Enlargement.   The capacity to synthesize DNA and hence make new myocytes is not completely lost, even in the adult. In some species, notably primates (including humans), DNA can replicate so that myocytes may contain more than two sets of chromosomes (*polyploid nuclei*), without necessarily being associated with cell division. Compensatory growth is accompanied by a marked shift to nuclei with a high degree of ploidy (Adler, 1976). Linzbach (1952) proposed that cardiac enlargement above a certain critical size could be supplemented by the addition of new cells, involving the splitting of polyploid nuclei. That stage is reached when the heart has about doubled its weight to reach 500 g, and the LV free wall weight is about 250 g (Astorri et al., 1977). At about that weight, the cell diameter reaches a peak and then declines because of myocyte division. Cell length, on the other hand, keeps on increasing. Thus, in extremely large hearts, there is both hyperplasia and hypertrophy.

RNA Transcription in Hypertrophy.   When the heart responds to a hemodynamic overload through an acute increase in protein synthesis, there are increases in RNA transcription, in nuclear export, in the proportion of actively translating heart ribosomes, and a decrease in the relative rate of protein degradation (Fig. 13-4). An important question is whether there are specific new mRNAs invoked by the hypertrophy process or whether there is simply an amplification of the existing mechanisms. The latter is by far the major event in rats with hypertrophy caused by aortic stenosis (Boheler and Dillmann, 1988). In other words, part of the basic response during hypertrophy consists of an increased rate of turnover of the existing mechanisms. In addition, however, fetal phenotypes emerge.

SIGNALING IN HYPERTROPHY

The size of the heart is closely and effectively matched to changes in the hemodynamic requirements of an individual. Functional demands—ultimately reflected in the activity of myosin crossbridges—must provide some kind of growth-regulating signal. Despite numerous hypotheses, however, the exact link between hemodynamic function and cardiac growth remains elusive. At least three types of signal systems appear to be involved (Fig. 13-5). First, stretch acts in several complex ways to be of prime importance. Second, there is a group of agonists such as angiotensin II (AII), α_1-catecholamines, and endothelin that act on heptahelical receptors (seven transmembrane spans) to link to protein kinase C (PKC). Third, growth factors such as insulinlike growth factor (IGF) and transforming growth factor (TGF) are linked to receptor tyrosine kinases (RTK) that in turn transmit the signal by phosphorylation of steps further down the line.

Stretch-Activated Signals

The enhanced preload and afterload of the overloaded myocardium results in the stretch of muscle cells. Stretch induces compensatory growth.

Cytoskeletal changes provide part of the response to stretch. The microtubular network of the cell may be involved in linking mechanical stress on the sarcolemma to the formation of new proteins because an increased density of the network follows acute mechanical overload. Two constituent components, *desmin* and *tubulin,* change their spatial orientation (Fig. 13-6) and may link the stretched sarcolemma to the nucleus.

If stretch were the prime signal, protein synthesis should be higher in those parts of the heart with the greater mechanical load. Thus, the turnover of myosin is greater in the hemodynamically loaded left than in the unloaded right ventricle (Samarel, 1989). Additional evidence is that the mRNA for the new myosin isoform (V_3) also is increased in the left but not in right ventricle of pressure-overloaded hearts (Imamura et al., 1990).

An increased tension can be separated from increased stretch by varying the tension in isometric conditions (Peterson and Lesch, 1972). The distinction between tension and stretch could be important. Stretch may be the prime signal to elongation of the fibers in volume overload, whereas tension could be the signal in pressure overload (Fig. 13-2).

Stretch-Activated Ion Channels. Such observations can be explained by the existence of a *stretch-activated ion channel,* an example of a mechanoreceptor. Thereafter, multiple further signals appear to be involved. One proposal is that the stretch channel is linked to PKC via phospholipase C (Crozatier, 1996; von Harsdorf et al., 1989), eventually to stimulate the production of proto-oncogenes (Komuro et al., 1990). Stretch-activated tyrosine kinases may mediate a response

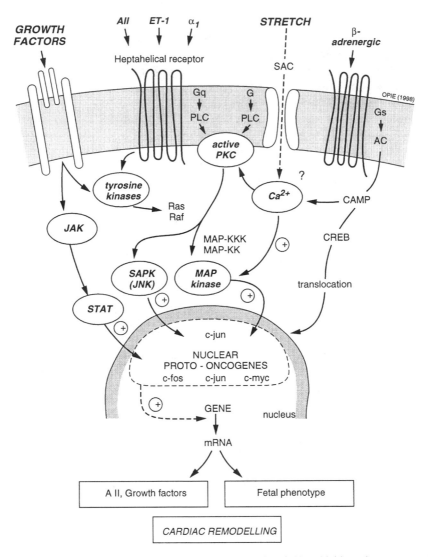

FIG. 13-5. Cell signals in response to hypertrophic stimuli. Note highly active postreceptor cross-talk. For clarity some pathways are omitted, e.g., AII receptor linking to JAK. AII, angiotensin 11; JAK, Janus Kinase (see Berk and Corson, *Circ Res* 1997;80:607); STAT, signal transducers and activators of transcription; JNK, SAPK, where JNK = c-JUN NH$_2$-terminal kinase; SAPK, stress-activated protein kinase (see Kudoh et al., *Circ Res* 1997;80:139); ET-1, endothelin-1; α_I, α_I-adrenergic activity; SAC, stretch activated channel; PLC, phospholipase C; CREB, cyclic AMP response element binding protein (see Goldspink and Russell, *Circ Res* 1994;74:1042); MAP, mitogen-activated protein; MAP kinase is also called ERK, extracellular signal related kinase; MAPKK, MAP kinase kinase, also called MEK, where EK = ERK kinase.

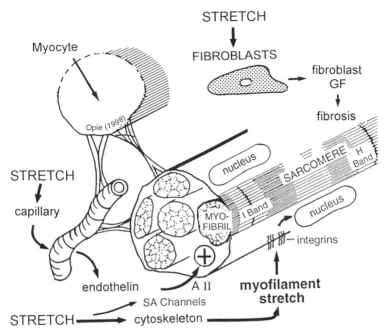

FIG. 13-6. Pressure transduction of nucleus. Schematic representation of connections between the extracellular matrix and the nucleus in the cardiac myocyte. Note proposed role of tubulin and desmin in linking mechanical stress on the sarcolemma to formation of new proteins in the nucleus. SA, stretch activated. Modified from Samuel et al. (1990).

similar to that of IGF (Kijima et al., 1996) (Fig. 13-5). Another proposal is that a deformation-dependent sodium influx is converted into a calcium signal by first promoting sodium–calcium exchange and thereby increasing intracellular calcium, which then governs several key steps in the growth cascade (Fig. 13-5). Additionally, stretch appears directly to promote opening of the L-calcium channels, thereby further increasing internal calcium (Crozatier, 1996).

If an *increased cytosolic calcium* were an important signal to hypertrophy, then calcium could both mediate the early acute inotropic response and play a continued role in the slower process of hypertrophy. Such a proposal would link with a similar concept for vascular smooth muscle (VSM), where a variety of agents, including AII, promote both contraction and hypertrophy (Khairallah and Kanabus, 1983; Geisterfer et al., 1988). Another similarity between the two types of muscle is that stretch may stimulate the synthesis of growth factors both in the myocardium and in vessels (Tomanek, 1990). Calcium also may have a permissive role in the action of AII (Sadoshima and Izumo, 1993).

Release of Angiotensin II. In response to stretch, isolated myocytes liberate AII (Sadoshima et al., 1993). Furthermore, the signaling response to AII is enhanced during stretch so that more IP$_3$ forms (Fig. 13-7). Thus, stretch sensi-

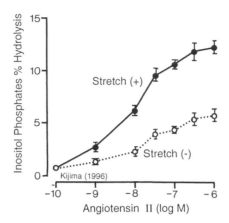

FIG. 13-7. Stretch and angiotensin II. Effects of myocyte stretching on the inositol phosphate response to AII. Cardiac myocytes were stretched for 12 hours. AII-mediated inositol phosphate production was then determined. Each point represents the percentage hydrolysis of ^{3}H-labeled inositol phosphate from the total labeled pool. From Kijima et al. (1996) with permission of the American Heart Association.

tizes the cell to effects of AII (Kijima et al., 1996). "Angiotensin II fulfils the criteria as a critical mediator of the stretch-induced adaptive response in cardiac myocytes" (Sadoshima et al., 1993). The origin of the AII appears to be from a local endogenous renin-angiotensinogen-AII system, which feeds back on the myocardium in an autocrine manner to promote growth. This system is upregulated during cardiac hypertrophy (Kijima et al., 1996).

Stretch and Nonmyocardial Cells. The extracellular AII formed in response to stretch of myocyctes may be expected to act on endothelial and VSM cells to stimulate growth (Fig. 13-8). Endothelin, released from endothelial cells in response both to AII and increased stretch, further promotes the activity of the PKC system in VSM cells, already stimulated by AII and by stretch. Endothelin and AII both release other growth factors, such as *TGF-β* from VSM cells and *fibroblastic growth factor (FGF)* from fibroblasts. All these stimuli promote growth of matrix cells such as fibroblasts, as well as causing myocytes to grow, beyond and in addition to the direct effects of stretch on these cells. Therefore, the ultimate effects of stretch, both direct and indirect, lead to very complex dynamic events in the heart in response to an increased load (Fig. 13-8).

Atrophy as Reverse Stretch. If stretch promotes growth, then disuse should promote atrophy, as it does. In isolated nonbeating myocyctes, there is repression of the growth of myosin heavy chains and the myofibrils are minute in size (Decker et al., 1991). The key factor may be contractile activity, which induces active tension development. Thus, in isolated neonatal myocytes, where stretch

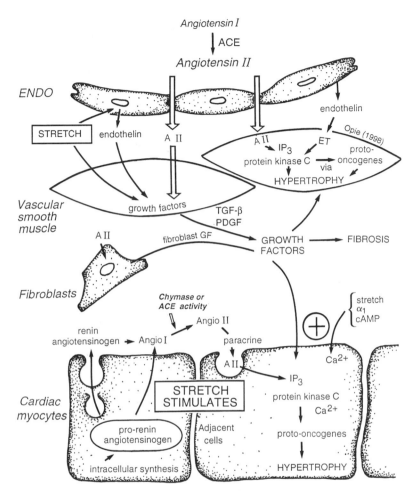

FIG. 13-8. Stretch and cardiac growth. Some proposals for a multicellular interactive renin-angiotensin system involving cardiac myocytes, fibroblasts, VSM and endothelin. Although these systems are postulated to have an important function regulating vascular and myocardial hypertrophy, proof of this significance is still awaited.

and hemodynamic load can be excluded, protein synthesis is higher in contractile than in noncontractile cells (Sharp et al., 1993).

Factors Other Than Stretch and Tension.   There may be growth-inducing factors other than stretch and tension. The evidence is as follows. When the rat heart is subjected to a severe load by thoracic binding, there is increased expression of the mRNAs for two types of protein isoforms: one for myosin (β-myosin heavy chain) and one for actin (α-skeletal actin). Yet only one of these, that of the myosin isoform, follows the distribution of increased wall tension, being found to a greater degree in the subendocardium (Schiaffino et al., 1989), where wall tension is probably higher. Furthermore, when the fetal rat ventricle is transplanted into the anterior eye chamber and there is no hemodynamic workload at all, it is still possible to induce proliferation and differentiation of cells (Bishop et al., 1990). These observations focus on the role of growth-inducing hormones and factors.

Role of Angiotensin II and Protein Kinase C in Growth

Both indirect and direct evidence links PKC to growth. In general, those agonists such as AII, endothelin, and α_1-adrenergic activity that link to PKC via a heptahelical receptor and the G_q protein (Fig. 13-5) are also able to activate proto-oncogenes and to promote growth. The phorbol esters, which activate PKC directly, also promote formation of proto-oncogenes and gene expression (Komuro et al., 1988). Of the three receptor agonists, it is AII that is now attracting most attention because (1) it is released from isolated myocyctes in response to stretch, and then feeds back on the same myocyctes in an autocrine manner (Sadoshima et al., 1993); (2) such release is accompanied by increased activity of MAP kinase (Yamazaki et al., 1995); (3) AII stimulation induces proto-oncogenes within 15 minutes both in cardiac myocytes and nonmyocytes (Kent and McDermott, 1996; Sadoshima et al., 1995); (4) the AII receptor (AT_1) is upgraded in response to stretch in neonatal myocytes and in association with the growth of viable myocytes surviving coronary artery ligation (Meggs et al., 1993); (5) the tissue renin-angiotensin system is upgraded in response to external pressure (Bardy et al., 1996); and (6) AII is also implicated in the growth of fibroblasts (Schorb et al., 1993).

Of the other two agonists interacting with the PKC system, α_1-adrenergic stimulation is discussed in the next section, and endothelin may be most active in the failing heart, when its synthesis is induced in the myocardium (see Chapter 16).

Adrenergic Factors.   Cardiac enlargement can be induced by chronic infusion of norepinephrine in doses that do not lead to hypertension, acting at least in part through α_1-receptor stimulation. In neonatal tissue, such α_1-receptor stimulation appears to play an important role in acting as a growth factor receptor and in regulating RNA transcription (Simpson, 1988). In the adult myocardium the role of α_1-receptors is not clear, although still potentially active (Kawaguchi et al., 1993). Nonetheless, hypertrophy can be induced by a hemodynamic load even in the presence of α-blockade (Cooper et al., 1985). Furthermore, in hypertensive patients with LVH, the pure β-blocker propranolol is more effective in regressing LVH than the combined α-β-blocker, labetalol (Szlachcic et al., 1990).

Protein kinase A may be involved in the component of the adrenergic response that is linked to β- rather than to α-receptors (Fig. 13-5). When an isolated rat heart is subjected to a mechanical overload, even for a short time, there is an increase in the myocardial cyclic adenosine monophosphate (cAMP) level, which can be linked to increased activity of cAMP-dependent protein kinase A, to CREB, and to enhanced rates of protein synthesis (Xenophontos et al., 1989). In some instances, the mechanical load appears to act by direct activation of adenylate cyclase.

Exchangers. Sodium–proton exchange is stimulated by AII and by endothelin, with intracellular alkalinization (Ito et al., 1997). As protons move out, sodium moves in, and sodium-calcium exchange is enhanced so that intracellular calcium can be expected to increase, to promote growth signaling. The mRNA for the sodium–calcium exchanger increases when a load is applied to cardiac myocytes (Kent and McDermott, 1996).

Mitogen-Activated Protein Kinase. This enzyme, mitogen-activated protein (MAP) kinase, is a crucial enzyme in the growth cascade (Force et al., 1996). Upon activation it undergoes translocation to the nucleus, where it stimulates the immediate-early response mediated by proto-oncogenes. Because this kinase is ultimately linked to extracellular growth factors and peptides, it is also called the extracellular signal-related protein kinase (ERK). MAP kinase is only active when phosphorylated in response to another kinase, MAP kinase kinase, also called MEK (MAP/ERK) kinase. This kinase in turn requires yet another kinase, MAP kinase kinase kinase (MAPKKK), also called MEKK, for phosphorylation into activity. Hence, there is a three-kinase cascade (Cobb and Goldsmith, 1995). To limit overactivity of this cascade of phosphorylation, there are the appropriate phosphatases, which are little understood. The major upstream signal to this cascade is Ras-Raf, with probably a variety of other inputs.

Growth Factors and Their Signal Systems

By analogy with the concept of agonists such as AII interacting with their receptors and producing intracellular signals that then act on a specific effector such as PKC, there is another chain of intracellular events in response to soluble molecules called growth factors. This term sometimes includes all the extracellular signals for growth, including those agents such as AII interacting with the PKC system. Nonetheless this term is especially suited for those growth factors that do not link in with PKC, as for example IGF-1, TGF-β, platelet-derived growth factor (PDGF), and FGF. Such growth factors interact with a membrane-associated growth factor receptor, similar to the insulin model, and generally also linked to tyrosine or serine-threonine kinase (see Fig. 11-6). Interaction with such receptors stimulates intracellular transducers, such as tyrosine kinases. The latter, including JAK-STAT (Fig. 13-5), in turn phosphorylate a variety of intracellular proteins, thereby activating proto-oncogenes and various nuclear growth factors. The latter include the transcription factors that bind to DNA and regulate the rate of RNA transcription (Fig. 13-4).

The signal systems working downstream from the receptors for the growth factors are not fully clarified. Taking IGF-1 as an example, it interacts with the insulin receptor (Fig. 13-5) to initiate a series of events linking via the early guanosine triphosphate (GTP)-binding protein called Ras to form Raf and to stimulate the kinases that activate MAP kinase. PDGF, originating from damaged platelets and best documented for its effects on VSM, can likewise stimulate Raf and MAP kinase (Liao et al., 1996). In the case of TGF-β only some steps are similar to those of other growth factors.

TGF-β comprises a powerful superfamily that regulates many vital growth processes (Brand and Schneider, 1995; Niehrs, 1996), besides having ill-understood functions such as immunosuppression and protection for ischemic-reperfusion damage and heat shock (Flanders et al., 1997). Members of this family bind to the extracellular component of one of the three receptor complexes, which then transmit a transmembrane signal by activating serine-threonine kinases, which then phosphorylate intracellular proteins. Downstream from this ligand–receptor interaction, several cytoplasmic signal systems may be involved, including the so-called *Mad* proto-oncogenes that when phosphorylated by the serine/threonine kinases can move into the nucleus to activate a previously undescribed class of transcription factors (Niehrs, 1996). In the heart, a specific feature of the activity of an isoform of this family, TGF-β_1, is that it eventually activates (transforms) fibroblasts to make collagen (Sigel et al., 1996). Hypothetically, an excess of collagen in ventricular hypertrophy is associated with adverse effects on myocardial compliance and with irreversible damage. Of interest is that growth factors such as PDGF and TGF-β_1 also activate other pathways involved in growth such as that involving PKC (see section on Shared Signal Systems, below).

Growth Hormone. Secreted by the pituitary gland, growth hormones promote myocyte growth without fibrosis (Cittadini et al., 1996). The intracellular signaling paths are not established but are presumably similar to those of insulin. The terms "growth hormone" and "growth factors" have different meaning, despite the probable overlap in the intracellular signal systems. Clinically, the disease acromegaly is accompanied by cardiomegaly and LV dysfunction. Growth hormone is not thought to play a role in stretch-induced hypertrophy.

Shared Signal Systems. At first sight it would seem that there should be a clear separation between those agonists such as AII that link to PKC via G_q and those linked via tyrosine (or serine-threonine) kinases to activation of Ras-Raf and the downstream effects. Yet in the myocardium, AII also activates tyrosine kinase and MAP kinase (Sadoshima and Izumo, 1993). In VSM, the unexpected observations are that AII activates Raf, whereas PDGF activates PKC (Liao et al., 1996). Thus, starting from very different agonists such as AII and PDGF, and their equally different receptors, there appear to be shared and interlinked signal systems (van Biesen et al., 1996). MAP kinase appears to be the common signal to these paths, and it may also respond to cross-talk originating in stretch.

Evaluation of Hypotheses.   Although all these hypotheses represent reasonable interpretations of an impressive volume of experimental data, none of them fully explains all aspects of cardiac growth. The fact that the heart is able to translate the signals generated by hemodynamic activity into growth, and that stretch appears to involve an ion channel, puts the emphasis on mechanoreceptors. Not only do stretch and tension result in increased protein synthesis, but conversely when these factors are removed, the muscle undergoes atrophy to become relatively overburdened with collagen (Kent et al., 1985). In addition to stretch, there are clearly other factors involved, of which the best documented is AII, which probably magnifies the stretch signal. The common downstream signal in response to diverse hypertrophic signals appears to be MAP kinase.

PROTO-ONCOGENES AND GENE EXPRESSION

A hemodynamic load may act on several steps in this growth signal cascade. In the rat heart, 10 of 400 individual cardiac mRNAs respond rapidly to a pressure overload, some as early as within 30 minutes (Komuro et al., 1988). Most of these mRNAs also exist in the fetal heart when growth rates are high. Thus, the cell hypertrophy of adult hearts and fetal cell division may have at least some features in common. Included in the early response to a hemodynamic load are increases in the proto-oncogenes, such as *c-fos* and *c-myc*, and the heat shock protein gene, hsp 70 (Izumo et al., 1988). These complex findings can be understood within the general hypothesis that myocardial hypertrophy mimics the growth response of other cell types (Izumo et al., 1988).

Oncogenes are defined as genes causing cancer (Greek *onkos,* tumor) and constitute about 20 among the total human repertoire of about 100,000 genes. Oncogenes, or c-oncs, have names such as *ras, myc,* and others. In normal healthy cells including heart cells, similar genes also exist and are often called proto-oncogenes (Greek *protos,* early form) because they can give rise to tumor-producing oncogenes in certain circumstances. Whereas in the lungs these law-abiding proto-oncogenes can be converted to cancer-causing oncogenes by carcinogens such as tobacco smoke, in the myocardium proto-oncogenes have only a physiologic function not related to cancer. The term "proto-oncogene," therefore, is sometimes (incorrectly) replaced by oncogenes, abbreviated as c-oncs.

A *proto-oncogene* increases the activity of a growth factor, a receptor, an intracellular signaling molecule, or a protein that regulates transcription (Simpson, 1988). Increased activity of proto-oncogenes can be elicited without the need for new protein synthesis. Because they can accelerate the early stages of the growth process, they are also called *immediate-early genes*. Proto-oncogenes may be divided into three classes by their putative sites of action (Frohlich et al., 1992). Class I encodes growth factors, class 2 encodes the second messengers, and class 3 (including *c-myc*, *c-fos*, and *c-jun*) encodes nuclear proteins. Their final effects depend on the cellular and molecular context in which they operate. For example, proto-oncogenes may regulate RNA transcription by binding to certain sequences in the genes (Fig. 13-5). Others seem to be G proteins. They are "key players in the regulatory network that extends from the cell surface to the nucleus" (Simpson, 1988).

Proto-oncogenes in Hypertrophy.   The proto-oncogene model emphasizes that regulation of cell growth can be understood in terms of a limited number of critical regulatory proteins or peptides, including growth factors, growth factor receptors, transducing proteins, and transcription factors. This model remains the most plausible explanation for the early transitory changes in gene expression after cardiac overload (Table 13-1). Nonetheless, association does not equal causation, and it has been difficult specifically to link increased protein synthesis in myocardial hypertrophy with increased activity of proto-oncogenes.

Heat Shock Proteins.   These appear in the cell in response to a variety of nonspecific stresses, including an acute pressure load. Heat shock proteins, such as hsp 68 and 70 (molecular weight 68 or 70 kilodaltons) may help the myocardial cell to withstand and overcome that stress. At present, their real role is believed to be related to the control of protein folding and unfolding (chaperone function).

Polyamines are derivatives of the amino acid, ornithine, that stimulates several enzymes involved in protein synthesis. The content of polyamines in myocardial cells is elevated in practically all models of hypertrophy.

Growth Inhibitors.   In some systems, inhibition of some aspects of growth is required for other aspects to proceed. Then TFG-β can have inhibitory effects, as in angiogenesis (Brand and Schneider, 1995). Heparan sulfate, a proteoglycan found in the extracellular matrix, inhibits growth of both cardiac and vascular

TABLE 13-1. *Sequence of changes in growth controlling signals, proto-oncogenes, and genes in response to sustained pressure overload*

Time after onset of load	Response
30 min	Immediate-early proto-oncogenes are induced (*c-fos, c-jun, c-myc, egr-1,* hsp 70)
6–12 hr	Induction of genes normally only expressed in fetus. Contractile genes include β-myosin heavy chain, skeletal α-actin, β-tropomyosin. Noncontractile genes include ANP and BNP.
12–24 hr	Upregulation of constitutively expressed genes, such as myosin light chain-2, cardiac α-actin.
More than 24 hr	General increase in protein and RNA content; increase in cell size but not number.

Adapted from Glennon et al. *Br Heart J* 1995;73:496, with permission.

myocytes, as does the closely related compound heparin that is clinically used (Akimoto et al., 1996).

Altered Gene Expression During Hypertrophy

To recapitulate, the coordinated increase in protein synthesis, mainly due to stimulation of the transcription process, results in a multiplication of the number of contractile units. In this way, the myocardium becomes thicker in response to a pressure load, and the wall stress or tension becomes less, so that the oxygen demand decreases despite the myocardium having to do the extra work of overcoming the increased afterload by the Laplace law (see Chapter 16).

In addition, chronic hemodynamic load results in quantitative changes in gene expression, so that (1) different protein *isoforms* are made (isoforms have the same function but with a slightly different molecular structure) and (2) there is the expression of a more fetal phenotype, with, for example, the increased synthesis of atrial natriuretic peptide (ANP) by the ventricles. The basic mechanisms are ill-understood.

Isoenzymes: Isoforms of Contractile Proteins. The rate of shortening of the myofibril (unloaded shortening velocity, V_{max}) is decreased through isoform replacement, which allows the heart to produce normal tension at a lower cost by reaching the required tension more slowly (Fig. 13-9). This adaptation is best clarified in small species, such as the rat, when there is a shift of the type of myosin (isomyosin) to V_3, the slow myosin isoform (Fig. 13-10). The isoforms are also called $\alpha\alpha$-MHC (myosin heavy chain, V_1) and $\beta\beta$-MHC (V_3). A rapid induction of the mRNA that encodes for $\beta\beta$-MHC precedes the appearance of the new isoform in the rat.

In ventricles of species that are predominantly V_3 in the adult stage, such as dog, cat, pig, guinea pig, and particularly humans, this isoform change cannot occur. In humans, the isoform shift occurs only in the atria, which are normally predominantly V_1 and can change to V_3. Conceivably, this change helps the atria to cope with the increased pressure load during their contraction phase.

Membrane Changes. Myosin isoenzyme changes do not occur in the overloaded human ventricle. Nonetheless, there are membrane changes. For example, the number of calcium channels per unit area of membrane is unchanged, yet the cell has undergone hypertrophy. That means that the gene for production of the calcium channel has had its degree of expression stimulated in a concordant way together with the contractile apparatus. In contrast, β-adrenergic receptor density decreases in man and in rats, one explanation being that the gene for β-receptor synthesis is not stimulated during the hypertrophy process. It seems as if a variety of membrane changes, some of which still await description, are part of the explanation for the depressed contractile

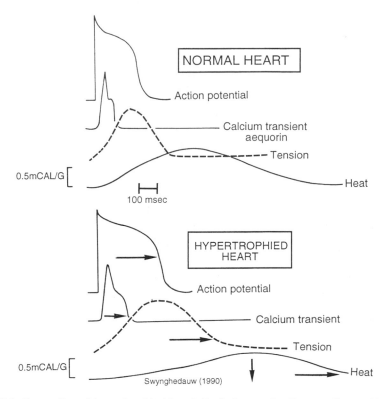

FIG. 13-9. Properties of hypertrophied heart. Excitation–contraction coupling and heat production in the hypertrophied heart compared with the normal heart. The lengthening of the action potential in the hypertrophied myocardium is not due to any increase in the density of the inward calcium channels. Note that in the hypertrophied heart, the calcium transient measured by aequorin is prolonged in the relaxation phase and that the rate of onset of physiologic systole and the length of physiologic diastole are both prolonged (Gwathmey and Morgan, 1985). Hypothetically, it is proposed that the hypertrophied heart works more economically, which can be seen from the reduced rate of heat production. See Swynghedauw et al. (1990).

function in the failing human myocardium. Experimentally, the rate of calcium uptake by isolated sarcolemmal vesicles or homogenates from failing hearts is diminished, the relative density of the Ca^{2+}-ATPase (the calcium uptake pump of the SR) is decreased, and the level of mRNA for the Ca^{2+}-ATPase also is lowered (de la Bastie et al., 1990). The release of calcium from the sarcoplasmic reticulum is decreased. Swynghedauw (1989) has proposed that diminished expression of genes for the Ca^{2+}-ATPase of the sarcoplasmic reticulum, for sodium–calcium exchange, and for β_1-receptors may all be adaptation changes that contribute to slowing of the contraction–relaxation cycle.

Changes in Action Potential and Ionic Currents. A constant finding during chronic mechanical pressure overload is the increase in the *action potential*

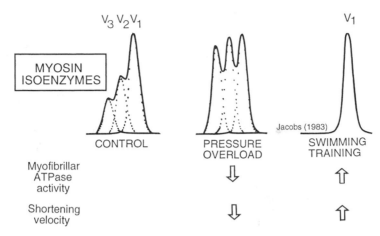

FIG. 13-10. Pressure versus dynamic exercise. Contrasting effects of pressure overload and swimming training on myosin isoenzyme patterns of rat heart. Swimming training is better able to increase adrenergic activity in the rat than is running. From Jacob et al. *Adv Myocardiol* 1983;4:70.

duration (Fig. 13-9). This lengthening is not related directly to changes in the calcium current, nor does the number of channels or dihydropyridine receptors change in relation to the degree of hypertrophy (Charlemagne et al., 1990). The increased action potential duration may be due to an impaired flow of the outward repolarizing current, I_{to}, due to decreased density of this channel (Tomita et al., 1994). In the pressure-overloaded heart, the hypertrophied muscles have a prolonged period of isometric contraction, but with a low peak value, corresponding to a similar prolongation of the calcium transient with a decreased peak calcium value (Bailey and Houser, 1993). These data suggest that the rate of sequestration and release of calcium by the sarcoplasmic reticulum is decreased in hypertrophy (Gwathmey and Morgan, 1985).

T-type Calcium Channels. T-type calcium channels are normal in fetal and neonatal ventricular myocytes, but not in the adult. T-channels are, however, induced in hypertrophy (Nuss and Houser, 1993). Hypothetically, the ensuing T-currents could promote arrhythmias in partially depolarized hypertrophic myocytes.

Thyroid-Induced Hypertrophy. The expression of ventricular myosin isoenzymes is affected not only by the workload. The thyroid status of the animal also is important. In rats, hyperthyroidism induces the V_1 form and hypothyroidism the V_3 form. These changes are regulated by mRNA transcription. Going back further, the thyroxine receptor, when activated by the hormone, binds to part of the enhancer gene encoding for the α-myosin heavy chain to activate expression of this gene. The resultant cardiac hypertrophy is better than that induced by mechanical hypertrophy, being more able to withstand ischemia (Buser et al., 1990), possibly because the coronary circulation in the thyrotoxic heart is normal or supranormal. A further reason is that thyroxine stimulates mitochondria to increase their size relative to that of the myofibrils so that the rate of energy production is potentially higher. A third reason is that thyroxine does not produce interstitial fibrosis, as does the pressure overload model (Weber et al., 1989). On the other hand, the hypermetabolic state leads to a high oxygen demand that, coupled with the hypertrophy, poses the risk of oxygen imbalance (see Chapter 17).

Fetal Phenotype Reprogramming. The hypertrophic response does not just produce a thicker heart that compensates for the increased wall stress. In addition, proto-oncogenes also induce a number of embryonic-fetal type genes, for example those of atrial and brain natriuretic peptides (ANP and BNP), skeletal α-actin, β-myosin heavy chain (Sadoshima et al., 1992), troponin T isoforms (Anderson et al., 1991), and the mRNAs that program for endothelin (Sakai et al., 1996). These changes seem to occur especially in the failing heart, and hypothetically could help the circulation to adapt, for example by increase sodium excretion as result of increased activity of ANP and BNP, and increased peripheral vasoconstriction in response to endothelin (see Chapter 16).

ULTRASTRUCTURAL CHANGES IN HYPERTROPHIC HEART

When the myocardium undergoes hypertrophy, the myocytes increase considerably in size. Capillaries and interstitial cells, the latter containing collagen, increase to a lesser extent by the process of hyperplasia. The myocyte increases basically by an increase in cell diameter and a much smaller increase in cell length, at least in response to pressure overload (Fig. 13-11). However, the capillary surface area remains relatively unchanged, increasing by only a small amount. Therefore, the ratio of the capillary surface area to the total cell volume decreases. The distance between capillaries also increases until the slower growth of the capillary bed catches up at a later stage (Fig. 13-12). Whether or not a completely normal situation is reached is a matter of dispute.

Some of the cellular changes of importance are as follows (Fig. 13-12). When the cell volume increases by about 60%, β-receptor density (sites per unit surface area) decreases by about 33%, the sodium–calcium exchange rate decreases, as does the density of the calcium-ATPase pump in the sarcoplasmic reticulum. Complex changes occur in the sodium–potassium pump that are difficult to understand. In the rat, the activity of the low-affinity form decreases, whereas that of the high-affinity form increases by about 60% (sites per unit surface area). There are relative increases in the size of the T-tubules and of the sarcoplasmic reticulum surface area. Possibly, these may compensate for the

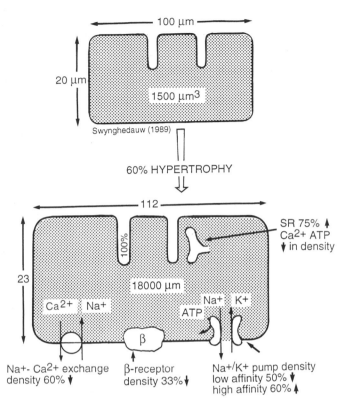

FIG. 13-11. Hypertrophic rat heart cell compared with normal. The data shown are for a 60% increase in cell volume. Note decreased β-receptor density, decreased activity of sodium–calcium exchange, decreased sarcoplasmic reticulum calcium-ATPase activity, and increased density of the high affinity sodium–potassium pump. For further details, see Swynghedauw (1989). SR, sarcoplasmic reticulum.

MYOCARDIUM

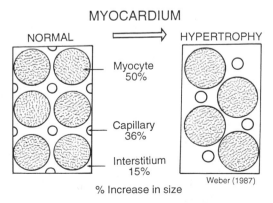

FIG. 13-12. Ultrastructure of hypertrophied myocardium. Note increase of size of myocytes relative to capillaries and interstitium. Adapted from Weber et al. (1987).

decreased density of the sarcolemmal calcium pump. At least some of the changes in the hypertrophic cell suggest a lower rate of calcium release and uptake (decreased β-receptor density, decreased sodium exchange, and decreased calcium ATPase of the sarcoplasmic reticulum), changes that in the rat heart would add to the abnormalities of contraction associated with the decreased myosin ATPase activity.

Collagen and Interstitial Fibrosis

The myocardium is composed of cardiac myocytes and of connective tissue cells. An accumulation of collagen in the myocardium is termed fibrosis. Collagen exists in several genetically distinct types, of which type I and III are found in the myocardium (Weber et al., 1989), type I being dominant and having a tensile strength greater than that of steel. Collagen is chiefly located in the interstitial (between cell) spaces and increases in amount during LV pressure overload. There is first a *reactive fibrosis* with an increase of interstitial collagen, which increases the stiffness of the myocardium both in systole and in diastole. The former increase may improve myocardial force generation (Weber et al., 1989), whereas the latter may contribute to impaired relaxation rates (Brilla et al., 1991). If linkage of the crossbridges binding collagen and elastin fibers is prevented by a specific inhibitor (a lathyrogen), hypertrophy develops without increased stiffness.

Hypothetically, increased collagen formation, with an increase in the ratio of type III to type I, may occur in response to a variety of growth signals, of which stretch acting on the fibroblasts might be the most important (Carver et al., 1991), followed by AII, TGF and FGF. In addition, Weber's group has emphasized the possible role of aldosterone (Brilla et al., 1993). At a cellular level, TGF-β_1 acts on fibroblasts to promote the synthesis of collagen.

VASCULAR REMODELING

Just as the ventricles remodel and hypertrophy in response to a sustained pressure load, so do the arterial blood vessels in response to hypertension. Similar questions are posed: How much is due to pressure (or stretch) and how much results from renin-angiotensin activation? What role do the other growth factors play? What are the signal systems? In the aorta, an increased transmural pressure stimulates the local renin-angiotensin system, with net production of AII (Bardy et al., 1996). The angiotensin-1 (AT$_1$) receptors of the arterial tissue respond to both stretch and to AII. Both an increased pressure and AII act synergistically to induce the expression of *fibronectin,* one of the components of the extracellular matrix of the aorta.

However, growth in VSM is different from that in myocardium in that both hyperplasia and hypertrophy occur in the early stages of VSM growth, whereas there is only hypertrophy in the early response of the myocardium (Fig. 13-1). As a generalization, the growth factors promote hyperplasia, whereas the receptor agonists linked to PKC promote vascular hypertrophy. For example, PDGF causes hyperplasia, whereas AII causes hypertrophy (Liao et al., 1996). Yet the signal systems downstream from the receptors do not differ much, both converging on MAP kinase, albeit through somewhat different intermediate steps. Thus, it remains unclear what the significant differences between AII and PDGF signalling might be. Hypothetically, all the agonists linked to PKC (including AII) should also increase cytosolic calcium and promote vasoconstriction, with an increase in wall tension that should promote hyperplasia as in myocardial cells.

VSM growth might be a step on the way to atherosclerosis. As in the case of the myocardium, proto-oncogenes such as *c-myc* help to promote growth. The hypothesis is that *c-myc* therefore could be downregulated to prevent excess growth of VSM cells (Bennett et al., 1994).

CLINICAL APPLICATION: REGRESSION OF LEFT VENTRICULAR HYPERTROPHY

LVH is now recognized as an independent risk factor for cardiovascular disease, a logical proposition bearing in mind that LVH is a step on the way to heart failure, and that coronary vascular reserve is impaired in the hypertrophic heart (see Chapter 16). Thus it makes sense to remedy those factors predisposing to pressure overload, such as hypertension or aortic stenosis, and those that cause a volume overload, such as mitral or aortic valve regurgitation (see Chapter 16). Once there is LVH with fibrosis, it is not certain that normality can be regained despite relief of the overload.

An additional question is whether there is any specific means of achieving regression of the LVH. The basic data reviewed in this chapter show that AII is increasingly seen as crucial in growth promoting pathways, providing apparent logic for the clinical use of angiotensin converting enzyme (ACE) inhibitor drugs to regress LVH. Do these agents act like any other antihypertensive to decrease stretch, and thereby to reduce growth, or do they have a unique role? Controversial data suggest that low doses of ACE inhibitors are able to induce regression of LVH without reducing the blood pressure. But the weight of evidence shows that ACE inhibitors cannot regress LVH until the LV systolic pressure decreases (Böhm et al., 1995; Brilla et al., 1993; Zierhut et al., 1991). Furthermore, when isolated myocytes are loaded, overall protein synthesis can be found even when there is blockade of the AII receptors (Kent and McDermott, 1996). If it is stretch that is the fundamental signal that in the first instance induces the upregulation of tissue renin-angiotensin and the release of AII, then any other antihypertensive (including a diuretic) that brings down the blood pressure to relieve stress in the LV wall should be equally effective. Perhaps the answer to this conflict is that although AII can promote growth even in nonstretched cells, it is much more effective in stretched cells (Fig. 13-7). Therefore, reduction of LV stretch by whatever means that is effective should be the primary goal of therapy aimed at regression of LVH.

SUMMARY

1. *Mechanoreceptors* translate a mechanical signal, such as a prolonged pressure overload, into growth signals. Calcium ions may be important in this sequence.
2. *Protein kinase C* (PKC) links with several important agonists, including angiotensin II, via phospholipase C. Further controlling steps in the growth cascade involve several steps leading up to mitogen-activated protein kinase (MAP kinase), which sets a further chain of events in motion.
3. *Angiotensin II* is the most important of the PKC-linked agonists. It is released from myocytes in response to stretch and acts in an autocrine manner to promote cell growth. However, the rationale for preferential use of ACE inhibitors in the clinical therapy of regression is not firmly based on experimental evidence.
4. *Growth factors* such as insulinlike growth factor (IGF-1), transforming growth factor β (TGF-β_1), and others linked to receptors form a group that includes the insulin receptor.
5. *MAP kinase.* Mitogen activated protein kinase is an important enzyme on which most but not all of the growth-promoting pathways converge. Through a further sequence of signals, it activates proto-oncogenes.
6. *Proto-oncogenes.* The events subsequent to the above initiating events are not entirely clear. Part of the biochemical response is increased activation of proto-oncogenes (also called early-immediate genes) that speed up the growth process at three levels: the receptors, the second messengers, and nuclear events.
7. *Isozyme changes.* In small animals, an important change is from rapidly contracting myosin (V_1) to one that contracts slowly (V_3), a change not found in humans.
8. *Ionic changes.* The action potential duration is prolonged, possibly the result of inhibition of the repolarizing current I_{to}. The calcium transients have a low peak with delayed recovery.
9. *Fetal phenotype.* Especially in the failing hypertrophied heart, there is expression of the fetal phenotype with, for example, the capacity of the ventricles to manufacture atrial natriuretic peptide, brain natriuretic peptide, and endothelin. These might be protective changes in the context of the failing circulation.
10. *Nonmyocytic cells.* In contrast to myocyctes, the basic response of which is to undergo hypertrophy in response to a load, there is an actual increase in the number of capillary cells and in those of the extracellular matrix. The increased collagen, in response to transforming growth factor (TGF-β) causes fibrosis, which when it is significant not only disturbs systolic and diastolic function, but causes the LV hypertrophy to become irreversible.

STUDENT QUESTIONS

1. What is a growth factor? Describe the signal systems that link the sarcolemmal receptor to the nuclear synthetic processes.
2. Describe the signal system linking angiotensin II occupancy of its receptor to nuclear proto-oncogenes.
3. What is meant by cross-talk? Gives examples.
4. What role if any does free cytosolic calcium play in the regulation of growth?
5. What is the three kinase cascade? Why is the most distal component of this cascade so important in the regulation of growth?

CARDIOLOGIST-IN-TRAINING QUESTIONS

1. What are the differences between hypertrophy and hyperplasia? When and why can cardiac myocytes undergo hyperplasia?
2. Which are the agonists coupling to protein kinase C (PKC), and which are some of the downstream signals involved between PKC and nuclear events?
3. Do you think that angiotensin II has a specific role in the response to stretch? If so, is it mandatory to use ACE inhibitors in the therapeutic management of left ventricular hypertrophy?
4. What is vascular remodeling, and which are the signals involved in this condition?
5. Myocardial fibrosis is hypothesized as being an irreversible step in the development of left ventricular hypertrophy. What are the major growth signals involved in the production of fibrosis, and how may these steps be interrupted by therapeutically active agents?

REFERENCES

1. Adler CP. DNA in growing hearts of children. Biochemical and cytophotometric investigations. *Beitr Pathol* 1976;158:173–202.
2. Akimoto H, Ito H, Tanaka M, et al. Heparin and heparan sulfate block angiotensin II-induced hypertrophy in cultured neonatal rat cardiomyocytes. A possible role of intrinsic heparin-like molecules in regulation of cardiomyocyte hypertrophy. *Circulation* 1996;93:810–816.
3. Anderson PWA, Malouf NN, Oakeley AE, et al. Troponin T isoform expression in humans. A comparison among normal and failing adult heart, fetal heart and adult and fetal skeletal muscle. *Circ Res* 1991;69:1226–1233.
4. Astorri E, Bolognesi B, Colla B, et al. Left ventricular hypertrophy: a cytometric study on 42 human hearts. *J Mol Cell Cardiol* 1977;9:763–775.
5. Bailey BA, Houser SR. Sarcoplasmic reticulum-related changes in cytosolic calcium in pressure-overload-induced feline LV hypertrophy. *Am J Physiol* 1993;265:H2009–H2016.
6. Bardy N, Merval R, Benessiano J, et al. Pressure and angiotensin II synergistically induce aortic fibronectin expression in organ culture model of rabbit aorta. Evidence for a pressure-induced tissue renin-angiotensin system. *Circ Res* 1996;79:70–78.
7. Bennett MR, Evan GI, Newby AC. Deregulated expression of the c-myc oncogene abolishes inhibition of proliferation of rat vascular smooth muscle cells by serum reduction, interferon-γ, heparin and cyclic nucleotide analogues and induced apoptosis. *Circ Res* 1994;74:525–536.

8. Bishop SP, Anderson PG, Tucker DC. Morphological development of the rat heart growing in oculo in the absence of hemodynamic work load. *Circ Res* 1990;66:84–102.
9. Boheler KR, Dillmann WH. Cardiac response to pressure overload in the rat: the selective alteration of in vitro directed RNA translation products. *Circ Res* 1988;63:448–456.
10. Böhm M, Castellano M, Agabiti-Rosei E, et al. Dose-dependent dissociation of ACE-inhibitor effects on blood pressure, cardiac hypertrophy, and β-adrenergic signal transduction. *Circulation* 1995;92: 3006–3013.
11. Brand T, Schneider MD. The TGFβ superfamily in myocardium: ligands, receptors, transduction and function. *J Mol Cell Cardiol* 1995;27:5–18.
12. Brilla C, Janicki JS, Weber KT. Impaired diastolic function and coronary reserve in genetic hypertension. Role of interstitial fibrosis and medial thickening of intramyocardial coronary arteries. *Circ Res* 1991;69:107–115.
13. Brilla CG, Matsubara LS, Weber KT. Anti-aldosterone treatment and the prevention of myocardial fibrosis in primary and secondary hyperaldosteronism. *J Mol Cell Cardiol* 1993;25:563–575.
14. Buser PT, Wikman-Coffelt J, Wu ST, et al. Postischemic recovery of mechanical performance and energy metabolism in the presence of left ventricular hypertrophy. A 31P-MRS study. *Circ Res* 1990;66:735–746.
15. Carver W, Nagpal ML, Nachtigal M, et al. Collagen expression in mechanically stimulated cardiac fibroblasts. *Circ Res* 1991;69:116–122.
16. Charlemagne D, Mayoux E, Scamps F, et al. Ion channels in the hypertrophied myocardium: electrophysiological studies and molecular aspects. In: Swynghedauw B (ed). *Research in Cardiac Hypertrophy and Failure.* London: INSERM/John Libbey Eurotext, 1990;199–211.
17. Cittadini A, Stromer H, Katz SE, et al. Differential cardiac effects of growth hormone and insulin-like growth factor-1 in the rat. A combined in vivo and in vitro evaluation. *Circulation* 1996;93: 800–809.
18. Cobb MH, Goldsmith EJ. How MAP kinases are regulated. *J Biol Chem* 1995;270:1483–1486.
19. Cooper G, Kent RL, Uboh CE, et al. Hemodynamic versus adrenergic control of cat right ventricular hypertrophy. *J Clin Invest* 1985;75:14843–14846.
20. Crozatier B. Stretch-induced modifications of myocardial performance: from ventricular function to cellular and molecular mechanisms. *Cardiovasc Res* 1996;32:25–37.
21. de la Bastie D, Levitsky D, Rappaport L, et al. Function of the sarcoplasmic reticulum and expression of its Ca^{2+}-ATPase gene in pressure overload-induced cardiac hypertrophy in the rat. *Circ Res* 1990;66:554–564.
22. Decker ML, Behnke-Barclay M, Cook MG, et al. Morphometric evaluation of the contractile apparatus in primary cultures of rabbit cardiac myocytes. *Circ Res* 1991;69:86–94.
23. Flanders KC, Bhandiwad AR, Winokur TS. Transforming growth factor-β block cytokine induction of catalase and xanthine oxidase mRNA levels in cultured rat cardiac cells. *J Mol Cell Cardiol* 1997; 29:273–280.
24. Force T, Pombo CM, Avruch JA, et al. Stress-activated protein kinases in cardiovascular disease [Mini Review]. *Circ Res* 1996;78:947–953.
25. Frohlich ED, Apstein C, Chobanian AV, et al. The heart in hypertension [Review]. *N Engl J Med* 1992;327:998–1008.
26. Geisterfer AAT, Peach MJ, Owens GK. Angiotensin II induces hypertrophy, not hyperplasia, of cultured rat aortic smooth muscle cells. *Circ Res* 1988;62:749–756.
27. Gwathmey JK, Morgan JP. Altered calcium handling in experimental pressure-overload hypertrophy in the ferret. *Circ Res* 1985;57:836–843.
28. Imamura S, Matsuoka R, Hiratsuka E, et al. Local response to cardiac overload on myosin heavy chain gene expression and isoenzyme transition. *Circ Res* 1990;66:1067–1073.
29. Ito N, Kagaya Y, Weinberg EO, et al. Endothelin and angiotensin II stimulation of Na^+-H^+ exchange is impaired in cardiac hypertrophy. *J Clin Invest* 1997;99:125–135.
30. Izumo S, Lompre A-M, Matsuoka R, et al. Myosin heavy chain messenger RNA and protein isoform transitions during cardiac hypertrophy. *J Clin Invest* 1987;79:970–977.
31. Izumo S, Nadal-Ginard B, Mahdavi V. Protooncogene induction and reprogramming of cardiac gene expression produced by pressure overload. *Proc Natl Acad Sci USA* 1988;85:339–343.
32. Kawaguchi H, Sano H, Iizuka K, et al. Phosphatidylinositol metabolism in hypertrophic rat heart. *Circ Res* 1993;72:966–972.
33. Kent RL, McDermott PJ. Passive load and angiotensin II evoke differential responses of gene expression and protein synthesis in cardiac myocytes. *Circ Res* 1996;78:829–838.

34. Kent RL, Uboh CE, Thompson EW, et al. Biochemical and structural correlates in unloaded and reloaded cat myocardium. *J Mol Cell Cardiol* 1985;17:153–165.
35. Khairallah PA, Kanabus J. Angiotensin and myocardial protein synthesis. In: Tarazi RC, Dunbar JB (eds). *Perspectives in Cardiovascular Research.* New York: Raven, 1983;337–347.
36. Kijima K, Matsubara H, Murasawa S, et al. Mechanical stretch induces enhanced expression of angiotensin II receptor subtypes in neonatal rat cardiac myocytes. *Circ Res* 1996;79:887–897.
37. Komuro I, Kaida T, Shibazaki Y, et al. Stretching cardiac myocytes stimulates proto-oncogene expression. *J Biol Chem* 1990;265:3595–3598.
38. Komuro I, Katoh Y, Kaida T, et al. Mechanical loading stimulates cell hypertrophy and specific gene expression in cultured rat cardiac myocytes. *J Biol Chem* 1991;266:1265–1268.
39. Komuro I, Kurabayashi M, Takaku F, Yazaki Y. Expression of cellular oncogenes in the myocardium during the developmental stage and pressure-overloaded hypertrophy of the rat heart. *Circ Res* 1988; 62:1075–1079.
40. Liao D-F, Duff JL, Daum G, et al. Angiotensin II stimulates MAP kinase kinase kinase activity in vascular smooth muscle cells. Role of Raf. *Circ Res* 1996;79:1007–1014.
41. Linzbach AJ. Die Anzahl der Herzmuskelkerne in normalen, uberlasteten, atrophischen und mit Corhomon behandelten Herzkammern. *Z Kreislaufforsch* 1952;41:641–658.
42. Meerson FZ. The failing heart. In: Katz AM (eds). *Adaptation and Deadaptation.* New York: Raven, 1983.
43. Meggs LG, Coupet J, Huang H, et al. Regulation of angiotensin II receptors on ventricular myocytes after myocardial infarction in rats. *Circ Res* 1993;72:1149–1162.
44. Morgan HE, Rannels DE, McKee EE. Protein metabolism of the heart. In: Berne R (ed). *Handbook of Physiology: Circulation.* Washington, DC: American Physiology Society, 1979;845–871.
45. Niehrs C. Mad connection to the nucleus. *Nature* 1996;381:561–562.
46. Nuss HB, Houser SR. T-type Ca^{2+} current is expressed in hypertrophied adult feline left ventricular myocytes. *Circ Res* 1993;73:777–782.
47. Peterson MB, Lesch M. Protein synthesis and amino acid transport in the isolated rabbit right ventricular papillary muscle. Effect of isometric tension development. *Circ Res* 1972;31:317–327.
48. Sadoshima J, Qui Z, Morgan J, Izumo S. Angiotensin II and other hypertrophic stimuli mediated by G protein-coupled receptors activate tyrosine kinase, mitogen-activated protein kinase and 90-kD S6 kinase in cardiac myocytes. The critical role of Ca^{2+}-dependent signalling. *Circ Res* 1995; 76:1–15.
49. Sadoshima J-I, Izumo S. Signal transduction pathways of angiotensin II-induced c-fos gene expression in cardiac myocytes in vitro. Roles of phospholipid-derived second messengers. *Circ Res* 1993; 73:424–438.
50. Sadoshima J-I, Jahn L, Takahashi T, et al. Molecular characterization of the stretch-induced adaptation of cultured cardiac cells. An in vitro model of load-induced cardiac hypertrophy. *J Biol Chem* 1992;267:10551–10560.
51. Sadoshima J, Xu Y, Slayter HS, Izumo S. Autocrine release of angiotensin-II mediates stretch-induced hypertrophy of cardiac myocytes in vitro of cardiac myocytes in vitro. *Cell* 1993;75:977–984.
52. Sakai S, Miyauchi T, Kobayashi M, et al. Inhibition of myocardial endothelin pathway improves long-term survival in heart failure. *Nature* 1996;384:353–355.
53. Samarel AM. Regional differences in the in vivo synthesis and degradation of myosin subunits in rabbit ventricular myocardium. *Circ Res* 1989;64:193–202.
54. Samuel JL, Schiaffino S, Rappaport L. Myocardial cells: early changes in the expression and distribution of proteins or their mRNAs during the development of myocardial hypertrophy in the rat. In: Swynghedauw B (ed). *Research in Cardiac Hypertrophy and Failure.* London: INSERM/John Libbey Eurotext, 1990;277–292.
55. Schiaffino S, Samuel JL, Sassoon D, et al. Nonsynchronous accumulation of alpha-skeletal actin and beta-myosin heavy chain mRNAs during early stages of pressure-overload-induced cardiac hypertrophy demonstrated by in situ hybridization. *Circ Res* 1989;64:937–948.
56. Schorb W, Booz GW, Dostal DE, et al. Angiotensin II is mitogenic in neonatal rat cardiac fibroblasts. *Circ Res* 1993;72:1245–1254.
57. Sharp WW, Terracia L, Bork TK, Samarel AM. Contractile activity modulates actin synthesis and turnover in cultured neonatal rat heart cells. *Circ Res* 1993;73:172–183.
58. Sigel AV, Centrella M, Eghbali-Webb M. Regulation of proliferative response of cardiac fibroblasts by transforming growth factor-β_1. *J Mol Cell Cardiol* 1996;28:1921–1929.
59. Simpson PC. Role of proto-oncogenes in myocardial hypertrophy. *Am J Cardiol* 1988;62:13G–19G.

60. Swynghedauw B. Remodelling of the heart in response to chronic mechanical overload. *Eur Heart J* 1989;10:935–943.
61. Swynghedauw B, Moalic JM, Delcayre C. The origins of cardiac hypertrophy. In: Swynghedauw B (ed). *Research in Cardiac Hypertrophy and Failure.* London: INSERM/John Libbey Eurotext, 1990; 23–50.
62. Szlachcic J, Hall WD, Tabau JF, et al. Left ventricular hypertrophy reversal with labetalol and propanolol: a prospective, randomized, double-blind study. *Cardiovasc Drug Ther* 1990;4:427–434.
63. Tomanek RJ. Response of the coronary vasculature to myocardial hypertrophy. *J Am Coll Cardiol* 1990;15:528–533.
64. Tomita F, Bassett AL, Myerburg RJ, Kimura S. Diminished transient outward currents in rat hypertrophied ventricular myocytes. *Circ Res* 1994;75:296–303.
65. van Biesen T, Luttrell LM, Hawes BE, Lefkowitz RJ. Mitogenic signalling via G protein-coupled receptors. *Endocr Rev* 1996;17:698–714.
66. von Harsdorf R, Lang RE, Fullerton M, Woodcock EA. Myocardial stretch stimulates phosphatidyl-inositol turnover. *Circ Res* 1989;65:494–501.
67. Weber KT, Clark WA, Janicki JS, Shroff SG. Physiologic versus pathologic hypertrophy and the pressure-overloaded myocardium. *J Cardiovasc Pharmacol* 1987;10(suppl 6):37–49.
68. Weber KT, Jalil JE, Janicki JS, Pick R. Myocardial collagen remodeling in pressure overload hypertrophy. *Am J Hypertension* 1989;2:931–940.
69. Xenophontos XP, Watson PA, Chua BHL, et al. Increased cyclic AMP content accelerates protein synthesis in rat heart. *Circ Res* 1989;65;647–656.
70. Yamazaki T, Komuro I, Kudoh S, et al. Angiotensin II partly mediates mechanical stress-induced cardiac hypertrophy. *Circ Res* 1995;77:258–265.
71. Zierhut W, Zimmer H-GM, Gerdes AM. Effect of angiotensin converting enzyme inhibition on pressure-induced left ventricular hypertrophy in rats. *Circ Res* 1991;69:609–617.

PART V

The Circulation

14

Blood Pressure
and Peripheral Circulation

Cardiovascular homeostasis is achieved by the
orchestration of neural and hormonal systems.
T.D. Giles, 1990

The arterial blood pressure (usually abbreviated to blood pressure or BP) is strictly given by the peak and trough pressures found on direct arterial puncture. These are the systolic and diastolic values in millimeters of mercury (mm Hg), yet cannot be regarded as physiologic values because invasive monitoring is an impractical procedure in abnormal circumstances. Rather, less precise but widely available noninvasive determination is standard—using the sphygmomanometer and stethoscope—taking the systolic value as the detection of the first Korotkoff sounds and the diastolic as the disappearance of all the sounds. Physiologically, although BP varies considerably from an early morning high to a nocturnal low (see Fig. 1-9), certain limits are recognized. When BP is consistently too high, with the majority of daytime readings exceeding 140/90 mm Hg, the condition is called hypertension. Because BP is such an important regulator of cardiovascular function and indicator of disease, it should be emphasized that there are large variations in BP in response to temporary events such as exercise or emotional stress.

PHYSIOLOGY OF BLOOD PRESSURE CONTROL

The control of BP is mediated through complex, overlapping mechanisms that interact to produce appropriate responses in a wide variety of circumstances. The arterial BP, although subject to large diurnal variations, is relatively tightly controlled (Fig. 14-1). It should be recalled that

$$BP = CO \times PVR$$

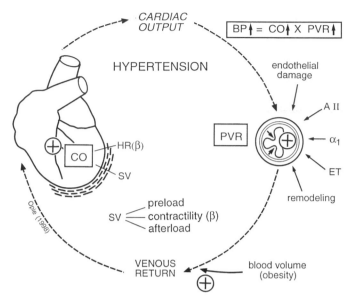

FIG. 14-1. Basic mechanisms in hypertension. In younger hypertensive patients, the cardiac output (CO) is generally increased, whereas in older hypertensive patients, it is the systemic vascular resistance (SVR) that is increased (see Fig. 14-2). SV, stroke volume; HR, heart rate; α_1, α_1-adrenergic; ET, endothelin.

Thus, as the cardiac output (CO) increases (e.g., during exercise), a decreased peripheral vascular resistance (PVR) can prevent BP from increasing excessively. Such acute regulation of the PVR over minutes and hours is achieved largely by (1) neuronal regulation, which through pressure receptors and autonomic reflexes provides rapid responses of the circulation to minute-by-minute BP variations, and (2) regulation of the peripheral arteriolar tone by both local metabolic factors such as nitric oxide (NO) and adenosine, and by variations in the outflow of adrenergic or cholinergic signals. Longer term BP control over days and weeks depends more on regulation of blood volume and renal factors such as the renin-angiotensin system, with changes in the PVR being an important regulator of the BP equation.

Autonomic Control and Baroreflexes

The *vasomotor center* at the base of the brain brings together signals from the body as a whole and then transmits afferent impulses through vasoconstrictor or vasodilator fibers to the arterioles. Some of the afferent stimuli traveling to the vasomotor center originate in the baroreceptors in the walls of the arch of the aorta and at the origin of the internal carotid artery. In this way the high-pressure side of the circulation is constantly monitored and the BP regulated. Likewise, there are low-pressure receptors. Both high- and low-pressure receptors respond to stretch.

Baroreceptors. Baroreceptors, or high-pressure receptors, are situated on the arterial side of the circulation in the carotid sinus and aortic arch (Fig. 14-2). Despite their name (Greek *baros,* weight), these are stretch receptors that respond to distension of the vessels rather than to pressure. These mechanoreceptors form the first line of defense against acute hypertension or hypotension, adjusting both vagal tone and sympathetic outflow against the level of receptor input. The baroreceptors respond both to the rate of pressure-induced stretch-mediated deformation and have static responses to sustained BP changes. Baroreflexes supply afferents via the vagus and glossopharyngeal nerves to the nucleus tractus solitarius, which is part of the *vasomotor center* in the medulla oblongata. Impulses from these receptors are inhibitory in nature. Thus, in response to acute hypertension, the baroreflexes engender increased neuronal

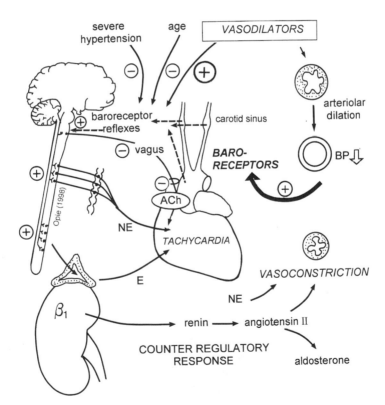

FIG. 14-2. High-pressure receptors and baroreflexes. In response to acute drug-induced vasodilation and hypotension, baroreflexes inhibit vagal outflow and stimulate adrenergic outflow to mediate counter-regulation and vasoconstriction. For effects of hypertension, see Fig. 2-1.

traffic to the vasomotor center, with consequent inhibition of sympathetic outflow and increase of vagal tone. These changes in autonomic outflow decrease the heart rate, contractility, and cardiac output, as well as inducing a decrease in the PVR. Thus, the acute increase in BP induces self-correcting changes.

In response to acute *hypotension,* there is a decrease in the distending pressure in the baroreceptors, resulting in a decreased frequency of discharge, lessened signals to the vasomotor center, and a consequent increase in sympathetic outflow and inhibition of vagal tone. The α-mediated reflex response will increase heart rate and contractility, so that the cardiac output increases. Simultaneously, the α-mediated increase in PVR will also help to elevate BP.

Sometimes BP decreases abruptly after painful or psychological stimuli, probably in response to inhibitory input into the vasomotor center from higher centers such as the hypothalamus and the cerebral cortex. Excitatory stimuli, increasing BP, are received from chemoreceptors in the carotid bodies and the aorta, from muscles during isometric exercise, from pain pathways, and from higher centers. Any such BP changes will then automatically induce baroreflexes that revert BP toward normal.

Low Pressure Receptors. Distending volumes on the venous side of the circulation are sensed by *cardiopulmonary receptors,* which are stretch receptors in the atria, pulmonary arteries, and ventricular endocardium (Fig. 14-3). These receptors respond primarily to alterations in the filling volumes of the venous side of the heart (Giles, 1990; Roddie and Shepherd, 1958). Thus, an increase in blood volume (e.g., by a transfusion) will send signals along vagal afferent fibers

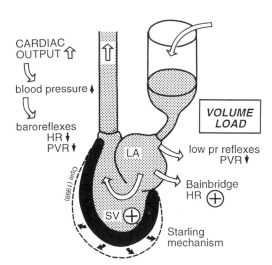

FIG. 14-3. Low pressure and Bainbridge reflexes in response to volume load. Note that once BP increases, high-pressure baroreflexes tend to reduce heart rate (HR) and PVR.

to the brain to inhibit the sympathetic outflow and to decrease the release of renin (Mancia et al., 1975). Such inhibitory signals act to decrease the PVR and to lessen the BP increase. Thus, at the onset of exercise, when the venous return is increased and the cardiac output increases by Starling's law, the decrease in the PVR helps to avoid a large increase in BP.

Bainbridge Reflex. This reflex increases the heart rate in response to an increased atrial pressure (Fig. 14-3) and is mediated by stretch receptors in the atrium at the junction with the pulmonary veins (Kappagoda et al., 1979). The result is that an increased venous return not only increases the stroke volume by the Starling mechanism, but increases the heart rate to increase the cardiac output. In some circumstances, such as in a recumbent resting conscious dog, the heart rate effect can account for all of the increase in the cardiac output in response to a volume infusion (Vatner and Boettcher, 1978). Normally, in response to exercise in the erect posture, both the Starling and the heart rate effects are important. Whatever the mechanism, the increase in cardiac output tends to increase BP, which evokes an inhibitory baroreflex response and tends to slow the heart rate, especially because the cardiopulmonary reflexes also promote vagal activity. This expected decrease in heart rate does not happen because as the atrial pressure is increased by a volume infusion, the baroreflex sensitivity lessens (Vatner et al., 1975). The overall result is an increased cardiac output with tachycardia and less than the expected increase in BP.

Integrated Control of Peripheral Vascular Resistance. It must not be supposed that the baroflexes and low pressure receptors invoke only reflex autonomic changes. The response of the kidneys is also important. Whenever there is decreased sympathetic outflow, the kidneys respond by less renin release, thereby attenuating angiotensin-mediated vasoconstriction. A converse sequence occurs with increased sympathetic outflow. For example when *standing,* a reflex increase in the PVR restores BP to the normal range. This increase is obtained by (1) reflex stimulation of the vasoconstrictive α_1-adrenergic receptors as a result of baroreflex activation, and (2) stimulation of renin release from the kidneys, both by the low renal artery pressure and by a β_1-adrenergic mediated effect, facilitated by the activity of the low-pressure reflexes. Conversely, if BP rises too high, as when cold evokes vasoconstriction, the protective mechanisms include (1) baroreflex inhibition of the adrenergic system and (2) endothelial regulation of BP. Provided that the endothelium is normal, a rise in BP increases shear forces that release vasodilatory NO. In the presence of damaged endothelium (repetitive elevation of BP), stimulation of the endothelium releases vasoconstrictory endothelin.

Neurohumoral Control of Blood Pressure

Renin-Angiotensin System. Angiotensin II (AII) is powerfully vasoconstrictive and is the end product of a coordinated neurohormonal cascade that plays a central role in the control of fluid and electrolyte balance, blood volume, and BP regulation. The first event is release of *renin* from the juxtaglomerular apparatus in the kidney (Fig. 14-4). Renin is a glycoprotein enzyme that catalyzes the conversion of *angiotensinogen* to angiotensin I, which in turn is converted to *AII* by the angiotensin-converting enzyme (ACE), primarily found in vascular endothelial cells. Renin is released from the kidneys in response to three major stimuli: increased β_1 adrenergic stimulation; a decreased renal artery pressure (hypotension); and decreased tubular reabsorption of sodium, as, for example, in response to a low sodium diet or diuretic therapy (Fig. 14-4). Release of renin is inhibited by negative feedback from AII. It also stimulates the release of aldosterone from the adrenal cortex, thereby increasing sodium reabsorption in the kidney and decreasing release of renin. *Angiotensin III,* the major metabolite of AII, is less powerful as a vasoconstrictor.

AII has several other important effects besides vasoconstriction (Table 14-1). First, it regulates sodium and water balance at several levels. It promotes the release of the sodium-retaining hormone aldosterone from the adrenal cortex.

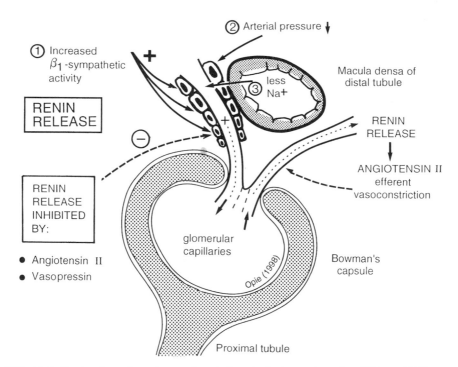

FIG. 14-4. Mechanisms for release of renin from juxtaglomerular cells of kidney: (1) β_1-sympathetic activity, (2) hypotension or decreased renal blood flow, and (3) decreased tubular reabsorption of sodium, as, for example, during a low-sodium diet or diuretic therapy. Note that renin, by forming AII, maintains efferent arteriolar vasoconstriction and, therefore, the intraglomerular pressure.

TABLE 14-1. *Role of angiotensin II in maintaining blood pressure during hypotension*

Site of action of AII	Effect
Vascular smooth muscle	Constriction; increase of PVR
Renal efferent arteriole	Constriction; maintenance of GFR
Proximal renal tubule	Na^+ reabsorption ↑
Adrenal cortex	Aldosterone secretion ↑
Central adrenergic activation	Increased release of NE
Ganglionic facilitation	Increased release of NE
Presynaptic receptors	Increased release of NE; decreased re-uptake
Baroreflexes	Withdrawal of vagal tone

GFR, glomerular filtration rate; NE, norepinephrine.

Next, it acts on the renal circulation to constrict the efferent renal arterioles, thereby increasing the intraglomerular pressure. Thus, during arterial hypotension, renal filtration function can be preserved. AII also acts on the proximal renal tubules to stimulate the Na^+/H^+ exchanger to promote sodium reabsorption. In addition, AII stimulates the thirst center in the hypothalamus, resulting in increased water intake.

AII also has an *indirect permissive adrenergic effect,* stimulating the sympathetic nervous system at several levels (Fig. 14-5), by acting on (1) the brain stem to promote central adrenergic activation; (2) autonomic ganglia, to facilitate neurotransmission; (3) presynaptic AII receptors of sympathetic nerve terminal neurons, to stimulate the release of norepinephrine and to lessen its re-uptake; and (4) the endothelium, to promote release of endothelin. By all these many actions, AII helps to maintain blood volume and BP in the face of arterial hypotension.

AII also interacts with the *baroreflexes,* which would normally set in motion a series of events that would tend to counteract all the multiple mechanisms whereby AII increases BP. For example, it would be expected that the heart rate would decrease as BP increased. This does not happen because AII acts on central receptors to reset the baroreflexes and to lessen the anticipated bradycardia (Reid, 1996).

The *local tissue renin-angiotensin* is also important, and all components of the system have been identified in tissues such as heart and blood vessel walls. Locally produced AII, acting via the IP_3 path, is vasoconstrictive by increased intracellular Ca^{2+} concentrations and is also probably implicated in the growth process in myocardial hypertrophy (see Chapter 13).

Catecholamines. The endocrine function of the catecholamines is primarily related to acute responses such as the fight or flight response. Whether, in addition, these agents are major factors affecting day-to-day or longer term BP control, as postulated by the neurogenic theory of hypertension, is still open to dispute. Under normal circumstances, circulating norepinephrine does not exert significant vascular effects because the concentrations in plasma are too low, whereas epinephrine concentrations are within the active range. Nonetheless,

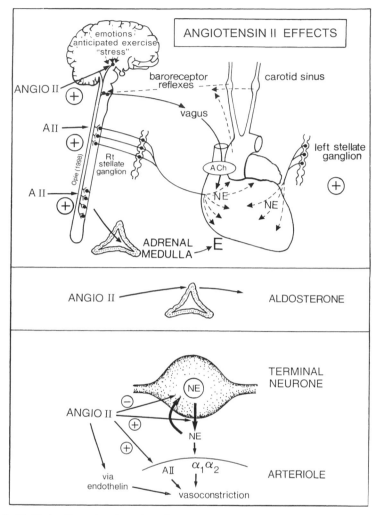

FIG. 14-5. Multiple sites of action of angiotensin II (angio II) including central activation, facilitation of ganglionic transmission, release of aldosterone from the adrenal medulla, release of norepinephrine (NE) from terminal sympathetic varicosities with inhibition of reuptake, and direct stimulation of vascular angiotensin II receptors. Angiotensin II also releases vasoconstrictory endothelin from the endothelium. The major net effect is powerful vasoconstriction.

norepinephrine released from the terminal neurons into the synaptic cleft is locally active to promote α_1-mediated vasoconstriction.

Antidiuretic Hormone.   Antidiuretic hormone (ADH) is secreted by the posterior pituitary gland in response to stimulation of osmoreceptors by a decrease in blood volume, BP, or β-adrenergic stimulation and helps to control blood volume. ADH increases the reabsorption of water in the kidney, acting on V_2 receptors located in the collecting duct of the nephron. ADH is also a potent vasoconstrictor, acting at V_1 receptors found throughout the body (hence the alternate name, arginine vasopressin). By both actions and in large doses, ADH elevates BP, but under physiologic conditions its central action depresses cardiac output so that there is little overall effect on BP.

Atrial Natriuretic Peptide. Atrial natriuretic peptide (ANP, also called atrial natriuretic factor) is released in response to atrial distension as in volume overload or left heart failure. It acts on vascular smooth muscle cells to promote vasodilation via the cyclic guanosine monophosphate (cGMP) system (see Fig. 16-26). ANP also has a diuretic action both by a direct renal effect and by inhibition of secretion of aldosterone. ANP is an endogenous antagonist to AII, and binding sites for these two compounds overlap (Giles, 1990). During physical exercise, release of ANP may be important in counteracting the undesirable effects of vasoconstrictor norepinephrine. In patients with congestive cardiac failure, circulating levels of ANP are increased to counter the prevailing sodium and volume overload, but the ANP receptors become resistant to its effects (Giles, 1990).

Control of Peripheral Vascular Resistance

How is the PVR generated? It will be recalled that the high systolic and diastolic pressures in the aorta decrease abruptly at the level of the arterioles. The diameter of the arterioles therefore controls the PVR according to Poiseuille's law (see Fig. 12-15), which can be simplified into the following statement: *The resistance is inversely related to the fourth power of the radius.* Halving the radius will therefore increase the PVR by 16 times. The major mechanisms controlling the PVR depend on two major signalling systems and on the vascular endothelium (Table 14-2).

TABLE 14-2. *Contrasting regulation of contraction in myocardium and vascular smooth muscle*

	Myocardium	Vascular smooth muscle
Major agonists	β-adrenergic	α-adrenergic, AII, ET, β2
Major messengers	cAMP	IP$_3$ and cyclic nucleotides
Histology	Striated	Smooth, nonstriated
Metabolic rate	High	Low
Rate of contraction and relaxation	Fast	Slow; maintains tone: latch mechanism
Site of calcium effect	Troponin-C	Myosin light-chain kinase
cAMP effects	Contract	Relax
cGMP effects	Inhibitory (modest effect)	Relax (powerful effect)

IP$_3$, inositol trisphosphate; ET, endothelin; β2, β2-adrenergic.

1. *IP₃-dependent vasoconstrictory system.* There are three major vascular receptors linked to the formation of inositol-1,4,5-trisphosphate (IP_3). These receptors respond to agonists that reflect neurogenic, neurohumoral, and endothelial function (Fig. 14-6). First, the α_1-adrenergic vasoconstrictor system operates via norepinephrine (NE) released from terminal neurons in response to adrenergic stimulation. Second, AII, the end product of renin release, is a major constrictor in its own right in addition to its indirect actions via norepinephrine. Third, endothelin is another powerfully vasoconstrictory peptide, released from the damaged endothelium. The apparently contradictory properties of endothelin as a physiologic vasodilator and pathophysiologic constrictor are discussed in Chapter 9.

2. *Cyclic nucleotide vasodilatory system.* Although the inhibition of vascular contraction by cyclic adenosine monophosphate (cAMP) and cGMP is complex in its mechanism, a useful simplification is that they both inhibit myosin light-chain kinase (see Fig. 9-5) and thereby promote vasodilation. cAMP increases in response to β-adrenergic vasodilation. There are vasodilatory β-receptors (β_2 and to a lesser extent β_1 in nature) in arterioles, especially in skeletal muscle but also in the coronary arterioles. These respond to circulating epinephrine released from the adrenal gland in response to severe stress or emotion. For reasons not well understood, NE released from the nerve terminals predominantly stimulates the vasoconstrictory α_1 receptors. cGMP increases in response to stimulation of the NO messenger system, as is thought to occur during exercise. Therefore, the endothelium has potentially both vasoconstrictory and vasodilatory functions, which will now be considered.

3. *Endothelial control of vascular resistance.* The established concept is that the healthy endothelium releases vasodilatory NO and the damaged

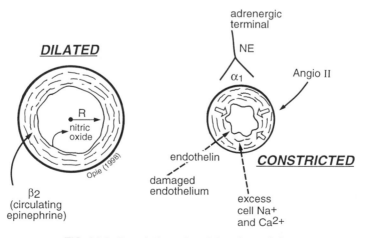

FIG. 14-6. Regulation of peripheral arterioles.

endothelium releases vasoconstrictory endothelin (see Fig. 9-2). Hence, endothelial integrity is important in maintenance of coronary and peripheral vascular tone. Endothelin is so well known as a vasoconstrictor that it was surprising to find that, in a mouse knock-out model, the total absence of endothelin led not to hypotension but rather to hypertension (Kurihara et al., 1994). The revised concept is that endothelin in low physiologic concentrations can vasodilate, acting on the vasodilatory ET_B receptors on the endothelium to release NO. In contrast, the vasoconstrictory receptors on the vascular smooth muscle cells are thought to be ET_A in nature, though these distinctions are not absolute (see Chapter 9).

Besides NO, other vasodilators that are synthesized include prostacyclin (PGI_2) and endothelium-derived hyperpolarizing factor, the latter still awaiting identification. A wide range of other vasoactive substances acts through endothelium-derived factors or through metabolic activity of the endothelium. These include acetylcholine, bradykinin, arachidonic acid, histamine, 5-hydroxy-tryptamine (serotonin), substance P, and vasopressin. Hypoxia, thrombin, and oxygen-derived free radicals inhibit the activity of vasodilator endothelial substances or increase the release of endothelin. Physiologic and pathologic effects on shear stress need to be distinguished. Physiologically, shear stress, as during increased blood flow, leads to release of NO and flow-induced vasodilation, but excess shear stress, as in sustained arterial hypertension, can damage the endothelium, with impaired release of NO and excess release of endothelin.

Myogenic Properties.   Quite independently of the autonomic input, the arterioles respond to an increase in transmural pressure, as in hypertension or acute BP elevation, by contracting, which is to some extent a counterproductive response that will further increase the PVR and hence BP. Nonetheless, this increase in the wall tension is mechanically required to offset the tendency of the increased intraluminal pressure to split the arteriole open (two halves forced apart).

Response of Skin to Heat and Cold.   Vascular tone can be viewed as a balance between the vasoconstrictory and vasodilatory influences, the balance resulting in the degree of tone that in turn governs the arteriolar diameter and the PVR. Nonetheless, vasoconstriction as an overall concept includes three separate events of which only one determines arteriolar tone: first, an increase of arteriolar tone (resistance vessels); second, an increase of venous tone (capacitance vessels); and, third, increased cutaneous constriction as in response to cold. Not all of these may happen at the same time: the old adage recalls the combination of "warm heart, cold hands" in response to adrenergic stimulation, the cold hands resulting from constrictor cutaneous fibers.

By means of specific drugs (e.g., calcium channel blockers) or β_2-receptor stimulation, peripheral arteriolar vasodilation can be obtained independently of exercise. Such vasodilation is not the same as heat-induced vasodilation, where physiologic necessity diverts blood to the skin. There may be such marked cutaneous vasodilation that blood can even be diverted from the muscles and the central blood volume can decrease, decreasing the left ventricular (LV) filling pressure (right atrial pressure) and making exercise in such conditions impossible. By contrast, in standard conditions where an excessively increased ambient temperature is not the dominant factor and where maintenance of central blood volume is possible, cutaneous vasodilation can occur without adverse redistribution of the circulation. Thus, the balance between the PVR and the cardiac output is maintained so that BP is as close to normal as possible.

Other Regional Circulations.   Organs such as brain and heart that need continuous perfusion have circulations that are relatively independent of circulatory control mechanisms, and autoregulation becomes more important. During exercise, up to 90% of the cardiac output may be diverted to the working muscles, and prominent vasodilation is required. Thus, sympathetic vasoconstriction that dominates at rest gives way to metabolic vasodilation. On the other hand, the blood flow to the splanchnic circulation is not essential during states of fight or flight, so that vasoconstriction and diversion of blood to the exercising muscle and myocardium is achieved.

DIFFERENT BLOOD PRESSURE RESPONSES

Diurnal Blood Pressure Variation

BP is not static over 24 hours but highly variable. The nocturnal decrease in BP is associated with vagal activity. Upon awakening, withdrawal of vagal tone and adrenergic "spurt" lead to early morning hypertension (Fig. 1-9). Thereafter, BP usually decreases gradually throughout the day, but may increase during occupational stresses. Usually heart rate and BP vary together, yet BP changes relatively less than heart rate because of reflex compensatory variations in the PVR.

Mental Stress

In normal subjects, mental stress increases plasma epinephrine and norepinephrine. Heart rate increases considerably and BP only modestly (Fig. 14-7). The probable explanation for the relatively small increase in BP is that adrenergic activation causes both muscular vasodilation (β-receptors in arterioles) and vasoconstriction in the splanchic bed. In hypertensive or prehypertensive patients, the PVR increases as does the cardiac output, and there appears to be little or no decrease in the resistance in muscular arterioles. In other words, there is a greater tendency toward vasoconstriction (α greater than β effects). This is the basis of the neurogenic theory of hypertension whereby repetitive transient BP increases become fixed.

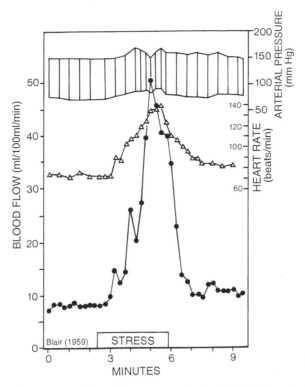

FIG. 14-7. Effect of severe emotional stress on systemic arterial BP, heart rate (Δ) and fore-arm blood flow (•) in a normal medical student. The marked increase in heart rate is due to increased sympathetic nerve activity to the sinus node and to circulating epinephrine released from the adrenal medulla. The striking increase in forearm blood flow is due to the circulating epinephrine stimulating vasodilatory β_2-adrenergic receptors in the skeletal muscle resistance vessels. The increase in BP is caused by a greater increase in cardiac output than decrease in PVR. From Blair et al. (1959) with permission.

Acute Exercise

BP increases during exercise, with different patterns for static and dynamic exercise (see Fig. 15-2). This acute increase is followed by some hours of BP decrease, depending on the intensity of the exercise. There may be different responses to exercise in normal individuals and in hypertensive patients, and between younger and older individuals. In normal individuals, it is chiefly the systolic BP that increases during exercise because concomitant metabolically driven peripheral vasodilation will decrease diastolic BP, which would otherwise increase as the stroke volume increased (Fig. 14-8).

Effects of Age on Blood Pressure

With increasing age, the systolic BP increases so that values over 140 mm Hg become common (Fig. 14-9). This physiologic pressure increase is now regarded

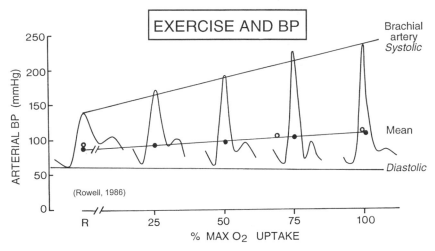

FIG. 14-8. Effect of exercise on BP in the brachial artery and aorta. Note increased systolic blood pressure. Modified from Rowell, *Human Circulation,* Oxford University Press, New York, 1986.

as an adverse response and is treatable. The two major factors are (1) loss of the buffer function of the aorta as its elasticity decreases (Fig. 14-10) and (2) the increased intraluminal aortic pressure resulting from the increase of PVR with age (Tonkin and Wing, 1994). The stiffened aorta conducts the pulse wave faster in both directions, forward and backward, so that the characteristic abrupt increase and decrease of the pulse wave in the elderly can be explained (Fig. 14-11).

In a unique study, Lund-Johansen (1991) observed a selected number of normal and hypertensive subjects for 20 years and studied them invasively during

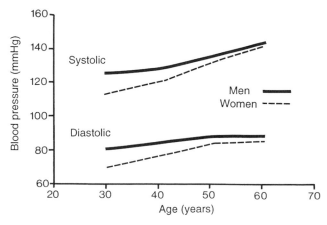

FIG. 14-9. Blood pressure with age. Note progressive increase in systolic BP. From Whelton, *Lancet* 1994;344:102, with permission.

EARLY-SYSTOLE   MID-SYSTOLE   END-SYTOLE

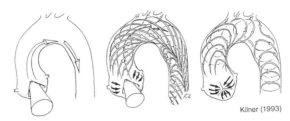

Kilner (1993)

FIG. 14-10. Aortic hemodynamics during systole. With increasing age, the elasticity of the aorta decreases. Aortic impedance is one important component of the afterload, the other being the arterial BP (see Fig. 12-10). From Kilner, *Circulation* 1993;88:2235. Copyright American Heart Association.

exercise. The striking feature was that in the younger hypertensive patients, cardiac output and heart rate were higher than normal, in agreement with the increased adrenergic drive postulated by the neurogenic theory. With aging, the PVR increased and the stroke volume decreased (Fig. 14-12). The increase in PVR was presumably due to degenerative changes in the arterioles caused by loss of elasticity or endothelial damage, and the decreasing stroke volume possibly due to increasing myocardial fibrosis with age.

Physiologic Versus Pathologic Changes in the Elderly. It could be argued that the systolic hypertension that is common with aging is physiologic in origin, whereas true hypertension with elevations of both systolic and diastolic pressure is pathologic, as in younger ages. As a group, the elderly are high-risk patients, and treatment is about 40 times more effective in avoiding cardiovascular complications than in the middle-aged. The frequent therapeutic response to low-dose diuretics suggests that this type of hypertension is low renin and salt sensitive, so that by implication a low-salt diet becomes desirable with aging. Systolic hypertension, even though physiologic in origin, also should be treated.

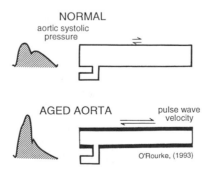

FIG. 14-11. The aged aorta. Effect on pulse wave velocity. Modified from O'Rourke, *The Arterial Pulse,* Lea and Febinger, Philadelphia, 1992.

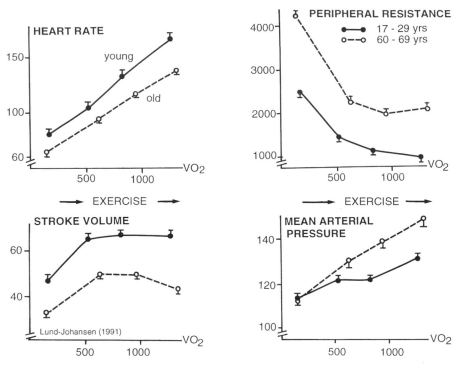

FIG. 14-12. Exercise effects on young and old hypertensive patients. Note increased stroke volume and heart rate in younger subjects and increased peripheral resistance in older group. From Lund-Johansen (1991) with permission. Copyright American Heart Association.

Pseudohypertension. Pseudohypertension of the elderly is a condition in which BP as measured by the cuff overestimates the true arterial BP. Supposedly this problem can be avoided if Osler's maneuver is used, which means that when systolic BP is increased to 50 mmHg above the systolic value during the cuff procedure, the wall of the artery should be impalpable (Osler negative). If it stays palpable (Osler positive), then pseudohypertension may be suspected. This test did not work when invasively evaluated (Kuwajima et al., 1990).

BLOOD PRESSURE AND AFTERLOAD

During systole, the left ventricle contracts against the afterload (the load after the onset of contraction, against which the left ventricle contracts during LV ejection). In the simplified model of the circulation, it is the PVR against which the heart contracts (see Fig. 2-14). When this resistance increases, BP increases and the afterload increases. Generally, in clinical practice, it is a sufficient approximation to take the arterial BP as a measure of the afterload, provided there is no significant aortic stenosis or change in arterial compliance. Nonetheless, this approximation can be wrong, as when arterial compliance decreases in the elderly.

Wall Stress and Afterload. The afterload, being the load on the contracting myocardium, is also the wall stress after the onset of systole. Increased afterload means that an increased intraventricular pressure has to be generated first to open the aortic valve and then to eject the blood during the ejection phase. These increases will translate themselves into an increased myocardial wall stress, which can be measured either as an average value throughout systole or at a given phase of systole, such as end-systole. *Systolic wall stress* reflects the two major components of the afterload, namely arterial BP and arterial compliance. Decreased arterial compliance and increased afterload can be anticipated when there is aortic dilation, as in severe systemic hypertension or in the elderly.

Aortic Impedance. Aortic impedance (arterial input impedance) gives another accurate measure of the afterload. The aortic impedance is the aortic pressure divided by the aortic flow at that instance, so this index of the afterload varies at each stage of the contraction cycle. Factors reducing aortic flow, such as a high arterial BP, aortic stenosis, or loss of aortic compliance, will increase impedance and hence the afterload. During systole, when the aortic valve is open, an increased afterload will communicate itself to the ventricles by increasing wall stress. In LV failure, aortic impedance is augmented not only by peripheral vaso-constriction but by decreases in aortic compliance (Eaton et al., 1993). The problem with the clinical measurement of aortic impedance is that invasive instrumentation is required. An approximation can be found by using transesophageal echocardiography to determine aortic blood flow, for example, at the time of maximal increase of aortic flow just after aortic valve opening.

Anrep Effect. When the afterload is abruptly increased by rapid elevation of the aortic pressure, then a positive inotropic effect follows within 1 or 2 minutes. This change used to be called homeometric autoregulation (Greek *homoios,* the same; *metric,* length), because it was apparently independent of muscle length and by definition a true inotropic effect. A reasonable speculation would be that increased LV wall tension could act on myocardial stretch receptors to increase cytosolic sodium and then by sodium–calcium exchange elevate the cytosolic calcium (Kent et al., 1989). Thus, this effect would be different from that of an increase in preload (which acts by length–activation). Physiologically and in normal humans, a sudden increase in BP is compensated for by an increased force of contraction, here described as the Anrep effect, and by a reflex decrease of the PVR, mediated by the baroreflexes.

HYPERTENSION: A GREATER THAN NORMAL BLOOD PRESSURE LEVEL

In systemic arterial hypertension there is an upset of the complex regulation of the circulation so that BP consistently runs above the normal range. Because BP is so variable and there is a spectrum of values from normal to abnormal, any cut-off point must be arbitrary. A sustained (taken frequently) BP value of the resting seated subject exceeding 140/90 mm Hg is generally regarded as too high. Only 5% of all hypertensive patients present with secondary hypertension caused by another abnormality such as an endocrine or renal disease. The remainder have *essential hypertension,* a complex condition of variable etiology. Either the PVR is too high in absolute terms (as in most middle-aged or elderly hypertensive patients) or the PVR fails to decrease when the cardiac output increases (as in younger hypertensive patients). The mechanism for the absolute or relative failure of peripheral vasodilation is complex and still not fully clarified.

Multifactorial Origin of Essential Hypertension

In most cases, several different factors acting over many years contribute to the development of essential hypertension, which is a heterogeneous disease that is multifactorial in origin. The basic concept is a resetting of control mechanisms at a higher than normal BP level. For BP to increase requires a sustained increase in either the cardiac output or the PVR, because $BP = CO \times PVR$. Normally the baroreflexes would compensate for any increase in either cardiac output or PVR; therefore, there is impaired baroreflex sensitivity in hypertension (Zanchetti and Mancia, 1991). An increase in cardiac output is more commonly observed in younger hypertensive patients, and an increase in PVR is more commonly observed in the older group (Lund-Johansen, 1991).

Neurogenic Theory. The *neurogenic theory* for hypertension takes into account that the early phase of hypertension is often characterized by features suggestive of enhanced adrenergic activity, such as tachycardia and an increased cardiac output (Julius and Nesbitt, 1996) (Fig. 14-12). Over the years, there is a transition from the high cardiac output to an increased PVR, which could hypothetically be the result of several factors, such as increased vasoconstriction (AII- or adrenergic-mediated), damage to the endothelium resulting from BP surges, and loss of elasticity in the arterioles with age. Hypothetically, decreased formation of NO and increased formation of endothelin could increase PVR as a result of chronic pressure-induced damage to the endothelium.

Abnormalities of Sodium Handling. *Abnormalities of sodium handling by the kidneys* explain why, in all forms of hypertension, the normal pressure-induced excretion of sodium in the urine (natriuresis) is reset to a higher BP level (Stanley et al., 1994). An interesting hypothesis attempts to link decreased natriuresis by the kidney of hypertensive patients to excess retention of intracellular sodium in vascular smooth muscle (Fig. 14-13). The operation of sodium–calcium exchange then promotes an increased cytosolic calcium and vasoconstriction. Alternatively or additionally, there may be a membrane defect in sodium transport so that vascular cells retain too much sodium. These hypotheses would also

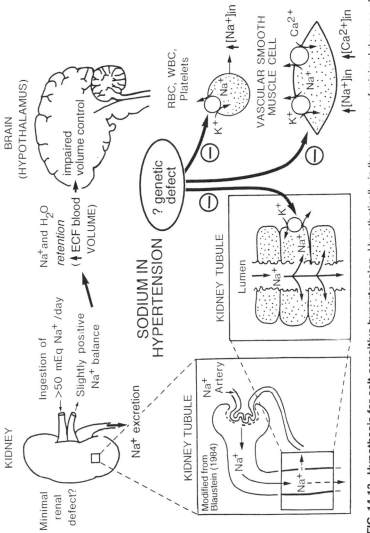

FIG. 14-13. Hypothesis for salt-sensitive hypertension. Hypothetically, in the presence of minimal degrees of a genetically determined renal defect, small amounts of sodium are retained so that the extracellular fluid (ECF) volume is increased with release of the proposed natriuretic hormone natriuretic from the hypothalamus. This hormone inhibits sodium–potassium exchange in vascular smooth muscle. Cell sodium in the myocyte increases to increase calcium via the sodium–calcium exchange to enhance vascular tone. Modified from Blaustein (1984) with permission.

explain the antihypertensive effect of a low salt diet and of diuretic compounds. But not all forms of hypertension are salt sensitive.

Salt-Sensitive Hypertension.   Certain individuals are more prone than others to develop hypertension when their diet is salt loaded, and there is a broad relationship between the salt intake of a population and mean BP levels. Logically, there should be abnormalities of renal handling of sodium in salt-sensitive hypertensive patients, with delayed salt excretion, as more commonly found in African-Americans and in the elderly (Campese et al., 1991; Luft et al., 1991).

Obesity.   Although obesity is commonly associated with hypertension, the mechanism remains ill defined. Because of the greater body mass of the obese, the blood volume is also greater and the cardiac output tends to increase. For reasons not well understood, there may be activation of the adrenergic system in obesity (Hall et al., 1996), so that in some ways the circulation resembles that of the hyperkinetic younger hypertensive patients. Two other factors are involved: increased intra-abdominal fat and pressure that impair renal function, as well as insulin resistance.

Insulin Resistance.   *Metabolic cardiovascular syndrome, Reaven's syndrome, and Syndrome X* are all names for the clinical manifestations of insulin resistance as a pentad of hypertension, obesity, maturity-onset type II diabetes, arte-

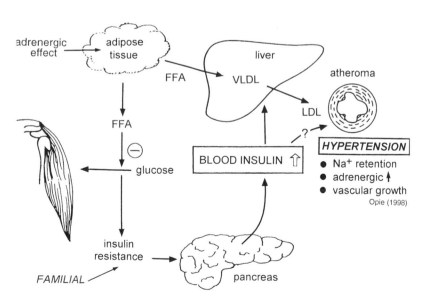

FIG. 14-14. Insulin resistance. Proposed sequence of events leading to insulin resistance. Based on inhibition of uptake of glucose by circulating free fatty acids. VLDL, very low density lipoproteins.

riosclerosis, and blood lipid disorders. This condition is present when the ability of insulin to stimulate the uptake and metabolism of glucose by muscle is impaired (Fig. 14-14). As a group, hypertensive patients suffer from insulin resistance, although the links are more marked in the obese than in the non-obese (Reaven et al., 1996). Insulin resistance is also associated with increased adrenergic activity, either being the cause of the increase (Meehan et al., 1994) or the consequence (Jamerson et al., 1994). Insulin resistance also may account for the increased tendency toward abnormalities of blood lipid profile in hypertensive patients and especially in the obese.

Low Renin Hypertension in Specific Population Groups.   The elderly and black patients are thought, as a group, to have relatively low renin values and to be prone to salt-sensitive hypertension. Normally, salt loading leads to increased tubular reabsorption of sodium, with inhibition of renin release, less formation of AII, and less constriction of the efferent renal arterioles (Fig. 14-4). In low renin groups, this compensatory mechanism is impaired. These observations have therapeutic implications, because salt restriction and diuretics work best in low renin states.

Endothelium-Derived Factors in Hypertension.   Do endothelin or NO play a role in hypertension? One popular hypothesis asserts that the increased intraluminal pressure damages the endothelium to allow release of endothelin and to inhibit the release of NO. The ensuing vasoconstriction helps to perpetuate the hypertension. Nonetheless, the evidence is not clear cut. Whereas physiologic levels of endothelin are probably vasodilatory, pathophysiologically, as in human hypertension, there is incomplete evidence that endothelin could contribute to arteriolar constriction and an increase in PVR (Schiffrin, 1995). NO is an extremely evanescent compound, suggesting that it primarily mediates rapid vasodilation. This does not mean that the role of the endothelium is inconsequential in hypertension. The injection of inhibitors of NO in experimental ani-

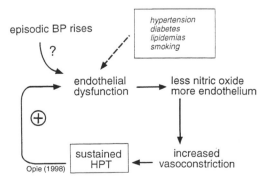

FIG. 14-15. Endothelial dysfunction and its hypothetical role in perpetuation of hypertension.

mals produces immediate and sustained increases in BP, which is reversible by administration of the NO precursor L-arginine. An attractive hypothesis is that endothelial dysfunction could result in decreased release of NO (Dominiczak and Bohr, 1995). Either hypertension causes endothelial dysfunction, or endothelial dysfunction promotes hypertension—the exact scenario involving the endothelium and the increased BP is unclear (Fig. 14-15).

LIFE-STYLE AND BLOOD PRESSURE

Besides genetic and other predisposing factors, some aspects of life-style can contribute to the development of hypertension. *Obesity* is often associated with "essential" hypertension, possibly acting through insulin resistance. In population studies, increasing dietary *salt* is associated with increasing BP levels. Excess *alcohol* (more than two or three drinks per day) appears to provoke hypertension, possibly acting through release of aldehydes that stimulate the adrenergic system. Although regular *smoking* alone does not alter resting diastolic BP (taken when the patient is not actually smoking), ambulatory BP measurements show that smoking, via its vasoconstrictive effects, is likely to increase BP swings and, possibly, to help promote endothelial damage and thereby the hypertensive state. *Emotional stress* promotes temporary BP increases and could therefore in the long-term contribute to the development of hypertension. Stress may act indirectly via excess smoking, smoking plus coffee, lack of exercise, and poor nutrition.

Conversely, *endurance exercise training* by regular isotonic aerobic exercise may help to reduce resting BP, in addition to promoting weight reduction, improving the sense of well-being, and lessening cardiovascular risk. Such training appears to enhance vagal activity and to decrease sympathetic activity. *A monastic environment* also protects. Nuns living in a stress-free environment characterized by silence, meditation, and isolation from society avoid the otherwise inevitable increase of BP with age (Timio et al., 1988).

CARDIAC COMPLICATIONS OF HYPERTENSION

Whatever its cause, hypertension significantly increases both morbidity and mortality. The incidence of coronary artery disease, stroke, and renal dysfunction are all increased. There is no simple relationship between arterial BP level and the complications of hypertension, except for BP and stroke. All vital organs can be affected except those protected by special circulations such as the liver and lungs. Cardiovascular complications are described below.

Left ventricular hypertrophy (LVH) is the consequence of a sustained pressure overload. It is often associated with diastolic dysfunction. In contrast, systolic failure with congestive heart failure may be the end result of sustained overload (see Chapter 16). Another disadvantage of LVH is that the coronary vascular reserve is diminished, possibly the result of endothelial dysfunction.

Coronary artery disease is the most common cause of death in hypertensive patients in the western world. BP lowering in trials has not yielded the expected reduction in coronary disease, perhaps because its multifactorial etiology would mandate simultaneous reduction of blood lipids, as well as smoking cessation.

Coronary endothelial dysfunction can occur even in the absence of angiographically visible coronary disease, as shown by the decreased coronary dilation in response to exercise in hypertensive patients (Frielingsdorf et al., 1996).

Aortic aneurysm is often preceded by marked aortic unfolding. Its presence indicates a marked loss of aortic elasticity and therefore an increased afterload on the heart. Other vascular complications include the spectrum of cerebrovascular disease and renal artery stenosis.

VASCULAR RESPONSE IN PATHOPHYSIOLOGIC STATES

The possible role of the endothelium in disease states is currently under intense scrutiny. There are several disease states characterized by poor vasodilatory responses to acetylcholine, implying the existence of endothelial damage. These states include systemic hypertension, coronary artery disease, congestive heart failure, and vein graft rejection (Ishii et al., 1993). The endothelium, by its potent vasodilatory and antiaggregatory platelet effects, may have an important role in delaying the progress of these different types of arterial disease. This protective role of the endothelium draws attention to the number of vasoconstrictory conditions in which excess vasoconstriction predominates to exert potentially harmful effects on the heart and circulation. Such states include hypertension, congestive heart failure, and ischemic reperfusion.

SUMMARY

1. *Baroreflexes* are high-pressure mechanoreceptors that are important in the acute buffering of blood pressure (BP) changes. For example, an acute increase in BP evokes a baroreflex-mediated decrease in cardiac output and decrease in peripheral vascular resistance (PVR), as a result of increased vagal and decreased sympathetic outflows.
2. *Low-pressure cardiopulmonary receptors* react to changes in blood volume by altering autonomic discharge rate in such a way that fluid overload is accompanied by a decreased PVR, with converse changes when the blood volume is too low and the receptors not normally stimulated.
3. *Renin-angiotensin system.* Both high- and low-pressure receptors couple to the renin-angiotensin systems. During acute hypertension or fluid overload, adrenergic discharge rate is decreased, the PVR decreases, and release of renin from the kidneys is diminished. Conversely, during hypotension or too low a circulating blood volume, increased adrenergic discharge induces a β_1-mediated release of renin, which leads to increased angiotensin II and peripheral vasoconstriction. Angiotensin II increases BP by multiple mech-

anisms beyond peripheral vasoconstriction, including adrenergic facilitation and baroreflex inhibition.

4. *Peripheral vascular resistance.* The PVR is an important regulator of BP. Vasoconstriction or vasodilation by altering the PVR increases or decreases BP because $BP = CO \times PVR$, where CO is the cardiac output. The PVR is regulated by at least three factors: (1) autonomic control with α_1-mediated constriction in contrast to vagally or β_2-mediated vasodilation; (2) vasoconstrictory neurohormones such as angiotensin II; and (3) endothelial control (endothelin versus nitric oxide).

5. *Hypertension* is a state of chronically elevated BP, usually multifactorial in origin, with an increased cardiac output playing an important role in younger subjects and an increased PVR being more important in the older group.

6. *Role of aorta.* The aorta has a dual role in relation to BP control. First and physiologically, it is an important part of the afterload, which is therefore not only composed of the PVR and reflected in BP. Second, systolic hypertension in the elderly is the direct result of decreased compliance of the aorta.

7. *Role of endothelium.* Although no simple relationship exists between circulating endothelin levels and chronic hypertension, an attractive hypothesis is that the mechanical strains imposed by the high intravascular pressure could damage the endothelium to release more endothelin and less nitric oxide. This change may explain the impaired coronary dilation found in hypertensive patients.

STUDENT QUESTIONS

1. Outline the major differences in the regulation of the contraction in the myocardium and in vascular smooth muscle.
2. Describe the defense mechanisms of the body against hypotension.
3. What is Poiseuille's law, and describe how operation of this law could influence the blood pressure.
4. Describe in detail how the peripheral vascular resistance (total peripheral resistance) increases in response to standing.
5. What changes may be found in the afterload in chronic arterial hypertension?

CARDIOLOGIST-IN-TRAINING QUESTIONS

1. What is the neurogenic theory for hypertension? How can it explain the increase in the peripheral vascular resistance with age, as found in hypertensive patients?
2. When a subject enters a cold environment, the blood pressure increases. Describe in detail the physiologic changes involved.

3. Why does the systolic blood pressure increase with age but the diastolic tend to remain the same? What is the reason for the characteristic pattern of the peripheral pulse in the elderly?
4. In hypertensive patients, there may be impaired coronary vascular dilation. Why is this?
5. Describe the role of the renin-angiotensin system in blood pressure control.

REFERENCES

1. Blair DA, Glover WE, Greenfield ADM, Roddie IC. Excitation of cholinergic vasolidator nerves to human skeletal muscles during emotional stress. *J Physiol* 1959;148:633–647.
2. Blaustein MP, Hamlyn JM. Sodium transport inhibition, cell calcium and hypertension. The natriuretic hormone/Na^+-Ca^{2+} exchange/hypotension hypothesis. *Am J Med* 1984;77(suppl A4):45–59.
3. Campese VM, Parise M, Karubian F, Bigazzi R. Abnormal renal hemodynamics in black salt-sensitive patients with hypertension. *Hypertension* 1991;18:805–812.
4. Dominiczak AF, Bohr DF. Nitric oxide and its putative role in hypertension. *Hypertension* 1995;25:1202–1211.
5. Eaton GM, Cody RJ, Binkley PF. Increased aortic impedance precedes peripheral vasoconstriction at the early stage of ventricular failure in the paced canine model. *Circulation* 1993;88:2714–2721.
6. Frielingsdorf J, Seiler C, Kaufmann P, et al. Normalisation of abnormal coronary vasomotion by calcium antagonists in patients with hypertension. *Circulation* 1996;93:1380–1387.
7. Giles TD. Defining the role of atrial natriuretic factor in health and disease. *J Am Coll Cardiol* 1990;15:1331–1333.
8. Hall JE, Zappe DH, Alonso-Galicia M, et al. Mechanisms of obesity-induced hypertension. *News Physiol Sci* 1996;11:255–261.
9. Ishii T, Okadome K, Komari K, et al. Natural course of endothelium-dependent and independent responses in autogenous femoral veins grafted into the arterial circulation of the dog. *Circ Res* 1993;72:1004–1010.
10. Jamerson KA, Smith SD, Amerena JV, et al. Vasoconstriction with norepinephrine causes less forearm insulin resistance than a reflex sympathetic vasoconstriction. *Hypertension* 1994;23:1006–1011.
11. Julius S, Nesbitt S. Sympathetic overactivity in hypertension. A moving target. *Am J Hypertens* 1996;9(suppl):113–120.
12. Kappagoda CT, Linden RJ, Sivananthan N. The nature of the atrial receptors responsible for a reflex increase in heart rate in the dog. *J Physiol* 1979;291:393–412.
13. Kent RL, Hoober K, Cooper G. Load responsiveness of protein synthesis in adult mammalian myocardium: role of cardiac deformation linked to sodium influx. *Circ Res* 1989;64:74–85.
14. Kurihara Y, Kurihara H, Suzuki H, et al. Elevated blood pressure and craniofacial abnormalities in mice deficient in endothelin-1. *Nature* 1994;368:703–710.
15. Kuwajima I, Hoh E, Suzuki Y, et al. Pseudohypertension in the elderly. *J Hypertens* 1990;8:429–432.
16. Luft FC, Miller JZ, Grim CE, et al. Salt sensitive and resistance of blood pressure. Age and race as factors in physiological responses. *Hypertension* 1991;17(suppl I):102–108.
17. Lund-Johansen P. Twenty-year follow up of hemodynamics in essential hypertension during rest and exercise. *Hypertension* 1991;18:54–61.
18. Mancia G, Romero JC, Shepherd JT. Continuous inhibition of renin release in dogs by vagally innervated receptors in the cardiopulmonary region. *Circ Res* 1975;36:529–535.
19. Meehan WP, Buchanan TA, Hsueh W. Chronic insulin administration elevates blood pressure in rats. *Hypertension* 1994;23:1012–1017.
20. Reaven G, Lithell H, Landsberg L. Hypertension and associated metabolic abnormalities—the role of insulin resistance and the sympathoadrenal system. *N Engl J Med* 1996;334:374–381.
21. Reid IA. Angiotensin II and baroreflex control of heart rate. *News Physiol Sci* 1996;11:270–274.
22. Roddie IC, Shepherd JT. Receptors in the high-pressure and low-pressure vascular systems. Their role in the reflex control of the human circulation. *Lancet* 1958;493–496.
23. Schiffrin EL. Endothelin: Potential role in hypertension and vascular hypertrophy. *Hypertension* 1995;25:1135–1143.

24. Stanley WC, Hall JL, Smith KR, et al. Myocardial glucose transporters and glycolytic metabolism during ischemia in hyperglycaemic diabetic swine. *Metabolism* 1994;43:61–69.
25. Timio M, Verdecchia P, Venanzi S, et al. Age and blood pressure changes. A 20-year follow-up study. *Hypertension* 1988;12:457–461.
26. Tonkin AL, Wing LM. Effects of age and isolated systolic hypertension on cardiovascular reflexes. *J Hypertens* 1994;12:1083–1088.
27. Vatner SF, Boettcher DH. Regulation of cardiac output by stroke volume and heart rate in conscious dogs. *Circ Res* 1978;42:557–561.
28. Vatner SF, Boettcher DH, Heyndrickx GR, McRitchie RJ. Reduced baroreflex sensitivity with volume loading in conscious dogs. *Circ Res* 1975;37:236–242.
29. Zanchetti A, Mancia G. Cardiovascular reflexes and hypertension. *Hypertension* 1991;18:III-13–III-21.

15

Cardiac Output and Exercise

The cardiac output is the volume of blood pumped by the heart. During dynamic exercise the increase in cardiac output is obligatory; otherwise, the exercising myocardium and skeletal muscle cannot obtain the required oxygen and nutrients. During emotional stress the increase of cardiac output is not essential but is a physiologic side effect of sympathetic stimulation.

The *definition of the cardiac output* is the product of the stroke volume (SV) and the heart rate (HR):

$$\text{Cardiac output (Q)} = \text{SV} \times \text{HR (units = liters per minute)}.$$

The normal value is about 6 to 8 L/min, doubling or sometimes even tripling during peak aerobic exercise. An Olympic athlete might reach 25 L/min. Of the four major factors determining the cardiac output (Fig. 15-1), the most important is the heart rate. The other three factors, namely the preload, the afterload, and the contractile state of the myocardium, all influence the stroke volume (for definitions see Table 15-1).

During dynamic exercise, it is the increased heart rate that provides most of the adaptation. In addition, there is an increased venous return, which acts by the Frank-Starling mechanism, and increased contractility, which stimulates the force of contraction. Regarding the afterload, the systolic blood pressure increases during exercise despite the peripheral vasodilation. Thus, the healthy heart can readily deal with all the hemodynamic changes occurring during exercise. By contrast, the failing myocardium cannot cope with the increased peripheral resistance that results from angiotensin II and other vasoconstrictors.

There are important conceptual distinctions between an increased cardiac output and increased work of the heart, although these two entities are easy to confuse. An increased cardiac output is the result of external cardiac work, whereas internal work can be much increased, as in the case of the hypertrophied myocardium, without an obligatory increase in external work. When the work of the heart increases considerably during isometric exercise, the cardiac output increases relatively little. Another conspicuous difference between heart work

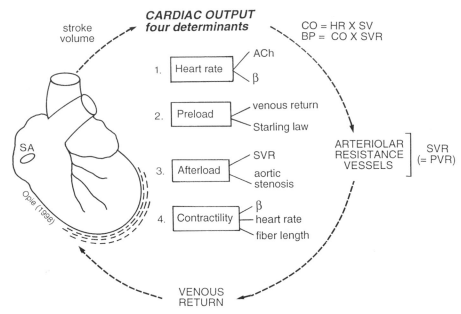

FIG. 15-1. Major factors regulating cardiac output (CO). Heart rate is regulated chiefly by the relative inputs of cholinergic (ACh) and β-adrenergic (β) stimulation. Preload is regulated by the venous return and also increases when the left ventricle fails to empty fully. Afterload increases when the peripheral vascular resistance (PVR) increases or when there is aortic stenosis. Contractility increases with β-stimulation or with increased fiber lengths. SV, stroke volume; HR, heart rate. SVR = systemic vascular resistance = PVR.

and cardiac output is found in the failing heart, which is afterload dependent (see Chapter 16). In this serious situation, further increases in the peripheral resistance decrease the cardiac output even though the work of the heart is increased. In other words, the oxygen demand increases even though the cardiac output decreases. These distinctions emphasize the potential differences between the effects of increased cardiac output and increased heart work on myocardial oxygen uptake.

TABLE 15-1. *Definition of determinants of cardiac output*

Term	Definition
Heart rate	Number of heart beats per minute (complete cardiac cycle).
Preload	The LV volume at the end of diastole; this is frequently approximated as the LV end-diastolic pressure, assuming normal compliance and pressure-volume relations.
Afterload	The resistance against the ejection of blood, including the peripheral vascular resistance, any aortic valve stenosis, the aortic impedance, and the blood distending the left ventricle at the end of diastole.
Contractility	The inherent capacity of the myocardium to contract independently of changes in preload and afterload.

CARDIAC OUTPUT, BLOOD PRESSURE, AND EXERCISE

The cardiac output is related to the blood pressure and peripheral vascular resistance by the following equation (see Chapter 14):

$$BP = \text{cardiac output} \times PVR$$

Therefore,

$$BP = SV \times HR \times PVR$$

The two contrasting types of exercise, dynamic and static, have different consequences on these parameters (Fig. 15-2). *Dynamic exercise* (aerobic or isotonic) includes running, walking, and related sports: regular muscular activity occurs, but against a light load. Static (isometric) exercise includes such activities as carrying a suitcase or weightlifting: muscle tension develops, but there is little or no displacement of the object worked against. During dynamic running, the heart rate increases due to an early withdrawal of the normal vagal inhibition followed by β-adrenergic stimulation. The latter also increases contractility. The cardiac

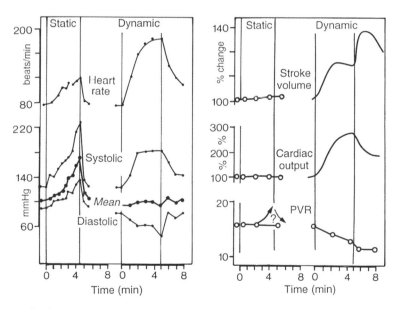

FIG. 15-2. Static versus dynamic exercise. Static exercise, at 30% of maximum voluntary contraction (MCV), caused a much larger increase in mean blood pressure than did dynamic exercise, for the first three minutes at oxygen consumption values of 28.5 ml/kg/min and then at 43.8 ml/kg/min. Conversely, dynamic exercise increased heart rate much more. For original data, see Lind and McNicol (1967). Data on stroke volume are extrapolated from Flamm et al. (1990). Peripheral vascular resistance (PVR) for 0 to 2 minutes is based on the data of Waldrop et al. (1996), and for 2 to 4 minutes on those of Lind and McNicol (1967), shown above, in which the blood pressure increases markedly at 2 to 4 minutes of static exercise even when the increase in heart rate has leveled off; therefore, the PVR must have increased.

output increases substantially because both the heart rate and the stroke volume increase. The total peripheral resistance decreases as a result of exercise-induced metabolic dilation of arterioles in skeletal muscle, so that the diastolic blood pressure decreases to a variable extent. In contrast, the systolic blood pressure increases because increased contractility means that the blood is ejected more rapidly from the left ventricle to hit the elasticity of the major blood vessels, which expand more, to elevate the systolic pressure. There is concurrent splanchnic vasoconstriction, so that the distribution of the cardiac output moves from the abdominal viscera to the exercising muscles and the heart.

In contrast, during *static exercise,* both systolic and diastolic blood pressure increase, with the heart rate increasing only modestly (Fig. 15-2). Stroke volume is unchanged, so that cardiac output increases only in proportion to the heart rate. The peripheral vascular resistance increases relatively little at low loads with variable increases at high loads. The increase in both systolic and diastolic blood pressure is accounted for by a combination of (1) the increase in cardiac output and (2) *pressor reflexes* originating in the exercising muscles. For example, when the muscle mass involved in static exercise is ischemic, the blood pressure can increase while the heart rate is relatively unchanged (Gandevia and Hobbs, 1990). All of these factors increase the myocardial oxygen demand during static exercise relatively more than the increase in the amount of external work performed. In contrast, during dynamic exercise the large increase in heart rate causes both the oxygen uptake and the cardiac output to increase substantially, as does the external work.

HEART RATE AND CARDIAC OUTPUT

The example of exercise shows that heart rate is among the most important variables influencing cardiac output. During dynamic exercise, the maximal

TABLE 15-2. *Factors increasing the heart rate, cardiac output, and the myocardial oxygen uptake*

β-adrenergic stimulation
   Exercise
   Emotional stress
   Early morning increase in heart rate
Decreased vagal inhibition
   Early morning increase in heart rate
   Initiation of exercise
Disease states
   Cardiac conditions (cardiac output may not increase): congestive heart failure, arrhythmias, acute myocardial infarction
   Extracardiac conditions influencing the heart: thyrotoxicosis, anemia
   Fevers
Drug-induced tachycardia
   Sympathomimetic drugs such as bronchodilators (cardiac β_2-receptors)
   Vasodilators (reflex tachycardia, β_2-agonists)

heart rate that can be reached is given by the following arbitrary but widely used formula:

$$\text{Max HR} = 220 \text{ beats/min, minus age in years.}$$

Two other physiologic factors that most consistently increase heart rate and hence cardiac output are waking up in the morning and emotional stress, both of which are associated with increased β-adrenergic stimulation.

Each cycle of contraction and relaxation performs a certain amount of work and takes up a certain amount of oxygen. The faster the heart rate, the higher the cardiac output and the higher the oxygen uptake (Table 15-2). Exceptions occur (1) when the heart rate is extremely fast, as may occur during a paroxysmal tachycardia, because an inadequate time for diastolic filling decreases the cardiac output; (2) in the presence of coronary artery disease when a less severe tachycardia decreases the stroke volume because of transient ischemic failure of the left ventricle; and (3) in left ventricular failure (LVF), when the cardiac output increases only transiently before decreasing (Fig. 15-3).

Therefore, the heart rate can have both positive and negative influences on cardiac output (Fig. 15-3). In nonexercising normal subjects, an initial increase of heart rate by the sudden onset of a supraventricular tachycardia yields the

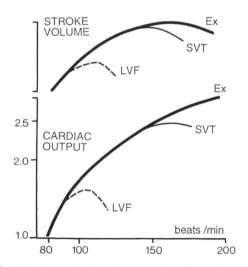

FIG. 15-3. Effect of heart rate on stroke volume and cardiac output. During dynamic exercise (Ex), an initial increase of stroke volume is followed by a near plateau and then a small decline. Note the steep increase of cardiac output with only slight leveling off at maximal heart rates, despite the decrease in stroke volume, associated with a decreasing PVR (Fig. 15-2). In supraventricular tachycardia (SVT), in the absence of the adrenergic stimulation and peripheral dilation found in exercise, stroke volume and cardiac output both decrease due to decreased diastolic filling time. In subjects with LVF, there is a rapid decline in both stroke volume and cardiac output. Data for dynamic exercise were adapted from Flamm et al. (1990). Curves for SVT and LVF are hypothetical.

expected increase in cardiac output. Thereafter, the increase in heart rate comes to be balanced by a decrease in stroke volume as the time for ventricular filling declines, producing a flat, near-plateau phase. As the heart rate increases even further, cardiac output decreases, perhaps because of the very limited time for diastolic filling. In myocardial failure, the onset of the downward slope (Fig. 15-3) occurs much sooner, so that any plateau is lost. In dynamic exercise, in contrast, for any given heart rate, there is a greater cardiac output, probably because of the accompanying adrenergic stimulation with a contractility increase and peripheral vasodilation (Pierard et al., 1987). As the heart rate reaches extreme values of, say over 170 beats/min, the cardiac output still increases but the stroke volume declines.

During dynamic exercise in humans, therefore, an increased heart rate provides most of the increased cardiac output. The Starling mechanism also contributes (Flamm et al., 1990). The mechanism of the increase in heart rate during these stimuli is a combination of withdrawal of inhibitory vagal tone and increased adrenergic β-receptor stimulation. The signals for these changes come from the vasomotor center in the brain stem, which coordinates several types of input: one is from the cerebral cortex (e.g., the runner's readiness to go at the start of exercise), the second arises from the exercising muscles (Gandevia and Hobbs, 1990), and the third is the Bainbridge reflex, stimulated by the increased venous return during exercise (see Fig. 14-3). This reflex seems less powerful in humans than expected from experimental data. An increase in venous return by evoking a tachycardia can further invoke a positive inotropic effect by the Bowditch effect, quite apart from and in addition to the operation of the Starling mechanism. In addition, the low-pressure receptors reduce the afterload by decreasing peripheral vasoconstriction (see Chapter 14).

Force–Frequency Relationship. An increased heart rate progressively increases the force of ventricular contraction even in an isolated papillary muscle preparation (*Bowditch staircase phenomenon*). In isolated human ventricular strips, increasing the stimulation rate from 60 to about 160 per minute stimulates force development (see Fig. 12-11). In samples from failing hearts, there is no such increase.

OTHER DETERMINANTS OF CARDIAC OUTPUT

Preload. At the start of exercise, as the skeletal muscle squeezes out blood, the venous return augments, the right atrial pressure increases, and stroke volume increases in part by the Starling mechanism (Rowell et al., 1996). Increased depth of breathing will reduce the intrathoracic pressure and help the venous return to flow to the right atrium.

Afterload. In general, when the afterload decreases, the cardiac output increases. Physiologic examples of this principle exist during peripheral vasodilation induced by a hot bath or sauna or by a meal (Yi et al., 1990). In these conditions, however, there is also an accompanying tachycardia, as during drug-induced vasodilation. Conversely, when the afterload increases, there is initially a compensatory mechanism to maintain the stroke volume. If the afterload keeps increasing, compensatory mechanisms cannot adapt, and the stroke volume eventually decreases. In dynamic exercise, the peripheral vascular resistance decreases to explain the decrease in diastolic blood pressure. Yet, because the systolic blood pressure increases, so does the impedance to systolic ejection, so that the afterload against which the ventricle works actually increases. Thus, at really high rates of upright exercise, the stroke volume begins to decrease even though the cardiac output continues to increase, the

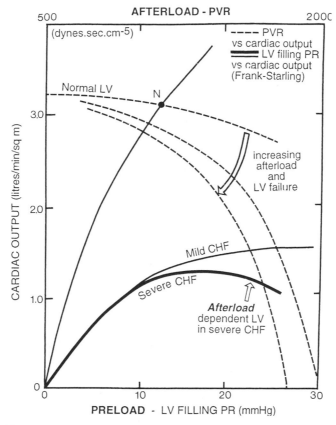

FIG. 15-4. Effect of preload and afterload on cardiac output. Normally cardiac output increases with an increased preload and decreases very little as the afterload increases (a three-factor relationship). In mild congestive heart failure (CHF), the increased afterload reduces stroke volume to balance the effect of increasing the preload so that the curve plateaus. In severe CHF, the afterload is high and the function of the left ventricle is poor, so that cardiac output decreases (descending limb of the Starling curve). PVR, peripheral vascular resistance.

latter as a result of the heart rate increases (Flamm et al., 1990). In congestive heart failure with a failing left ventricle, the stage at which the stroke volume and hence the cardiac output starts to decrease in response to the compensatory peripheral arteriolar constriction is much sooner than with the normal left ventricle (Fig. 15-4).

Contractility.   During β-adrenergic stimulation or exercise, the contractile state is enhanced to contribute to the increased cardiac output. Conversely, during congestive heart failure or therapy with β-adrenergic blockade, decreased contractility means a decreased stroke volume.

MEASUREMENT OF CARDIAC OUTPUT

The *Fick principle* has been the classic method for deriving cardiac output. The arteriovenous difference of oxygen is obtained by arterial puncture and a mixed central venous sample. The oxygen uptake is determined by spirometry. Cardiac output is the volume of blood needed to account for oxygen uptake. The defect of this procedure is its invasive nature.

The *indicator-dilution* method uses a dye, such as indocyanine green, which is injected centrally into the superior vena cava. Turbulence mixes the dye with blood within the ventricles, and the rate of appearance and disappearance of the dye in the aorta depends on the cardiac output. During exercise, the peak concentration of dye in the arterial circulation is less, and the dye appears and disappears more rapidly. *Lithium chloride* is the basis of a new indicator-dilution technique that is potentially noninvasive (Band et al., 1997).

Thermodilution is part of the invasive technique of *Swan-Ganz catheterization* (see Fig. 16-9). A known amount of ice-cold saline is injected into the central venous circulation. The rate of temperature decrease at the tip of the catheter further along depends on the cardiac output.

Doppler determinations of cardiac output have the great advantage of being noninvasive, although still under development. An ultrasound beam is directed onto the stream of blood passing through the mitral valve. The signal returning to the sound-receiving crystal is shifted in frequency in response to the velocity of flow. The area of the mitral valve orifice is determined by two-dimensional echocardiography. The cardiac output is calculated from the mean velocity of blood flow and the diastolic mitral valve area (Fisher et al., 1983). Using such techniques, the cardiac output during exercise can increase from the normal resting value of 6 to 7 L/min to 14 L/min in mild exercise, and 25 L/min during severe exercise in highly trained athletes. In congestive heart failure, the cardiac output is low (Fig. 15-4), with inadequate tissue perfusion during exercise. In cardiogenic shock (as in severe myocardial infarction), the cardiac output is so low that the tissues are inadequately perfused even at rest, and life is threatened.

WORK AND CARDIAC OUTPUT

In general, when the heart rate increases, so does the cardiac output, the work of the heart, and the myocardial oxygen uptake (Fig. 15-5). Cardiac output correlates with *external work,* which is done when a mass is lifted a certain distance. In terms of the heart, the cardiac output is the mass moved, and the resistance against which it is moved is the blood pressure.

$$\text{Minute work} = \text{systolic or mean BP} \times \text{CO}$$

The difference between external work and increased wall stress can be epitomized by the man standing and holding a heavy suitcase, doing no external work yet becoming very tired, compared with the man lifting a much lighter suitcase, doing external work yet not becoming tired. Another situation where internal work is relatively high is pressure work (Fig. 15-6). In contrast, when the heart is volume loaded, the increased oxygen uptake is spent in performing external rather than internal work.

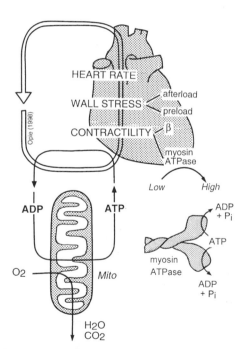

FIG. 15-5. Myocardial oxygen demand can be related to the load on the heart (wall stress), heart rate, and contractility. The last is related to several factors, including cytosolic calcium and the myosin ATPase activity. Mitochondrial metabolism increases to augment the oxygen uptake. The link between the determinants of oxygen demand and the oxygen uptake by the mitochondria is the breakdown of ATP to ADP. The latter is an important signal for mitochondrial (mito) oxygen uptake.

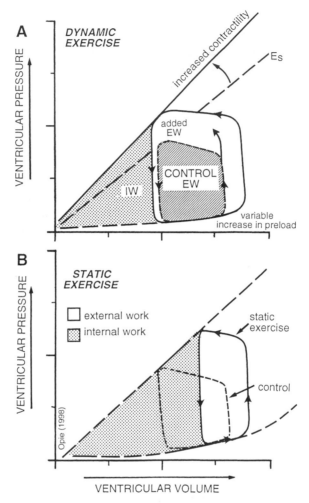

FIG. 15-6. Dynamic versus static exercise: effects on PV loop. During dynamic exercise, sympathetic stimulation increases contractility to displace the end-systolic pressure–volume relationship (E_s). The much greater venous return increases the preload to a variable extent, depending on the posture and the contractile response (for the dog, see Fig. 15-7). The result is that external work is increased relatively more than internal work (IW in stipples). During static exercise, afterload greatly increases (see BP and PVR in Fig. 15-2), so that inefficient and more oxygen-demanding internal work is much greater. See also contrasting effects of volume and pressure work (Fig. 12-17). For further concepts, see Suga et al. (1982).

Increased ventricular wall stress is the factor common to both external and internal work. It is wall stress (Fig. 12-15) that correlates with the myocardial oxygen uptake. The overall concept of wall stress includes the effects of changes in afterload because an increased afterload requires an increased systolic wall stress. Wall stress also includes changes in the preload, which generates end-diastolic wall stress. Wall stress allows for energy required for generation of muscular contraction that does not result in external work. Furthermore, in states of enhanced contractility, systolic wall stress increases faster. Thus, thinking in terms of wall stress provides a comprehensive approach to the problem of myocardial oxygen uptake. Wall stress accounts for most of the clinically relevant changes in myocardial oxygen uptake. There may be an additional metabolic component, usually small, which may be prominent in certain special circumstances, such as when circulating free fatty acids are abnormally high. Thus, at a fixed heart rate, the myocardial wall stress is the major determinant of the myocardial oxygen uptake. When the heart rate changes and the wall stress does not, then the heart rate becomes the major determinant of the myocardial oxygen uptake. Several clinical indices indirectly reflect oxygen uptake (Table 15-3).

In *tight aortic stenosis,* there is a marked discrepancy between cardiac output, which tends to be low, and heart work, which is considerably increased for three reasons. First, pressure work increases because of the greater intraventricular pressure required to eject the blood past the tightly narrowed aortic valve. Second, kinetic work, normally low enough to ignore, increases sharply as the cross-sectional area narrows. Third, the hypertrophied ventricle requires much more internal work for the same stroke volume (Fig. 15-6). Thus, it is not surprising that in patients with severe aortic stenosis and LV hypertrophy, the oxygen demand is much higher than normal, and that ischemia with angina pectoris can occur during exercise even in the absence of coronary artery disease.

TABLE 15-3. *Some indices of myocardial oxygen uptake[a]*

Index	Advantage	Comment
Heart rate	Extremely simple	Fairly good correlation[b]
Double product[b]		
Rate-pressure (RPP) Systolic pressure × heart rate	Noninvasive, easy	No allowance for contractile state
Triple product[a]		
Above × systolic ejection time	Noninvasive, more difficult	Some allowance for contractile state
Time-tension index[a]	Little advantage, requires invasive methods	Should be called "time-pressure" index; little used
Pressure-volume area[c]	Direct from pressure-volume loop, requiring no assumptions	Clinically validated in humans but is invasive
Pressure-work index[d] (SBP × HR × SV)	Noninvasive approximation	Should strictly be the integral of pressure and flow during ejection period

[a]For cautions, see Baller et al. (1981).
[b]Gobel et al. (1978).
[c]Takaoka et al. (1993).
[d]Rooke and Feigl (1982).

EXERCISE

Dynamic and static exercise have contrasting effects on the pressure-volume (PV) loop (Fig. 15-6). The greatly increased venous return of dynamic exercise increases the preload, whereas the increased contractility displaces upward the end-systolic point (see Fig. 12-6). Thus, the increase in external work is large, and that in internal work is small. Static exercise greatly increases afterload (see BP and PVR in Fig. 15-2), so that inefficient internal work increases. Thus, static work is much more oxygen demanding than might be expected.

During dynamic exercise, the cardiac output must increase manyfold. Hence, either stroke volume or heart rate or both must increase. The major adaptation to dynamic exercise is generally held to be the increased heart rate. In addition, there are changes in the PV loop. Both systolic and diastolic components of the PV loop enlarge to increase the external work (Fig. 15-7). The early diastolic part of the PV loop moves downward, so that LV filling augments even without an increase in left atrial pressure (Cheng et al., 1992). The mechanism involved is complex and associated with sympathetic stimulation and tachycardia. This exercise-induced change in the PV loop means that much more external work is being done during exercise, but slightly less internal work is being done, which resembles the effects of β-adrenergic stimulation (see Fig. 12-18).

The expected increase in end-diastolic volume as a result of the increased venous return may be annulled in part by increased contractility (increased adrenergic discharge, which allows the heart to increase the stroke volume without any

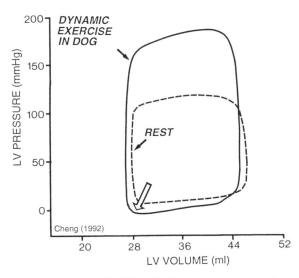

FIG. 15-7. Exercise promotes early LV filling. During exercise in dogs, the early diastolic portion of the LV pressure–volume loop moves downward (*open arrow*). This decrease in early diastolic pressure increases the transmural filling pressure and flow to compensate for shortened diastole during exercise. Modified from Cheng et al. (1992) by permission of the American Heart Association.

change in the diastolic fiber length). Animal experiments have suggested that the increased fiber length of the Starling relationship is shown most readily at very low filling pressures (hemorrhagic shock, dehydration) or as a beat-to-beat regulatory mechanism in response to respiratory variation in the intrathoracic pressure or during strenuous exercise (Vatner et al., 1972). Therefore, tachycardia should contribute more than does altered venous filling pressure to the normal response to dynamic exercise. Similar patterns are held to be correct for human subjects exercising in both the recumbent and supine positions. The erect position, when compared with the supine, decreases venous return, so at rest there is a lower LV end-diastolic pressure, a lower stroke volume, and a higher heart rate (Poliner et al., 1980). In these circumstances, an increased venous return could be expected to play a more major role than in recumbent exercise. This expectation is true, but in practice, the difference between upright and recumbent exercise is modest, and the major adaptation remains that of an increased heart rate with a lesser contribution from the Starling mechanism (Poliner et al., 1980).

An initial withdrawal of vagal tone and then increased adrenergic drive soon after the start of vigorous exercise can explain why the heart rate may double (Fig. 15-8). Even when the β-adrenergic receptors are blocked by β-blocking drugs, the

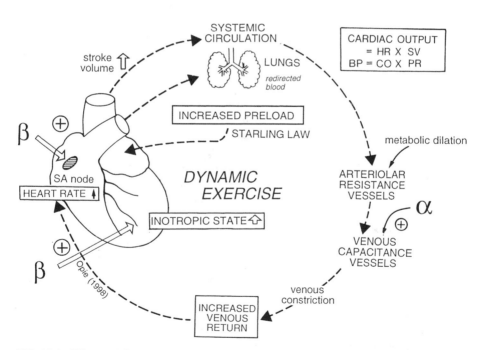

FIG. 15-8. Effects of dynamic exercise on circulation. The major factor in the increased cardiac output of dynamic exercise is tachycardia, with contributions from increased preload (Starling mechanism) and increased inotropic state (contractility). β-adrenergic stimulation (β) increases heart rate (HR) and the inotropic state. α-adrenergic stimulation (α) contracts venous capacitance vessels to increase the venous return and to redirect blood from the abdominal organs to the lungs.

heart rate can still double during maximal exercise because of the principle of competitive antagonism whereby the enhanced adrenergic drive can displace the β-blocking drug from the receptor. However, the absolute heart rates reached are much reduced. In dogs with cardiac denervation (Donald and Shepherd, 1963), the heart rate can still increase, although it does so more slowly and less than in controls because there is no vagal withdrawal. Increased circulating rather than locally released catecholamines are the major stimulus to the tachycardia. Another consequence of adrenergic discharge is redistribution of blood from abdominal organs (α-adrenergic vasoconstriction) to the heart and lungs (Flamm et al., 1990).

Response to Running

The circulatory and cardiac changes in response to dynamic exercise (Fig. 15-8) can now be traced out, taking the example of a runner and making some simplifying assumptions. When running exercise starts, the leg muscles contract to increase the venous return, which evokes the Starling mechanism and, by stimulating the atrial mechanoreceptors, the Bainbridge reflex (see Fig. 13-3). The major stimulus to the all-important tachycardia of exercise comes chiefly from altered activity of the autonomic nervous system, in response to central arousal mechanisms, which are activated by the runner's readiness to go. Initially there is withdrawal of vagal tone (Fig. 15-9). Then the release of norepinephrine into the synaptic clefts within the heart stimulates the β_1-adrenergic receptors around the sinus node, the pacemaker currents respond, and the heart rate increases further. Release of epinephrine from the adrenal gland also contributes to the cardiac β_1-adrenergic response. Sustained exercise leads to release of catecholamines from both the terminal neurons and the adrenal gland, and the blood catecholamine levels increase. The increase in heart rate is a major factor governing the increase in the myocardial oxygen uptake during exercise. The required peripheral vasodilation is complex in origin, partly autonomic, and partly related to the metabolites formed by skeletal muscle exercise (see next section). Nonetheless, the systolic blood pressure will increase because of the increase in the cardiac output, and the systolic afterload will increase.

That there is adrenergic stimulation during exercise is proved by the doubling of the plasma value of norepinephrine (Chidsey et al., 1962) and by the discharge of norepinephrine from the heart into the coronary sinus (Cousineau et al., 1977). Not surprisingly, when β-adrenergic blocking agents are given, the degree of exercise activity that can be reached is impaired, so that when normal subjects are exercised to their limit, the cardiac output is about 25% lower after β-blockade.

In summary, during vigorous dynamic exercise in humans, the following hemodynamic changes occur: the cardiac output increases up to three times, the heart rate nearly doubles, end-diastolic volume (Starling effect) enlarges by about one fourth, the ejection fraction increases, and there is a marked predominantly systolic blood pressure elevation (Flamm et al., 1990). End-systolic volume, an index of contractility (see Table 12-5), decreases throughout exercise,

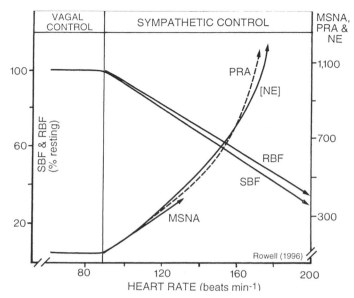

FIG. 15-9. Effects of dynamic exercise on vagal and sympathetic control. When the heart rate approaches 100 beats/min, vagal withdrawal is nearly complete and sympathetic effects start. There is an increase of circulating norepinephrine (NE) and of plasma renin activity (PRA), as well as in directly measured muscle sympathetic nerve activity (MSNA). Concurrently, there are decreases in splanchnic blood flow (SBF) and renal blood flow (RBF). Modified from Rowell et al. (1996).

and decreases dramatically to half just when exercise ends, presumably because of the combination of high circulating catecholamine levels and a low work load. During intense exercise in dogs, the major changes lie in contractility and in heart rate (Vatner et al., 1972).

Neurohumoral Response in Dynamic Exercise

During graded dynamic exercise, there is not only the expected increase in plasma catecholamines, but also in renin activity, angiotensin II, and neuropeptide Y (Rowell et al., 1996). These start to be evident at about 140 beats/min and increase rapidly thereafter (Fig. 15-9). Proof of an increase of sympathetic nerve outflow to exercising muscle comes from direct measurements by microelectrode techniques. Such activity increases in relation to the amount of dynamic exercise (Rowell et al., 1996). The importance of the overall increase in sympathetic activity may be summarized as follows: (1) heart rate and cardiac output increase; (2) there is redistribution of blood from splanchnic organs and kidneys; and (3) decreased renal blood flow and increased β-adrenergic stimulation lead to activation of the renin-angiotensin system, which is both vasoconstrictive and contributes to the increased contractility by facilitating neurotransmission and release of norepinephrine (see Fig. 14-5).

Peripheral Resistance During Dynamic Exercise

During dynamic exercise, there is marked peripheral arteriolar vasodilation with an increased blood flow (exercise hyperemia) to the exercising muscles. Both autonomic and local metabolic factors are involved. Normally, α-mediated vasoconstriction contributes to the resting arteriolar tone. During exercise, the increased venous return will stimulate the low-pressure receptors to lessen peripheral vasoconstriction. As exercise increases in intensity, other vasoconstrictive factors such as angiotensin II and neuropeptide Y come into play. Metabolic products of exercise lead first to inhibition of the distal α_2-mediated vasoconstriction in the smaller arterioles, and then at more intense levels of exercise to relief of α_1-mediated control of the larger arterioles (Anderson and Faber, 1991). Simultaneous β_2-mediated vasodilation, in response to increased circulating levels of epinephrine, probably also contributes. As in the case of the coronary vasodilation that also occurs during exercise, the vasodilatory metabolites are not fully clarified, but include formation of adenosine and nitric oxide, as well as others such as protons, carbon dioxide, and potassium. *Nitric oxide* appears to play more of a role in control of the blood flow to muscles during rest than in exercise (Endo et al., 1994). Of interest, nitric oxide can increase the glucose uptake of exercise skeletal muscle, probably by enhanced formation of cyclic guanosine monophosphate (Young et al., 1997). The nitric oxide may be formed in vascular endothelium in response to the increased blood flow.

Static Exercise and Central Integration of Reflex Stimuli

The origin of the blood pressure increase during static exercise is not immediately evident because the peripheral vascular resistance may remain relatively flat and the cardiac output only increases modestly. Central *neural command* must play a role because during total paralysis of subjects by neuromuscular blockade, attempted contraction of the paralyzed muscles still increases heart rate and blood pressure (Gandevia et al., 1993). This indicates that a central feed-forward mechanism alone can drive the cardiovascular system in a manner independent of peripheral feedback from muscle. The chain of command goes from cerebral cortex to hypothalamus to the vasomotor center in the medulla, and thence along the sympathetic outflow. However, during intense static exercise, when the muscle becomes ischemic, C fibers in the muscle are stimulated to cause a reflex increase in the arterial blood pressure (*muscle pressor reflex*). The afferent arm of this reflex conveys stimuli to the nucleus solitarius (solitary tract nucleus) in the medulla, from where they travel to a very restricted hypothalamic region, which when stimulated gives a very similar BP response to those found during exercise (Eldridge et al., 1981). This hypothalamic site links to both the cerebral cortex and the cardiovascular control centers in the medulla. In the case of static exercise, efferent stimuli travel from the hypothalamus to the sympathetic vasomotor center in the medulla, which coordinates the sympathetic responses that increase the blood pressure chiefly by increasing the cardiac output.

In the case of dynamic exercise, central command conveys messages from the cortex to the hypothalamus and thence to the medulla, initially to decrease vagal outflow. This inhibitory vagal response is mediated by the vagal nuclei in the medulla, previously called the cardioinhibitory center. Later, as the heart rate increases, sympathetic outflow from the vasomotor center in the medulla is increased (Fig. 15-9) in response to a variety of stimuli, including continued central command, removal of the normal inhibition exerted by the vagal nucleus on the sympathetic vasomotor center with decreased sensitivity of the baroreflexes to the increase in systolic pressure, and other poorly understood factors, which may include reflexes arising in the exercising muscles.

It must not be supposed that the three cardiovascular control centers located in the hypothalamus, the vagal nuclei, and the sympathetic vasomotor center all act in isolation. Rather, there is a constant stream of messages between them. It also should be stressed that the control centers are not as clearly defined as previously thought, so the details remain controversial.

Despite these reservations, the overall picture that emerges includes a role for both straight-down feed-forward control of heart and blood vessels, especially during dynamic exercise, and for integration of signals incorporating reflexes originating in the muscles, especially during static exercise (Fig. 15-10).

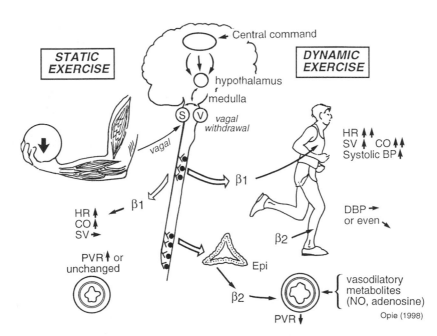

FIG. 15-10. Combined central and peripheral control during exercise. During dynamic exercise, central command is thought to play a major role, whereas during static exercise, reflexes from the exercising muscle become more important. The drawing of static exercise on the left is modeled on the work of Shepherd et al. (1981), and the rest of the figure was designed by L.H. Opie. HR, heart rate; CO, cardiac output; SV, stroke volume; PVR, peripheral vascular resistance; β_1, β_1-adrenergic; epi, epinephrine; DBP, diastolic blood pressure.

Cardiac Energy Metabolism in Exercise

Patterns of substrate metabolism of the human heart during exercise can be defined by the use of coronary sinus catheterization. There is a marked increase of the contribution of lactate to the oxidative metabolism of the heart during a short burst of exercise. Thus, the heart takes up and oxidizes the lactate, which is being produced by the peripheral muscles.

During exercise, the oxygen uptake of the myocardium must increase as each of the determinants increases: heart rate, contractility, and wall stress (Fig. 15-5). Wall stress increases in response to the increased afterload as the blood pressure increases. Cellular metabolic signals are set off by increased work to ensure that an adequate flow of substrates is ultimately metabolized by the citrate cycle to produce enough adenosine triphosphate (ATP). As cytosolic ATP is rapidly converted by contraction to ADP, mitochondrial oxygen uptake and ATP formation are stimulated, $NADH_2$ is converted to NAD, the citrate cycle is stimulated, and the uptake of glucose, lactate, and free fatty acids is enhanced (see Fig. 11-12). The mechanism whereby increased heart work stimulates glucose uptake is unknown, although it involves increased glucose transport across the sarcolemma. An increase of cyclic adenosine monophosphate (cAMP) in response to nitric oxide may contribute to the increased glucose uptake (Young et al., 1997). Lactate uptake increases because transfer of pyruvate into mitochondrial pathways is enhanced after increased availability of NAD and activation of pyruvate dehydrogenase. The mechanism of the increased uptake of free fatty acids is linked to increased mitochondrial metabolism and increased removal of acetyl CoA and $NADH_2$ to stimulate the β-oxidation spiral. The stimulus to increased mitochondrial respiration is not fully understood but appears to be a combination of increased ADP from increased myocardial work and increased mitochondrial calcium levels (see Chapter 11).

The exercising heart, like the normal heart, consumes what it is given. Therefore, early on, when blood lactate is high, lactate dominates, whereas during prolonged exercise when blood lactate is used up and the levels of free fatty acids increase, the latter become dominant. At the onset of severe exercise, when the heart is not given enough external substrate, glycogen is broken down and used in preference to external glucose (Goodwin et al., 1996).

Dynamic (Aerobic) Exercise Training and the Heart

With aerobic training, the resting heart rate decreases (Blumenthal et al., 1990) as a result of an alteration of the balance between the sympathetic and parasympathetic neural stimulation to the heart. Reduction of the resting heart rate and of the heart rate during submaximal exercise are two of the basic signs of exercise training. After training, β-adrenergic blockade has less effect in reducing the heart rate both at rest and during exercise (Ekblom et al., 1973). Thus, exercise training has some effects similar to β-adrenergic blockade (Brundin et al., 1976), except that the level of exercise reached is much higher in trained than in β-blocked individuals.

The Athlete's Heart. Bradycardia is one explanation for the apparent increased size of the heart found in highly conditioned athletes, the mechanism being an increased diastolic filling time (Fig. 15-11). True *physiologic hypertrophy* occurs and must be distinguished from the rare diseases causing pathologic hypertrophy (Ikaheimo et al., 1979), which can cause sudden death in young athletes. It is not known whether the stimulus to hypertrophy in endurance athletes is prolonged work load (both a volume and a pressure load), or prolonged stimulation by catecholamines. Physiologic LV hypertrophy differs from pathologic LV hypertrophy by the setting in which it occurs, the accompanying bradycardia, and by

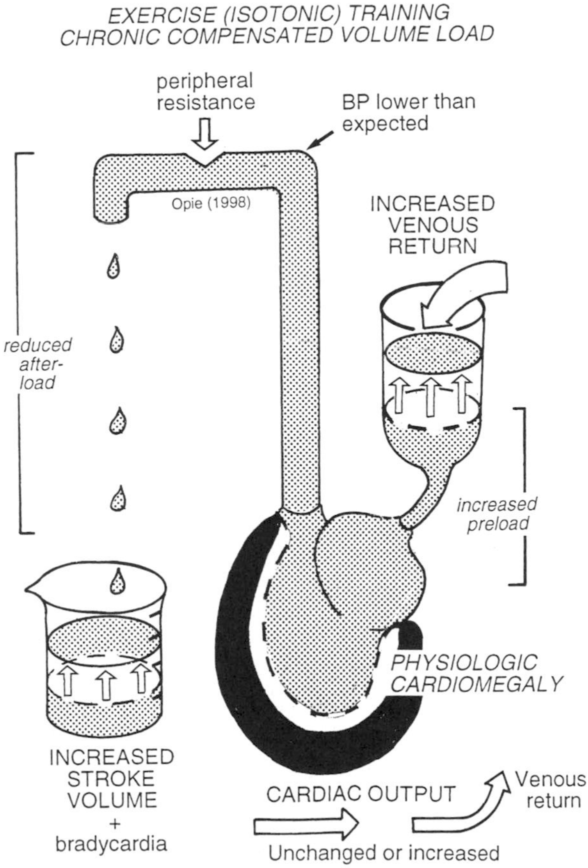

EXERCISE (ISOTONIC) TRAINING
CHRONIC COMPENSATED VOLUME LOAD

FIG. 15-11. The athlete's heart. As a simplification, the adaptations involved in dynamic exercise training may be regarded as compensatory responses to a chronic volume load, including physiologic cardiomegaly.

improved rather than impaired early diastolic filling on the Doppler echocardiogram. The increased vagal tone (either absolute or relative) of the athlete can give rise to *excess bradycardia* with prolonged conduction between atria and ventricles (prolonged PR-interval) and abnormalities of repolarization. In some rare cases, the sinus node function is suppressed, so that some heart beats fail to develop and hypotensive episodes result. Sometimes conduction through the atrioventricular node is so delayed that the *Wenkebach phenomenon* develops (see Fig. 5-20). Such effects of overtraining can be cured by less exercise.

There may be crucial differences between such physiologic hypertrophy and the pathologic variety (see Chapter 13). Scheuer and Buttrick (1987) compared the effects of hypertrophy induced by repetitive catecholamine stimulation with those of exercise in rats. They found that pathologic hypertrophy impaired myocardial relaxation, whereas physiologic hypertrophy allowed the heart to contract and relax better.

Exercise as Prophylaxis for Cardiac Protection.   Lack of exercise is now recognized as a major independent risk factor for cardiovascular disease. Conversely, exercise training is associated with a lower all-cause mortality in middle-aged and older men (Paffenberger et al., 1993). Explanations for the apparent beneficial effect of dynamic exercise in preventing ischemic heart disease are as follows. First, exercise training could act in a nonspecific way to modify the risk factors, such as by favorably altering blood lipoprotein patterns (Heath et al., 1983) or by decreasing the blood pressure (Martin et al., 1990). Second, exercise training need have no direct effect on the development of coronary artery disease but rather on the response of the myocardium to a given extent of coronary disease. For example, the arrhythmogenic effect of coronary artery occlusion could be decreased (Posel et al., 1989). The decreased release of catecholamines from the heart after exercise training (Cousineau et al., 1977) is the sort of change that could be operating. Third, exercise training promotes overall vagal activity, as assessed by beat-to-beat heart period variability (Goldsmith et al., 1992). Such an increase is protective against ischemia and cardiac ventricular arrhythmias (Lubbe et al., 1992). A slow heart rate at rest is in general a sign of greater longevity than a faster rate. From this point of view, it is likely that dynamic rather than static exercise training would be more protective because such training is associated with a greater increase of heart rate during exercise than is static exercise (Martin et al., 1990). Fourth, exercise training may open coronary collateral vessels. In dogs, it is only the epicardial collaterals that develop, and their functional significance is open to question (Neil and Oxendine, 1979). Fifth, exercise training may augment the degree of coronary vasodilation in response to testing by nitroglycerin, suggesting improved endothelial function (Haskell et al., 1993). Sixth, exercise by enhancing the rate of glucose transport across the muscle membranes helps to lessen insulin resistance and thereby may improve a variety of conditions, including obesity and maturity-onset diabetes, which in turn predispose to cardiovascular disease.

Exercise-Induced Arrhythmias. One concern is that exercise may precipitate arrhythmias. In a large majority of cases, such arrhythmias are related to coronary heart disease, where exercise amplifies the negative cardiac effects of ischemia. In addition, systemic circulatory changes could play a role. Blood catecholamine levels may increase as much as 15-fold during exercise, plasma potassium can double, and the blood pH may decrease by 0.4 units (Paterson, 1996). Each of these exercise-induced changes could induce arrhythmias at rest, yet in normal subjects they are paradoxically well tolerated. The proposal is that adrenergic stimulation offsets the harmful effects of an increased external potassium level, and vice versa. This principle of mutual antagonism is explained by the capacity of adrenergic stimulation to increase the inward calcium current during K^+-induced depolarization, and for a high external K^+ to shorten the action potential and thereby to lessen the risk of calcium-induced afterdepolarizations (Paterson, 1996). The major risk of arrhythmias may arise postexercise, when the blood potassium transiently decreases to hypokalemic levels but the catecholamines stay high. There are interactive effects of these extracardiac chemical changes associated with exercise and cardiac ischemia, which attenuates the protective effects of norepinephrine and amplifies the adverse effects of changes in blood potassium and pH (O'Neill et al., 1997). Thus, in the presence of pre-existing coronary disease, vigorous exercise can occasionally trigger sudden death, especially in untrained sedentary individuals in whom vagal tone is likely to be low (Mittelman et al., 1993). In contrast, regular aerobic exercise training is protective against cardiovascular disease and sudden cardiac death.

EMOTIONAL STRESS, BRAIN, AND HEART

Emotional stress, like dynamic exercise, is a potent source of catecholamine discharge (Fig. 15-12). Closely related is intense cerebral activity, such as forced fast mental arithmetic. Central distress, acting via the hypothalamus and the medullary centers, leads to enhanced activity of the adrenergic system, including increases in circulating epinephrine, so that β-adrenergic activity is enhanced. The increased β-adrenergic discharge also leads to a series of events that enhance myocardial oxygen uptake: tachycardia, increased contractility, and increased cardiac output (Freyschuss et al., 1988).

Psychological stress generally causes the peripheral vascular resistance to decrease (Freyschuss et al., 1988; Schmieder et al., 1987), with an increase in splanchnic vasoconstriction (Fig. 15-11). There can even be a marked increase in forearm blood flow, reflecting brisk peripheral vasodilation, and a relatively small increase in blood pressure (see Fig. 14-7). These responses partly resemble those of dynamic exercise (Table 15-4). It seems likely that in certain individuals there is a tendency toward increased peripheral vascular resistance, perhaps through excess $α_1$-adrenergic-mediated vasoconstriction (Ruddel et al., 1988). Such individuals might be at greater risk for the development of subsequent hypertension (Santangelo et al., 1989). In normotensive individuals it is

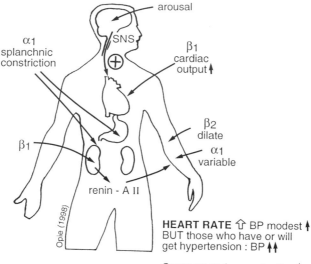

FIG. 15-12. Acute emotional stress reaction. Note some similarities to dynamic exercise (Fig. 15-10). During severe emotional stress, release of epinephrine and β2-mediated peripheral vasodilation prevent a major rise in diastolic blood pressure. In contrast, in hypertensives or those destined to become hypertensive, such stress may cause peripheral vasoconstriction with a substantial rise in blood pressure. SNS/Sympathetic nervous system.

chiefly plasma epinephrine that increases during mental stress, epinephrine being predominantly vasodilatory by β2-stimulation (Freyschuss et al., 1988; Grossman et al., 1989). Borderline hypertensive individuals, however, experience an increase of both epinephrine and norepinephrine secretion, the latter being vasoconstrictory. The greater increase in circulating catecholamines in

TABLE 15-4. *Comparative effects of exercise, mental stress, volume, and pressure loading on hemodynamic parameters*[a]

	HR	SV	CO	PVR	BP
Volume load	++[b]	0 or +	++	0 or −	0
Pressure load (hypertension)	+	0	+	++	++
Exercise, dynamic erect	+++	+	+++	− − −	+SBP, −DBP
Exercise, static	+	0	+	0 or +	++
Mental stress	++	+	++	−	+
Epinephrine infusion	++	+	++	−	+SBP, −DBP
Norepinephrine infusion	±	±	±	++	++
Acetylcholine	−	−	−	−	−

[a]Data sources: Erect bicycle exercise: Iskandrian et al. (1983); static exercise: Lind et al. (1967), Shepherd et al. (1981); mental stress: Freychuss et al. (1988), Schulte and Neus (1983); infusion of epinephrine: Stratton et al. (1985); infusion of norepinephrine: Barcroft and Swan (1953).

[b]+, increased effect; −, decreased effect; SBP, systolic blood pressure; DBP, diastolic blood pressure; HR, heart rate; SV, stroke volume; PVR, peripheral vascular resistance.

borderline hypertensive individuals can be correlated with the increase in blood pressure during mental stress (Nestel, 1969). Hypothetically, repeated episodes of elevated blood pressure can damage the vascular endothelium and facilitate the development of chronic hypertension (see Chapter 14). In true hypertensive individuals, the peripheral resistance increases rather than decreases during mental stress (Schmieder et al., 1987).

Psychological stress may play a role in the precipitation of sudden cardiac death. For example, on the day of an earthquake in Los Angeles, there was a sharp increase in the number of sudden deaths from cardiac causes (Leor et al., 1996). Emotional upset may trigger acute myocardial infarction in about 20% of cases (Tofler et al., 1990). The newly described personality trait, type D (D for distress), in which emotional distress is suppressed, predicts a fourfold increase of death in patients with coronary heart disease (Denollet et al., 1996). A hypothetical chain of events starts with central distress and arousal and leads through the hypothalamus and medulla to cardiovascular adrenergic activation (Skinner et al., 1985) and a potentially lethal increase in myocardial levels of the arrhythmogenic second messenger, cAMP (Lubbe et al., 1992).

SUMMARY

1. *Cardiac output.* This is the product of the stroke volume and the heart rate. The dominant factor governing cardiac output during dynamic exercise is the heart rate. Other factors include preload, afterload, and contractility. Cardiac output is an important component of the external work of the heart. In general, the same factors that increase cardiac output increase the myocardial oxygen uptake, but there are important differences depending on the amount of internal work done, which is much increased during a pressure load including static exercise. In contrast, during a volume load (similar to dynamic exercise), internal work increases little and external work and oxygen uptake increase in proportion to the heart rate.

2. *Wall stress and oxygen uptake.* Both increased internal and external work augment wall stress. The oxygen demands of internal work can be high (the man holding the heavy suitcase) even when in strictly physical terms no work is done (because the mass is not moved). Internal work requires development of wall stress that can increase even when the chamber size of the heart is unchanged, because stress depends on the product of pressure and radius. Wall stress increases as the heart dilates (heart failure), so that heart size is a major determinant of the oxygen uptake of the heart. Therefore, the concept of wall stress allows a unitary approach to the complexities of myocardial oxygen uptake.

3. *Exercise: dynamic versus static.* Exercise is an example of a physiologic increase in oxygen uptake. There are important contrasting differences between dynamic and static exercise. The increased cardiac output of dynamic exercise is mediated by a combination of increased venous return,

increased heart rate (the dominant factor), and increased contractility. In addition, the systolic but not diastolic pressure increases. In contrast, in static exercise both systolic and diastolic pressures increase, probably as a result of reflexes arising in the muscles and conveyed by C fibers to cardiovascular centers in the medulla and hypothalamus. During dynamic exercise, increased cortical command and feed-forward to increased sympathetic adrenergic activity are the prime control mechanisms.

4. *Myocardial response to exercise.* As the heart rate and blood pressure increase, more external work and more oxygen uptake is required. A higher rate of myocardial oxygen uptake reflects increased production of ATP. Mitochondrial metabolism is driven by a greater rate of formation of ADP and an increased mitochondrial calcium concentration. Glycogen may play a special role in the energy metabolism of the exercising heart, especially at the onset of increased heart work.

5. *Emotional stress.* In this case the increased myocardial oxygen demand is mediated by a combination of β- and α-adrenergic activity. In normal individuals, secretion of epinephrine dominates, and the tachycardia is accompanied by an increased stroke volume, peripheral vasodilation, and surprisingly modest changes in the blood pressure. However, in hypertensive or borderline hypertensive individuals, emotional stress can induce substantial blood pressure increases.

6. *Athlete's heart.* In this condition, bradycardia and physiological left ventricular hypertrophy go together. Distinction from pathologic left ventricular hypertrophy is determined by the setting in which each occurs, and by the improved diastolic filling in the physiologic variety.

7. *Endurance training* by repetitive aerobic exercise counters lack of exercise, which is an independent risk factor for cardiovascular disease. The mechanisms involved are multiple, including enhanced vagal tone.

ACKNOWLEDGMENT

Dr. D. Paterson at the University Laboratory of Physiology, Oxford, England, is thanked for advice and assistance.

STUDENT QUESTIONS

1. List and define each of the major determinants of the cardiac output.
2. What differences do you expect between static (isometric) and dynamic (isotonic or aerobic) exercise in relation to (a) heart rate; (b) cardiac output; and (c) the blood pressure?
3. What is the relationship between wall stress and myocardial oxygen uptake?
4. During static exercise, both systolic and diastolic blood pressure increase. Trace out the reflex pathways involved.

5. How do exercise and emotional stress, both of which increase catecholamine discharge, differ in their hemodynamic effects?

CARDIOLOGIST-IN-TRAINING QUESTIONS

1. What determines the myocardial oxygen uptake in (a) dynamic exercise in a normal subject; (b) static (isometric) exercise; (c) severe aortic stenosis; and (d) left ventricular failure?
2. Can heart work be increased without major changes in the myocardial oxygen uptake? If so, describe the mechanisms involved and speculate on any therapeutic potential.
3. Exercise (endurance) training may have beneficial cardiovascular effects. What are they, and which mechanisms may be involved?
4. What is the athlete's heart? How can it be distinguished from pathologic left ventricular hypertrophy?
5. During an earthquake, a man of 65 dies suddenly after a brief period of a central chest pain diagnosed as acute myocardial infarction. Speculate on the mechanisms involved.

REFERENCES

1. Anderson KM, Faber JE. Differential sensitivity of arteriolar α_1- and α_2-adrenoreceptor constriction to metabolic inhibition during rat skeletal muscle contraction. *Circ Res* 1991;69:174–184.
2. Baller D, Bretschneider HJ, Hellige G. A critical look at currently used indirect indices of myocardial oxygen consumption. *Basic Res Cardiol* 1981;76:163–181.
3. Band DM, Linton RAF, O'Brien TK, et al. The shape of indicator dilution curves used for cardiac output measurement in man. *J Physiol* 1997;498:225–229.
4. Barcroft H, Swan HJC. In: *Sympathetic Control of Human Blood Vessels.* London: Edward Arnold and Co, 1953.
5. Blumenthal JA, Frederikson M, Kuhn CM, et al. Aerobic exercise reduces levels of cardiovascular and sympathoadrenal responses to mental stress in subjects without prior evidence of myocardial ischemia. *Am J Cardiol* 1990;65:93–98.
6. Brundin T, Edhag O, Lundman T. Effects remaining after withdrawal of long term beta-receptor blockade. *Br Heart J* 1976;38:1065–1072.
7. Cheng C-P, Igarashi Y, Little WC. Mechanism of augmented rate of left ventricular filling during exercise. *Circ Res* 1992;70:9–19.
8. Chidsey CA, Harrison DC, Braunwald E. Augmentation of the plasma norepinephrine response to exercise in patients with congestive failure. *N Engl J Med* 1962;267:650–654.
9. Cousineau D, Ferguson RJ, de Champlain J, et al. Catecholamines in coronary sinus during exercise in man before and after training. *J Appl Physiol* 1977;43:801–806.
10. Denollet J, Sys SU, Stroobant N, et al. Personality as independent predictor of long-term mortality in patients with coronary heart disease. *Lancet* 1996;347:417–421.
11. Donald DE, Shepherd JT. Response to exercise in dogs with cardiac denervation. *Am J Physiol* 1963;205:393–400.
12. Ekblom B, Kilblom A, Soltysiak J. Physical training bradycardia and autonomic nervous system. *Scand J Clin Lab Invest* 1973;32:251–256.
13. Eldridge FL, Millhorn DE, Waldrop TG. Exercise hypernea and locomotion: parallel activation from the hypothalamus. *Science* 1981;211:844–846.
14. Endo T, Imaizumi T, Tagawa T, et al. Role of nitric oxide in exercise-induced vasodilation of the forearm. *Circulation* 1994;90:2886–2890.

15. Epstein SE, Robinson BF, Kahler RL, Braunwald E. Effects of beta-adrenergic blockade on the cardiac response to maximal and submaximal exercise in man. *J Clin Invest* 1965;44:1745–1753.
16. Fisher DC, Sahn DJ, Friedman MJ, et al. The mitral valve orifice method for noninvasive two-dimensional echo Doppler determinations of cardiac output. *Circulation* 1983;67:872–877.
17. Flamm SD, Taki J, Moore R, et al. Redistribution of regional and organ blood volume and effect on cardiac function in relation to upright exercise intensity in healthy human subjects. *Circulation* 1990; 81:1550–1559.
18. Freyschuss U, Hjemdahl P, Juhlin-Dannfelt A, Linde B. Cardiovascular and sympathoadrenal responses to mental stress: influence of β-blockade. *Am J Physiol* 1988;255:H1443–H1451.
19. Gandevia SC, Hobbs SF. Cardiovascular responses to static exercise in man: central and reflex contributions. *J Physiol* 1990;430:105–117.
20. Gandevia SC, Killian K, McKenzie DK, et al. Respiratory sensations, cardiovascular control, kinaesthesia and transcranial stimulating during paralysis in humans. *J Physiol* 1993;470:85–107.
21. Gobel FL, Nordstrom LA, Nelson RR, et al. The rate-pressure product as an index of myocardial oxygen consumption during exercise in patients with angina pectoris. *Circulation* 1978;57:549–556.
22. Goldsmith RL, Steinman RC, Fleiss JL. Comparison of 24-hour parasympathetic activity in endurance-trained and untrained young men. *J Am Coll Cardiol* 1992;20:552–558.
23. Goodwin GW, Ahmad F, Taegtmeyer H. Preferential oxidation of glycogen in isolated working rat heart. *J Clin Invest* 1996;97:1409–1416.
24. Grossman E, Oren S, Garavaglia G, et al. Disparate hemodynamic and sympathoadrenergic responses to isometric and mental stress in essential hypertension. *Am J Cardiol* 1989;64:42–44.
25. Haskell WL, Sims C, Myll J, et al. Coronary artery size and dilating capacity in ultradistance runners. *Circulation* 1993;87:1076–1082.
26. Heath GW, Ehsani AA, Hagberg MM, et al. Exercise training improves lipoprotein lipid profiles in patients with coronary artery disease. *Am Heart J* 1983;105:889–895.
27. Ikaheimo MJ, Palatsi IJ, Takkunen JT. Noninvasive evaluation of the athletic heart: sprinters versus endurance runners. *Am J Cardiol* 1979;44:24–30.
28. Iskandrian AS, Hakki AH, DePace NL, et al. Evaluation of left ventricular function by radionuclide angiography during exercise in normal subjects and in patients with chronic coronary heart disease. *J Am Coll Cardiol* 1983;1:1518–1529.
29. Leor J, Poole WK, Kloner RA. Sudden cardiac death triggered by an earthquake. *N Engl J Med* 1996;334:413–419.
30. Lind AR, McNicol GW. Muscular factors which determine the cardiovascular responses to sustained and rhythmic exercise. *Can Med Assoc J* 1967;96:703–713.
31. Lubbe WH, Podzuweit T, Opie LH. Potential arrhythmogenic role of cyclic adenosine monophosphate (AMP) and cytosolic calcium overload: implications for prophylactic effects of beta-blockers in myocardial infarction and proarrhythmic effects of phospodiesterase inhibitors. *J Am Coll Cardiol* 1992;19:1622–1633.
32. Martin JE, Dubbert PM, Cushman WC. Controlled trial of aerobic exercise in hypertension. *Circulation* 1990;81:1560–1567.
33. Mittelman MA, Maclure M, Tofler GH, et al. Triggering of acute myocardial infarction by heavy physical exertion. Protection against triggering by regular exertion. *N Engl J Med* 1993;329:1677–1683.
34. Neill WA, Oxendine JM. Exercise can improve coronary collateral development without improving perfusion of ischemic myocardium. *Circulation* 1979;60:1513–1519.
35. Nestel PJ. Blood pressure and catecholamine excretion after mental stress in labile hypertension. *Lancet* 1969;1:692–694.
36. O'Neill M, Sears CL, Paterson DJ. Interactive effects of K^+, acid, norepinephrine and ischemia on the heart: implications for exercise. *J Appl Physiol* 1997;82:1046–1052.
37. Paffenberger RS, Hyde RT, Wing AL, et al. The association of changes in physical activity level and other lifestyle characteristics with mortality among men. *N Engl J Med* 1993;328:538–545.
38. Paterson DJ. Antiarrhythmic mechanisms during exercise [Review]. *J Appl Physiol* 1996;80: 1853–1862.
39. Pierard LA, Serruys PW, Roelandt J, Melzer RS. Left ventricular function at similar heart rates during tachycardia induced by exercise and atrial pacing: an echocardiographic study. *Br Heart J* 1987;57:154–160.
40. Poliner LR, Dehmer GJ, Lewis SE, et al. Left ventricular performance in normal subjects: a comparison of the responses to exercise in the upright and supine positions. *Circulation* 1980;62:528–534.
41. Posel D, Noakes T, Kantor P, et al. Excercise training after experimental myocardial infarction

increases the ventricular fibrillation threshold before and after the onset of reinfarction in the isolated rat heart. *Circulation* 1989;80:138–145.

42. Rooke GA, Feigl EO. Work as a correlate of canine left ventricular oxygen consumption and the problem of catecholamine oxygen wasting. *Circ Res* 1982;50:273–286.

43. Rowell LR, O'Leary DS, Kellogg DL. Integration of cardiovascular control systems in dynamic exercise. In: Rowell LB, Shepherd JT (eds). *Handbook of Physiology.* Section 12. New York: Oxford University Press, 1996;730–838.

44. Ruddel H, Langewitz W, Schachinger H, et al. Hemodynamic response patterns to mental stress: diagnostic and therapeutic implications. *Am Heart J* 1988;116:617–628.

45. Santangelo KL, Falkner B, Kushner H. Forearm hemodynamics at rest and stress in borderline hypertensive adolescents. *Am J Hypertens* 1989;2:52–56.

46. Scheuer J, Buttrick P. The cardiac hypertrophic responses to pathologic and physiologic loads. *Circulation* 1987;75(suppl I):63–68.

47. Schmieder RE, Rueddel H, Neus H, et al. Disparate hemodynamic responses to mental challenge after antihypertensive therapy with beta-blockers and calcium entry blockers. *Am J Med* 1987;82:11–16.

48. Schulte W, Neus H. Hemodynamics during emotional stress in borderline and mild hypertension. *Eur Heart J* 1983;4:803–809.

49. Shepherd JT, Blomqvist CG, Lind AR, et al. Static (isometric) exercise. *Circ Res* 1981;48(suppl1):179–188.

50. Skinner JE. Regulation of cardiac vulnerability by the cerebral defense system. *J Am Coll Cardiol* 1985;5:88B–94B.

51. Stratton JR, Pfeifer MA, Ritchie JL, Halter JB. Hemodynamic effects of epinephrine: concentration-effect study in humans. *J Appl Physiol* 1985;58:1199–1206.

52. Suga H, Hisano R, Hirata S, et al. Mechanism of higher oxygen consumption rate: pressure-loaded vs volume-loaded heart. *Am J Physiol* 1982;242:H942–H948.

53. Takaoka H, Takeuchi M, Odake M, et al. Comparison of hemodynamic determinants for myocardial oxygen consumption under different contractile states in human ventricle. *Circulation* 1993;87:59–69.

54. Tofler GH, Stone PH, Maclure M, et al. Analysis of possible triggers of acute myocardial infarction (The MILIS Study). *Am J Cardiol* 1990;66:22–27.

55. Vatner SF, Franklin D, Higgins DB, et al. Left ventricular response to severe exertion in untethered dogs. *J Clin Invest* 1972;51:3052–3060.

56. Waldrop TG, Eldridge FL, Iwamoto GA, Mitchell JH. Central neural control of respiration and circulation during exercise. In: Rowell LB, Shepherd JT (eds). *Handbook in Physiology.* Section 12. New York: Oxford University Press, 1996;333–380.

57. Yi JJ, Fullwood L, Stainer K, et al. Effects of food on the central and peripheral haemodynamic response to upright exercise in normal volunteers. *Br Heart J* 1990;63:22–25.

58. Young ME, Radda GK, Leighton B. Nitric oxide stimulates glucose transport and metabolism in rat skeletal muscle in vitro. *Biochemistry* 1997;322:223–228.

16

Heart Failure and Neurohumoral Responses

There are basically three mechanisms for myocardial failure (Table 16-1): pressure overload, volume overload, and primary myocardial disease (cardiomyopathy). In each case, through different mechanisms, the myocardium attempts to compensate for the primary defect before the stage of overt myocardial failure develops. Meerson described three stages of myocardial reaction to the load: (1) the initial hemodynamic load and its effects; (2) myocardial hypertrophy, compensating for the load; and (3) overload and overt ventricular failure (Fig. 16-1). In addition, there are complex neurohumoral changes in the circulation that attempt to maintain normal organ perfusion in the face of decreasing myocardial function. These changes involve activation of the renin-angiotensin and other systems that cause peripheral vasoconstriction, thereby helping to maintain the blood pressure.

MYOCARDIAL REACTION TO PRESSURE OR VOLUME OVERLOAD

In response, for example, to aortic stenosis or sustained severe hypertension, left ventricular (LV) pressure that is developed must increase (first phase of Meerson) to overcome the resistance to the ejection of blood (Fig. 16-1). The mechanism for the increase at a cellular level is probably a stretch-induced increase in the inotropic state, involving mechanoreceptors. The result is that the LV systolic pressure increases, the obstruction to the outflow of blood from the left ventricle is overcome, and the cardiac output is maintained. The disadvantage of this mode of adaptation is that *LV wall stress* is greatly increased. In other words, the transmural force acting on the left ventricle will tend to dilate the heart, which further increases the wall stress, and LV failure would rapidly becomes more and more inevitable. However, with a sustained pressure load, the myocardium adapts by concentric hypertrophy, which means that it becomes

TABLE 16-1. *Causes of left-sided heart failure*

Excessive pressure load
    Aortic stenosis
    Hypertrophic obstructive cardiomyopathy
    Arterial hypertension
Excessive volume load
    Aortic or mitral regurgitation
    High-output states (thyrotoxicosis)
    Some types of congenital heart disease
Primary myocardial disease
    Hypertrophic (nonobstructive) cardiomyopathy
    Hypertrophic obstructive cardiomyopathy
    Dilated cardiomyopathy
    Cardiomyopathy of the elderly
    Myocarditis
    Metabolic heart disease
    Endocrine heart disease
Impaired LV filling
    Tight mitral stenosis
    Constrictive pericarditis
    Restrictive cardiomyopathy

thicker without increasing in radius, and the wall stress normalizes (second phase, Fig. 16-1). The mechanism whereby the myocardial cells undergo transverse hypertrophy and become fatter in shape is not known, although evidently the mechanical pattern of increased transmural wall stress elicits an appropriate signal system. The result in concentric hypertrophy is that the abnormally increased wall stress resulting from the pathologically high intraventricular pres-

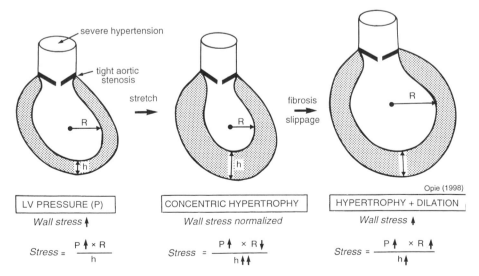

Opie (1998)

LV PRESSURE (P)	CONCENTRIC HYPERTROPHY	HYPERTROPHY + DILATION
Wall stress ↑	*Wall stress normalized*	*Wall stress ↑*

$$Stress = \frac{P{\uparrow} \times R}{h}$$
$$Stress = \frac{P{\uparrow} \times R{\downarrow}}{h{\uparrow}{\uparrow}}$$
$$Stress = \frac{P{\uparrow} \times R{\uparrow}}{h{\uparrow}}$$

FIG. 16-1. Pressure load and overload. During severe aortic stenosis or hypertension, initial concentric hypertrophy normalizes wall stress, but when dilation develops, wall stress increases. R, radius; h, wall thickness; P, pressure.

sure is reduced or even normalized, so that systolic function at rest is normal. However, such compensatory hypertrophy is bought at the double cost of greater susceptibility to ischemia and of abnormal diastolic function.

Diastolic Dysfunction in Left Ventricular Hypertrophy

Left ventricular hypertrophy (LVH) is characterized by an increased LV wall thickness and mass, with abnormal diastolic properties. There is a triad of loss of distensibility (so that the ventricle is stiffer), impaired relaxation, and decreased early diastolic filling. Characteristically, the echocardiogram shows a decrease or reversal of the normal E/A ratio (see Fig. 12-23). These abnormalities of relaxation may in part result from the mechanical properties of the hypertrophied ventricle, such as increased interstitial connective tissue (Cuocolo et al., 1990). Yet at least some of the functional changes can reverse upon acute administration of an angiotensin-converting enzyme (ACE) inhibitor, enalapril, to patients with LVH resulting from severe aortic stenosis (Friedrich et al., 1994). At a cellular level, hypertrophic myocyctes have abnormal calcium cycles, including prolonged calcium transients and impaired relaxation (Friedrich et al., 1994). The proposal is that such functional abnormalities may have been induced in part by the local activity of angiotensin II, perhaps in part acting through its indirect permissive action in promoting adrenergic activity (see Fig. 14-5), and hence cytosolic calcium overload.

Systolic Function in Compensated Left Ventricular Hypertrophy

According to the Meerson hypothesis, the third stage of overt LV failure, with poor systolic function, is only reached when compensated hypertrophy degenerates into myocardial dilation.* In accord with this proposal, systolic function in the hypertrophied heart should be and often is normal despite diastolic deterioration. Yet in response to exercise, systolic abnormalities may develop, especially in the presence of more severe LVH (Cuocolo et al., 1990). The proposal is that marked diastolic abnormalities of filling and decreased distensibility lead to inadequate end-diastolic stretch of the ventricular myocytes so that the Frank-Starling mechanism does not operate as it should during exercise. Exercise brings out such defects because tachycardia diminishes the time for diastolic filling and further increases the myocardial oxygen demand.

Volume Overload and LV Function

The initial event in a volume load is again hemodynamic, being valvular regurgitation (incompetence) of either the mitral valve or the aortic valve. Some investigators include the effects of severe and prolonged exercise training as a

---

*"Dilation" versus "dilatation." I do not see any reason for the longer tongue-twister, although it is preferred by the Oxford English Dictionary, and has etymologic evidence in its favor (*Lancet* 1993;341:867).

volume load, but it seems better to distinguish between a pathologic and a physiologic origin for the load. Exercise training can in no true sense be equated with an organic regurgitant valve lesion. *Regurgitation* means that with every contraction there is more of the stroke volume recycled, so that a greater volume of blood must be dealt with per stroke (Fig. 16-2). To deal with this volume load, there are both changes in the loading conditions and in ventricular size. First, the volume load means that the preload increases and that the heart is functioning at the length limit of the Frank-Starling curve. Second, Grossman et al. (1975) have proposed that a volume load could cause "longitudinal hypertrophy" (see Fig. 13-2), thereby increasing the size of the LV cavity, which in turn could increase the chamber size without increasing the wall thickness. Some increase in chamber volume also may be attained by slippage of cells (same number of cells, wall is thinned). The result of the volume overload is that there is enhanced early diastolic filling and decreased LV stiffness (Zile et al., 1993), so that diastolic function improves rather than deteriorates as in a pressure overload. Nonetheless, as the chamber size increases, wall tension must increase. The consequence is some hypertrophy, which will allow the LV cavity to regain a normal wall stress by the modest and proportional degree of LVH.

Volume Versus Pressure Load. Extremely severe degrees of hypertrophy, 100% or more, as found in marked concentric hypertrophy, do not occur in volume hypertrophy, possibly because the greater systolic wall stress of the pres-

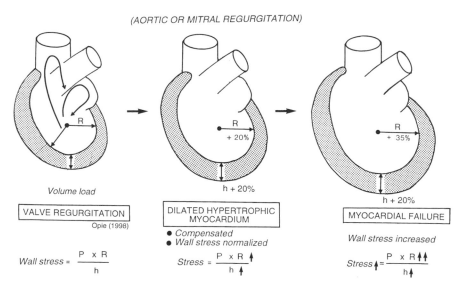

FIG. 16-2. Volume load and overload as occurs in mitral or aortic regurgitation initially leads to a dilated myocardium with some hypertrophy normalizing wall stress. When myocardial failure sets in, the degree of dilation exceeds the degree of hypertrophy.

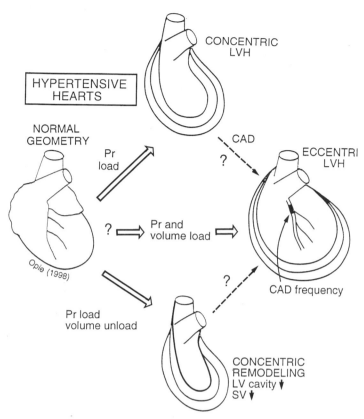

FIG. 16-3. Hypertension and the heart. A chronically elevated blood pressure causes a compensatory concentric hypertrophy, thereby lessening the effect of the increased afterload on wall tension (see Fig. 12-15). Concentric remodeling, without increase of LV mass but with a smaller than normal LV cavity size, may reflect combined pressure loading and volume unloading. Eccentric hypertrophy might reflect combined pressure and volume loading. Different types of hypertension have different circulating volumes, which might hypothetically account for these ill-understood differences in LV response. CAD, coronary artery disease.

sure load is a more potent stimulus to myocyte hypertrophy (Fig. 16-3). Because of the lesser degree of increase in the thickness of the LV free wall and less internal work with a volume load (see Fig. 12-17), the oxygen supply/demand ratio is likely to be better maintained in a volume load than in a pressure load. Also, diastolic function improves in a volume load and deteriorates in a pressure load.

PRIMARY MYOCARDIAL FAILURE: CARDIOMYOPATHY

In primary myocardial failure (Fig. 16-4), there is no initial defect in the loading conditions of the left ventricle, so both volume and pressure load are initially

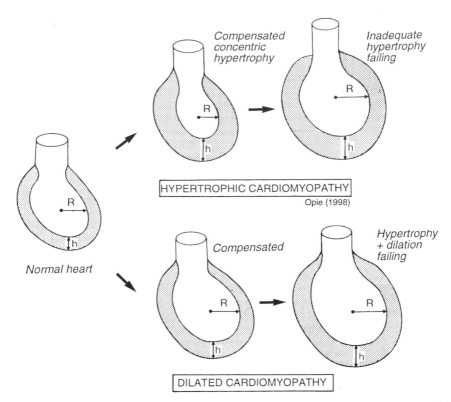

FIG. 16-4. Cardiomyopathy. Note contrast between the two types of cardiomyopathy in the initial phases. Compensated concentric hypertrophy leads to a normal relationship between wall thickness and wall stress, whereas the development of dilation leads to myocardial failure. In dilated cardiomyopathy, there may be an initial compensated phase when hypertrophy is proportional to the degree of chamber enlargement, followed by excessive chamber enlargement and inadequate hypertrophy.

normal. For a given end-diastolic volume (and, therefore, sarcomere length), tension generation is inadequate due to the primary myocardial disease or cardiomyopathy (*myopathy*, muscle degeneration). Sometimes the cause of the disease is known (secondary cardiomyopathy), and sometimes it is unknown (primary cardiomyopathy). For practical purposes, whenever the origin of the myocardial disease is obscure, it is useful to think of a state of primary cardiomyopathy.

In *hypertrophic cardiomyopathy,* the ventricular wall is abnormally thick and the cavity size small. There are some similarities between the early stages of compensated concentric hypertrophy of this type of cardiomyopathy and the first phase of hypertrophy in response to a pressure load. The state of marked concentric hypertrophy found in primary hypertrophic cardiomyopathy causes a high systolic ejection fraction, and diastolic dysfunction predominates. Here the major problem lies in the small size of the LV cavity, virtually obliterated by the hypertrophy, with consequent inability to fill normally during diastole. The obstructive subvariety of hypertrophic cardiomyopathy, *hypertrophic obstructive cardiomyopathy,* is characterized by an excessively thick interventricular septum, which during systole actually obstructs the LV outflow to cause a pressure gradient between the LV cavity and the aorta, thereby increasing the pressure that has to be generated within the left ventricle. Thus, the systolic wall stress increases, theoretically to exaggerate the degree of hypertrophy.

Genetic defects may underlie *hypertrophic cardiomyopathy.* The muscle cells undergo excess growth in size in response to a genetic abnormality of the contractile proteins. Three abnormal genes have been found, encoding for β-myosin heavy chain or α-tropomyosin or cardiac troponin T (Watkins, 1994).

In primary *dilated cardiomyopathy,* the initial event is myocardial failure due to an unknown cause but often thought to be viral infection, with poor pressure generation, so that the ejection fraction decreases, and now a self-induced volume overload takes place accompanied by a marked increase in wall stress. There is usually a certain degree of compensatory hypertrophy, inadequate to normalize wall stress. Dilated cardiomyopathy also can develop as a secondary phenomenon, whenever a large mass of myocardium is damaged, as in alcoholic damage or after a large myocardial infarct or with severe generalized coronary artery disease.

The *cardiomyopathy of the elderly* is basically the result of fewer myocytes. Starting with about 10^9 cells in the heart of a young adult, the cells diminish at the rate of 38 million per year (Olivetti et al. 1991). In compensation, there is modest hypertrophy of the remaining cells, but without being able to maintain a normal myocardial mass. Therefore, there is overall loss of contractile power, accounting for impaired effort tolerance of the elderly. Also contributing to exertional dyspnea is a decreased myocardial compliance with diastolic heart failure.

Tumor Necrosis Factor and Nitric Oxide.   An interesting hypothesis relates virus infection to impaired contractile function in dilated cardiomyopathy by the newly described nitric oxide messenger system (Fig. 16-5). The proposal is that a virus infection, which might be occult, elicits a macrophage response that produces *tumor necrosis factor-α,* a cytokine that then induces the enzyme nitric oxide synthase in the myocytes. The resulting excess production of nitric oxide has a negative inotropic effect by increasing the level of cyclic guanosine monophosphate (cGMP), thereby limiting calcium ion influx.

Mechanical Restriction of the Myocardium

Restrictive cardiomyopathy is a rare disease in which the chief problem is that the ventricle is mechanically prevented from relaxation, for example, by an infiltrative disease process. In this condition, the cardiomyopathic process replaces normal ventricular myocardium by an infiltrate that stiffens the ventricular wall

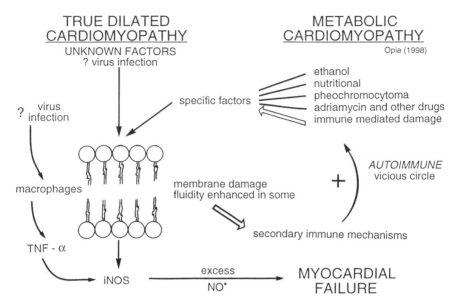

FIG. 16-5. Postulated cellular mechanisms in cardiomyopathy. Note role of tumor necrosis factor alpha (TNF-α), thought to induce nitric oxide synthase (iNOS), to produce excess nitric oxide (NO), thereby increasing the degree of myocardial failure. For cardiac overexpression of TNF-α, see Kubota et al., *Circ Res* 1997;81:627.

to restrict filling and emptying. Alternatively, there can be mechanical obstruction to the LV filling, from disease of the pericardial sac, such as constrictive pericarditis (Table 16-1).

COMMON VALVE LESIONS

Four prototypical valve lesions are induced by aortic stenosis and regurgitation, and mitral stenosis and regurgitation. Each of these causes a typical type of hemodynamic lesion, with a pressure load in the case of aortic stenosis, and volume load in the regurgitant lesions. Tight mitral stenosis limits flow from the left atrium to the left ventricle and causes left-sided heart failure even in the presence of normal myocyte function because it restricts both the inflow and hence the outflow of blood from the left ventricle.

Specific Aspects of Mitral Regurgitation. The apparent benefits of regurgitation—improved diastolic function and reduced afterload—all revert back to normal after mitral valve replacement (Zile et al., 1993). The crucial benefit is that the enlarged ventricular cavity becomes smaller. Whereas in aortic regurgitation the afterload is increased by systolic hypertension, in mitral regurgitation the volume overload is ejected into the atrium during systole, thereby decreasing rather than increasing the afterload. These may be among the reasons why mitral regurgitation may be so well tolerated for so long and why it often seems a less serious lesion than that produced by aortic regurgitation.

Hypertensive Patterns.   Although hypertension is often thought of as posing a pure pressure load on the myocardium, and therefore causing concentric LVH, eccentric hypertrophy may be caused in some patients by an associated volume load (increased blood volume) (Fig. 16-3). *Concentric remodeling* (Ganau et al., 1992) could result from the combination of pressure overload and volume underload. In this condition the LV mass is normal, the cavity size reduced, the wall thickness increased, and the stroke volume diminished. These findings are "surprising and counterintuitive from the vantage point of most clinical cardiologists" (Reichek, 1992).

PROGRESSION FROM HYPERTROPHY TO FAILURE

The third stage of overload with overt systolic failure develops when either pressure or volume overload is no longer compensated for by the appropriate degree of hypertrophy, and the radius increases excessively with increase in wall stress. It should be emphasized that overt systolic failure is always accompanied by diastolic dysfunction. Thus, in response to a sustained pressure or volume load, the myocardium passes from a compensated phase to a dilated failing phase. The mechanism whereby hypertrophy develops into myocardial failure is not known. One reasonable hypothesis is that the hypertrophied myocardium is prone to an imbalance between the oxygen supply/demand ratio (Fig. 16-6) by a variety of mechanisms, including the following.

The Myocardium Outstrips Its Blood Supply.   Gross and Spark, writing in 1937, were among the first to suggest that the hypertrophied myocardium failed

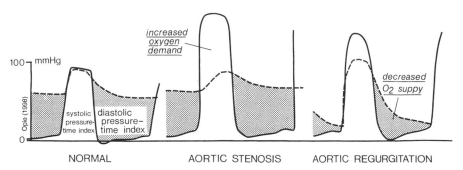

FIG. 16-6. Oxygen demand versus supply in aortic valve disease. Note contrasting effects of pressure overload in aortic stenosis and volume overload in aortic regurgitation. In the LVH of aortic stenosis, there is increased systolic pressure with increased oxygen demand, but coronary vascular reserve is reduced. In the volume overload of aortic regurgitation, there is a reduced diastolic perfusion pressure, with a decreased oxygen supply.

because of a "disturbed relationship between muscle fiber size and the volume of blood flow through the capillary bed." Linzbach (1960) saw concentric hypertrophy when the normal myocardial response that persisted until a critical limit was reached at which the hypertrophied heart would outstrip its blood supply, leading to focal necrosis and myocardial failure. This *critical limit* for myocardial hypertrophy may be about 500 g, that is, about twice the normal heart weight. Not only is the myocardial oxygen demand increased because the individual cells are hypertrophied, but the myocardium outgrows its blood supply. During myocardial hypertrophy, the capillary surface area decreases in relation to the myocyte volume, and the distance between the capillaries increases (Tomanek et al., 1982).

Impaired Coronary Vascular Reserve.   Coronary reserve is the ratio of coronary resistance at rest to that following maximum coronary dilation by dipyridamole (see Fig. 10-5). The coronary reserve is much decreased when there is coronary artery disease. Even in its absence, there is decreased coronary reserve in LVH, especially in the endocardial zones, which are subject to the greater wall stress (Hittinger et al., 1990). Thus, especially during exercise, when the much thicker muscle mass requires a much higher myocardial oxygen uptake, the coronary circulation is inadequate. Repeated bouts of ischemia could eventually lead to fibrosis by stimulation of the collagen synthesis. Once fibrosis sets in, it tends to strangulate the normal myocardial cells (Jalil et al., 1989). Even when the myocardial hypertrophy regresses by therapeutic relief of the pressure load, the collagen that has formed does not disappear, so there is a permanent defect in the left ventricle (Krayenbuehl et al., 1983). Thus, excess collagen formation could signal the transition to irreversible myocardial failure.

Role of Angiotensin II and Aldosterone.   Angiotensin II is also potentially a stimulus to fibrosis (see Fig. 17-12), as is aldosterone. Thus, the renin-angiotensin system may not only play a crucial role in the hypertrophic process but also in irreversible damage. The proposal is that at least some of the angiotensin II originates locally within the myocytes, possibly in response to stretch and/or ischemia.

Increased Collagen Tissue and Decreased Myocardial Compliance.   In physiologic amounts, collagen may help to limit ventricular dilation, when it is increased in proportion to the degree of myocardial hypertrophy. In contrast, when there is an excessive collagen response to ischemia or metabolic signals such as angiotensin II, then compliance decreases with an increase in *chamber stiffness* or a decrease in *distensibility.* On the pressure–volume loop, the pressure increases more than it should for any given volume increase (see Fig. 12-18). That is because the thicker the wall of the ventricle, the more the intraluminal pressure is required to make it stretch. Thus, the wall tension increases more than expected, with a corresponding increase in the oxygen demand. This, in turn, contributes to relative ischemia of the hypertrophied myocardium and promotes interstitial fibrosis.

Apoptosis. The left ventricle undergoes progressive dilation and thinning during the development of severe heart failure. A current hypothesis is that apoptosis, a form of programmed cell death, may contribute to the attrition. Apoptosis, as more fully described in Chapter 18, is a gene-directed process that results in predictable cell death, as recognized by a number of indirect markers of DNA damage such as laddering. There is new gene expression, for example of the *Fas* gene, and inactivation of the anti-apoptotic gene, *bcl-2*. Only a low incidence of apoptotic cells is found in severe heart failure. Yet if only 0.2% of the entire population of cells were lost per day, then, because the apoptotic cycle is so short, up to 50% of the total pool of myocardial cells could be lost over one year (Colucci, 1996). Despite the fascination of the subject and its major implications, the true role of apoptosis in progression of heart failure is not yet evident.

WHAT IS THE BASIC BIOCHEMICAL DEFECT?

Apart from the proposed consequences of oxygen imbalance, a more fundamental biochemical defect has been suspected since at least 1913, when Clark found that the hypodynamic frog's heart "loses its power of combining with calcium." Since then, studies too numerous to analyze have delineated defects in oxidative phosphorylation, high-energy phosphate metabolism, calcium ion movements, contractile proteins, protein synthesis and breakdown, and catecholamine metabolism. It is apparent though that there is no unifying hypothesis to explain divergent findings. Much of the confusion increases because models of congestive heart failure differ from each other and from the situation in real life, where congestive failure is the end-product of numerous different chronic processes, such as ischemic heart disease, valvular heart disease, hypertension, cardiomyopathy, and high-output states such as thyrotoxicosis.

The earlier hope that there would be a unitary molecular explanation for congestive heart failure has not been supported. There is no firm evidence that the final common path in congestive heart failure is decreased availability of energy for cellular integrity and function. It seems, instead, that each type of experimental failure involves different mechanisms. The final end result reflects earlier specific changes, together with added nonspecific changes resulting from molecular stretch and distortion. Biochemical studies of particular interest can be analyzed as follows.

Oxygen Uptake. As long as no reasonable consensus can be reached on basic observations, such as the oxygen uptake of the muscle and the state of mitochondria in congestive heart failure, it would be fair to conclude that any such abnormalities found are not the basic defect in congestive failure. From the clinical point of view, no therapy has been evolved based on correcting possible defects of mitochondrial metabolism. The major clinical problem relates to the increased oxygen uptake (relative to the mechanical function) required by the large dilated heart and the benefits obtained by changing the position of the heart on the Frank-Starling curve (see Fig. 12-5) by altering either preload or afterload.

Energy Starvation.   In some experimental conditions, there appears to be an enhanced uptake of oxygen per gram of active tension developed, that is, a variety of oxygen-wastage (Fig. 16-7) (Gunning and Coleman, 1973). The mechanism for this is not known. Speculatively, cytosolic calcium overload could result, for example, from abnormalities of mitochondrial or sarcoplasmic function. The corresponding situation in patients may be the increased oxygen consumption per unit mass of heart, even when LV function is impaired (Strauer, 1983). In patients with LV hypertrophy, myocardial oxygen uptake per 100 g of tissue is almost 50% greater in normals, and intermediate values are found in essential hypertension. The increasing LV wall stress out of proportion to the LV mass explains the abnormal increase in the myocardial oxygen uptake. On the basis of this or other changes in the myocardial oxygen supply/demand ratio, foci of myocardial ischemia result with, it is proposed, the formation of fibrous tissue and consequences for the compliance of the myocardium. The

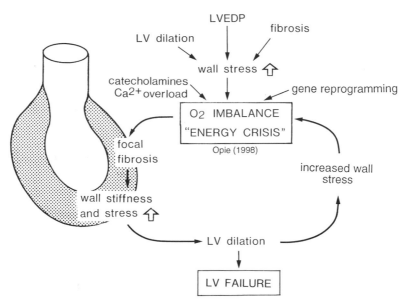

FIG. 16-7. Proposed energy crisis in the failing heart. Note role of oxygen imbalance. The onset of focal fibrosis by collagen growth may be a critical feature in the progression from the compensated hypertrophic state to the dilated failing myocardium. LV, left ventricle; LVEDP, left ventricular end-diastolic pressure.

imbalance between energy production and use in the failing heart leads to Katz's (1989) proposal that there is a state of energy starvation. Of interest, in relation to this metabolic hypothesis, is that activation of a gene-regulating pathway is associated with a defect of the fatty acid oxidizing enzymes (Sack et al., 1996).

Contractile Proteins in Experimental Failure.   There could be either abnormal myocardial proteins with normal calcium ion movements or abnormal interaction of calcium ions with normal proteins (or combinations of these changes). Increasing attention is being directed to the links between the contractile state of the myocardium and the myosin adenosine triphosphate (ATP)ase activity. The hypothesis has been postulated and probably proven that abnormal myosin isoenzymes are formed in experimental congestive heart failure (Lompre et al., 1979). The decreased ATPase values and depressed mechanical function are seen as beneficial compensatory (Pagani et al., 1988). High-pressure low-speed work is more easily managed by the hypertrophied, failing heart in contrast to its poor ability to cope with the high-volume load temporarily created by exercise.

Myosin ATPase Activity in Human Hearts.   Most of these results are based on experimental aortic or pulmonary stenosis in animals. Such overloading does not increase the heart weight by more than about 50%, whereas in human heart hypertrophy the heart may enlarge by 200% to 300%. In humans, shifts of isoenzyme pattern (from V_1 to V_3, see Fig. 13-11) do not seem to occur. There must be another explanation for decreased myosin ATPase activity (Mercadier et al., 1983), which decreases abruptly when the heart weight exceeds a critical value of 500 g (Leclerq and Swynghedauw, 1976). This critical value is reminiscent of the concept that above a similar critical mass, the capillary supply is outstripped (Linzbach, 1960) and myocytes increase in number as well as size. Myosin ATPase activity is markedly depressed in the failing human heart and may be a crucial feature in the development of end-stage heart failure (Pagani et al., 1988).

Sarcomere Length in Heart Failure.   It used to be thought that in congestive heart failure the sarcomeres were overstretched, thereby removing myosin crossbridges from their interactive sites on the actin. However, this concept has been laid to rest by direct measurements of sarcomere length in human heart failure (Fig. 16-8). Sarcomere length does not exceed 2.2 µm or slightly longer in length. Although these fibers are near the limit of their length, they can still stretch a little more without decreasing and possibly even increasing force development (Holubarsch et al., 1996). Because of the associated low ejection fraction and the increased end-diastolic volume caused by the low inotropic state, there is an increase in subendocardial wall stress with a relative ischemia and fall-off in LV performance.

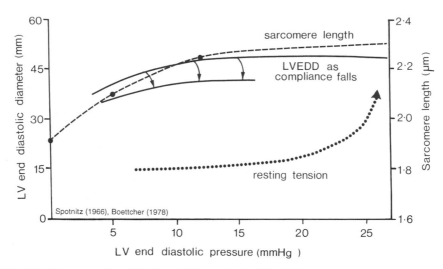

FIG. 16-8. Sarcomere length in heart failure. As the LV end-diastolic pressure increases, the LV end-diastolic volume (here measured as LV end-diastolic diameter, LVEDD) increases over low pressures but rapidly reaches a maximum. Similarly, sarcomere length also reaches a maximum. If the LV end-diastolic pressure is increased beyond the physiologic limit of about 12 mm Hg, resting tension starts to increase and will impair subendocardial myocardial perfusion. If the compliance of the ventricle is decreased, as after myocardial infarction, dV/dP decreases, and there is a lesser volume increase for a given pressure increase (see Fig. 12-25). These relationships can explain some aspects of the Frank-Starling curve in heart failure. Data based on Spotnitz et al. (1966) and Boettcher et al. (*Am J Physiol* 1978;234:H338).

TRANSGENIC MODELS

Specific knock-out models delineate certain factors that could precipitate heart failure. For example, LVH can be found in knock-out models of α-myosin heavy chain, interleukin-6, a subtype of the α-1 receptor, P-21 ras, the glucose transporter GLUT 4, or β-adrenergic receptor kinase (β-ARK) (Jaber et al., 1996). It is not always readily apparent why a specific knock-out model should be associated with LV hypertrophy, pointing to a role for other poorly understood growth signals.

THE CLINICAL SYNDROME OF CONGESTIVE HEART FAILURE

There is no entirely satisfactory definition of heart failure. The clinical picture of fully developed congestive heart failure is an admixture of three separate components. First, as a result of *diastolic failure,* there is imperfect filling of the left ventricle so that features of pulmonary congestion and increased venous pressure develop. Second, there is *systolic failure* with impaired contractile behavior of the heart and decreased force development, so that the myocardium is on a lower Frank-Starling curve than normal (Fig. 16-9). Stroke volume and cardiac output increase less than they should during exercise, and peripheral perfusion is impaired and muscular fatigue develops. Third, there are important *neurohumoral changes* that increase peripheral vascular resistance and afterload: the sympathetic tone is increased, the renin-angiotensin-aldosterone system is activated, and there is fluid retention with peripheral congestion and edema so that the preload is also increased.

Definitions of congestive heart failure are often tautologically flawed (Harris, 1983). Some investigators hold that heart failure may be defined as a state in which the heart fails to maintain an adequate circulation for the needs of the body despite a satisfactory venous pressure. In brief, heart failure is then illogically defined as a state in which the heart fails. Another defective definition dates back to Lewis (1933): "There is but one meaning to the term cardiac failure—it signifies the inability of the heart to discharge its contents adequately."

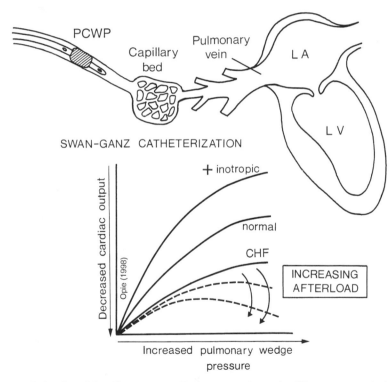

FIG. 16-9. A family of Starling curves. Each curve relates the filling pressure (pulmonary wedge pressure) to the LV stroke output and to the cardiac output. Note that the depressed inotropic state of the myocardium causes an abnormally low curve and that the downward limb can be related to an increased afterload. Clinically the measurements relating filling pressure to cardiac output are obtained by Swan-Ganz catheterization, which measures the preload on the left ventricle as the pulmonary wedge pressure and the afterload as the peripheral vascular resistance (PVR), from the equations BP = CO × PVR, and PVR = BP/CO. Note the close association between LV diastolic dysfunction and pulmonary congestion.

Except during the phase of increasing pulmonary edema, the left ventricle must be discharging as much blood as enters; therefore, this definition is far from perfect.

In relation to the Frank-Starling curve, congestive heart failure is a state in which the heart is overloaded, so that further elevation of the venous pressure fails to increase the cardiac output as expected (Wood, 1952). The problem with this definition is the difficulty in obtaining measurements of the LV filling pressure and cardiac output without invasive Swan-Ganz catheterization, and even then the further problem of having to increase the filling pressure. Besides which, limits of normality are not well defined.

For clinical purposes, heart failure is a clinical syndrome characterized by exertional symptoms and caused by heart disease. This simple definition, verbally proposed by Packer some years ago, allows the bedside diagnosis of heart failure. *Congestive heart failure* is the term that encompasses fluid and sodium retention (congestion) sufficiently severe to cause increased jugular venous pressure, or systemic edema or liver enlargement. The New York Heart Association has proposed a widely used classification of heart failure into four grades, based on the severity of dyspnea, thus emphasizing the clinical relevance of the diastolic failure that causes such symptoms.

For the experimentalist, however, clinical definitions are inadequate, and it must be considered that the dominant hemodynamic basis of heart failure is either diastolic or systolic, or both. Diastolic failure may occur on its own and often precedes systolic failure, whereas systolic failure is always accompanied by diastolic failure. The crucial issue is that the contraction–relaxation cycle of the myocardium is depressed as the result of a disease state. In an area where very many definitions have already been offered, it may be appropriate to put forth yet one more: *LV failure exists when the venous filling pressure is increased because of relaxation abnormalities or when myocardial ejection is impaired because the inotropic state is depressed.*

Modern View of Backward and Forward Failure

The distinctions between the forward and backward aspects of congestive heart failure have been recognized for many years (Harrison, 1935; McMichael, 1952; McMichael and Sharpey-Schafer, 1944). Even today, with our sophisticated understanding of hemodynamic and neurohumoral abnormalities, this division is useful (Figs. 16-10 and 16-11). Basically, the critical hemodynamic events are (1) backward failure with an increased pulmonary capillary pressure, (2) depressed myocardial contractility with forward failure, and (3) increased systemic vascular resistance with an increased afterload with worsening of LV function and exaggeration of forward failure.

Backward failure has the following clinical consequences (Table 16-2): increased pulmonary wedge pressure (Fig. 16-10), pulmonary crackles, a tendency toward pulmonary edema, pulmonary arterial hypertension, right ventric-

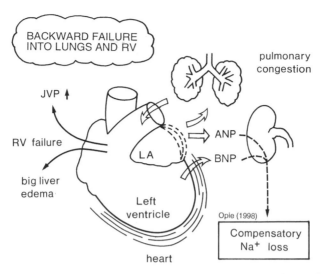

FIG. 16-10. Backward failure. Note association with pulmonary congestion and abnormalities of left atrial emptying or LV relaxation. α_1, α-adrenergic; β, β-adrenergic; aldo, aldosterone; RV, right ventricle; LA, left atrium; JVP, jugular venous pressure; ANP, atrial natriuretic peptide; BNP, brain natriuretic peptide.

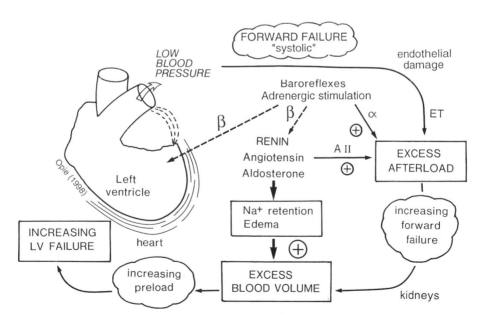

FIG. 16-11. Forward failure. Note association of forward failure with hypotension and neurohumoral activation with consequent afterload increase to which increased angiotensin II (AII) and endothelin (ET) contribute.

TABLE 16-2. *Common symptoms and signs of congestive heart failure and their mechanisms*

Symptoms/signs	Mechanism
Backward failure	
Exertional dyspnea	Increased back pressure with exercise; impaired diastolic relaxation
Pulmonary crepitations (crackles, extra lung sounds)	Increased LV end-diastolic pressure with back pressure
Right ventricular failure, elevated jugular venous pressure,[a] distended liver	Features of increasing back pressure
Forward failure	
Exertional limb fatigue	Forward failure with low cardiac output
Cold extremities	Peripheral vasoconstriction; sympathetic and renin-angiotensin activation
Tachycardia	Sympathetic activation; Bainbridge reflex
Edema and fluid retention	Aldosterone activation
Metabolic-endocrine	
Impaired renal function	Backward and forward failure
Oliguria (low urine volume)	Severe fluid retention; poor renal perfusion
Low serum sodium	Aldosterone and vasopressin secretion
Low serum potassium	Usually drug-induced (diuretics, sympathomimetic agents), sometimes effect of excess aldosterone

[a]Correlates with pulmonary wedge pressure (Butman et al., 1993).

ular failure, jugular venous pressure elevation, hepatic distention and dysfunction, and increased renal vein pressure and renal dysfunction. Of all these features, it is breathlessness, or dyspnea, that is the most sensitive index of backward failure. "The first indication of cardiac failure is to be found in diminished tolerance to exercise. Of the very numerous tests of cardiac efficiency . . . there is none that approaches in delicacy the symptom breathlessness" (Lewis, 1933).

Such breathlessness can best be related to an increased pulmonary capillary wedge pressure, which in turn signifies either abnormal LV filling or decreased left atrial emptying. In other words, backward failure and diastolic dysfunction are the same entity. Both effort intolerance and diastolic dysfunction can be an early feature of LV hypertrophy, and both have the same hemodynamic explanation.

Forward failure is best explained by poor systolic ejection (Fig. 16-11). Poor muscle perfusion causes impaired exercise capacity with muscle fatigue on exertion. The onset of tachycardia, increased peripheral vasoconstriction, and sodium retention with edema all result from forward failure. Sodium retention results from increased aldosterone secretion, impaired glomerular filtration rate, and renal dysfunction (the latter resulting in part from decreased renal perfusion and also from backward failure). Aldosterone is a sodium-retaining hormone secreted by the adrenal gland. A critical event in the progression of forward failure is the activation of a series of neurohumoral abnormalities (so-called because the adrenergic nervous system is activated to evoke the renin-angiotensin humoral response).

Clinical Detection of Myocardial Dysfunction. Besides the symptoms of effort intolerance, there will be sinus tachycardia (Table 16-3), cardiomegaly (cardiac enlargement detected by clinical examination or by chest x-ray), and added heart sounds, such as the third heart sound that results from ventricular dilation. There is now increasing evidence that patterns of diastolic function are abnormal at an early stage when, for example, the predominant cardiac findings are LVH and sustained systolic function. A major problem is the complexity of the echocardiographic techniques required to interpret diastolic dysfunction and conflicting interpretations of the observations made. However, it is widely agreed that when diastolic function is depressed, there are abnormal patterns of filling that are associated with symptoms of pulmonary congestion.

The myocardial inotropic state is defective, and systolic function is decreased, as shown by a low ejection fraction and a pressure-volume loop that is small in area (decreased heart work) and depressed to the right. As heart failure advances, diastolic dysfunction is progressive and correlates better with the patient's functional status than does the extent of systolic failure (Packer, 1990; Vanoverschelde et al., 1990).

CATECHOLAMINES AND β-RECEPTORS IN HEART FAILURE

Just when along the course of development of congestive heart failure the *sympathetic adrenergic stimulation* starts is not clear. Experimentally, it is closely associated with failure of myocardial contractility (Legault et al., 1990). We know that in severe heart failure, plasma norepinephrine is elevated. The degree of elevation bears a relation to the severity of heart failure. The plasma level of norepinephrine is powerfully related to the prognosis (Kaye et al., 1995), as is the increase in heart rate or decrease in heart work. Therefore, it is reasonable to suppose that myocardial failure results in sympathetic activation and that such activation has adverse consequences. A possible mechanism is that impaired myocardial function results in relative hypotension that stimulates the baroreceptors to activate the sympathetic nervous system.

Excess Catecholamine Stimulation. Excess catecholamine stimulation, such as that found in severe congestive heart failure, could have a direct toxic effect on the failing myocardium, but proof of this proposal is still lacking. It could be argued, for example, that β-adrenergic receptor downgrading is a protective mechanism that allows a lesser inotropic response while preserving the myocardium from the adverse effects of catecholamines. However, as β_1-adrenergic receptors are downgraded, β_2 and (possibly) α_1-adrenergic receptors become more prominent and may mediate other adverse catecholamine effects (Bristow et al., 1985). The sum total of the potential harm of excess catecholamine stimulation is serious and includes (1) enhanced sarcolemmal permeability, (2) intracellular calcium overload and a delayed diastolic decrease in calcium, (3) arrhythmogenic mechanisms that follow excess cAMP or calcium

TABLE 16-3. *Pathophysiologic mechanisms in congestive heart failure*

Change	Mechanism	Advantages	Disadvantages
Hypotension	Depressed inotropic state	Conserves oxygen	Evokes adrenergic activation supply
Tachycardia	Baroceptor-mediated, reflex adrenergic	Helps to maintain cardiac output as stroke volume ↓	MVO_2 increased
Arteriolar vasoconstriction	1. Adrenergic drive increased 2. Renin-angiotensin ↑ 3. Endothelin release	Helps to maintain blood pressure	Cardiac output decreased
LV volume increased	Mitral regurgitation, fiber slippage	Helps to maintain stroke volume by Starling mechanism	MVO_2 increased wall tension ↑
Atrial stretch	ANP secretion	Vasodilatory and diuretic	ANP receptor downgrading
Myosin ATPase ↓	Gene reprogramming. Altered isoenzymes in animals	High pressure, low speed work	Slower rate of contraction inotropic state ↓
Catecholamine depletion of heart	Unknown. Decreased uptake and synthesis	Protects myocardium from calcium overload	May contribute to inotropic state ↓
Liver enlargement	Hepatic congestion	None	May cause hepatic failure
Renal congestion	Poor renal perfusion	None	May precipitate prerenal failure
Congested lungs	Increased pulmonary wedge pressure; LV diastolic dysfunction	Limits exercise, conserves MVO_2	Dyspnea, pulmonary edema
Gene resetting, neonatal phenotype	Chronic LV failure	LV makes ANP, BNP, adrenomedullin	Fatty acid enzymes ↓, energy production ↓

MVO_2, myocardial oxygen uptake; CO, cardiac output; ↓, decreased; ↑, increased.

stimulation, (4) impaired mechanical function, possibly with impaired diastolic relaxation, and (5) myocardial oxygen wastage (Opie et al., 1979). The ultimate effects of excess catecholamines and of calcium overload are likely to be harmful and contribute to the process of accelerating myocardial failure.

The *major hemodynamic consequences of sympathetic stimulation* include (1) β-mediated sinus tachycardia and α-mediated peripheral vasoconstriction (Table 16-3), both of which have potentially harmful effects on the failing myocardium, the former by decreasing the diastolic filling time and the latter by increasing the afterload; and (2) a potential positive inotropic effect, which only in part compensates for decreased stroke volume and the inherent contractile failure of the myocardium, because of β-receptor downregulation (Fig. 16-12). It is not clear whether such excessive and prolonged myocardial sympathetic stimulation leads directly to β₁-adrenergic receptor downgrading or whether genetic reprogramming is involved; the end result is a lesser degree of inotropic response to catecholamines (Arai et al., 1995; Bristow et al., 1982). This impaired response to catecholamines is relatively specific to the myocardium so that increased sympathetic stimulation of the kidneys leads to increased renin release with consequent formation of vasoconstrictive angiotensin II.

β₁-Adrenergic Receptor Downregulation.   During the development of congestive heart failure, circulating catecholamine levels increase, especially during exercise. Chronic high-level exposure to such catecholamines should lead to a marked decrease in myocardial responsiveness through the process of desensiti-

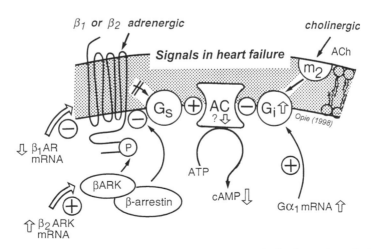

FIG. 16-12. Receptors in heart failure. Proposed changes in β-adrenergic and cholinergic receptor signal systems in severe congestive heart failure (CHF), with depressed levels of cAMP and decreased contractility. For concepts, see Lohse (1995). AC, adenylate cyclase; β₁AR, β₁-adrenergic receptor; β₂AR, β₂-adrenergic receptor; βARK, β-adrenergic receptor kinase; M₂, muscarinic receptor; ACh, acetylcholine; Gᵢ, inhibitory G protein; Gₛ, stimulatory G protein.

zation (Fig. 16-8). The rate of development of such changes is not known, although desensitization is found after several days of catecholamine treatment (Brodde et al., 1990). Such changes in receptor density differ from a molecular change in the receptor, whereby, for example, β-agonist catecholamines induce or stabilize a high-affinity form of the β-adrenergic receptor, which is specific for agonists and binds antagonists rather weakly (Lefkowitz and Hoffman, 1980). Possible changes in the β-adrenergic receptor affinity in conditions of excess catecholamine stimulation have not been well studied.

Compensatory Role of β₂-, α₁-Adrenergic, and Vasoactive Intestinal Peptide Receptors. Sizeable amounts of *β₂-adrenergic receptors* are found in the non-failing human ventricle, amounting to about 15% of the combined β_1- plus β_2-adrenergic receptor population. These β_2-adrenergic receptors may (1) phys-iologically help to sustain the full and maximal inotropic response to cate-

---

TABLE 16-4. *Receptors and signaling systems in severe congestive heart failure*[a]

---

1. *Receptors*
   β_1-adrenergic receptors downgraded, i.e., density and activity decreased[b]
   β_2-adrenergic receptor density unchanged, functional uncoupling[b]
   α_1-adrenergic receptors relatively increased in density[b]
   VIP receptors decreased in density but affinity considerably more[c]
2. *G-proteins*
   G_i increased with inhibition of adenylate cyclase[d–f]
   G_s normal[g] or decreased[h]
3. *Adenylate cyclase*
   Decreased cyclase activity with less production of cAMP, related to G_i increase[e]; still responds directly to forskolin[i]
4. *cAMP*
   Production impaired, presumably due to adenylate cyclase inhibition[j]
5. *Calcium transients*
   Impaired transients with low peak and delayed decrease in diastole[j]
   Calcium uptake by SR unchanged[j] or decreased in situ[i,k]
   Calcium release by SR decreased[l]
   Single calcium channel activity normal[k,m]
   Amount of calcium entry via calcium channel may be abnormal[l]

---

[a]For review see Lohse. *Trends Cardiovasc Med* 1995;5:63. Note that most data in human congestive heart failure have been obtained on patients with cardiomyopathy coming to transplantation. In other diseases, different findings may hold as, for example, the concordant decrease in β_1- and β_2-adrenergic receptor activity in mitral valve disease (Brodde et al., 1990).
[b]Bristow et al. (1989).
[c]Hershberger et al. (1989).
[d]Eschenhagen (1992).
[e]Böhm et al. (1994).
[f]Feldman et al. (1988).
[g]Schnabel et al. (1990).
[h]Feldman et al. (1990).
[i]Morgan et al. (1990).
[j]Böhm et al. (1994).
[k]Movsesian et al. (1989).
[l]D'Agnolo et al. (1992).
[m]Holmberg and Williams (1989).

cholamine stimulation and (2) pathologically come into greater prominence as the β_1-adrenergic receptors are downgraded in severe congestive heart failure. Nonetheless, the β_2-adrenergic receptors are also not normal in that they are uncoupled from G proteins (Table 16-4). Thus, β_2-agonist stimulation does not have the expected inotropic result.

α_1-Adrenergic receptor stimulation, in general, helps to mobilize internal calcium (Homcy and Graham, 1985) and enhances trans-sarcolemmal calcium influx, so that α_1-adrenergic receptor stimulation plays an additional inotropic role (Bruckner et al., 1985), independently of cAMP. In severe congestive heart failure (cardiomyopathy), there is a relative increase in α_1-adrenergic receptor density (Bristow et al., 1989).

Vasoactive intestinal peptide (VIP, a 28–amino acid peptide neurotransmitter) acts on receptors that are coupled to adenylate cyclase. In the failing human heart, ventricular VIP receptors become much more sensitive to VIP. This may therefore be one mechanism to help maintain contractility despite the downgraded β_1-adrenergic receptors.

G Proteins and Adenylate Cyclase.   Studies on G proteins are still actively in progress. Nevertheless, there is agreement that the content of the inhibitory G_i protein increases, whereas G_s is either unchanged or decreased in tissues from human heart failure (Table 16-4). In general, the increase in G_i is accompanied by a decreased activity of adenylate cyclase.

cAMP Generation in Heart Failure.   Another serious abnormality in end-stage heart failure is poor generation of cAMP (Fig. 16-13) in response both to β-agonist agents and also (unexpectedly) to the phosphodiesterase inhibitors, agents that inhibit the breakdown of cAMP (Feldman et al., 1987; Morgan et al., 1990). Whereas the failure of β-agonists to work can be explained by receptor downgrading and the inhibition of adenylate cyclase by G_i, the explanation for the failure of phosphodiesterase inhibition to increase cAMP is obscure. Possibly, intracellular compartmentation of cAMP could be invoked (Rapundalo et al., 1989).

Calcium Transients.   There are a number of possible factors that are likely to cause calcium overload in congestive heart failure: sarcolemmal damage and enhanced membrane permeability (Dhalla, 1976), microfoci of ischemia, excess circulating catecholamines and microvascular spasm (Factor et al., 1982), besides the consequences of therapeutic procedures, such as sodium pump inhibition by digitalis, β-agonist stimulation, and phosphodiesterase inhibition (Fig. 16-13). Calcium overload occurs in a model of hereditary heart failure, the golden Syrian hamster (Jasmin and Bajusz, 1975). Cellular calcium overload can be expected to contribute to the adverse mechanical changes of the failing or hypertrophied myocardium. For example, in the myopathic heart, there is less of an increase of internal calcium, followed by a prolonged calcium transient (Fig. 16-14), reflecting multiple abnormalities of the regulation of internal calcium

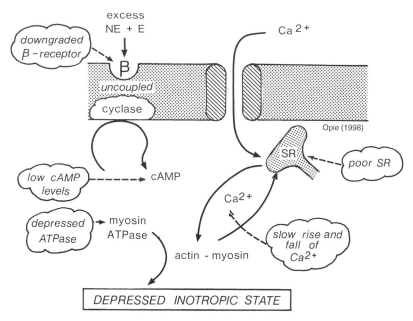

FIG. 16-13. **Calcium in severe heart failure.** Note multiple mechanisms for depressed inotropic state. For receptor changes, see Fig. 16-12. NE, norepinephrine; E, epinephrine; SR, sarcoplasmic reticulum; β, β-adrenergic; cAMP, cyclic AMP.

(Table 16-4). Particularly when the heart rate is fast, there is not enough time for the internal calcium to decrease to baseline levels (Morgan et al., 1990), which may explain why tachycardia is so badly tolerated in heart failure.

β₃-Adrenergic Receptors.   Besides their important role in adipose tissue, these receptors may have a cardiac function (Gauthier et al., 1996). The proposal is

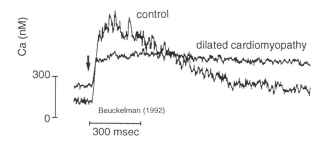

FIG. 16-14. **Calcium transients in heart failure cells.** Note in cells from dilated cardio-myopathy that the calcium transients increase less than in controls, and then stay abnormally elevated. From Beuckelman et al. *Circulation* 1992;85:1046 by permission of the American Heart Association.

that they respond to adrenergic stimulation by an unexpected negative inotropic response, which leads to the further suggestion that they could contribute to the poor mechanical function of the failing heart.

ANGIOTENSIN II AND OTHER VASOCONSTRICTIVE PEPTIDES

In severe heart failure, an increased afterload is a prominent adaptation (Figs. 16-15 and 16-16). Both a low renal perfusion pressure and increased β-adrenergic stimulation contribute to renin release (Fig. 16-17). The result is ultimately an angiotensin-mediated vasoconstriction to add to that mediated by the activated sympathetic nervous system (Fig. 16-11). Angiotensin II both directly constricts the peripheral vessels and enhances the degree of sympathetic activation (see Figs. 9-4 and 14-5). Angiotensin II also evokes the release of aldosterone with an increase of body fluid volume, as well as retention of sodium and water. The latter process is clinically manifest as excess volume of the legs, detected by pitting in response to finger pressure (edema). Sodium and water retention resulting from aldosterone secretion tends to reverse the low renal perfusion pressure and also, by maintaining the blood pressure, lessens the reflex sympathetic stimulation. The causes of increased renin secretion therefore are subject to feedback, which may explain why in nearly half of patients with severe cardiac edema the renin and aldosterone levels are normal (Anand et al., 1989). In some severe cases, the low blood sodium resulting from excess volume retention sends out the wrong signals to the pituitary gland (at the base of the brain) and

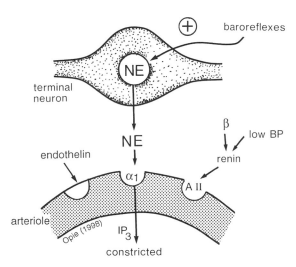

FIG. 16-15. Afterload increase in heart failure. NE, norepinephrine; β, β-adrenergic; BP, blood pressure; IP_3, inositol trisphophate; α_1, α_1-adrenergic; AII, angiotensin II.

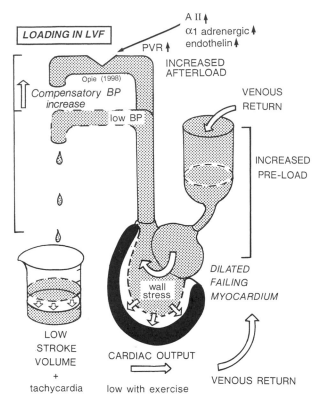

FIG. 16-16. Loading conditions in severe heart failure. Wall stress is increased as a result of increased preload, ventricular dilation, and increased peripheral vascular resistance (PVR). α_1, α_1-adrenergic; AII, angiotensin II; BP, blood pressure.

causes an inappropriate secretion of the *antidiuretic hormone.* Antidiuretic hormone is also called *vasopressin* (Greek *vas,* vessel; *pressin,* pressure) and may further increase the afterload by peripheral vasoconstriction. It also decreases renal loss of water, with more retention of extracellular fluid and an exaggeration of the low blood sodium (hyponatremia). In contrast, there is overall sodium retention. The increased fluid retention increases cardiac work by causing volume overload.

Sodium Retention and Edema. An overall retention of water (fluid) and sodium is characteristic of congestive heart failure, and this state is termed "edema," which is one of the cardinal clinical signs of congestive heart failure. The overall retention of sodium is the combined result of excess aldosterone secretion and poor renal blood flow. It should be stressed that there can be a combination of a low serum sodium together with marked overall sodium retention, reflecting the respective consequences of vasopressin and aldosterone secretion.

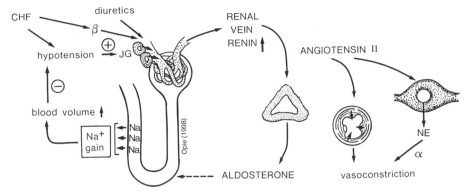

FIG. 16-17. Renin-angiotensin system in congestive heart failure increases renin secretion from the juxtaglomerular (JG) cells in the kidney by two mechanisms: hypotension and increased β-adrenergic stimulation (β). Circulating renin then stimulates a plasma substrate to convert circulating angiotensinogen to angiotensin I, which is converted to angiotensin II in the tissue to cause vasoconstriction. Angiotensin II also increases release of norepinephrine (NE) further to promote vasoconstriction. Angiotensin II releases aldosterone from the adrenal glands, thereby causing sodium and water retention, which helps to maintain the blood pressure and renal perfusion. There is thus a feedback loop on the kidney to diminish renin secretion. Note the role of diuretic therapy in promoting renin release. CHF, congestive heart failure; α, α-adrenergic.

Endothelin in Heart Failure

Circulating levels of endothelin are increased in severe heart failure, the source of the endothelin being at least in part from the myocardium, in which there are increased levels of pre-pro-endothelin-1 (Sakai et al., 1996). Endothelin, by promoting myocardial calcium overload, has a direct toxic effect and induces hypertrophy and increases contractility (Sakai et al., 1996). Administration of an endothelin receptor antagonist lessens mortality in experimental heart failure and improves hemodynamics in humans (Kiowski et al., 1995).

Cytokines in Heart Failure

Cytokines are locally acting autocoid polypeptide mediators (Greek *autos,* self; *akos,* remedy). This group of still poorly understood agents interacts with receptors that are phospholipase C linked and mediates vasoconstriction through release of calcium from the sarcoplasmic reticulum. Cytokines act locally in one of several manners: autocrine (active on the cells of origin), paracrine (acting on neighboring cells), or juxtacrine (acting on adjacent cells). Examples are the inflammatory cytokines, such as the interleukins, derived from macrophages and leukocytes. Such cells are especially found in the myocardium in infective cardiomyopathies, but also after myocardial infarction and reperfusion. *Tumor necrosis factor-α* and another cytokine, interleukin-6, increase the formation of soluble ICAM-I (intercellular adhesion molecule-1). They also appear to be linked, as does interleukin-1, to the myocardial nitric oxide signaling system, which is upregulated in response to inflammatory mediators (Kelly and Smith, 1997). In this way, cytokines are thought to exert excess negative inotropic influences by formation of myocardial cGMP (Tsutamoto et al., 1995). Although this sequence seems to be established in the case of septic shock with heart failure, the importance of cytokines in standard heart failure is still being researched.

ATRIAL AND BRAIN NATRIURETIC PEPTIDES

Thus far, many of the adaptations discussed have been potentially harmful to the failing myocardium, either directly or by increasing the afterload and preload. However, release of *atrial natriuretic peptide* (ANP) from the atria has properties beneficial for the circulation in heart failure (Fig. 16-18). ANP has diuretic activity (increases urine flow), vasodilates, and inhibits aldosterone secretion. ANP is an endogenous antagonist to angiotensin II, and binding sites for these two compounds overlap (Giles, 1990). ANP inhibits release of norepinephrine from terminal neurons, which also leads to vasodilation (Ferrari and Agnoletti, 1989). Circulating levels of ANP are increased in congestive heart failure in proportion to the atrial pressure (Raine et al., 1986). Furthermore, the

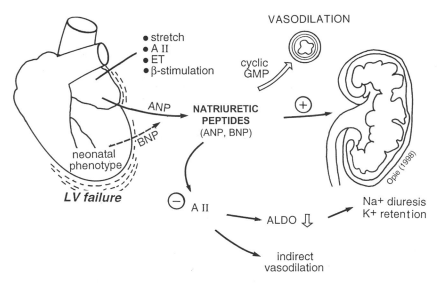

FIG. 16-18. Atrial natriuretic peptide (ANP) is released from the atria in response to stretch or β-adrenergic (β) stimulation, or angiotensin II (AII) or endothelin (ET). In congestive heart failure (CHF), there is increased release with increased blood levels of ANP. In CHF, some of the circulating ANP comes from the ventricles, as does brain natriuretic peptide (BNP). ANP has effects that oppose those of renin-angiotensin activation (see Fig. 16-17) and competes with angiotensin II for receptors. Adrenomedullin is a recently identified vasodilatory peptide. Generally the beneficial effects of ANP secretion are outweighed by vasoconstrictory stimuli and excess sodium retention. ALDO, aldosterone secretion from the adrenals.

higher the levels of ANP, the more serious the severity of the congestive heart failure is likely to be (Gottlieb et al., 1989). It may well be asked why the beneficial effects of increased ANP are not apparent.

The increased levels of ANP in congestive heart failure are overcome by the drives toward vasoconstriction and sodium retention resulting from renin-angiotensin-aldosterone activation. In addition, the atrial stretch receptors involved in the secretion of ANP become downgraded, and vascular ANP receptors decrease their reaction to circulating ANP stimulation (Ferrari and Agnoletti, 1989; Tsutamoto et al., 1995). That ANP does have potentially beneficial effects in congestive heart failure is shown by the worsening of signs when monoclonal anti-ANP antibodies are given in experimental heart failure (Giles, 1990).

Release of ANP from Atria.   It is clear that atrial stretch, not pressure, regulates such release, presumably acting via mechanoreceptors. A number of facilitatory factors promote or inhibit the release of ANP. Increased ANP released during ventricular tachycardia or supraventricular tachycardia is thought to be the cause of the polyuria associated with those conditions. The chief stimulus to such ANP release in these conditions is probably atrial distention, with the tachycardia itself being an additional independent factor (Ferrari and Agnoletti, 1989). The ultimate signal to ANP release could involve calcium, elevated, for example, after mechanoreceptor or β-adrenergic stimulation or after a rapid tachycardia with insufficient time for calcium re-uptake into the sarcoplasmic reticulum. Other factors increasing cell calcium, such as phorbol esters that stimulate protein kinase C, as well as angiotensin, vasopressin, and endothelin, also facilitate ANP release (Ruskoaho et al., 1989, ref. 71). Conversely, in response to acetylcholine, there is a gradual decline in ANP secretion. The actual release process from the atrial storage granules in response to increased atrial tension involves the movement within seconds of the granules from the center to the periphery of the cell. It is this process that seems to become exhausted with repetitive stretch, and there is less ANP release (Ferrari and Agnoletti, 1989). Such movements occur along the microtubules and are accelerated by monensin, a sodium ionophore that increases cell sodium and calcium (Iida et al., 1988). The release of ANP is either as such or as pro-ANP (126 amino acids), the latter then being cleaved by a serum protease to ANP, which consists of 28 amino acids in humans (Genest and Cantin, 1987).

At a cellular level the major effect of ANP is stimulation of guanylate cyclase, which increases cGMP, causing vascular dilation closely resembling that induced by nitrates, although there are some differences (see Fig. 9-2). The mechanism of the diuresis is still unclear and appears to be more than could be explained by simple increased renal blood flow. Experimentally, a simple marker for heart failure is increased urinary levels of cGMP.

ANP and BNP Release from Failing Ventricles.   Besides being secreted from the atria, ANP can also be formed and secreted from diseased ventricles. *ANP* *gene reprogramming* may occur at the onset of ventricular hypertrophy (Pasternac and Cantin, 1990). In the LV, it appears to be that volume or pressure overload promotes release of ANP or its precursors, especially from the endocardial layers (Ruskoaho et al., 1989, ref. 70). Ventricles are also a source of ANP in severe experimental heart failure, the model being hereditary hamster cardiomyopathy (Thibault et al., 1989). In general, however, it remains true that it is the atria and not the ventricles that are the major source of ANP. Besides ANP, brain natriuretic peptide is also released from the atria and especially from failing ventricles (Ogawa et al., 1991). The proposal is that BNP has effects similar to those of ANP in heart failure.

Adrenomedullin.   This newly identified peptide, first found in extracts of human pheochromocytoma, has potent vasorelaxing and natriuretic properties, and in this way it resembles ANP. Furthermore, in severe human heart failure, it is found in the circulation and secreted by the heart (Jougasaki et al., 1996). Presumably it joins ANP and BNP as self-protecting peptides made by the failing myocardium.

PRINCIPLES OF THERAPY FOR CONGESTIVE HEART FAILURE

The principles of *conventional therapy* are fourfold. First, diuretic therapy, by increasing output of urine and sodium, relieves the fluid retention and pulmonary congestion, thereby reducing the preload on the heart (Fig. 16-19). Unfortunately, diuretic therapy promotes the secretion of renin, which helps to cause angiotensin-induced vasoconstriction. Second, ACE inhibition has several

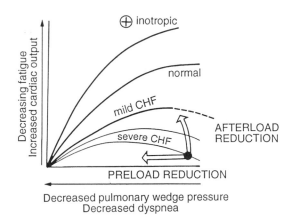

FIG. 16-19. Load reduction in heart failure. Theoretical Starling curves are shown for congestive heart failure (CHF). Note effects of preload reduction on dyspnea and pulmonary wedge pressure and afterload reduction on cardiac output and muscle fatigue. For example, nitrates reduce the preload, and angiotensin-converting enzyme inhibitors reduce both preload and afterload.

benefits. Most obviously, it relieves the vasoconstriction and excess afterload resulting from excess activation of the renin-angiotensin system. More hidden benefits might lie in the improvement of diastolic function and in countering the tendency to excess fibrosis. These compounds improve exercise capacity, probably in part through improving diastolic properties. In patients with severe congestive heart failure, added therapy by ACE inhibition decreases mortality. Besides the ACE inhibitors, other vasodilators decrease the preload by dilating the venous system or decrease the afterload by acting on the arterial dilators. Third, positive inotropic agents, including digitalis, stimulate the myocardium to contract and move it to a higher Starling curve (Fig. 16-9). In general, inotropes act by either increasing cytosolic calcium or increasing the sensitivity of the contractile proteins to calcium. Such agents have not decreased mortality, and in some cases have lessened survival, perhaps because of the adverse effects of an increased cytosolic calcium level. Fourth, vasodilators such as nitrates and hydralazine relieve the preload and the afterload, respectively.

Novel therapies are being developed. Endothelin antagonists are under test and should indirectly improve prognosis by relief of peripheral vasoconstriction. Currently, full therapy increasingly includes the use of β-adrenergic blocking agents to counter some of the effects of excess circulating β-adrenergic stimulation.

Surgical options for reduction of heart volume are also available. The dilated ventricle is subject to abnormal wall stress, which could theoretically be relieved by surgical removal of part of the ventricular wall, an operation under study. Relief of load on the ventricle could be achieved by a variety of artificial heart or pumping devices, which leave the ailing heart in place but allow it to recover as the load is lessened. One such device pumps blood from the dilated ventricles to the aorta. Also novel is cardiomyoplasty, whereby skeletal muscle is placed around the dilated ventricle to help it contract. In every case, the concept is that there is mechanical assistance to the left ventricle, providing it with a bridge to recovery.

SUMMARY

1. *An excessive pressure load* is initially compensated for by concentric hypertrophy. Hypertension is an example of an excess pressure load and may lead to left ventricular hypertrophy (LVH), impaired LV diastolic function, and eventually LV dilation. The mechanism of the change from the compensated hypertrophic to the dilated myocardium is still under evaluation, but impaired coronary vascular reserve with focal hypoxia and fibrosis may be a crucial factor.

2. *An excessive volume load* causes the myocardial chamber size to enlarge by mechanisms not fully understood, possibly including longitudinal hypertrophy and fiber slippage. Some radial hypertrophy also takes place. The resulting compensated state can exist for a long time. However, the longitudinally

enlarged cell appears not to compensate well to demands for further hypertrophy, and eventually failure occurs.

3. *In primary myocardial disease* (cardiomyopathy), the cause of the defect is unexplained. In dilated cardiomyopathy, the diseased myocardium causes the cavity size to enlarge, thereby increasing wall tension. In hypertrophic cardiomyopathy, the cause of the hypertrophy is genetic. The extreme degree of hypertrophy sensitizes the myocardium to a series of abnormalities that eventually cause myocardial fibrosis and thereby myocardial failure.

4. *The coronary vascular reserve* of the hypertrophied myocardium is impaired, which makes it especially sensitive to the possibility of an oxygen supply/demand imbalance, most notably in the subendocardial zones.

5. *Focal fibrosis* may be the consequence of focal hypoxia and causes an increased chamber stiffness and permanent damage. Excess circulating catecholamines, as found in patients with established congestive heart failure, can have further adverse effects on the myocardium through calcium overload, thereby increasing myocardial oxygen demand and decreasing myocardial mechanical performance.

6. *The sarcomere lengths* are at or close to a maximum in myocardial failure, and any increase in LV end-diastolic pressure leads to increased endocardial wall tension, with a defect in the oxygen supply/demand ratio. Increasingly, the myocardium functions at the limits of the Starling curve, and any further increase in LV end-diastolic pressure is not matched by an increase in performance. Rather, as subendocardial wall tension increases and afterload increases, LV performance fails to increase despite the increase in the LV diastolic pressure.

7. *Diastolic dysfunction* is closely linked to abnormalities of LV filling and LV relaxation. The result is increased left atrial and pulmonary wedge pressure, closely linked to the severity of the shortness of breath.

8. *The clinical picture of severe heart failure* is intimately linked to the concomitant development of a series of myocardial metabolic and circulatory neurohumoral abnormalities, including renin-angiotensin-aldosterone activation. These abnormalities serve to aggravate the severity of heart failure by increasing myocardial mechanical impairment and by systemic effects, such as sodium retention, volume overload as a result of fluid retention, and an increased afterload on the heart by virtue of increased peripheral vascular resistance.

9. *Cytokines* such as interleukins 1 and 6, and tumor necrosis factor α, may contribute to peripheral vasoconstriction. In addition, acting through the myocardial nitric oxide system and cGMP, they are thought to have a negative inotropic effect.

10. *Novel therapies* include cautious β-adrenergic blockade and mechanical assist devices that relieve the excessive wall stress on the left ventricle, and thereby unload the heart.

11. *Atrial natriuretic peptide* (ANP) is released by increased pressure acting on atria and to a lesser extent on ventricles. ANP stimulates vascular guanylate cyclase to cause vasodilation and by an unknown mechanism increases diuresis. Part of the molecule is similar to angiotensin II, and ANP antagonizes effects of angiotensin II, including vasoconstriction and release of aldosterone. Brain natriuretic peptide is also released from the failing left ventricle and has similar properties to those of ANP. Adrenomedullin is another recently identified vasodilating and natriuretic peptide. In established heart failure, these benefits of the three vasodilating peptides are overcome by opposing vasoconstrictory and sodium-retaining stimuli, such as angiotensin II, endothelin, vasopressin, and aldosterone.

STUDENT QUESTIONS

1. Compensated hypertrophy: describe the molecular mechanism governing myocardial growth in the development of this condition.
2. Describe typical calcium transients in advanced heart failure. How do these patterns come about?
3. What is the role of the renin-angiotensin-aldosterone system in the evolution of congestive heart failure.
4. What are cytokines and how might they play a role in heart failure?
5. Atrial and brain natriuretic peptides: what is their physiologic function and their role in heart failure?

CARDIOLOGIST-IN-TRAINING QUESTIONS

1. What are the patterns of left ventricular response in chronic hypertension? Specifically describe how these conditions differ in respect of left ventricular wall thickness and cavity size. What differences in wall stress do you expect?
2. Cardiomyopathy. In which types are molecular mechanisms involved in the etiology?
3. What factors are thought to be involved in the transition from compensated left ventricular hypertrophy to failure?
4. Can the Starling relationship explain the changes in contractile function of the dilated failing left ventricle? Include an evaluation of the changes of sarcomere length found in this condition.
5. What roles do catecholamine stimulation and β-adrenergic receptors have in the evolution of the syndrome of advanced heart failure?
6. A patient severely short of breath and with a central chest pain thought to be due to acute myocardial infarction, and with acute pulmonary edema not responding to conventional therapy by a loop diuretic, is subject to Swan-Ganz catheterization. What can be measured, and what information can be

obtained about (a) the preload and (b) the afterload on the left ventricle? What are the principles of acute therapeutic intervention?

REFERENCES

1. Alpert NR, Mulieri LA. Increased myothermal economy of isometric force generation in compensated cardiac hypertrophy induced by pulmonary artery constriction in the rabbit. *Circ Res* 1982;50: 491–500.
2. Anand IS, Ferrari R, Kalra GS, et al. Edema of cardiac origin. Studies of body water and sodium, renal function, hemodynamic indexes, and plasma hormones in untreated congestive cardiac failure. *Circulation* 1989;80:299–305.
3. Arai AE, Grauer SE, Anselone CG, et al. Metabolic adaptation to a gradual reduction in myocardial blood flow. *Circulation* 1995;92:244–252.
4. Böhm M, Eschenhagen T, Gierschik P, et al. Radioimmunochemical quantification of Giα in right and left ventricles from patients with ischaemic and dilated cardiomyopathy and predominant left ventricular failure. *J Mol Cell Cardiol* 1994;26:133–149.
5. Böhm M, Reiger B, Schwinger RH, Erdmann E. cAMP concentrations, cAMP dependent protein kinase activity, and phospholamban in non-failing and failing myocardium. *Cardiovasc Res* 1994;28: 1713–1719.
6. Bristow MR, Ginsburg R, Minobe W, et al. Decreased catecholamine sensitivity and beta-adrenergic receptor density in failing human hearts. *N Engl J Med* 1982;307:205–211.
7. Bristow MR, Kantrowitz NE, Ginsburg R, Fowler MB. Beta-adrenergic function in heart muscle disease and heart failure. *J Mol Cell Cardiol* 1985;17(suppl 2):41–52.
8. Bristow MR, Port JD, Gilbert EM. The role of adrenergic receptor regulation in the treatment of heart failure. *Cardiovasc Drug Ther* 1989;3:971–978.
9. Brodde OE, Daul A, Michel-Rehner M, et al. Agonist-induced desensitization of β-adrenoceptor function in humans. Subtype-selective reduction in β_1- or β_2-adrenoceptor-mediated physiological effects by xamoterol or procaterol. *Circulation* 1990;81:914–921.
10. Brodde OE, Zerkowski HR, Doetsch N, et al. Myocardial beta-adrenoceptor changes in heart failure: concomitant reduction in β_1- and β_2-adrenoceptor function related to the degree of heart failure in patients with mitral valve disease. *J Am Coll Cardiol* 1989;14:323–331.
11. Bruckner R, Mugge A, Scholz H. Existence and functional role of alpha$_1$-adrenoceptors in the mammalian heart. *J Mol Cell Cardiol* 1985;17:639–645.
12. Butman SM, Ewy GA, Standen JR, et al. Bedside cardiovascular examination in patients with severe chronic heart failure: importance of rest or inducible jugular venous distension. *J Am Coll Cardiol* 1993;22:968–974.
13. Colucci WS. Apoptosis in the heart. *N Engl J Med* 1996;335:1224–1226.
14. Cuocolo A, Sax FL, Brush JE, et al. Left ventricular hypertrophy and impaired diastolic filling in essential hypertension. Diastolic mechanisms for systolic dysfunction during exercise. *Circulation* 1990;81:978–986.
15. D'Agnolo A, Luciani GB, Mazzucco A, et al. Contractile properties and Ca^{2+} release activity of the sarcoplasmic reticulum in dilated cardiomyopathy. *Circulation* 1992;85:518–525.
16. Dhalla NS. Involvement of membrane systems in heart failure due to intracellular calcium overload and deficiency. *J Mol Cell Cardiol* 1976;8:661–667.
17. Eschenhagen T, Mende U, Nose M, et al. Increased messenger RNA level of the inhibitory G protein α subunit $G_{i\alpha-2}$ in human end-stage heart failure. *Circ Res* 1992;70:688–696.
18. Factor SM, Minase T, Cho S, et al. Microvascular spasm in the cardiomyopathic Syrian hamster: a preventable cause of focal myocardial necrosis. *Circulation* 1982;66:342–354.
19. Feldman AM, Cates AE, Veazey WB, et al. Increase of the 40,000-mol wt pertussis toxin substrate (G-protein) in the failing human heart. *J Clin Invest* 1988;82:189–197.
20. Feldman AM, Tena RG, Kessler PD, et al. Diminished beta-adrenergic receptor responsiveness and cardiac dilation in hearts of myopathic Syrian hamsters (BIO 53.58) are associated with a functional abnormality of the G stimulatory protein. *Circulation* 1990;81:1341–1352.
21. Feldman MD, Copelas L, Gwathmey JK, et al. Deficient production of cyclic AMP: pharmacologic evidence of an important cause of contractile dysfunction in patients with end-stage heart failure. *Circulation* 1987;75:331–339.

22. Ferrari R, Agnoletti G. Atrial natriuretic peptide: its mechanism of release from the atrium. *Int J Cardiol* 1989;24:137–149.
23. Friedrich SP, Lorell BH, Rousseau MF, et al. Intracardiac angiotensin-converting enzyme inhibition improves diastolic function in patients with left ventricular hypertrophy due to aortic stenosis. *Circulation* 1994;90:2761–2771.
24. Ganau A, Devereux RB, Roman MJ, et al. Patterns of left ventricular hypertrophy and geometric remodeling in essential hypertension. *J Am Coll Cardiol* 1992;19:1550–1558.
25. Gauthier C, Tavernier G, Charpentier F, et al. Functional β_3-adrenoreceptor in the human heart. *J Clin Invest* 1996;98:556–562.
26. Genest J, Cantin M. Atrial natriuretic factor. *Circulation* 1987;75(suppl I):118–124.
27. Giles TD. Defining the role of atrial natriuretic factor in health and disease. *J Am Coll Cardiol* 1990;15:1331–1333.
28. Gottlieb SS, Kukin ML, Ahern D, Packer M. Prognostic importance of atrial natriuretic peptide in patients with chronic heart failure. *J Am Coll Cardiol* 1989;13:1534–1539.
29. Gross H, Spark C. Coronary and extracoronary factors in hypertensive heart failure. *Am Heart J* 1937;14:160–182.
30. Grossman W, Jones D, McLaurin L. Wall stress and patterns of hypertrophy in the human left ventricle. *J Clin Invest* 1975;56:56–64.
31. Gunning JF, Coleman HN. Myocardial oxygen consumption during experimental hypertrophy and congestive heart failure. *J Mol Cell Cardiol* 1973;5:25–38.
32. Harris P. Origins of congestive cardiac failure. *Cardiovasc Res* 1983;17:440–445.
33. Harrison TR. In: *Failure of the Circulation*. Baltimore: Williams & Wilkins, 1935.
34. Hershberger RE, Anderson FL, Bristow MR. Vasoactive intestinal peptide receptor in failing human ventricular myocardium exhibits increased affinity and decreased density. *Circ Res* 1989;65:283–294.
35. Hittinger L, Shannon RP, Kohin S, et al. Exercise induced subendocardial dysfunction in dogs with left ventricular hypertrophy. *Circ Res* 1990;66:329–343.
36. Holmberg SRM, Williams AJ. Single channel recordings from human cardiac sarcoplasmic reticulum. *Circ Res* 1989;65:1445–1449.
37. Holubarsch C, Ruf T, Goldstein DJ, et al. Existence of the Frank-Starling mechanism in the failing human heart. Investigations on the organ, tissue and sarcomere levels. *Circulation* 1996;94:683–689.
38. Homcy CJ, Graham RM. Molecular characterization of adrenergic receptors. *Circ Res* 1985;56:635–650.
39. Iida H, Barron WM, Page E. Monensin turns on microtubule-associated translocation of secretory granules in cultured rat atrial myocytes. *Circ Res* 1988;62:1159–1170.
40. Jaber M, Koch WJ, Rockman H, et al. Essential role of β-adrenergic receptor kinase 1 in cardiac development and function. *Proc Natl Acad Sci USA* 1996;93:12974–12979.
41. Jalil JE, Janicki JS, Pick R, et al. Fibrosis-induced reduction of endomyocardium in the rat after isoproterenol treatment. *Circ Res* 1989;65:258–264.
42. Jasmin G, Bajusz E, Solymoss B. Selective prevention by verapamil and other drugs of hamster hereditary cardiomyopathy. In: Bradley WS, Gardner D, Medum D, Walton NJ (eds). *Recent Advances in Myology.* New York: Elsevier, 1975;413–417.
43. Jougasaki M, Rodeheffer RJ, Redfield MM, et al. Cardiac secretion of adrenomedullin in human heart failure. *J Clin Invest* 1996;97:2370–2376.
44. Katz AM. Changing strategies in the management of heart failure. *J Am Coll Cardiol* 1989;13:513–523.
45. Kaye DM, Lefkovits J, Jennings GL, et al. Adverse consequences of high sympathetic nervous activity in the failing human heart. *J Am Coll Cardiol* 1995;26:1257–1263.
46. Kelly RA, Smith TW. Cytokines and cardiac contractile function. *Circulation* 1997;95:778–781.
47. Kiowski W, Sutsch G, Hunziker P, et al. Evidence for endothelin-1-mediated vasoconstriction in severe chronic heart failure. *Lancet* 1995;346:732–736.
48. Krayenbuehl HP, Hess OM, Schneider J, Turina M. Physiologic or pathologic hypertrophy. *Eur Heart J* 1983;4(suppl A):29–34.
49. Leclerq JF, Swynghedauw B. Myofibrillar ATPase, DNA and hydroxyproline content of human hypertrophied heart. *Eur J Clin Invest* 1976;6:27–33.
50. Lefkowitz RJ, Hoffman BB. Adrenergic receptors. *Adv Cycl Nucleotide Res* 1980;12:37–47.
51. Legault F, Rouleau JL, Juneau C, et al. Functional and morphological characteristics of compensated and decompensated cardiac hypertrophy in dogs with chronic infrarenal aorto-caval fistulas. *Circ Res* 1990;66:846–859.

52. Lewis T. In: *Diseases of the Heart.* London: Macmillan, 1933.
53. Linzbach AJ. Heart failure from the point of view of quantitative anatomy. *Am J Cardiol* 1960;5: 370–382.
54. Lohse MJ. G-protein-coupled receptor kinases and heart. *Trends Cardiovasc Med* 1995;5:63–68.
55. Lompre AM, Schwartz K, D'Albis A, et al. Myosin isoenzymes redistribution in chronic heart over-loading. *Nature* 1979;282:105–107.
56. McMichael J. Dynamics of heart failure. *Br Med J* 1952;2:525–529.
57. McMichael J, Sharpey-Schafer EP. The action of intravenous digoxin in man. *Q J Med* 1944;13: 123–135.
58. Mercadier J-J, Bouveret P, Gorza L, et al. Myosin isoenzymes in normal and hypertrophied human ventricular myocardium. *Circ Res* 1983;53:52–62.
59. Morgan JP, Erny RE, Allen PD, et al. Abnormal intracellular calcium handling, a major cause of systolic and diastolic dysfunction in ventricular myocardium from patients with heart failure. *Circulation* 1990;81(suppl III):21–32.
60. Movsesian MA, Bristow MR, Krall J. Ca^{2+} uptake by cardiac sarcoplasmic reticulum from patients with idiopathic dilated cardiomyopathy. *Circ Res* 1989;65:1141–1144.
61. Ogawa Y, Nakao K, Mukoyama M, et al. Natriuretic peptides as cardiac hormones in normotensive and spontaneously hypertensive rats. *Circ Res* 1991;69:491–500.
62. Olivetti G, Melissari M, Capasso JM, Anversa P. Cardiomyopathy of the ageing human heart. Myocyte loss and reactive cellular hypertrophy. *Circ Res* 1991;68:1560–1568.
63. Opie LH, Thandroyen FT, Muller CA, Bricknell OL. Adrenaline-induced "oxygen-wastage" and enzyme release from working rat heart. Effects of calcium antagonism, beta-blockade, nicotinic acid and coronary artery ligation. *J Mol Cell Cardiol* 1979;11:1073–1094.
64. Packer M. Abnormalities of diastolic function as a potential cause of exercise intolerance in chronic heart failure. *Circulation* 1990;81(suppl III):78–86.
65. Pagani ED, Alousi AA, Grant AM, et al. Changes in myofibrillar content and Mg-ATPase activity in ventricular tissues from patients with heart failure caused by coronary artery disease, cardiomyopathy, or mitral valve insufficiency. *Circ Res* 1988;63:380–385.
66. Pasternac A, Cantin M. Atrial natriuretic factor: a ventricular hormone. *J Am Coll Cardiol* 1990;15: 1446–1448.
67. Raine AEG, Erne P, Burgisser E, et al. Atrial natriuretic peptide and atrial pressure in patients with congestive heart failure. *N Engl J Med* 1986;315:533–537.
68. Rapundalo ST, Solaro RJ, Kranias EG. Inotropic responses to isoproterenol and phosphodiesterase inhibitors in intact guinea pig hearts: comparison of cyclic AMP levels and phosphorylation of sar-coplasmic reticulum and myofibrillar proteins. *Circ Res* 1989;64:104–111.
69. Reichek N. Patterns of left ventricular response in essential hypertension. *J Am Coll Cardiol* 1992; 19:1559–1560.
70. Ruskoaho H, Kinnunen P, Taskinen T, et al. Regulation of ventricular atrial natriuretic peptide release in hypertrophied rat myocardium. Effects of exercise. *Circulation* 1989;80:390–400.
71. Ruskoaho H, Vakkuri O, Arjamaa O, et al. Pressor hormones regulate atrial-stretch-induced release of atrial natriuretic peptide in the pithed rat. *Circ Res* 1989;64:482–492.
72. Sack MN, Rader TA, Park S, et al. Fatty acid oxidation enzyme gene expression is downregulated in the failing heart. *Circulation* 1996;94:2837–2842.
73. Sakai S, Miyauchi T, Kobayashi M, et al. Inhibition of myocardial endothelin pathway improves long-term survival in heart failure. *Nature* 1996;384:353–355.
74. Schnabel P, Bohm M, Gierschik P, et al. Improvement of cholera toxin-catalyzed ADP-ribosylation by endogenous ADP-ribosylation factor from bovine brain provides evidence for an unchanged amount of G in failing human myocardium. *J Mol Cell Cardiol* 1990;22:73–82.
75. Spotnitz HM, Sonnenblick EH, Spiro D. Relation of ultrastructure to function in the intact heart. *Circ Res* 1966;18:49–66.
76. Strauer BE. Left ventricular dynamics, energetics and coronary hemodynamics in hypertrophic heart disease. *Eur Heart J* 1983;4(suppl A):137–142.
77. Thibault G, Nemer M, Drouin J, et al. Ventricles as a major site of atrial natriuretic factor synthesis and release in cardiomyopathic hamsters with heart failure. *Circ Res* 1989;65:71–82.
78. Tomanek RJ, Searls JC, Lachenbruch PA. Quantitative changes in the capillary bed during developing, peak and stabilized cardiac hypertrophy in the spontaneously hypertensive rat. *Circ Res* 1982;51: 295–304.
79. Tsutamoto T, Hisanaga T, Fukai D, et al. Prognostic value of plasma soluble intercellular adhesion

molecule-1 and endothelin-1 concentration in patients with chronic congestive heart failure. *Am J Cardiol* 1995;76:803–808.
80. Vanoverschelde J-L, Raphael DA, Robert AR, Cosyns JR. Left ventricular filling in dilated cardiomyopathy: relation to functional class and hemodynamics. *J Am Coll Cardiol* 1990;15:1288–1295.
81. Watkins H. Multiple disease genes cause hypertrophic cardiomyopathy. *Br Heart J* 1994;72(suppl): 4–9.
82. Wood P. In: *Diseases of the Heart and Circulation.* London: Eyre & Spottiswoode, 1952;154–192.
83. Zile MR, Tomita M, Ishihara K, et al. Changes in diastolic function during development and correction of chronic LV volume overload produced by mitral regurgitation. *Circulation* 1993;87: 1378–1388.

PART VI

Pathophysiology

17

Oxygen Lack:
Ischemia and Angina

*Voluntary motion will soon be lost in the part thus
deprived of blood.*

J.E. Erichsen, 1842

Although there still is some argumentation about the definition of myocardial ischemia (Hearse, 1994), in the end the concept is simple: ischemia means that the blood supply to the myocardium is inadequate. The Greek *ischo* means "to hold back," and *haima* means "blood." The word "ischemia" was apparently first used by Rudolf Virchow in 1858:

> . . . so habe ich den neuen Ausdruck der Ischaemie vorgeschlagen, um damit die Hemmung der Blutzüfuhr, die Vermehrung der Widerstände des Einströmens zu bereichnen.

The approximate translation is that the word "ischemia" describes the limitation of the blood supply with an increased resistance to flow. The fundamental concept of supply/demand imbalance as a cause of ischemia came from observations on an exercising limb (Burns, 1809):

> In health when we excite the muscle action to more energetic action than usual, we increase the circulation in every part. If, however, we call into vigorous action a limb around which we with a moderate degree of tightness applied a ligature, we find then that the member can only support its action for a very short time; for now its supply of energy and its expenditure do not balance each other.

Myocardial ischemia therefore exists when the reduction of coronary flow is so severe that the supply of oxygen to the myocardium is inadequate for the oxygen demands of the tissue (Fig. 17-1). How can the myocardium survive such a severe insult? An emerging biological concept, based on general biological principles derived from liver and brain cells, proposes two phases of adaptation,

515

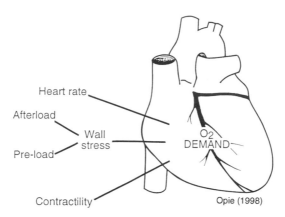

FIG. 17-1. Myocardial oxygen demand. The major determinants in the normal heart are heart rate, wall stress, and contractility. Wall stress is influenced both by preload and afterload.

namely short-term defense and longer term rescue (Hochachka et al., 1996). Applying these concepts to the oxygen-deficient heart, the aim of short-term defense is to achieve a new balance between the oxygen demand and supply, by a combination of downregulation of contraction and upregulation of anaerobic energy production by glycolysis. Long-term rescue is still poorly understood, but increasingly it seems that ischemia, perhaps acting through hypoxia, is able to induce a series of cellular signals that lead to protective genetic reprogramming (Knöll et al., 1994). When defense and rescue fail, because the ischemia is over-whelmingly severe and prolonged, then the result is cell necrosis. These long-term adaptations may account for unexpected protective reactions to ischemia, such as hibernation and preconditioning (see Chapter 19).

ACUTE ADAPTATION TO ISCHEMIA

Very rapidly after the onset of ischemia, there is an energy imbalance (Fig. 17-2) with a rundown of high-energy phosphate compounds, particularly phos-phocreatine, which protects the level of adenosine triphosphate (ATP) as long as possible, with an increase in intracellular inorganic phosphate. The latter is one of the main signals to the downregulation of contraction, which decreases within a few beats of the onset of coronary artery ligation. Simultaneously, the rundown in the energy status is probably the major signal to the increase in anaerobic glycolysis. The latter has as its initial source the acute onset of glycogen break-down, soon followed by an increase of glucose transport as a result of transloca-tion of the glucose transporters GLUT 1 and 4 to the sarcolemma (Young et al., 1997). Because of the ischemia, there is after a short delay the development of intracellular acidosis that also contributes to the decreased contraction. Thus, the ischemic myocardium can survive, for a limited time, by a combination of inhi-bition of contraction and initiation of anaerobic glycolysis. The result is that

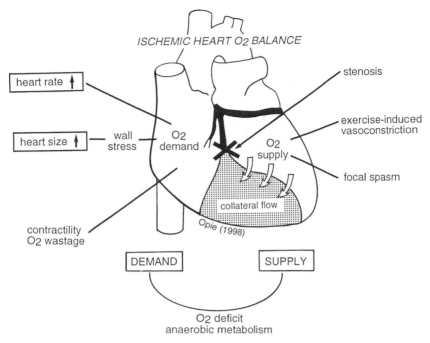

FIG. 17-2. Oxygen balance in the ischemic zone. Note important role of increased heart rate and increased heart size in increasing oxygen demand. Clinically, heart rate is one of the major determinants of myocardial oxygen uptake. Wall stress, much enhanced in the dilated heart, is increased when either preload or afterload increases.

upon reperfusion, there is rapid recovery of mechanical function (albeit to a somewhat lower level because of stunning), and reversal of the metabolic abnormalities (Fig. 17-3). The potential penalty is that the decreased contractile power may seriously threaten the well-being of the body as a whole, because the cardiac output will decrease if the ischemia involves enough myocardium.

Ischemic Contractile Failure

The major adaptation to ischemia is an abrupt decrease in the oxygen demand as contraction rapidly declines. Many theories have been advanced for such contractile failure (Table 17-1). The two basic mechanisms most frequently advanced relate to either (1) the effects of poor oxygen delivery or (2) the accumulation of inhibitory metabolites. The first factor results in depletion of high-energy phosphate compounds, including ATP and creatine phosphate. Many experiments have shown that contractile failure occurs before there is a major depletion of ATP, which is initially conserved because of the buffer function of creatine phosphate (Rauch et al., 1994). Such data cast doubt on the solitary role of the lack of ATP in contractile failure. Rather, the decrease

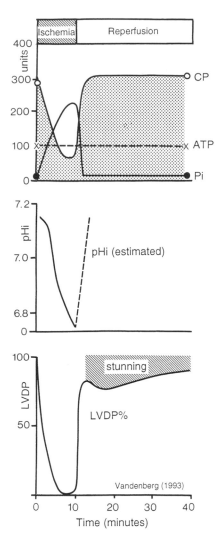

FIG. 17-3. Transient ischemia followed by reperfusion. Ten minutes of ischemia at 30°C results in a rapid decrease of creatine phosphate (CP) and increase of inorganic phosphate (Pi) while ATP is buffered. Internal pH decreases abruptly, as does left ventricular developed pressure (LVDP). Arbitrary concentration units for CP, ATP, and Pi. Modified from Vandenberg et al. (1993) by permission of the American Heart Association and Circulation Research.

of cytosolic creatine phosphate is sufficiently severe to suggest that the phosphocreatine (creatine phosphate) shuttle may be inhibited so that the problem may lie with energy transfer from the mitochondria. Nonetheless, careful repetitive measurements in very early ischemia show that there is some decrease of ATP preceding the start of contractile failure at about 10 seconds

TABLE 17-1. *Possible causes of early impairment of contractility in severe ischemia*

Proposed mechanism
Accumulation of metabolites
1. Intracellular acidosis with displacement of Ca^{2+} from intracellular binding sites on contractile proteins
2. Accumulation of inorganic phosphate with an interaction with calcium
3. Accumulation of neutral lactate
Changes in high-energy phosphate levels or availability
1. Decreased turnover of ATP
2. Decreased level of cytosolic phosphocreatine with impaired phosphocreatine shuttle[a]
3. Decreased ATP in a "contractile" subcompartment
4. Decreased free energy change (Δ_G) of ATP hydrolysis
Mechanical effects of decreased coronary flow
1. Loss of tissue turgor by reversed "garden hose" or "erectile" effect

[a]Phosphocreatine, creatine phosphate (Rauch et al., 1994).
For other references see Opie (1990).

(Hearse, 1979). If the ATP decline was localized to a contractile compartment, that could also explain the early impairment of diastolic relaxation shown by echocardiography. Cytosolic ATP seems to be required to regulate movement of sodium and hence calcium ions at the level of the cell membranes (Cross et al., 1996; Owen et al., 1990).

The second hypothesis, over 50 years old and currently much favored, is that it is the accumulation of products of ischemia that causes pump failure. In 1935 Tennant related early contractile failure to a buildup of lactic acid. In 1969 Katz and Hecht expanded this hypothesis in an influential editorial that proposed that an intracellular acidosis decreased contractility because protons displaced calcium from binding sites on the thin contractile filaments (Katz and Hecht, 1969). A very similar proposal stresses the retention of carbon dioxide during ischemia, also acting by the production of an intracellular acidosis (Cobbe and Poole-Wilson, 1980). There is now direct evidence that acidosis can impair contractility without decreasing cytosolic calcium levels (Lee and Allen, 1991). Nonetheless, intracellular acidosis can account for only about half the total decrease of contractile activity (Jacobus et al., 1982).

An alternate hypothesis is that the buildup of inorganic phosphate (Pi) released especially from creatine phosphate is the crucial factor (Kubler and Katz, 1977; Lee and Allen, 1991). The mechanism is still unclear, yet may involve a reversible Pi-sensitive step in the actomyosin crossbridge cycle (Kusuoka et al., 1986).

Whatever the mechanism (possibly a combination of the suggested proposals), the important point is that marked contractile failure and compensatory metabolic changes can occur within 10 to 120 seconds of the onset of severe ischemia. When contractile failure is very severe but localized, the ischemic myocardium actually bulges in systole (*dyskinesia*).

Effects of Poor Oxygen Delivery During Ischemia

Lack of adequate oxygen supply to the mitochondria rapidly decreases the energy available to the cytoplasm. The rapid rundown of high-energy phosphates, especially of creatine phosphate, stimulates glycolysis and glycogenolysis, and glycolytic flux is promoted to a greater extent than its end products (pyruvate and $NADH_2$) can enter the oxygen-deprived mitochondria. Potassium also escapes from ischemic cells, in part due to activation and opening of the potassium channels that are normally inhibited by ATP. Oxidation of fatty acids is reduced, and there is an accumulation of lipid metabolites with adverse detergent properties. There are important metabolic and mechanical differences between mild and severe ischemia (Table 17-2).

Lack of ATP.   Ultimately, all ion gradients depend on availability of ATP. Activity of the ATP-dependent potassium channel may be influenced specifically by the availability of glycolytic ATP. Likewise, provision of glycolytic ATP may play a role in the regulation of the sodium pump and hence of intracellular sodium and calcium levels.

Lack of oxygen is not the only cause of ATP depletion. Another cause lies in a variety of metabolic cycles that are ATP wasting, which have no apparent benefit for the ischemic myocardium and yet need ATP. An example is the excess

TABLE 17-2. *Mechanical and metabolic differences between mild and severe ischemia*

	Mild ischemia	Severe ischemia
Prototype	Demand ischemia with metabolic washout	Supply ischemia without metabolic washout
Animal model[a]	Low-flow global ischemia with added pacing	Coronary artery ligation
Human condition	Angina of effort or of pacing	Coronary occlusion; AMI, balloon inflation
Diastolic stiffness[b]	Increases	Decreases
Cytosolic calcium	Increases	Increases
Cause of increased cytosolic calcium	? Inhibited glycolysis, ?$Na^+/H^+/Ca^{2+}$ exchange	Tissue acidosis plus $Na^+/H^+/Ca^{2+}$ exchange
Factors opposing effect of increase of cytosolic calcium	None	Tissue acidosis, increased tissue inorganic phosphate
Coronary arteries in ischemic zone	Arteries normally distended, may contribute to stiff heart	Collapsed; loss of turgor with reversed garden hose effect
PV loop	End-diastolic point moves up	End-diastolic point may move rightward
LV systolic performance[c]	Moderately reduced	Markedly reduced
Reperfusion	Diastolic failure[d]	Systolic and diastolic failure

[a]Apstein and Grossman (1987).
[b]Apstein et al. (1997).
[c]De Bruyne et al. (1993).
[d]Serizawa et al. (1980).

TABLE 17-3. *Sources of proton formation and acidosis in the myocardium in anoxia–ischemia*

Process[a]	Mechanism of generation	Comment
Inhibition of mitochondrial oxidation of $NADH_2$	Inhibition of mitochondrial metabolism	$NADH_2$ formed by anaerobic glycolysis is regenerated to NAD by conversion of pyruvate to lactate; other processes must be responsible for increased cytosolic $NADH_2$/NAD ratio in ischemia
Anaerobic glycolysis	ATP breakdown	Anaerobic glycolysis results in no proton production; protons form during breakdown of ATP
Increased tissue CO_2	Continued residual respiration, poor washout	Only in ischemia, not in anoxia
Triglyceride-FFA cycle	Continued breakdown and resynthesis of TG; ATP lost with proton production	3 ATP used per cycle, 6–7 protons produced per cycle
Glycogen turnover	Excess recycling uses ATP and produces protons	1 ATP, 1 UTP, and 1 proton per cycle
Mitochondrial uptake of calcium	Counter transport of protons with calcium	Uptake of calcium by mitochondria uses ATP and therefore produces protons

[a]For assessment of relative roles of these cycles in production of protons, see Dennis et al. (1991). TG, triglyceride; UTP, uridine triphosphate.

internal cycling of excess levels of calcium, found in the ischemic-reperfused myocardium, in and out of the sarcoplasmic reticulum, a process that needs ATP for the uptake cycle. Other metabolic cycles provoked by ischemia and wasting ATP involve the breakdown of triglyceride and glycogen and their resynthesis. These processes may contribute to proton production in ischemia (Table 17-3).

Anaerobic Glycolysis. Ischemia has a biphasic effect on glycolysis depending on its severity (see Fig. 11-2). First, there is stimulation. Then, as the severity of ischemia increases, delivery of glucose decreases, glycogen becomes depleted, and inhibitory metabolites accumulate, so that the glycolytic rate decreases. During mild ischemia, glycolysis is stimulated at several levels, including translocation of the glucose transporters GLUT 1 and 4 to the sarcolemma (Young et al., 1997), while the activity of the key enzyme phosphofructokinase increases so that the glycolytic rate increases as the energy status declines (see Fig. 11-18). The major beneficial consequence of such anaerobic glycolysis is increased production of glycolytic ATP, quite inadequate in amount to replace the total energy needs of the contracting myocardium (see Fig. 11-19), yet possibly crucial in providing ATP strategically located near the sarcolemma and thus maintaining ion gradients. Although the existence of such a pool of membrane-related ATP is still controversial, the concept is useful in explaining some of the effects of the benefit of the provision of glucose to the ischemic myocardium (e.g., inhibition of enzyme loss when glucose is added to fatty acid perfusates).

Fatty Acid Metabolism in Ischemia.   There are two major changes in fatty acid metabolism. First, ischemic inhibition of fatty acid oxidation (basically by deprivation of blood flow and oxygen) leads to an accumulation of lipid metabolites, including intracellular free fatty acids, acyl CoA, and acyl carnitine. As the tissue contents of the metabolites increase, they are thought to inhibit various aspects of membrane function, such as the mitochondrial translocase, the sodium pump, and phospholipid cycles. Second, membrane phospholipids are broken down by the action of phospholipases, thought to be activated by an accumulation of calcium within the ischemic cell. High concentrations of the breakdown products accumulate to form micelles, which in turn are highly membrane active. It is proposed that such events may in part explain early ischemic ventricular arrhythmias (see Chapter 20).

Cytosolic Calcium in Ischemia.   Concordant data, obtained by several different methods, provide substantial evidence that cytosolic calcium can increase in ischemia (Leyssens et al., 1996). Experimentally, within seconds of complete arrest of coronary flow, left ventricular pressure decreases abruptly toward zero as cytosolic calcium increased rapidly and substantially (Meissner and Morgan, 1995).

    During prolonged ischemia or simulated ischemia, there is a consistent increase in cytosolic calcium either before (Allen et al., 1988), concurrently with the onset of ischemic contracture (Steenbergen et al., 1990), or just after the maximal depletion of ATP (Leyssens et al., 1996). The proposed adverse consequences of the increased calcium level include damage to contractile proteins, activation of phospholipases, increased depolarization, ischemic contracture, and mitochondrial damage (see Figs. 19-2 and 19-3).

Cytosolic Magnesium.   The affinity of ATP for magnesium is higher than that of ADP, so that cytosolic magnesium increases during ATP hydrolysis (Leyssens et al., 1996). By loading isolated myocytes with the magnesium-sensitive dye magnesium green (MgG), it is possible to establish a relationship between the depletion of ATP and other consequences of ischemia, such as contracture and the opening of the ATP-sensitive potassium channel (K_{ATP}).

Sodium and Sodium–Proton Exchange.   Internal sodium increases rapidly at about the time of onset of ischemic contracture, and the mechanism may be twofold (Fig. 17-4). First, as the ATP supply by anaerobic glycolysis becomes insufficient, the supply of membrane ATP is too low for the sodium pump, which then slows down with an increase in internal sodium and loss of potassium. Second, as acidosis develops, the sodium–proton exchange operates to eject protons

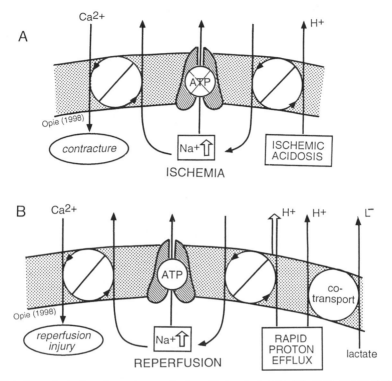

FIG. 17-4. Ions in ischemia and reperfusion. During ischemia (**A**), lack of glycolytic ATP inhibits the sodium pump, with an increase in internal sodium. Proton–sodium exchange contributes to the increase in sodium. Sodium–calcium exchange increases internal calcium, with enhanced risk of ischemic contracture. During reperfusion (**B**), rapid proton efflux by the cotransporter with lactate, and reverse sodium–proton exchange, indirectly mediates a transient increase in calcium despite restoration of energy needed for sodium pump activity.

and to gain sodium. In either event, an accumulation of sodium is potentially serious and leads to an increased osmotic pressure that can rupture the cell membrane with irreversible damage.

Effects of Poor Washout of Metabolites during Ischemia

The close links and an inverse relationship between the decrease of myocardial O_2 tension and the increase in CO_2 tension (Fig. 17-5) after the onset of ischemia mean that there is simultaneous onset of both poor oxygen delivery and poor metabolite washout. CO_2 accumulates in the ischemic zone partially as a result of continued residual respiration with formation of CO_2 and partially as a result of liberation of CO_2 from bicarbonate by protons. When the perfusate of an isolated heart is given an excessively high pCO_2, there is a rapid decrease of left ventricular pressure, which can be reversed by an increase of calcium in the

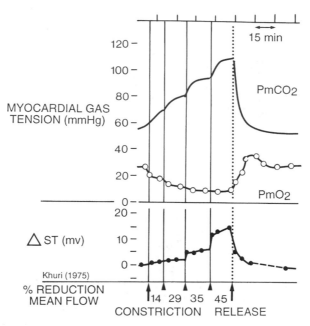

FIG. 17-5. Effects of increasing myocardial ischemia. Extent of reduction of mean coronary flow resulting from increasing coronary artery constriction is shown at bottom of figure, together with effects on ST-segment changes and myocardial CO_2 tension ($PmCO_2$) and myocardial oxygen tension (PmO_2). From Khuri (1985) with permission of American Heart Association.

perfusion fluid (Williamson et al., 1976). The tissue pCO_2 does not stay elevated indefinitely during prolonged myocardial ischemia. There is a late decrease in myocardial tissue pCO_2 and in the hydrogen ion concentration, probably a reflection of progressive irreversible cellular damage and loss of mitochondrial function (Khuri et al., 1985), so that the production of CO_2 by residual mitochondrial oxidative metabolism falls off.

Benefit Versus Harm of Acidosis. The combination of accumulation of CO_2 and of protons decreases the pH of the ischemic tissue considerably from the normal value of about 7.0 to 6.5 (Cross et al., 1995) or even lower. The consequent decrease of contractility should, theoretically, self-protect against ischemia by decreasing the oxygen demand. Furthermore, development of calcium-dependent ischemic contracture could be counteracted by acidosis. Direct evidence for protection by acidosis is that during ischemia a low pH inhibits the enzyme 5'-nucleotidase, which breaks down adenosine monophosphate so that during reperfusion there is a more rapid rate of resynthesis of ATP (Bak and Ingwall, 1994). Because of the heterogeneity of ischemia, the pH in some severely ischemic cells might decrease low enough to activate lysosomes, with irreversible tissue destruction. Thus, mild acidosis may be beneficial (Bing et al.,

1973) and severe acidosis may be harmful to the survival of the ischemic myocardium.

Lactate Accumulation. Increased neutral lactate in severe ischemia may have the following effects: decreased contractile activity in the ischemic zone (Tennant, 1935), promotion of mitochondrial damage (Armiger et al., 1974), decrease of the action potential duration (Wissner, 1974), and inhibition of glycolysis at the level of glyceraldehyde 3-phosphate dehydrogenase (Rovetto et al., 1975).

Are these really the effects of neutral lactate, or could it be that with the formation of large amounts of lactate, lactic acid could also be formed? Cairns et al. (1993) showed that 20 mmol/L external neutral lactate decreased internal myocyte pH by only 0.24 pH units, probably because of inhibition of the outward transport of protons as the high external lactate inhibited the lactate/proton cotransporter. The decrease in internal pH could, by Na^+/H^+ and Na^+/Ca^{2+} exchange, substantially increase cytosolic calcium with adverse consequences. Tissue lactate levels can increase to 30 to 50 μmol/g fresh weight after coronary ligation in the pig (Muller et al., 1986). Thus, adverse effects of high external levels of neutral lactate could well contribute to the overall mechanism of ischemic damage (Cross et al., 1995).

$NADH_2$ and Malate-Aspartate Shuttle. For glycolysis to proceed requires disposal of the $NADH_2$ (NADH + H^+) that is continuously generated. During normal oxygenation, cytoplasmic $NADH_2$ is removed by the malate-aspartate cycle, which depends on continued mitochondrial respiration and therefore slows down or stops in ischemia (see Figs. 10-18 and 10-19, previous edition of this book). In hypoxia or ischemia, $NADH_2$ is converted back to NAD as pyruvate forms lactate, so that the expected accumulation of $NADH_2$ is prevented. Nonetheless, the cytoplasmic $NADH_2$/NAD ratio will be forced toward $NADH_2$ as the tissue lactate increases in relation to the pyruvate level because of the equilibrium relationship. $NADH_2$ accumulation in the cytosol means more protons so that intracellular acidosis is promoted. Pyruvate dehydrogenase, located on the mitochondrial membrane, is inhibited by $NADH_2$ so that entry to the citrate cycle is inhibited, more lactate forms, and the ratio of $NADH_2$ to NAD increases further. $NADH_2$ also accumulates in the mitochondria with adverse effects: (1) there is inhibition of dehydrogenase enzymes at several sites so that any residual activity of the citrate cycle is decreased, and (2) intramitochondrial calcium increases, as proposed by Lehninger et al. (1978), probably because increased intramitochondrial H^+ influences exchange systems across the mitochondrial membrane in such a way that the internal calcium increases.

CLINICAL CONSEQUENCES OF ACUTE ISCHEMIA

Myocardial ischemia may be clinically manifest in at least five different ways: (1) contractile failure that may cause left-sided heart failure and shortness of breath, (2) chest pain, (3) characteristic electrocardiographic (ECG) changes, (4) arrhythmias, and (5) prolonged ischemia progressing to irreversible infarction. Myocardial ischemia is the product of an imbalance between the oxygen supply and demand. The severity and duration of the flow reduction governs the response pattern (Table 17-4).

Oxygen Balance in the Ischemic Zone. A useful hypothesis is that angina pectoris can be caused whenever the myocardial oxygen demand exceeds the supply to cause myocardial ischemia (e.g., when exercise increases the myocardial oxygen demand). The effects of some therapeutic agents, such as the β-adrenergic blocker propranolol, can be explained by alterations in the demand/supply ratio (Fig. 17-2) because propranolol reduces the increased heart rate normally found during exercise. Factors likely to precipitate angina of effort are all those that increase the oxygen demand in the face of a supply limited by coronary artery disease. During exercise, it is the increase of heart rate and blood pressure that precipitates effort angina, whereas an increase of heart rate (together with some increase of systolic blood pressure) is probably the major factor in emotion-provoked angina. The role of catecholamine-induced oxygen wastage as a factor increasing the oxygen demand has not been defined, nor has it been sought, apart from a specific experimental situation in which low-dose catecholamine infusion given to patients with coronary artery disease was able to evoke an increased oxygen uptake independently of hemodynamic changes (Simonsen and Kjekshus, 1978).

The overall metabolic changes in angina pectoris are well understood. The occurrence of lactate production during anginal attacks produced by pacing shows that angina is accompanied by anaerobic glycolysis. There is no reason to believe that the basic metabolic patterns found in human myocardial ischemia differ in any way from those in animal preparations. The release of inorganic

TABLE 17-4. *Relation between severity of coronary flow restriction and reported effects in ischemia*

Flow reduction	Effect
15%	Mid-zone pCO_2 increase, pO_2 decrease[a]
20%	Endocardial TQ-ST changes[b] transmural ATP relatively constant; after 5 hr drops by about 20%[c]
20–30%	Mid-zone external potassium increases, pH decreases, TQ-ST changes[d]
30–40%	Subepicardial external potassium increases[d]
40–50%	Segmental shortening impaired[d]; possible limit of myocardial hibernation
60–70%	Epicardial activation delay and TQ-ST changes[d]
80–85%	Epicardial action potential duration shortening[d]
90%	Transmural ATP reduced to 6% after 5 hr[c]

[a]Khuri et al. (1985).
[b]Maekawa et al. (1980).
[c]Neill et al. (1986).
[d]Watanabe et al. (1987).

phosphate and potassium proves that there is breakdown of high-energy phosphates and loss of potassium from ischemic cells in humans as in animals.

Supply Versus Demand Ischemia.   Thus, ischemia can be linked to myocardial contractile failure through a series of events that result ultimately from severe ischemia by a decreased blood supply. As the severity of coronary constriction increases, so does the myocardial O_2 tension decrease (Fig. 17-5). This condition was termed "supply ischemia" by Apstein and Grossman (1987). In contrast, when demand ischemia is produced by an increase of oxygen demand as occurs when the heart rate is increased during angina induced by pacing, the consequences for myocardial contraction are very different. The effects are those of inadequate tissue oxygenation without washout of metabolites. The major difference lies in the nature of the contractile defect, which in demand ischemia is an increased diastolic tension rather than systolic failure (De Bruyne et al., 1993). In demand ischemia, as found during pacing-induced angina, the basic defect may be the lack of supply of ATP and other high-energy phosphates, which hypothetically leads to a decreased movement of calcium against concentration gradients of the cell membranes, so that increased cytosolic calcium elevates the diastolic tension (Bricknell and Opie, 1978). The crucial event in supply ischemia, on the other hand, is the accumulation of metabolites, such as Pi and protons, leading to contractile failure with relaxation of the myofibrils despite any increase of intracellular calcium. In demand ischemia, the persisting coronary flow washes out protons and inorganic phosphate, and this sequence cannot occur. Nonetheless, these proposed differences between supply and demand ischemia may not be as clear cut as described because there are other factors, such as the duration and severity of ischemia, that are also important (Applegate et al., 1990).

In angina of effort, demand ischemia with excess cytosolic calcium is expected. If it occurs, recovery from angina should be delayed while the stiffened myocardium reverts to normal. Some evidence supports this proposed scenario, because effort angina is accompanied by predominant diastolic heart failure. Of interest, the recovery from angina may take 30 minutes or more, which may represent stunning (Ambrosio et al., 1996; Kloner et al., 1991).

Systolic Versus Diastolic Failure.   Supply ischemia can be linked to systolic failure, as in the early stages of developing myocardial infarction that is accompanied by features of forward failure (low cardiac output). However, there is also backward failure, with pulmonary congestion and shortness of breath caused by diastolic dysfunction. In severe ischemia, there are multiple abnormalities of diastolic function, including a reduced relaxation rate, upward shift of the diastolic pressure–volume curve, and an absence of any compensatory increase in late systolic filling, besides the expected systolic failure (Miyazaki et al., 1990). Demand ischemia should cause predominantly diastolic dysfunction with pulmonary congestion from the impaired return of blood from the lungs to the left side of the heart. In addition, the change of pressure–volume relationships means that systolic function will also be impaired (less pressure generated for a given diastolic volume).

Anginal Chest Pain and Silent Ischemia.   The origin of chest pain typical of angina pectoris is still not fully understood. Years ago, the legendary British cardiologist Lewis postulated the formation of the pain substance P. Lewis' P substance must be distinguished from the current concept of substance P (peptidergic), which is a powerful vasodilator acting by release of nitric oxide. The metabolite causing the pain must be formed readily in ischemia, must disappear as ischemia eases, and must be present for some hours in patients developing acute myocardial infarction. A recent postulate is that the pain is caused by adenosine, derived from ATP breakdown (see Fig. 17-10) as shown by the effects of adenosine infusion, which causes both an ischemic-like chest pain and forearm ischemic pain (Crea et al., 1990). In addition, adenosine exerts protective effects such as coronary vasodilation and negative inotropism (see Fig. 11-17).

Ischemia is not necessarily accompanied by pain. Painless or *silent ischemia* is shown by the development of typical ECG changes of ischemia as well as contractile failure on the echocardiogram in patients with coronary artery disease who at that time do not have any chest pain. Postulates are that (1) the ischemia is relatively mild and therefore does not stimulate the pain receptors or (2) the patients are less sensitive to painful stimuli than normal (perhaps because of a defect of the sensory nerves as in diabetics).

ELECTROCARDIOGRAPHIC FEATURES OF ISCHEMIA

Potassium Loss and Depolarization.   Potassium changes are fundamental in explaining the early ECG features of ischemia. Potassium is released into the local venous blood within seconds of the coronary artery ligation in a dog model, together with an increase in CO_2, lactate, and inorganic phosphate and a decrease in pH. Because there is ischemia, the potassium ions are not washed away, but accumulate on the outside of the ischemic cells. Thus, the transsarcolemmal gradient of potassium ions progressively decreases with membrane depolarization. The simultaneous loss of potassium can be linked to that of inorganic phosphate by the postulated role of the *ATP-dependent potassium channel*. It is proposed that depletion of cytosolic ATP leads to opening of the potassium channel normally inhibited by the intracellular level of ATP (Fig. 17-6). Breakdown products of ATP, such as ADP and adenosine, also help to open the channel. In isolated myocytes studied with the technique that controls the voltage of a small patch of the sarcolemma (patch-clamp technique), continued glycolysis is more effective than oxidative phosphorylation in preventing ATP-sensitive potassium channels from opening (Weiss and Lamp, 1987). Other mechanisms also mediate the loss of potassium from the ischemic cells (Wilde and Aksnes, 1995). Some proposals are (1) co-ionic loss as the positively charged potassium cation

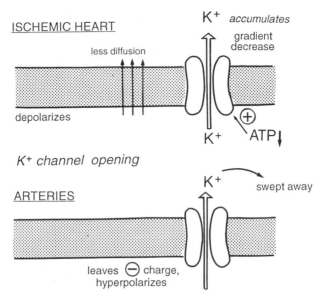

FIG. 17-6. Role of ATP-sensitive potassium channel in ischemia. Note major difference from vasodilatory role, which depends on hyperpolarization as potassium ions are removed from the extracellular site by the circulation. In ischemia, the poor blood flow leads to an accumulation of extracellular potassium ions, which cause depolarization.

leaves the myocardial cell in company with the negatively charged lactate and phosphate ions (Fig. 17-7), and (2) inhibition of the sodium-potassium pump as the local availability of ATP decreases sufficiently to inhibit the pump (Fig. 17-4).

Changes in Action Potential and ST Segment. If an exploring electrode is placed directly on the epicardial surface of the ischemic myocardium soon after coronary artery ligation, the action potential pattern undergoes characteristic changes largely caused by potassium ion loss from ischemic cells (Fig. 17-8). Topical applications of hyperkalemic solutions to the epicardium or intracoronary infusions provoke changes very similar to those of acute ischemia. The loss of only 1% of cellular potassium, raising the intracellular potassium from 4.0 to 9.6 mmol/L, can markedly decrease the resting membrane potential and the action potential duration (Holland and Brooks, 1977). If potassium loss were occurring to a significant extent through the K_{ATP} channel, then acute ischemic ST changes on the ECG should be much diminished in the presence of glibenclamimide, the blocker of this channel. Yet in reality, it is only the terminal part of the elevated ST segment that is so inhibited (Fig. 17-9), so that factors other than the opening of the K_{ATP} channel must be at work (Wilde and Aksnes, 1995).

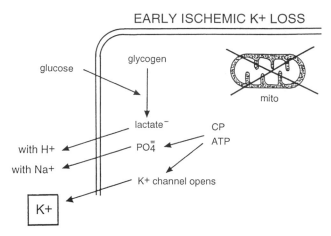

FIG. 17-7. Ischemic potassium loss. Some proposals for the mechanism of early potassium ion loss, which occurs right at the onset of myocardial ischemia, include (1) loss of membrane-related ATP with opening of the ATP-dependent potassium channel, and (2) co-ionic loss of K⁺ with negatively charged inorganic phosphate and lactate ions. The inhibition of the sodium pump follows somewhat later.

Current of Injury. During ischemia, a current of injury develops as depolarization causes the negative transmembrane potential found in diastole to decrease and become more positive than the surrounding normal tissue (Fig. 17-8). Therefore, in diastole the current flows from ischemic to normal tissue. This change appears to start with a modest reduction in coronary flow of about 20% (Table 17-3). If an electrode were to be placed directly on the ischemic zone (epicardial electrode), the current flowing away from the ischemic zone would produce diastolic (ST) depression. The net effect is elevation of the ST segment relative to the rest of the complex (ST elevation). Ischemia also decreases the amplitude of the action potential and shortens the action potential duration (possibly by enhanced K^+ channel activity), so that the ischemic zone is less negative in systole than is the normal myocardium. Hence, in systole current flows from the normal myocardium to the ischemic zone, and some true ST elevation is produced to add to the apparent elevation (produced by the diastolic, K^+-induced current). Exact measurement of the isoelectric line in patients shows that about 70% of the ST change is explained by diastolic currents and a lesser component by systolic currents (Cohen et al., 1983).

Epicardial Versus Endocardial Electrocardiogram. Whether ischemic depolarization will be evident as ST-segment elevation or ST-segment depression on the surface ECG depends on whether the ischemic zone is epicardial or endocardial. Apparent ST-segment elevation occurs in certain clinical conditions, such as epicardial ischemia or transmural ischemia, which may result from Prinzmetal's variant angina with severe spasm or early phase myocardial infarc-

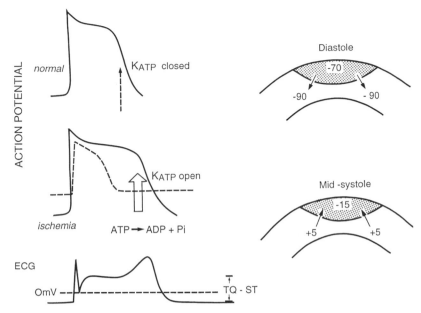

FIG. 17-8. Ischemic changes in action potential pattern and epicardial ECG. During the normal action potential (top left), the ATP-sensitive potassium channel is closed. During ischemia, the resting membrane potential is less negative, with a slow rate of depolarization and an early return to a higher resting level. Thus, there is shortening of the action potential duration and plateau. During diastole (top right panel), ischemic depolarization causes a less negative value in the ischemic zone (stipples). Current therefore flows from the ischemic to the nonischemic zone, causing depression of the TQ-segment. During mid-systole, however, the changes in the action potential duration mean that the ischemic zone is more negative than the nonischemic zone (compare dashed and solid lines in middle left panel). Therefore, during systole current flows from the nonischemic to the ischemic tissue. That is reflected as ST-segment elevation. Thus, as shown in the bottom left panel, there are two components for the apparent ST-segment elevation of the epicardial ECG, namely true TQ-depression (which is dominant) and true ST-elevation.

tion. In contrast, in effort angina, it is the subendocardial zone that chiefly is rendered ischemic, and the direction of current flow is away from the electrode that causes apparent ST-segment depression on the surface ECG.

ST Changes and Severity of Ischemia.   To summarize, ST deviations largely but not entirely reflect extracellular potassium ion accumulation as a result of acute ischemic injury. Thus, not surprisingly, attempts have been made to relate the degree of precordial ST deviation in early myocardial infarction to the magnitude of extracellular potassium accumulation and to the severity of myocardial ischemia. However, complex geometric factors influence just how a flow of current is recorded by an electrode (the solid angle theorem of Holland and Brooks, 1977). At best, measurements of early ST-segment deviations will give only an approximation of the severity of ischemia. Nonetheless, ischemic ST-segment

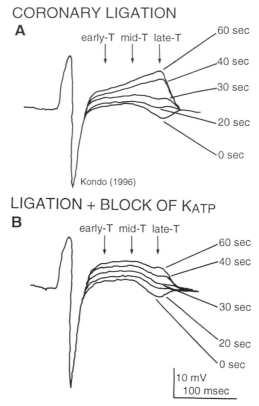

FIG. 17-9. Ischemic T waves on ECG. Note that the ATP-sensitive potassium channel, K_{ATP}, as defined by use of the blocker glibenclamide, largely centers on the terminal part of the ST-segment. With permission of Kondo et al. (1996).

depression during *effort testing* is a reliable end point if it is found. Generally, a horizontal depression of at least 1 mm of the ST segment is required for a positive effort test (Fig. 17-10). With 2 mm depression, there are fewer falsely positive results. Only about two thirds of patients with coronary artery disease have a positive effort test result, and sometimes features other than ST depression are the end point (chest pain, blood pressure decrease instead of the normal increase, arrhythmias, shortness of breath, fatigue).

T-Wave Inversion and Ischemia. Particularly confusing is the difference between acute metabolic ischemia, characterized by ST-segment deviation (as already argued) and the ischemia of some clinical electrocardiologists, who also include a chronically inverted T wave as part of the picture of ischemia. An acutely inverted T wave is thought to be a reflection of variations in the rate of repolarization throughout the myocardium and variations in the action potential

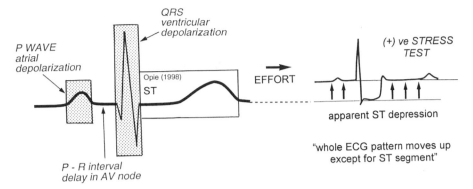

FIG. 17-10. Electrocardiogram in effort angina. The horizontal decrease in the ST segment of 1 mm or more is defined as a positive stress test. The quotation is the remark of a junior medical student.

duration, shortened by ischemia, possibly as a result of inadequate production of ATP at the cell membrane. Such ischemic T-wave changes generally are associated with ST-segment changes. However, a permanently inverted T wave in isolation usually does not indicate true metabolic ischemia. Rather, focal ischemia has probably progressed to fibrosis, so that the epicardium is repolarized differently from the endocardium.

RECOVERY FROM ISCHEMIA

Experimentally there is rapid recovery from ischemia that is not accompanied by contracture. For example, low flow ischemia can be withstood for hours, provided that the ischemic myocardium is supplied with external glucose. However, clinicians often have observed delayed recovery from exercise-induced angina, with systolic wall motion in ischemic segments taking 60 minutes to recover (Fig. 17-11) (Ambrosio et al., 1996), despite the return of coronary flow returns within 5 to 14 minutes (Camici et al., 1986). This delayed mechanical recovery is therefore a form of stunning, and one of the important metabolic derangements responsible could be an increase in cytosolic calcium levels (see Chapter 19). If so, it is important to trace out the metabolic events in the recovery period.

Normalization of Ions. At the end of a period of potentially reversible ischemia, there is an intracellular accumulation of protons, as well as sodium and calcium ions (Fig. 17-4). Numerous studies with inhibitors of sodium–proton exchange have shown a more rapid recovery from ischemia in the presence of these agents, suggesting the operation of this exchanger to help normalize the cell pH. The resultant decrease of the proton load during early reperfusion pro-

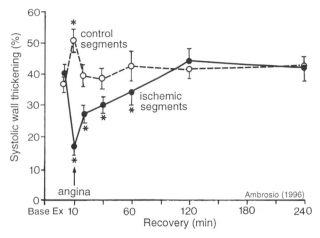

FIG. 17-11. Delayed postanginal recovery of systolic wall motion. Note that after cessation of angina, the previously ischemic segments take 60 minutes or more to recover when compared with controls. For further details see Ambrosio et al. (1996). Reproduced by permission of the American Heart Association and Circulation.

motes recovery (Liu et al., 1996). In addition, protons are extruded with lactate by the lactate–proton cotransporter (Vandenberg et al., 1993).

Energy Metabolism During Recovery from Ischemia. Several complex changes, not yet fully defined, occur during recovery from ischemia. A current hypothesis is that glycolysis is harmful because uncoupling of glycolysis from glucose oxidation can be harmful during recovery from ischemia (Lopaschuk and Stanley, 1997). Increased rates of glycolysis during postischemic recovery are accompanied by an inhibition of glucose oxidation (Lopaschuk and Stanley, 1997), the latter probably resulting from a relative increase of fatty acid metabolism. Overall, the rates of mitochondrial metabolism are depressed (Heyndrickx et al., 1993), and fatty acids appear to compete better than glucose for this residual metabolism. Measures to enhance glucose oxidation include replenishment of the citrate cycle intermediates by pyruvate (see Chapter 11); the agent dichloroacetate, which promotes pyruvate oxidation (Liu et al., 1996); and steps to decrease fatty acid oxidation. When there is an adequate amount of pyruvate from glycolysis, then glycolysis is beneficial and not harmful, presumably by supplying energy for the calcium uptake pump of the sarcoplasmic reticulum, thereby decreasing internal calcium (Jeremy et al., 1992). In humans, too, there are metabolic changes in the recovery phase of exercise-induced angina, with accelerated glucose extraction as monitored by ^{18}F-fluorodeoxyglucose (Camici et al., 1986); the fate of this glucose could be either glycogen formation or glycolysis or both. Of all the possible measures that could be tested in patients, inhibition of sodium–proton exchange might be most practical.

THERAPEUTIC MODIFICATION OF ISCHEMIA

Classic Antianginal Agents.   Both β-adrenergic blockers and calcium antagonist agents act beneficially by altering the supply-versus-demand equation. β-
adrenergic blockers act by decreasing the heart and contractile state of the
myocardium, whereas calcium antagonists act at least in part by relief of exercise-induced coronary vasoconstriction (Frielingsdorf et al., 1996). Both types
of agent also reduce the afterload by decreasing the blood pressure.

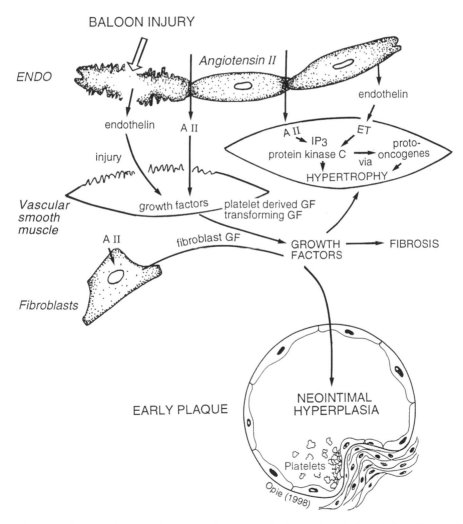

FIG. 17-12. Proposed molecular events in restenosis. Note role of balloon-induced injury of
endothelium, with release of endothelin (ET) and angiotensin II and stimulation of growth factors (GF)\. For IP$_3$ see Fig. 9-4.

Nitric Oxide.   Nitrates are thought to act in part as coronary dilators and in part as venodilators, thereby reducing the venous return to the heart and lessening the endocardial wall stress and its associated increase in oxygen demand. Because nitrates are nitric oxide donors, it is of interest that a further possible mechanism of action is as follows. Several studies have now shown that nitric oxide appears to inhibit mitochondrial metabolism, which will decrease the oxygen demand. Agents indirectly producing nitric oxide, such as the angiotensin-converting enzyme (ACE) inhibitors, which decrease the breakdown of bradykinin and stimulate the endothelium to form nitric oxide, may also reduce myocardial oxygen demand (Laursen and Harrison, 1997). In the case of nitrates, however, the decrease in oxygen uptake resulting from this mitochondrial action is probably more than balanced by the increased demand of the reflex tachycardia resulting from arterial dilation. This tachycardia can be countered by combining nitrates with β-adrenergic blockers.

Heart Size.   An enlarged heart means that the ventricular wall stress is increased by the Laplace law, so that the oxygen demand increases. Thus, treatment of cardiac failure becomes important because it will, in general, reduce the size of the ventricles. Besides conventional antianginal therapy, both diuretics and ACE inhibitors may be required in this situation.

Metabolic Mechanisms.   Although ischemia is basically a metabolic problem, so far no metabolic therapies have been truly successful for effort angina, unless the metabolic effects of β-adrenergic blockade are considered (see Fig. 11-20). A possible exception is the metabolically active antianginal agent trimetazidine, which has no hemodynamic action but may act by lessening intracellular acidosis or by limiting sodium–proton exchange.

Revascularization.   In the long run, ischemia can often be best decreased by coronary artery bypass grafting or by balloon angioplasty. Unfortunately, the latter procedure is very frequently followed by restenosis (Fig. 17-12).

SUMMARY

1. *Acute adaptation to ischemia.* The two major processes are (1) inhibition of the energy demand by decreased myocardial contraction and (2) an increase in anaerobic glycolysis to compensate in part for the decrease in oxidative metabolism.
2. *Metabolic consequences of myocardial ischemia.* These can be divided into those caused by inadequate oxygen supply and those caused by inadequate washout of metabolites. Common to both processes is an increase of cytosolic calcium.
3. *Supply versus demand equation.* Myocardial ischemia exists when the blood supply is inadequate (supply impaired) or when the demand is too great.

4. *Demand ischemia.* When there is an increased oxygen demand in the face of a fixed supply (as occurs during effort-induced angina), the myocardium becomes stiffer (decreased compliance), and the proposed explanation is that continued washout of metabolites, such as inorganic phosphate and protons, creates a situation where the increased cytosolic calcium leads to failure of relaxation.

5. *Supply ischemia.* On the other hand, during supply ischemia, when there is accumulation of inorganic phosphate and protons, the effects of the increased cytosolic calcium on contraction can be overridden, and contractile activity is inhibited with relaxation of the myocardium. An animal model of this type of ischemia is coronary artery ligation.

6. *Mild versus severe ischemia.* To some extent, similar differences exist between mild ischemia (like demand ischemia) and severe ischemia (which resembles supply ischemia). Glycolysis is stimulated by mild ischemia and inhibited in severe ischemia as the delivery of glucose decreases, glycogen becomes depleted, and products of glycolysis accumulate. On the other hand, fatty acid oxidation is depressed by all degrees of ischemia. When fatty acid metabolites accumulate, there are proposed adverse detergent effects on the ischemic cells.

7. *Survival of ischemic tissue.* This depends on both the severity and the duration of the ischemia, as well as on the myocardial oxygen demand.

8. *Effects of ischemia on cardiac action potential.* Fundamental in the causation of ischemic changes is potassium loss from the ischemic zone, with accumulation of potassium ions in the extracellular space. The mechanism of such loss is not fully understood, but opening of the ATP-sensitive potassium channel, K_{ATP}, plays a role. The result is ischemic depolarization and shortening of the action potential duration.

9. *Effort ECG test.* These changes in the action potential are reflected in ST-segment depression on the surface ECG, and during exercise, a sufficient degree of horizontal depression of 1 mm or more indicates a positive stress test result.

10. *Therapeutic procedures.* Established steps are to conserve the myocardial oxygen supply by decreased hart rate and contractility (β-adrenergic blockers) or to induce coronary vasodilation instead of vasoconstriction on exercise (calcium antagonists and nitrates). Angiotensin-converting enzyme inhibitors might have an indirect effect. They inhibit the breakdown of bradykinin, which in turn stimulates the formation of nitric oxide, which acts on mitochondria to decrease the myocardial oxygen demand.

STUDENT QUESTIONS

1. In ischemia, anaerobic glycolysis is accelerated. Do you see this as a beneficial or harmful process? What are the reasons for your choice?

2. Trace out the fate of $NADH_2$ (i.e., $NADH + H^+$) made by glycolysis during (a) normal oxygenation and (b) ischemia. What is the importance of these changes?
3. What are the changes in pathways of fatty acid metabolism found in ischemia? What is the potential significance in terms of the extent ischemic damage?
4. Describe how the lipids of the sarcolemma form micelles during ischemia.
5. Intracellular acidosis develops during ischemia. Where do the protons come from?

CARDIOLOGIST-IN-TRAINING QUESTIONS

1. Soon after the onset of severe ischemia, there is myocardial contractile failure. What are the metabolic processes involved?
2. Outline the metabolic and mechanical differences between mild and severe ischemia, and propose mechanism to explain these differences.
3. During an attack of angina pectoris caused by pacing, there is the acute loss of potassium ions into the extracellular space. Why is this? What are the consequences?
4. Describe the changes in the cardiac action potential found in ischemia. How do these relate to the changes in the surface electrocardiogram found during a positive effort stress test?
5. Describe the hypothesis that an imbalance between the myocardial oxygen supply and demand can cause angina pectoris. What are the therapeutic steps that can be taken to redress the imbalance?

REFERENCES

1. Allen DG, Lee JA, Smith GL. The effects of simulated ischaemia on intracellular calcium and tension in isolated ferret ventricular muscle. *J Physiol* 1988;401:81P.
2. Ambrosio G, Betocchi S, Pace L, et al. Prolonged impairment of regional contractile function after resolution of exercise-induced angina. Evidence of myocardial stunning in patients with coronary artery disease. *Circulation* 1996;94:2455–2464.
3. Applegate RJ, Walsh RA, O'Rourke RA. Comparative effects of pacing-induced and flow-limited ischemia on left ventricular function. *Circulation* 1990;81:1380–1392.
4. Apstein CS, Grossmann W. Opposite initial effects of supply and demand ischemia on left ventricular diastolic compliance: the ischemia-diastolic paradox. *J Mol Cell Cardiol* 1987;19:119–128.
5. Apstein CS, Varma N, Eberli FR. Ischemic diastolic dysfunction and postischemic diastolic stunning. In: Yellon DM, Rahimtoola SH, Opie LH (eds). *New Ischemic Syndromes. Beyond Angina and Infarction.* Philadelphia: Lippincott-Raven, 1997;106–135.
6. Armiger LC, Gavin JB, Herdson PB. Mitochondrial changes in dog myocardium induced by neutral lactate in vitro. *Lab Invest* 1974;31:29–33.
7. Bak MI, Ingwall JS. Acidosis during ischemia promotes adenosine triphosphate resynthesis in postischemic rat heart. *J Clin Invest* 1994;93:40–49.
8. Bing OHL, Brooks WW, Messer JV. Heart muscle viability following hypoxia: protective effect of acidosis. *Science* 1973;180:1297–1298.
9. Bricknell OL, Opie LH. Effects of substrates on tissue metabolic changes in the isolated rat heart dur-

ing underperfusion and on release of lactate dehydrogenase and arrhythmias during reperfusion. *Circ Res* 1978;43:102–115.

10. Burns A. In: *Observations on Some of the Most Frequent and Important Diseases of the Heart; on Aneurysm of the Thoracic Aorta; on Preternatural Pulsation in the Epigastric Region; and on the Unusual Origin and Distribution of Some of the Large Arteries of the Human Body.* Edinburgh, Scotland: Bryce, 1809.

11. Cairns SP, Westerblad H, Allen DG. Changes in myoplasmic pH and calcium concentration during exposure to lactate in isolated rat ventricular myocytes. *J Physiol* 1993;464:561–574.

12. Camici P, Araujo LI, Spinks T, et al. Increased uptake of ^{18}F-fluorodeoxyglucose in postischemic myocardium of patients with exercise-induced angina. *Circulation* 1986;74:81–88.

13. Cobbe SM, Poole-Wilson PA. The time of onset and severity of acidosis in myocardial ischaemia. *J Mol Cell Cardiol* 1980;12:745–760.

14. Cohen D, Savard P, Rifkin RD, et al. Magnetic measurement of S-T and T-Q segment shifts in humans. Exercise-induced ST-segment depression. *Circ Res* 1983;53:274–279.

15. Crea F, Pupita G, Galassi AR, et al. Role of adenosine in pathogenesis of anginal pain. *Circulation* 1990;81:164–172.

16. Cross HR, Clarke K, Opie LH, Radda GK. Is lactate-induced myocardial ischaemic injury mediated by decreased pH or increased intracellular lactate? *J Mol Cell Cardiol* 1995;27:1369–1381.

17. Cross HR, Opie LH, Radda GK, Clarke K. Is a high glycogen content beneficial or detrimental to the ischemic rat heart? *Circ Res* 1996;78:482–491.

18. De Bruyne B, Bronzwaer JGF, Heyndrickx GR, Paulus WJ. Comparative effects of ischemia and hypoxemia on left ventricular systolic and diastolic function in humans. *Circulation* 1993;88:461–471.

19. Dennis SC, Gevers W, Opie LH. Protons in ischemia: where do they come from and where do they go to? *J Mol Cell Cardiol* 1991;23:1077–1086.

20. Erichsen JE. On the influence of the coronary circulation on the action of the heart. *London Med Gazette NS* 1842;2:561–564.

21. Frielingsdorf J, Seiler C, Kaufmann P, et al. Normalisation of abnormal coronary vasomotion by calcium antagonists in patients with hypertension. *Circulation* 1996;93:1380–1387.

22. Hearse DJ. Oxygen deprivation and early myocardial contractile failure: a reassessment of the possible role of adenosine triphospate. *Am J Cardiol* 1979;44:1115–1121.

23. Hearse DJ. Myocardial ischaemia: can we agree on a definition for the 21st century? *Cardiovasc Res* 1994;28:1737–1744.

24. Heyndrickx GR, Wijns W, Vogelaers D, et al. Recovery of regional contractile function and oxidative metabolism in stunned myocardium induced by 1-hour circumflex coronary artery stenosis in chronically instrumented dogs. *Circ Res* 1993;72:901–913.

25. Hochachka PW, Buck LT, Doll CJ, Land SC. Unifying theory of hypoxia tolerance: molecular/metabolic defense and rescue mechanisms for surviving oxygen lack. *Proc Natl Acad Sci USA* 1996;93:9493–9498.

26. Holland RP, Brooks H. TQ-ST segment mapping: critical review and analysis of current concepts. *Am J Cardiol* 1977;40:110–129.

27. Jacobus WE, Pores IH, Lucas SK, et al. Intracellular acidosis and contractility in the normal and ischemic heart as examined by ^{31}P NMR. *J Mol Cell Cardiol* 1982;14(suppl 3):13–20.

28. Jeremy RW, Koretsune Y, Marban E, Becker LC. Relation between glycolysis and calcium homeostasis in postischemic myocardium. *Circ Res* 1992;70:1180–1190.

29. Katz AM, Hecht HH. The early "pump" failure of the ischemic heart. *Am J Med* 1969;47:497–502.

30. Khuri SF, Kloner RA, Karaffa SA, et al. The significance of the late fall in myocardial Pco2 and its relationship to myocardial pH after regional coronary occlusion in the dog. *Circ Res* 1985;56:537–547.

31. Kloner RA, Allen J, Cox TA, et al. Stunned left ventricular myocardium after exercise treadmill testing in coronary artery disease. *Am J Cardiol* 1991;68:329–334.

32. Knöll R, Arras M, Zimmermann R, et al. Changes in gene expression following short coronary occlusions studied in porcine hearts with run-on assays. *Cardiovasc Res* 1994;28:1062–1069.

33. Kondo T, Kubota I, Tachibana H, et al. Glibenclamide attenuates peaked T-wave in early phase of myocardial ischemia. *Cardiovasc Res* 1996;31:683–687.

34. Kubler W, Katz AM. Mechanism of early "pump" failure of the ischemic heart: possible role of adenosine triphosphate depletion and inorganic phosphate accumulation. *Am J Cardiol* 1977;40:467–471.

35. Kusuoka H, Weisfeldt ML, Zweier JL, et al. Mechanism of early contractile failure during hypoxia in intact ferret heart: evidence for modulation of maximal Ca-activated force by inorganic phosphate. *Circ Res* 1986;59:270–282.

36. Laursen JB, Harrison DG. Modulation of myocardial oxygen consumption through ACE inhibitors. NO effect? *Circulation* 1997;95:14–16.

37. Lee JA, Allen DG. Mechanisms of acute ischemic contractile failure of the heart. Role of intracellular calcium. *J Clin Invest* 1991;88:361–367.

38. Lehninger AL, Reynafarie B, Vercesi A, Tew WP. Transport and accumulation of calcium in mitochondria. *Ann NY Acad Sci* 1978;307:160–176.

39. Leyssens A, Nowicky AV, Patterson L, et al. The relationship between mitochondrial state, ATP hydrolysis, $[Mg^{2+}]_i$ and $[Ca^{2+}]_i$ studied in isolated rat cardiomyocytes. *J Physiol* 1996;496:111–128.

40. Liu B, Clanachan AS, Schulz R, Lopaschuk GD. Cardiac efficiency is improved after ischemia by altering both the source and fate of protons. *Circ Res* 1996;79:940–948.

41. Lopaschuk GD, Stanley WC. Glucose metabolism in the ischemic heart. *Circulation* 1997;95: 313–315.

42. Maekawa K, Yokoyama M, Katada Y, et al. A study on myocardial ischemia in the left ventricular wall with special reference to electrographic and metabolic changes. *Jpn Heart J* 1980;21:215–224.

43. Marban E, Kitakaze M, Koretsune Y, et al. Quantification of $[Ca^{2+}]_i$ in perfused hearts. Critical evaluation of the 5F-BAPTA and nuclear magnetic resonance method as applied to the study of ischemia and reperfusion. *Circ Res* 1990;66:1255–1267.

44. Meissner A, Morgan JP. Contractile dysfunction and abnormal Ca^{2+} modulation during postischemic reperfusion in rat heart. *Am J Physiol* 1995;268:H100–H111.

45. Miyazaki S, Guth BD, Miura T, et al. Changes of left ventricular diastolic function in exercising dogs without and with ischemia. *Circulation* 1990;81:1058–1070.

46. Muller CA, Opie LH, Hamm CW, et al. Prevention of ventricular fibrillation by metoprolol in a pig model of acute myocardial ischaemia: absence of a major arrhythmogenic role for cyclic AMP. *J Mol Cell Cardiol* 1986;18:375–387.

47. Neill WA, Ingwall JS, Andrews E, et al. Stabilization of a derangement in adenosine triphosphate metabolism during sustained, partial ischemia in the dog heart. *J Am Coll Cardiol* 1986;8:894–900.

48. Opie LH. Myocardial ischemia—metabolic pathways and implications of increased glycolysis. *Cardiovasc Drug Ther* 1990;4:777–790.

49. Owen P, Dennis S, Opie LH. Glucose flux rate regulates onset of ischemic contracture in globally underperfused rat hearts. *Circ Res* 1990;66:344–354.

50. Ralevic V, Milner P, Hudlicka O, et al. Substance P is released from the endothelium of normal and capsaicin-treated rat hind-limb vasculature, in vivo, by increased flow. *Circ Res* 1990;66:1178–1183.

51. Rauch U, Schulze K, Witzenbilcher B, Shultheiss HP. Alteration of the cytosolic-mitochondrial distribution of high energy phosphates during global myocardial ischemia may contribute to early contractile failure. *Circ Res* 1994;75:760–769.

52. Rovetto MJ, Lamberton WF, Neely JR. Mechanisms of glycolytic inhibition in ischemic rat hearts. *Circ Res* 1975;37:742–751.

53. Serizawa T, Carabello BA, Grossman W. Effect of pacing-induced ischemia on left ventricular diastolic pressure-volume relations in dogs with coronary stenosis. *Circ Res* 1980;46:430–439.

54. Simonsen S, Kjekshus JK. The effect of free fatty acids on myocardial oxygen consumption during arterial pacing and catecholamine infusion in man. *Circulation* 1978;58:484–491.

55. Steenbergen C, Murphy E, Watts JA, London RE. Correlation between cytosolic free calcium, contracture, ATP, and irreversible ischemic injury in perfused rat heart. *Circ Res* 1990;66:135–146.

56. Tennant R. Factors concerned in the arrest of contraction in an ischemic myocardial area. *Am J Physiol* 1935;113:677–682.

57. Vandenberg JI, Metcalfe JC, Grace AA. Mechanisms of pHi recovery after global ischemia in the perfused heart. *Circ Res* 1993;72:993–1003.

58. Virchow R. In: *Die Cellularpathologie in ihrer Begrundung auf physiologische und pathologische Gewebelehre.* Berlin: Hischwald, 1858;122.

59. Watanabe I, Johnson TA, Buchanan J, et al. Effect of graded coronary flow reduction on ionic, electrical, and mechanical indexes of ischemia in the pig. *Circulation* 1987;76:1127–1134.

60. Weiss JN, Lamp ST. Glycolysis preferentially inhibits ATP-sensitive K^+ channels in isolated guinea pig cardiac myocytes. *Science* 1987;238:67–70.

61. Wilde AAM, Aksnes G. Myocardial potassium loss and cell depolarisation in ischaemia and hypoxia. *Cardiovasc Res* 1995;29:1–15.

62. Williamson JR, Safer B, Rich T, et al. Effects of acidosis on myocardial contractility and metabolism. *Acta Med Scand* 1976;587:95–112.
63. Wissner SB. The effect of excess lactate upon the excitability of the sheep Purkinje fiber. *J Electrocardiol* 1974;7:17–26.
64. Young LH, Renfu Y, Russell R, et al. Low-flow ischemia leads to translocation of canine heart GLUT-4 and GLUT-1 glucose transporters to the sarcolemma in vivo. *Circulation* 1997;95:415–422.

18

Cell Death: Myocardial Infarction

In acute myocardial infarction (AMI), a clinical diagnosis, the primary event is most commonly an occlusive clot (thrombus) in an atherosclerotic coronary artery. The onset is characterized by severe persisting angina-like chest pain. If left untreated, the severity and duration of ischemia are sufficient to cause the condition to progress into ultimate cell necrosis (Fig. 18-1). The term "infarction" literally means "stuffed in" and refers to the swollen appearance of totally dead cells. The time taken for the whole sequence to develop is only 20 to 60 minutes when there is little or no collateral flow and the myocardial oxygen uptake is relatively high. In contrast, the time is extended to 2 to 6 hours when the collateral flow is high and the myocardial oxygen uptake low (Schaper et al., 1987).

How does ischemic damage progress? It can spread through the myocardial wall, often starting in the subendocardium, which is the most vulnerable site for several reasons. This zone lies furthest away from the source of the coronary blood supply via the epicardial arteries; there is more wall stress in the subendocardial zone after increase of ventricular pressure that results from ischemic contractile failure; and there are transmural metabolic differences that render the subendocardium more susceptible to ischemic damage. Once developed, subendocardial ischemia spreads toward the subepicardium, a process that constitutes an advancing wave-front (Reimer et al., 1977). The mechanism of the wave-front phenomenon may include a progressively increasing intraluminal ventricular pressure as the left ventricle progressively fails, transmitted through the flaccid ischemic myocardium to ever more subepicardial layers (Fig. 18-2). The larger the zone of initial ischemic damage, and the more rapid and severe the extent of contractile failure, the faster will the wave-front advance. Thus, it is not possible to lay down exact limits for the time that divides reversible and irreversible ischemic damage.

543

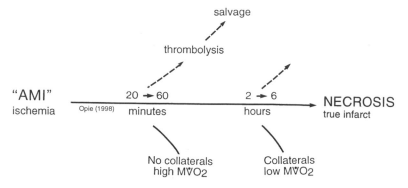

FIG. 18-1. Acute myocardial infarction is a clinical syndrome in which a significant number of ischemic cardiac cells eventually die. Although in the early stages the condition is reversible and constitutes ischemia and not necrosis, clinicians include such reversible early ischemia in the overall syndrome of AMI. If the thrombus is broken down by therapeutic thrombolysis, the threatened myocardium can be salvaged. The therapeutic window is that time between the onset of chest pain and irreversible ischemia. In the presence of collateral flow and a low myocardial oxygen uptake (MVO_2), animal data suggest an interval of 2 to 6 hours, whereas in the presence of no collateral flow and a high oxygen uptake, the interval is 20 to 60 minutes.

THE ATHEROSCLEROTIC PROCESS

The following brief summary of this complex process should be complemented by reference to the excellent review of Ross (1997). In essence, an intact vascular endothelium prevents the entry of lipoprotein molecules and protects the intima from invasion by cells such as macrophages. Endothelial damage is seen as the crucial event in the response-to-injury hypothesis (Ross, 1997). Each of the primary risk factors for coronary artery disease—hypercholesterolemia, hypertension, and cigarette smoking—leads through different events to endothe-

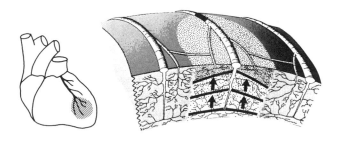

No lateral border zone (Hearse)
Advancing wave front (Reimer)

FIG. 18-2. The advancing wave front model. The progress to necrosis occurs across a transmural border zone, which may include a progression from endocardium to epicardium. See Hearse and Yellon (1984) and Reimer et al. (1977).

lial injury and dysfunction (Fig. 18-3). For example, in hypercholesterolemic patients, the normal endothelial-dependent vasodilator response to intra-arterial acetylcholine is changed into pathologic vasoconstriction (Zeiher et al., 1991). In hypertension, exercise causes vasoconstriction rather than normal vasodilation of coronary arteries, a change that is thought to reflect endothelial dysfunction (Frielingsdorf et al., 1996). Smoking acts synergistically with hypercholesterolemia to promote endothelial dysfunction (Heitzer, 1996). Other risk factors, such as diabetes mellitus, insulin resistance, and increased blood levels of homocysteine, as well as inflammatory processes, all promote endothelial damage.

The chain of events leading from endothelial damage to plaque formation is intricate but increasingly defined (Figs. 18-1 and 18-2). At least two cell types adhere to the damaged endothelium. Platelets aggregate and release platelet-

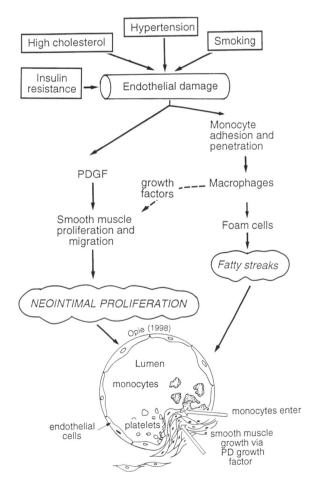

FIG. 18-3. Progression from endothelial damage to plaque. PDGF, platelet-derived growth factor.

derived growth factor (PDGF) and other growth factors that are thought to trigger the smooth muscle cell proliferation and migration, leading to neointimal hyperplasia (Fig. 18-4). Circulating monocytes roll on to the damaged endothelium at the site of various endothelial antigens, adhere, and transmigrate into the subendothelial space. There they become activated macrophages that contribute to growth of the lesion by producing an extraordinary number of biologically relevant molecules, including at least six growth factors that promote growth of smooth muscle cells (Ross, 1997). Macrophages themselves proliferate to be as important a component of neointimal growth as the smooth muscle cells. Macrophages are also scavenger cells, and they attempt to remove noxious molecules such as oxidized low-density lipoprotein (LDL), in the process being transformed into foam cells. Macrophages may accumulate large amounts of lipid.

Sources of growth factors are multiple, besides the macrophages and platelets. Vascular smooth muscle (VSM) cells secrete additional growth factors that stimulate themselves and their neighbors. The damaged endothelium contributes in several ways, for example, by release of endothelin and by decreased formation of nitric oxide (Cooke and Tsao, 1997). Such endothelium also releases fibroblastic growth factor and allows angiotensin II to activate PDGF (Dzau et al.,

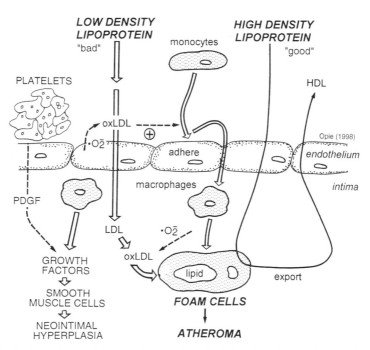

FIG. 18-4. Role of lipoproteins in atherosclerosis. When low-density lipoproteins become oxidized (oxLDL), they then are trapped in the intima of the arterial wall. High-density lipoproteins can re-export nonoxidized LDL. PDGF, platelet-derived growth factor.

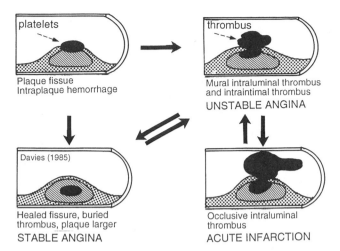

FIG. 18-5. Varieties of coronary artery disease. Some postulated events at the level of the diseased coronary artery underlying stable angina, unstable angina, and AMI. In the latter case, note complete transluminal occlusion setting in motion the sequences shown in the next figure. Adapted from Davies and Thomas (1985).

1991). Thus, growth factors derived from macrophages, the endothelium, and platelets all act on VSM cells, which develop the *synthetic phenotype* to enter the growth mode.

Next the collection of foam cells and the increased growth of VSM cells and macrophages set the scene for the atherosclerotic *fibrous plaque,* consisting of a variety of cells, some still growing, others becoming fibrous tissue, and others chiefly containing lipid. Hemodynamic shear forces are thought to trigger plaque rupture, the usual antecedent event leading to an occlusive thrombus and total coronary occlusion (Fig. 18-5). Just which fibrous plaques rupture is not clearly defined, and some evidence suggests that it is arteries that are not too severely narrowed that are at most risk of rupture, presumably because severe occlusion limits coronary perfusion and the hemodynamic stress required to precipitate the rupture.

Several of the important steps in atherogenesis are susceptible to dietary changes. Well known is the influence of diet on the blood levels of LDL. Recently described are the effects of dietary antioxidants such as vitamin C on the endothelium (Heitzer et al., 1996) and dietary arginine to promote the synthesis of nitric oxide, thereby possibly being a new therapy for atherosclerosis (Cooke and Tsao, 1997).

NECROSIS VERSUS APOPTOSIS

The struggle for survival is governed by both the severity and the duration of ischemia. Undoubtedly, prolonged severe ischemia leads to cardiac cell death.

Necrosis previously was regarded as the only mode of cell death, whereas now it is known that some cells also die by apoptosis (Fig. 18-6). Necrosis can be either coagulative or of the contraction band variety. *Coagulation necrosis* refers to progressive changes more prominent in the center of the developing infarct, whereby the myofilaments are broken and become indistinct as the cells swell and disintegrate, so that their contents appear to be coagulated. In more detail, the changes include (1) irreversible formation of amorphous dense bodies in the mitochondria, possibly derived from local lipids, so that ATP cannot be produced and the energy deficit becomes disastrous; (2) an increase in sarcolemmal permeability manifested by blebs and holes through which intracellular enzymes and proteins escape to become clinical markers of infarction; and (3) irreversible nuclear clumping so that protein synthesis is inhibited. *Contraction band necrosis* is more often found near the border of the infarct, and its chief feature is hypercontraction of the contractile elements. A proposed mechanism is that partially perfused cells take up a large amount of calcium ions, which cause lethal hypercontracture.

Apoptosis leads to cell death by a different route: there is a genetically programmed series of biochemical events that lead to shrinkage of the cell with intracellular degeneration yet with maintained sarcolemmal integrity. Mitochondria are relatively spared, whereas the entire nucleus is cleaved into two or more portions with the microscopic appearance of DNA fragmentation and formation of DNA ladders (Fliss and Gattinger, 1996). The whole process could be likened to dead leaves falling from the tree in autumn (James, 1994).

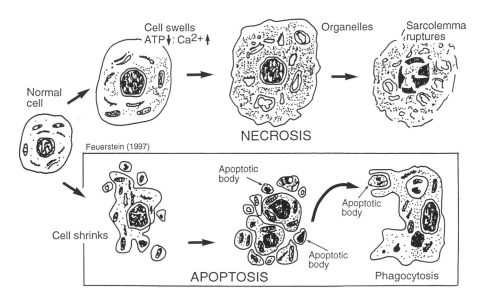

FIG. 18-6. Contrasts between necrosis and apoptosis. Courtesy of Dr. G Feuerstein, King of Prussia, Philadelphia.

The relative contributions of necrosis and apoptosis to cell death in ischemia and reperfusion is still open to debate, although necrosis appears to dominate during ischemia, and apoptosis may dominate during reperfusion. There is now evidence that apoptosis occurs both during prolonged sustained ischemia exceeding 2 to 3 hours and when reperfusion follows shorter periods of ischemia (Fliss and Gattinger, 1996). What controls apoptosis? *Tumor suppressor genes* promote apoptosis in a variety of tissues to lessen the risks of tumor formation. Such genes include p53, which is rapidly expressed in the reperfused myocardium to upregulate another gene called *Bax,* which in turn mediates apoptosis (Hayashida et al., 1996). Conversely, the bcl-2 protein inhibits apoptosis, and the Bax to bcl-2 ratio is increased in cells destined to die by apoptosis (Misao et al., 1996). There is emerging evidence for the role of apoptosis in human hearts with myocardial infarction (Misao et al., 1996).

Because necrosis and apoptosis have different underlying mechanisms, they could hypothetically respond to different therapeutic approaches. In the end, however, it is mitigation of ischemia that would prevent either mode of cell death.

INITIAL EVENTS IN ACUTE MYOCARDIAL INFARCTION

Animal models of AMI have generally used either acute occlusion by ligature of otherwise healthy coronary arteries or massive injections of catecholamines. The former procedure produces transmural myocardial infarction, and the latter procedure causes subendocardial infarction. The ideal model would be spontaneously occurring severe coronary atherosclerosis. Superimposed thereon would be the triggering event, which is now known to be an occlusive thrombus (Fig. 18-5), frequently associated with platelet/fibrin microemboli (Frink et al., 1988). In those patients with a sudden arrhythmic death, probably due to ventricular fibrillation, the initial event does not have to be an occlusive thrombus, although usually there is advanced coronary artery disease. Despite the defects of the various animal models, very early on both in animals and in humans there is a variable and possibly predominant element of reversibility (ischemia), with eventual irreversibility. Primary arterial occlusion is the initial event. Coronary arterial obstruction is the event initiating ischemia of sufficient severity to lead to AMI, and mechanical block is the most important cause of vascular obstruction. The cause of the block is usually thrombosis, the combined result of arterial wall pathology, platelet or fibrin aggregates, and vascular coagulation abnormalities. Less commonly, embolism or coronary artery spasm is the culprit. The occlusive theory is now known to be correct in the majority of patients with acute infarction, as proven by the results of very early coronary angiography in preparation for the introduction of thrombolytic agents into the occluded coronary artery.

Triggers to Myocardial Infarction. Emotional and physical stress may be identified as triggering factors in up to half of the cases of AMI in humans (Tofler et al., 1990). Probably closely related is the onset of AMI and sudden death soon after awakening (Muller et al., 1994). Increased adrenergic activation may be involved, originating from either intense central arousal or severe physical exercise. The mechanisms for the adverse adrenergic effects may include a series of events that may lead to plaque rupture with thrombosis in those with pre-existing coronary disease: (1) an increased heart rate and contractility increases the oxygen demand (MVO_2) and precipitates ischemia; (2) increased arterial blood pressure associated with the increased cardiac output and increased α-adrenergic–mediated peripheral vascular resistance exaggerates ischemia and damages the vascular endothelium; and (3) increased circulating free fatty acids have harmful effects on membranes and promote platelet aggregation. In addition, in high concentrations used experimentally, catecholamines may directly increase sarcolemmal permeability to cause the egress of intracellular enzymes. Although all these links to the onset of AMI are still speculative, they provide a challenging hypothesis. It also should be recalled that even when AMI is not triggered, there is an early increase in circulating catecholamine levels, especially in patients with large infarcts, and much evidence supports the concept that β-adrenergic activation can exaggerate the degree of myocardial ischemia.

MECHANISMS OF IRREVERSIBLE ISCHEMIC DAMAGE

The exact mechanism whereby reversible ischemia finally evolves into irreversible infarction is still controversial. Both the consequences of poor oxygen delivery and poor washout of metabolites may play a role, with the former probably being the predominant factor (Fig. 18-7). Five current theories for the development of irreversible ischemic damage are (1) loss of a critical amount of ATP, (2) membrane damage induced metabolically or mechanically, (3) formation of free radicals, (4) calcium overload, and (5) sodium pump inhibition.

A critical level of ATP can be excluded as the sole cause of irreversibility because of the different values for the critical level given by different investigators and because of the established concept of ATP compartmentation (mitochondrial versus cytoplasmic). It is impossible to say which compartment is depleted by measurements of overall ATP. However, the ATP theory is being revived and extended with the recent evidence that ATP produced by glycolysis may have a specific role in the prevention of membrane-related ischemic events, such as calcium influx (Owen et al., 1990) and potassium loss (Weiss and Hiltbrand, 1985). Inhibition of glycolysis markedly accelerates cell death in dogs with coronary occlusion (Sebbag et al., 1996). Thus, inhibition of glycolysis is postulated to be a crucial event in the progress to ischemic cell necrosis (Fig. 18-8).

Inhibition of the sodium pump may precipitate an excess of internal sodium, which in turn leads to an increased osmotic pressure, which helps to "pop" the cell membrane and to cause irreversible damage (Jennings et al., 1986). The proposed cause of the pump failure is inadequate synthesis of sufficient glycolytic ATP for the pump (Cross et al., 1995).

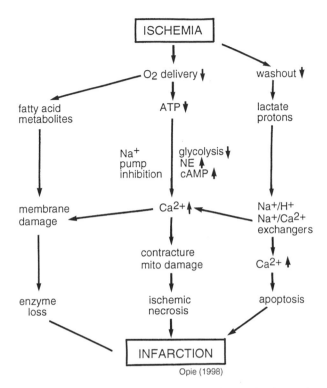

FIG. 18-7. Mechanisms of infarction. Proposed metabolic mechanisms whereby ischemia can produce infarction. The two major effects of ischemia are poor O_2 delivery (hypoxia) and poor washout of metabolites. Depressed mitochondrial metabolism results in decreased production of ATP and accumulation of fatty acid metabolites, which are normally metabolized in the mitochondria. Anaerobic metabolism causes accumulation of lactate and protons (the latter from breakdown of ATP), and continued residual respiration causes accumulation of CO_2. Decreased production of glycolytic ATP (a result of accumulation of lactate and/or protons) results in calcium accumulation. Inhibition of ion pumps by lack of ATP and by inhibition of fatty acid metabolites results in potassium loss, as well as sodium and water retention with cell swelling (shown at right). Fatty acid metabolites also cause membrane damage, which may result also from lysosomal activation by severe cellular acidosis. The final events leading up to infarction may be increasing ischemia caused by ischemic contracture, mitochondrial damage, enzyme loss as a result of membrane damage, and proteolysis from lysosomal activation.

Membrane damage is multifactorial in origin, and includes accumulation of free fatty acids inside and outside the ischemic cells and increased amounts of acyl CoA and acyl carnitine (Fig. 18-9). There may be a self-perpetuating cycle whereby part of the membrane damage results from the action of phospholipases that break down membrane lipids, with formation of lysophosphoglycerides, which further promote membrane damage.

Oxygen free radicals also may contribute to membrane damage by lipid peroxide formation. Free radicals are derived in part from neutrophils, particularly

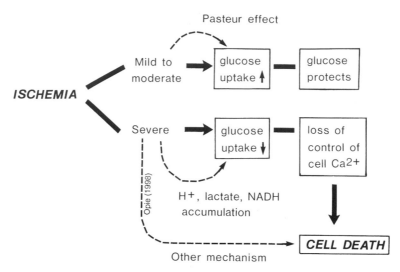

FIG. 18-8. Hypothesis relating the rate of glycolysis to cell death. During mild to moderate ischemia, glucose uptake is increased, providing the benefit of increased glycolytic ATP. During severe ischemia, the rate of glucose delivery becomes limiting (King et al., 1995). In addition, the accumulation of protons, lactate, and NADH inhibits glycolysis and glucose uptake. Consequently, there is a loss of control of intracellular calcium with the formation of ischemic contracture.

during the reperfusion phase of ischemic damage, and in part from damaged myocyte mitochondria (see Fig. 19-4).

The calcium overload concept of irreversibility has received special prominence in relation to conditions of massive calcium overload, such as catecholamine stimulation, severe reperfusion damage, or the very unusual experi-

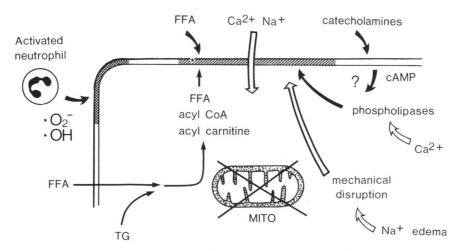

FIG. 18-9. Membrane damage in ischemia. FFA, free fatty acids; TG, triglyceride; MITO, mitochondrial metabolism; ·O_2^-, ·OH, oxygen-derived free radicals.

mental condition of the calcium paradox, whereby extracellular calcium is totally removed and then, when reintroduced, causes massive cellular damage. The basic concept of such severe degrees of calcium overload is that the mitochondria initially act as a buffer to take up calcium from the cytosol, which requires considerable energy. As a consequence, generalized cellular energy depletion is enhanced, the energy required for maintenance of ionic gradients becomes inadequate, and membrane integrity is lost. A modified form of this hypothesis is as follows. In ischemia, cytosolic calcium levels increase, possibly as a result of intracellular redistribution of calcium. Such cytosolic calcium increases can activate phospholipases, increase resting tension, and provoke fatal arrhythmias (Lubbe et al., 1992).

Irreversibility probably depends on no single metabolic event, but like the gradual death of a person, it may be a complex phenomenon resulting from the simultaneous operation of many diverse mechanisms (Fig. 18-7).

CLINICAL DIAGNOSIS OF IRREVERSIBILITY

It is often important to distinguish patients with true AMI from those who have other sources of chest pain, and among those with true AMI to diagnose irreversible damage. It is also important to know whether thrombolytic reperfu-

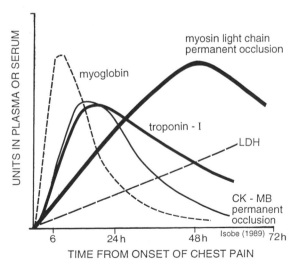

FIG. 18-10. Blood biochemical changes in acute myocardial infarction. Note early increase of myoglobin and slightly later increase of troponin-I and creatine kinase (CK-MB). These values are markedly influenced by reperfusion which causes an abrupt increase in plasma levels due to the washout of enzyme from the ischemic zone. Serum myosin light chain increases much later to attain a peak at about 48 hours (Isobe et al., 1989). Reperfusion does not increase the level of serum myosin light chain.

sion has taken place. The release of intracellular enzymes and contractile proteins into the circulation is helpful in these endeavors (Fig. 18-10).

Release of Creatine Kinase.   Creatine kinase of cardiac origin (CK-MB) is specific to the heart and can be detected within hours of the onset of AMI, but increased sensitivity and specificity is obtained by the assay of subforms of CK-MB. There is only one form of CK-MB in the heart, namely $CK-MB_2$, but this is converted in the blood to $CK-MB_1$, which can be detected within 6 hours of the onset of symptoms (Puelo et al., 1994).

Troponin T and Other Intracellular Proteins.   Increases in blood levels of myoglobin and troponin T are both candidates for the early diagnosis of AMI. For the purposes of ruling out AMI (often very important to cardiologists), early release of myoglobin is better (de Winter et al., 1995).

The release of cardiac myosin light chain is a much slower process, about two to four times slower than that of creatine kinase, and can be related to experimental infarct size (Isobe et al., 1989). Because of the slow release rate of this protein, with a much later peak than is the case with creatine kinase, the release of myosin light chain is not influenced by early reperfusion at 3 or 6 hours, whereas such reperfusion abruptly increases the rate of release of CK-MB, troponin T, and myoglobin. Therefore, release of myosin light chain helps in the late but not early diagnosis of AMI.

Diagnosis of Patency After Reperfusion.   After reperfusion, an important question is whether adequate patency has been achieved. The standard in invasive angiography and the degree of patency is arbitrarily classified according to the criteria in the TIMI study as TIMI grades 1 to 3, reflecting lesser to complete patency. Clearly noninvasive indices would be preferable. The logic for biochemical markers is that return of blood washes out markers such as myoglobin, troponin T, and CK-MB subforms (Laperche et al., 1995). A substantial increase in the blood values of these markers soon after reperfusion helps indicate patency.

Electrocardiographic Irreversibility

As ischemia is prolonged and irreversibility develops, so does a new series of electrocardiographic (ECG) changes, characterized by Q waves and an acute infarction pattern (Fig. 18-11). The very early ECG changes of *hyperacute infarction* during the stage of myocardial ischemia are those of ST-segment deviation, which is a positive deflection in the case of epicardial damage (Fig. 18-11A) and a negative deflection in the case of endocardial damage (Fig. 18-11B). The ST changes are those of depolarization caused by ischemic potassium ion shifts. Next, as the tissue undergoes necrosis, the electrode "sees" through the

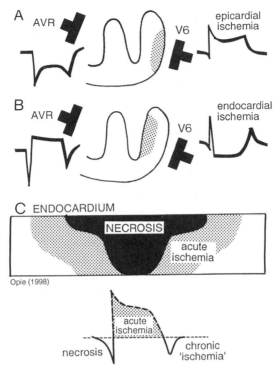

FIG. 18-11. ECG changes of the clinical syndrome of AMI. Patterns of ischemia and their contribution to the ECG changes of hyperacute (very early stage) developing myocardial infarction. **A:** A lead facing a zone of subepicardial ischemia (stipples), in this case lead V6, shows the expected ST-segment elevation. When monitored from the opposite side of the heart (lead AVR), there is an inverse picture, with ST-segment depression. **B:** A similar sequence is shown for endocardial ischemia. **C:** There is the introduction of a zone of necrosis surrounded by acute ischemia in developing infarction. Necrosis is reflected as Q-wave formation. Acute ischemia is reflected as ST elevation because it is transmural in this type of disease. T-wave inversion reflects different degrees of shortening of the action potential duration and may remain even after the ST segment has reverted to normal as the ischemic phase passes.

dead myocardium to look at the other wall of the ventricle, where the major electrical force moves in the opposite direction from the endocardium through the ventricular wall. Thus, the exploring electrode sees a negative deflection, that is, a Q wave. In this process, the R wave will first fall and decrease in magnitude before the Q wave becomes evident.

The extent of the change of the typical ECG pattern from early ST elevation to Q-wave formation 4 to 12 hours after the onset of ischemia provides an indirect index of myocardial necrosis. Theoretically, the efficacy of an intervention reducing experimental infarct size can be tested in humans by its capacity to lessen the development of ECG signs of necrosis, such as loss of frontal forces (decrease of R waves) and formation of Q waves, which occur over about 4 to

12 hours. Using this approach, early intravenous β-blockade diminishes the ECG features of infarction (Yusuf, 1980). The major factors preventing widespread use of the ECG technique are (1) the great individual variation in the evolution of the typical infarction pattern and (2) the difficulty of following the changes in inferior infarction, which requires special siting of the precordial electrodes.

INFARCT SIZE

In general, prognosis after myocardial infarction can be related to the amount of tissue irreversibly damaged by the infarct process, that is, the infarct size. However, this crucial measurement is not easy to undertake in humans. Enzymatic estimation of infarct size depends on many assumptions. The extent of ECG changes is only indirectly correlated with infarct size. Currently, a variety of imaging techniques are being investigated, including thallium scintigraphy, two-dimensional echocardiography (to detect the extent of impaired wall motion), computed tomography (CT) (to detect regional abnormalities of wall motion), and nuclear magnetic resonance (NMR) imaging. Such complex techniques have not come into general use, in part because the management of AMI in any case usually includes very early reperfusion and other feasible measures that are thought to reduce infarct size, such as reduction of heart rate by β-blockade, and in part because the techniques are so complex. The ideal scenario would be to delineate the extent of the total threatened myocardium (including area at risk) (Fig. 18-12) and then to assess the benefit of a specific intervention by its effect in preventing the conversion of the threatened zone to true infarction (Higgins, 1990). In the case of NMR imaging, the principle involved is that AMI is associated with an increased regional water content. The NMR signal can detect

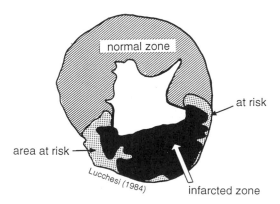

FIG. 18-12. Area at risk. The lateral and epicardial areas at risk can be saved from myocardial necrosis by appropriate intervention such as thrombolytic reperfusion. From Lucchesi et al. (1984).

the hydrogen nucleus by spin-echo imaging, so that the signal is increased in the infarct zone (Wesbey et al., 1984). More recently, the use of injected contrast media has helped to achieve better imaging and distinction between viable and nonviable tissue.

Infarct Size and Area at Risk.   When there is occlusion of a major coronary artery, the whole territory supplied by that vessel becomes the area at risk of infarction. Of this area, about 60% may undergo infarction in a typical rabbit heart experiment. Interventions that limit infarct size include preconditioning that reduces the infarct size to about 20% or even less of the area at risk (see Chapter 19). A large number of other experimental procedures reduce infarct size less strikingly. The principles are that either the blood supply to the infarcting tissue is improved, or the oxygen supply is conserved (e.g., by decreasing the heart rate). However, there are reservations about applying these therapeutic principles to humans. First, it is still difficult to measure infarct size and especially difficult to continuously monitor the evolution of the infarct process. Second, clinicians are increasingly demanding that new therapies should be designed to be additive in effect to those of thrombolysis, and that the end points of such studies should be mortality in mega-trials, which are hugely expensive. Of the many agents tested experimentally, it is only β-blockade that is currently in use. Such agents may not limit the true ultimate infarct size but rather reduce the rate of progression from ischemia to irreversible infarction.

POSTINFARCT REMODELING

After the onset of AMI, some patients undergo a progressive increase in left ventricular (LV) size manifested by a long-term increase in the end-diastolic and end-systolic volumes. The increase in LV volume is often observed in patients with large infarcts and clinical manifestations of heart failure. This process whereby the left ventricle progressively enlarges is called remodeling. One proposal is that the increased wall stress, resulting from LV damage and fewer contractile cells, stimulates the cardiac renin-angiotensin system (Yamagishi et al., 1993), as in the case of myocardial stretch caused by a pressure load (see Chapter 13). If left unchecked, this process will lead to left ventricular dilation and adverse remodeling. Therapy by angiotensin-converting enzyme inhibition (Fig. 18-13) appears to beneficially alter this process, acting by a combination of preload and afterload reduction, and inhibition of the cardiac renin-angiotensin system. Experimentally, growth hormone attenuates LV remodeling, presumably by inducing hypertrophy of noninfarcted myocytes (Cittadini et al., 1996). Clinically, patients may present with either predominantly diastolic or systolic heart failure (Fig. 18-14).

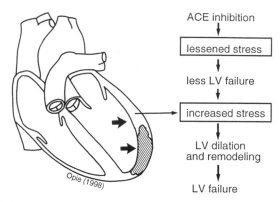

$$\text{WALL STRESS} = \frac{\text{Pressure x Radius}}{2 \text{ x (wall thickness)}}$$

ACE inhibition
↓
| lessened stress |
↓
less LV failure
↓
| increased stress |
↓
LV dilation
and remodeling
↓
LV failure

Opie (1998)

FIG. 18-13. Postinfarct remodeling. Role of large infarct in precipitation of left ventricular dilation by allowing increased wall stress as a result of fewer contractile cells. Therapy by angiotensin-converting enzyme (ACE) inhibition decreases preload and afterload, thereby lessening wall stress and helping to prevent left ventricular dilation and left ventricular failure.

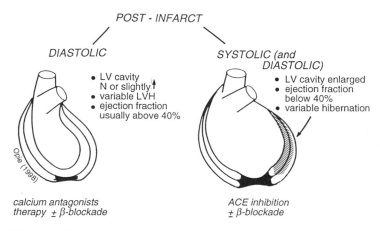

POST - INFARCT

DIASTOLIC

- LV cavity N or slightly↑
- variable LVH
- ejection fraction usually above 40%

calcium antagonists therapy ± β-blockade

SYSTOLIC (and DIASTOLIC)

- LV cavity enlarged
- ejection fraction below 40%
- variable hibernation

ACE inhibition ± β-blockade

Opie (1998)

FIG. 18-14. Varieties of postinfarct LV dysfunction. For further details see Opie (1996).

SUMMARY

1. *The mechanism of irreversible cell death by necrosis* is not simple and appears to be multifactorial. Although energy depletion, monitored by the level of ATP, cannot be related directly to outcome because of ATP compartmentation and multiple modes of generation of ATP, energy depletion may lead to an early redistribution of calcium ions in the cell, which in turn

could activate phospholipases to damage the sarcolemma. Membrane changes also result from the accumulation of unmetabolized lipid products, such as acyl CoA and acyl carnitine, as well as free radicals. These processes increase sarcolemmal damage, as does intracellular edema fluid formation consequent on sodium pump failure and increased internal sodium. Once membrane disruption occurs beyond a certain point, calcium ions enter from without, and such net gain of cellular calcium is associated with irreversible damage, large-scale release of enzymes, and the clinical point of no return.

2. *The time-scale for irreversible damage is highly variable.* Although severely or totally ischemic cells probably die after 20 to 60 minutes, in the presence of collateral flow and a low oxygen requirement the point of no return can be delayed for 2 to 6 hours.

3. *The ultimate extent of tissue necrosis* is important and highly variable from patient to patient, depending on the extent and number of sites of coronary artery occlusion, degree of spontaneous reperfusion, overall metabolic state of the patient including circulating catecholamines and free fatty acids, and, above all, pattern of pre-existing collateral flow. Infarct size is difficult to quantify, although modern imaging techniques may attain this goal in the near future. Infarct size limitation involves either relief of the coronary occlusion (e.g., by thrombolysis) or conservation of the oxygen supply (e.g., reduction of heart rate by β-blockade). Nonetheless, experimentalists point out that the effects of β-blockade may be merely to slow the rate of infarct development rather than to achieve a genuine reduction.

STUDENT QUESTIONS

1. Outline the major differences between necrosis and apoptosis. When may each play an important role in relation to (a) ischemia–reperfusion and (b) heart failure?

2. Give some current views on the cellular events that cause reversible ischemic injury to become irreversible.

3. After coronary occlusion, what is the area at risk of infarction, and what is infarct size?

CARDIOLOGIST-IN-TRAINING QUESTIONS

1. Describe in outline the atherosclerotic process as currently understood.

2. What are triggers to acute myocardial infarction and what is their pathophysiologic basis?

3. "Calcium overload causes necrosis in myocardial infarction." Critically consider this hypothesis.

4. What are the patterns of release (as a function of time) of relevant intracellular proteins after the onset of symptoms of acute myocardial infarction in patients? What mechanisms are involved?

5. Describe the typical electrocardiographic changes of early stage acute myocardial infarction and, in outline, the origin of such changes.
6. What is the basis for postinfarct remodeling? What are the possible consequences?
7. Distinguish between postinfarct diastolic and systolic heart failure.

REFERENCES

1. Cittadini A, Grossman JD, Katz SE, et al. Growth hormone attenuates LV remodeling and improves cardiac function in rats with large myocardial infarction [Abstract]. *J Am Coll Cardiol* 1996;27:12A.
2. Cooke JP, Tsao PS. Arginine: a new therapy for atherosclerosis. *Circulation* 1997;95:311–312.
3. Cross HR, Radda GK, Clarke K. The role of Na^+/K^+ ATPase activity during low flow ischemia in preventing myocardial injury: a ^{31}P, ^{23}Na and ^{87}Rb NMR spectroscopic study. *Magn Reson Med* 1995;34:673–685.
4. Davies MJ, Thomas AC. Plaque fissuring—the cause of acute myocardial infarction, sudden ischemic death and crescendo angina. *Br Heart J* 1985;53:363–373.
5. de Winter RJ, Koster RW, Sturk A, Sanders GT. Value of myoglobin, troponin T and CK-MB$_{mass}$ in ruling out an acute myocardial infarction in the emergency room. *Circulation* 1995;92:3401–3407.
6. Dzau VJ, Gibbons GH, Pratt RE. Molecular mechanisms of vascular renin-angiotensin system in myointimal hyperplasia. *Hypertension* 1991;18(suppl II):100–105.
7. Fliss H, Gattinger D. Apoptosis in ischemic and reperfused rat myocardium. *Circ Res* 1996;79: 949–956.
8. Frielingsdorf J, Seiler C, Kaufmann P, et al. Normalisation of abnormal coronary vasomotion by calcium antagonists in patients with hypertension. *Circulation* 1996;93:1380–1387.
9. Frink RJ, Rooney PA, Trowbridge JO, Rose JP. Coronary thrombosis and platelet/fibrin microemboli in death associated with acute myocardial infarction. *Br Heart J* 1988;59:196–200.
10. Hayashida W, Horiuchi M, Zhang L, Dzau VJ. Expression of p53 and Bax genes are induced in the ischemia-reperfused rat ventricle: potential roles in myocardial apoptosis. *Circulation* 1996;94(suppl I):1–225.
11. Hearse DJ, Yellon DM. Why are we still in doubt about infarct size limitation? The experimentalist's viewpoint. In: Hearse DJ, Yellon DM (eds). *Therapeutic Approaches to Myocardial Infarct Size Limitation.* New York: Raven, 1984;17–41.
12. Heitzer T, Just H, Münzel T. Antioxidant vitamin C improves endothelial dysfunction in chronic smokers. *Circulation* 1996;94:6–9.
13. Higgins CB. Nuclear magnetic resonance (NMR) imaging in ischemic heart disease. *J Am Coll Cardiol* 1990;15:150–151.
14. Isobe M, Nagai R, Yamaoki K, et al. Quantification of myocardial infarct size after coronary reperfusion by serum cardiac myosin light chain II in conscious dogs. *Circ Res* 1989;65:684–694.
15. James TN. Normal and abnormal consequences of apoptosis in the human heart. From postnatal morphogenesis to paroxysmal arrhythmias. *Circulation* 1994;90:556–573.
16. Jennings RB, Reimer KA, Steenbergen C. Myocardial ischemia revisited. The osmolar load, membrane damage, and reperfusion. *J Mol Cell Cardiol* 1986;18:769–780.
17. King LM, Boucher F, Opie LH. Coronary flow and glucose delivery as determinants of contracture in the ischemic myocardium. *J Mol Cell Cardiol* 1995;27:701–720.
18. Laperche T, Steg G, Dehoux M, et al. A study of biochemical markers of reperfusion early after thrombolysis for acute myocardial infarction. *Circulation* 1995;92:2079–2086.
19. Lubbe WH, Podzuweit T, Opie LH. Potential arrhythmogenic role of cyclic adenosine monophosphate (AMP) and cytosolic calcium overload: implications for prophylactic effects of beta-blockers in myocardial infarction and proarrhythmic effects of phospodiesterase inhibitors. *J Am Coll Cardiol* 1992;19:1622–1633.
20. Lucchesi BR, Romson JL, Jolly SR. Do leukocytes influence infarct size? In: Hearse DJ, Yellon DM (eds). *Therapeutic Approaches to Myocardial Infarct Size Limitation.* New York: Raven, 1984; 219–248.
21. Misao J, Hayakawa Y, Ohno M, et al. Expression of bcl-2 protein, an inhibitor of apoptosis and Bax, an accelerator of apoptosis, in ventricular myocytes of human hearts with myocardial infarction. *Circulation* 1996;94:1506–1512.

22. Muller JE, Abela GS, Nesto RW, Tofler GH. Triggers, acute risk factors and vulnerable plaques: the lexicon of a new frontier. *J Am Coll Cardiol* 1994;23:809–813.
23. Opie LH. The multifarious spectrum of ischemic left ventricular dysfunction: relevance of new ischemic syndromes. *J Mol Cell Cardiol* 1996;28:2403–2414.
24. Owen P, Dennis S, Opie LH. Glucose flux rate regulates onset of ischemic contracture in globally underperfused rat hearts. *Circ Res* 1990;66:344–354.
25. Puleo PR, Meyer D, Wathen C, et al. Use of a rapid assay of subforms of creatine kinase MB to diagnose or rule out acute myocardial infarction. *N Engl J Med* 1994;331:561–566.
26. Reimer KA, Lower JE, Rasmussen MM, Jenkins RB. The wavefront phenomenon of ischemic cell death. I. Myocardial infarct size vs duration of coronary occlusion in dogs. *Circulation* 1977;56: 786–794.
27. Ross R. The pathogenesis of atherosclerosis. In: Braunwald E (ed). *Heart Disease. A Textbook of Cardiovascular Medicine.* Philadelphia: WB Saunders, 1997;1105–1125.
28. Schaper W, Binz K, Sass S, Winkler B. Influence of collateral blood flow and of variations in MVO2 on tissue-ATP content in ischemic and infarcted myocardium. *J Mol Cell Cardiol* 1987;19:19–37.
29. Sebbag L, Reimer KA, Jennings RB. Elimination of glycolytically-derived ATP markedly accelerates the onset of transmural cell death during myocardial ischemia in vivo in dogs [Abstract]. *Circulation* 1996;94(suppl I):1–367.
30. Tofler GH, Stone PH, Maclure M, et al. Analysis of possible triggers of acute myocardial infarction (the MILIS Study). *Am J Cardiol* 1990;66:22–27.
31. Weiss J, Hiltbrand B. Functional compartmentation of glycolytic versus oxidative metabolism in isolated rabbit heart. *J Clin Invest* 1985;75:436–447.
32. Wesbey G, Higgins CB, Lanzer P, et al. Imaging and characterization of acute myocardial infarction in vivo by gated nuclear magnetic resonance. *Circulation* 1984;69:125–130.
33. Yamagishi H, Kim S, Nishikimi T, et al. Contribution of cardiac renin-angiotensin system to ventricular remodelling in myocardial-infarcted rats. *J Mol Cell Cardiol* 1993;25:1369–1380.
34. Yusuf S, Ramsdale D, Peto R, et al. Early intravenous atenolol treatment in suspected acute myocardial infarction: preliminary report of a randomized trial. *Lancet* 1980;2:273–276.
35. Zeiher AM, Drexler H, Wollschlager W, Just H. Endothelial dysfunction of the coronary microvasculature is associated with impaired coronary blood flow regulation in patients with early atherosclerosis. *Circulation* 1991;84:1984–1992.

19

Myocardial Reperfusion: New Ischemic Syndromes

Brief periods of coronary occlusion result in prolonged depression of myocardial function in the ischemic zone.

G.R. Heyndrickx et al., 1975

Myocardial reperfusion is no longer a laboratory event. Practicing cardiologists are now able to induce myocardial reperfusion after the onset of coronary thrombosis by the use of thrombolytic agents such as streptokinase or the tissue plasminogen activator (tPA). Despite promising findings with reperfusion, clinicians have noted that the results are not as positive as expected. Thus, sometimes even early restitution of blood flow leaves the function of the myocardium temporarily depressed, which has been termed the "stunned" myocardium (Braunwald and Kloner, 1982). Experimentalists have long been impressed by the finding that restitution of coronary flow to the ischemic myocardium may precipitate a sequence of events that presumably would have occurred either later or not at all (Hearse et al., 1975; Jennings et al., 1960; Opie, 1989). It is this spectrum of events, including reperfusion arrhythmias, stunning, microvascular damage, and accelerated death of the more severely damaged cells despite reperfusion, that is termed *reperfusion injury* (Opie, 1989).

The *new ischemic syndromes* include the novel aspects of ischemia, such as stunning, hibernation, and preconditioning (Table 19-1), in contrast to the classic conditions such as angina pectoris, unstable angina, and infarction. Stunning refers to postischemic impairment of myocardial function (Fig. 19-1). Hibernation occurs when the ventricle contracts poorly in the presence of severe coronary artery disease, but wakes up after revascularization by coronary artery surgery. Preconditioning is the protective state that lessens the severity of ischemic reperfusion when it follows one or more brief episodes of preceding

TABLE 19-1. *Proposed characteristics of conventional ischemia, stunning, hibernation, and preconditioning*

Parameter	Conventional ischemia	Acute stunning	Chronic stunning[a]	Hibernation	Preconditioning
Myocardial function	Reduced	Reduced	Reduced	Reduced	Protected during repeat ischemia by prior ischemia Brief ischemia → fully reperfused → test ischemia reperfused
Coronary blood flow	Severely reduced	Postischemic; fully restored	Partially restored	Modestly reduced or possibly normal at rest and repetitively reduced during exercise	
Myocardial energy metabolism	Reduced: increasingly severe as ischemia proceeds	Normal or excessive	Unknown but probably depressed	Reduced in relation to contractile decrease	Reduced ATP demand in test ischemic period
Duration	Minutes to hours	Hours to days	Days to weeks to months	Days to months	Protection lasts for hours; may return with "second window"
Outcome	Infarction if severe ischemia persists	Full recovery	Incomplete recovery	Recovery if revascularization	Decreased postischemic infarct size; decreased surrogate damage
Proposed changes in metabolic regulation of calcium	Insufficient glycolytic ATP to control cell calcium and to prevent reversibility	Cystolic overload and excess oscillations of calcium ions in early reperfusion	Prolonged calcium overload may have led to partial necrosis	Just enough glycolytic ATP to prevent contracture; chronic downregulation and ATP demand	Role of calcium not elucidated, except in hypothesis of repetitive stunning

[a]Distinguished from maimed myocardium (Boden et al., 1995), by potential for complete though delayed recovery. See Fig. 19-1.

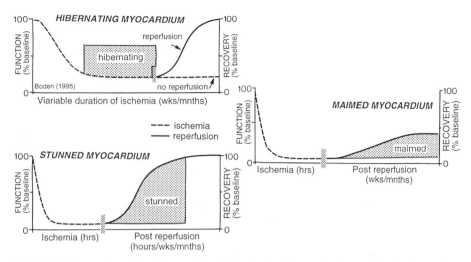

FIG. 19-1. Hibernation, stunning, and maiming. In the hibernating heart, chronic depression of function is relieved by revascularization. In the stunned heart, mechanical dysfunction results from reperfusion. In the maimed myocardium, there is some permanent damage resulting from prolonged ischemia, so that recovery is never complete. Modified with permission from Boden et al. (1995).

ischemia, each such episode being followed by reperfusion. Although the vast body of evidence favoring the entity of preconditioning has been found in experimental animals, current studies increasingly suggest that it also occurs in humans.

STUNNED MYOCARDIUM

Not all the mechanical recovery occurs rapidly after reperfusion; full recovery may be delayed by hours, days, or even weeks. Because myocardial function eventually recovers fully, it is *stunned* during the phase of delayed recovery (Braunwald and Kloner, 1982). In 1975, Heyndrickx and co-workers made the seminal discovery that regional ischemia in the dog heart when induced for only 5 minutes was followed by depressed mechanical function lasting for over 3 hours. Furthermore, 15 minutes of coronary occlusion resulted in more than 6 hours of left ventricular (LV) dysfunction. Of considerable importance was the point that the short periods of ischemia did not result in any residual necrosis. The impaired postischemic function could not be accounted for by any impairment of blood flow in the previously occluded vessel (Heyndrickx et al., 1978).

As reviewed by Braunwald (1991), myocardial stunning occurs in the following experimental conditions: (1) in the zones adjacent to necrotic tissue; (2) after myocardial oxygen demands have been transiently elevated in the presence of partial arterial stenosis; (3) after subendocardial ischemia in exercising dogs with LV hypertrophy, even without coronary occlusion; and (4) in isolated hearts when reperfused after global ischemia or reoxygenated after anoxia. Braunwald also noted that diastolic dysfunction is an important aspect of stunning.

Duration of Ischemia and Stunning

If the absence of necrosis is an essential part of the definition, as required by Bolli (1990, 1992), then it becomes clear that the longer and more severe the period of ischemia, the less the contribution of true stunning and the more the contribution of permanent damage to postinfarct dysfunction. Increasing the duration of severe ischemia from 30 to 90 minutes results in adverse events such as a further increase in postischemic diastolic pressure, with a marked gain in total tissue and mitochondrial calcium (Ferrari et al., 1986). These observations explain why 1 hour of coronary artery occlusion in the dog followed by 4 weeks of reperfusion does not yield complete recovery (Lavallee et al., 1983). This type of gradual and incomplete recovery over several days and even weeks, called the *maimed myocardium,* represents a mixture of chronic stunning and irreversible damage, so that there never will be full functional recovery (Boden et al., 1995). Chronic stunning, with much delayed but eventually full recovery, and the maimed myocardium probably merge into each other. In contrast, the typical duration of total ischemia that is soon followed by completely reversible stunning is 5 to 20 minutes (du Toit and Opie, 1994; Heyndrickx et al., 1975).

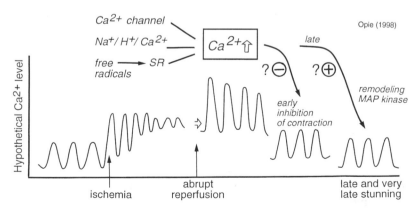

FIG. 19-2. Hypothetical cytosolic calcium levels. Note proposed role of increased cytosolic calcium in causing early stunning after reperfusion and in hypothetically playing a role in late remodeling by stimulation of protein synthesis, possibly at the level of MAP kinase (mitogen-activated protein kinase). $Na^+/H^+/Ca^{2+}$, sodium/proton and sodium/calcium exchange mechanisms (see Myers et al., 1995); SR, sarcoplasmic reticulum.

Mechanism of Stunning

Of the many theories to explain the development of stunning, the most plausible involve cytosolic calcium overload (Fig. 19-2) and the formation of oxygen-derived free radicals. Most logically, the delayed resynthesis of ATP, probably the consequence of loss of adenosine and related compounds during the ischemic period, could be blamed. Nonetheless, even when there is no decrease in ATP and rapid recovery of creatine phosphate after short periods of ischemia, there is already stunning (see Fig. 17-3).

Calcium. The fact that the stunned myocardium can respond well to inotropic stimulation by the catecholamine dopamine, isoproterenol, calcium infusion, epinephrine, or postextrasystolic potentiation suggests that stunning represents a lack of available intracellular calcium or a failure of uptake of calcium by the sarcoplasmic reticulum or a failure of the contractile proteins to respond to normal calcium concentration. Measurements of cytosolic calcium during early postischemic reperfusion show increased calcium levels and oscillations (Fig. 19-3) (Brooks et al., 1995; Gao et al., 1995; Meissner and Morgan, 1995). The concept could be that internal cytosolic calcium overload damages the contractile apparatus to impair the normal physiologic response to calcium so that there is mechanical stunning (Fig. 19-2).

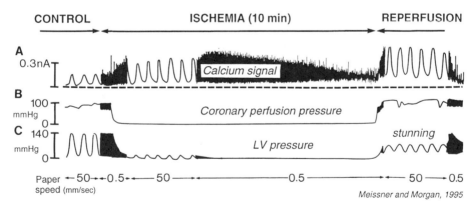

FIG. 19-3. Measured cytosolic calcium levels. Can LV mechanical failure during and after severe ischemia be explained by changes in the cytosolic calcium? These data show that when there is abrupt ischemic LV failure (LV pressure decreases to zero in C), then the calcium signal (A) increases before it decreases. Ischemia is designated by the abrupt decrease of coronary perfusion pressure to zero (B) in this isolated rat heart preparation. During reperfusion there is also a dissociation between the cytosolic calcium oscillations, which are augmented (right-hand panel of A) in contrast to LV contraction, which is decreased (right-hand aspect of bottom panel), so that there is mechanical stunning. It is thought that excess calcium oscillations damage the contractile proteins. Reproduced from Meissner and Morgan (1995) with permission of the authors and the American Physiological Society.

The source of the calcium could be external or internal. Calcium uptake during early reperfusion can result from sodium–calcium exchange or from calcium ion entry via the L-channels (du Toit and Opie, 1992). Calcium entering or leaving the sarcoplasmic reticulum is also important, as shown by inhibitors of the uptake or release mechanisms (du Toit and Opie, 1994).

Hypothetically, the effects of excess cytosolic calcium can be separated into two phases: it is proposed that in the first the damage is occurring and in the second the myocardium is dyfunctional as a result of the damage already done. This is the two-stage calcium model (Opie, 1991). The origin of the hypocontractile state differs according to the stage and so does the proposed therapy. In the first stage, it is hypothesized that all procedures leading to excess cytosolic calcium, including formation of free radicals, should be harmful and that the use of various agents including the calcium antagonists as well as Na^+/H^+ exchange inhibitors should be beneficial. In the second stage, calcium agonists such as β-adrenergic stimulants may be useful to stimulate the hypocontractile left ventricle (Becker et al., 1986; Ito et al., 1987). Cardiac surgeons have acknowledged this distinction by using low-calcium reperfusion solutions after cardiac arrest and coronary bypass surgery. Later, when LV failure is manifested in the early postoperative phase, calcium infusions or β-agonists are beneficial in sustaining the cardiac output.

It is crucial to distinguish between the present concept of cytosolic calcium overload and the earlier proposal that there is massive calcium overload leading to cell necrosis in the reperfusion period. Undoubtedly, such massive overload can occur, but a net excess of calcium uptake into cells that are already sufficiently damaged to be on their way to sure cell death is not really of fundamental interest. Such calcium overload is one lethal mechanism that accelerates the funeral of cells bound to die in any case. (For the role of calcium in lethal damage, see Chapter 18.) The concepts proposed in this chapter relate to a temporary cytosolic calcium overload with different possible sources, including decreased uptake into the sarcoplasmic reticulum (failure of availability of ATP), decreased extrusion from the cell (again failure of ATP), entry through the voltage-sensitive calcium channel (explaining inhibition of stunning by calcium antagonists at the time of reperfusion), and activity of sodium–calcium exchange. This early reversible cytosolic calcium overload does not exclude the possibility of later massive lethal overload, for example, when cell membranes have been damaged (see Chapter 18).

Role of Free Radicals in Stunning. Free radicals are highly reactive chemical species that differ from standard compounds in having unpaired electrons in their outer orbitals. Oxygen-derived free radicals include the superoxide radical $\cdot O_2^-$ (Fig. 19-4), where the dot indicates the free radical and the negative charge indicates the electron gained (superoxide anion). There is danger that the superoxide anion can react with hydrogen peroxide to form the even more highly reactive hydroxyl ion ($\cdot OH$), in which there is no charge

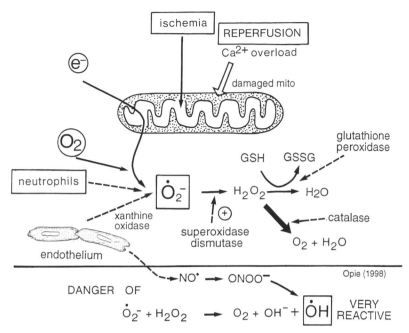

FIG. 19-4. Pathways for generation of oxygen free radicals with, in particular, the superoxide (·O_2^-) and hydroxyl (·OH) ions. GSH, reduced glutathione; GSSG, oxidized glutathione. Note formation of peroxynitrite from nitric oxide (·NO).

because normally the hydroxyl group carries the negative charge and gaining an electron confers a neutral compound. Nonetheless, this compound is highly reactive. Singlet oxygen (Table 19-2) is not, strictly speaking, a free radical but has two outer electrons spinning in opposite directions, which accounts for its instability.

Peroxidation of polyunsaturated lipids of the membranes (Meerson et al., 1982) can be caused by free radical formation and may contribute to reperfusion injury (Table 19-3). The key enzyme protecting against lipid peroxidation is

TABLE 19-2. *Potentially cytotoxic oxygen-derived species*

·O_2^-	Superoxide anion radical
H_2O_2	Hydrogen peroxide (not a free radical)
·OH	Hydroxyl radical
ROO·	Lipid peroxide radical (R = lipid chain)
$^1O_2$	Singlet oxygen[a]
ONOO⁻	Peroxynitrite

[a]In singlet oxygen, the two outer electrons occupy the same orbital and spin in opposite directions, hence being unstable. One mechanism for formation of singlet oxygen is by light activation on molecular oxygen in the presence of a photosensitizer, such as rose bengal. Another proposed mechanism is during superoxide dismutation.

TABLE 19-3. *Free radical generation: some essential equations*

1. Reduction of O_2 to H_2O
   $O_2 + e^- \rightarrow \cdot O_2^-$ (superoxide radical)
   $\cdot O_2^- + e^- + 2H^+ \rightarrow H_2O_2$ (hydrogen peroxide)
   $\cdot O_2^- + H_2O_2 + H^+ \rightarrow O_2 + H_2O + \cdot OH$ ($\cdot OH$ = hydroxyl radical)
   $\cdot OH + e^- + H^+ \rightarrow H_2O$
2. Iron-related reactions
   a. $Fe^{2+} + H_2O_2 \rightarrow Fe^{3+} + \cdot OH + OH^-$ (Fenton reaction)
   b. $Fe^{3+} + \cdot O_2^- \rightarrow Fe^{2+} + O_2$

   c. $\cdot O_2^- + H_2O_2 \xrightarrow[\text{catalyst}]{Fe} O_2 + \cdot OH + OH^-$ (Haber-Weiss reaction)
3. Lipid peroxidation
   Initiation: Lipid — H + $\cdot OH \rightarrow H_2O$ + lipid·
                    Lipid· + $O_2 \rightarrow$ lipid OO·
   Propagation: Lipid OO· + lipid — H $\rightarrow$ lipid—OOH + lipid·
   Termination: Lipid· + lipid· $\rightarrow$ lipid—lipid
4. Xanthine oxidase (XO) reaction[a]
   ATP $\rightarrow$ adenosine $\rightarrow$ xanthine
   Xanthine + H_2O + $2O_2 \xrightarrow{XO}$ uric acid + $2\cdot O_2^-$ + $2H^+$

[a]Xanthine oxidase is not found in the human myocardium, although it may be present in vascular endothelial cells (to be confirmed).

glutathione reductase, which uses reduced glutathione for H donation to the membrane lipids, thereby keeping them reduced. Once membranes are damaged by lipid peroxidation, increased permeability follows.

Antioxidant defense mechanisms occur naturally and protect against the formation of free radicals (Fig. 19-4, Table 19-4). It is when these mechanisms are overcome that the harmful effects of free radicals become evident, in which case a logical therapy is to remove excess free radicals by compounds that act as rad-

TABLE 19-4. *Naturally occurring defense systems against free radicals*

1. Superoxide dismutase
   $2\cdot O_2^- + 2H^+ \rightarrow H_2O_2 + O_2$
2. Catalase (peroxisome-bound)
   $2H_2O_2 \rightarrow O_2 + 2H_2O$
3. Glutathione peroxidase
   2 GSH + lipid—OOH $\rightarrow$ GSSG + lipid—OH + H_2O
   2 GSH + $H_2O_2 \rightarrow$ GSSG + $2H_2O$
4. Nonenzymatic scavengers
   α tocopherol
   β carotene
   Vitamin A
   Ascorbate
   Sulfhydryl group
   Thioether compounds

ical scavengers (Ambrosio et al., 1987). Thus far, no clinical tests with such drugs have been successful, which has dampened the interest of cardiologists in free radicals. By contrast, antioxidants are increasingly thought to play a preventative role in protection of the endothelium and in delaying the development of atheroma (see Chapter 18).

Interaction of Calcium and Free Radicals. It should not be supposed that evidence favoring free radical formation excludes a role for calcium (Bolli, 1992). Rather, the calcium-mediated and free radical–mediated components to the damage may be interactive (Fig. 19-5). A reasonable concept is that formation of free radicals increases cytosolic calcium by a variety of mechanisms: an effect on membrane phospholipids with an increase in cytosolic calcium, mitochondrial production of free radicals with mitochondrial injury, additive or parallel effects to calcium overload on ATP depletion, and activation of the calcium release channel of the sarcoplasmic reticulum with enhanced release of calcium. Free radicals also may (1) inhibit the uptake of calcium by the sarcoplasmic reticulum, (2) inhibit the sodium pump, (3) stimulate Na^+/Ca^+ exchange, and (4) decrease the rate of inactivation of the calcium current (Opie, 1991). Despite these important observations, therapy by

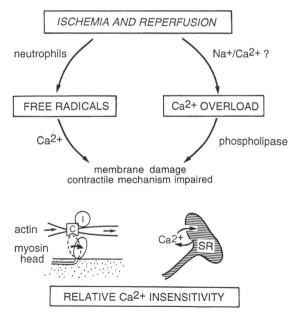

FIG. 19-5. Two major mechanisms for reperfusion injury: formation of free radicals and calcium overload. This scheme reconciles these apparently conflicting hypotheses, showing the proposed combined role of free radicals and calcium overload in causing membrane damage and relative calcium insensitivity of contractile mechanism (actin–myosin interaction on left and sarcoplasmic reticulum on right). From Opie (1989) with permission of the American Heart Association.

neither calcium antagonists nor by free radical scavengers has yet been established as a means of diminishing stunning in patients.

Stunning in the Clinical Setting

Postanginal Diastolic Failure.   Although the recovery from angina by cessation of exertion has been recognized for centuries, more recent work has shown that myocardial mechanical recovery is also delayed. For example, after the induction of pacing-induced angina, there is an increase in LV end-diastolic pressure and a stiffening of the myocardium with a decreased rate of LV wall thinning (Bourdillon et al., 1983). Similarly, regional wall motion abnormalities persist for at least 30 minutes after treadmill exercise testing (Kloner et al., 1991).

Bypass Surgery.   In another postischemic clinical situation, bypass surgery seems to promote diastolic dysfunction with an increase in LV diastolic chamber stiffness (McKenney et al., 1994). In more severe cases, the impairment in ventricular function also may be systolic, with clinical heart failure that responds to inotropic stimulation.

Postthrombolytic Chronic Stunning.   Delayed recovery (over days and weeks) of function is observed in postthrombolytic patients. Such chronic stunning may be a complex mixture of prolonged stunning, ventricular remodeling, and the benefits of the open artery that are not yet fully understood. The genesis of such chronic stunning is unclear, yet the protein synthetic changes probably involve mitogen-activated protein (MAP) kinase, a calcium-activated regulator of growth.

Therapeutic intervention is not yet clarified. Because stunning is by definition transient, it may be argued that there is no necessity to treat a self-healing condition. This argument becomes less acceptable when it is considered that repetitive stunning may be a cause of hibernation (Shen and Vatner, 1995) and may therefore contribute to critically impaired LV failure. Based on the calcium hypothesis for stunning, one small study with the calcium antagonist nisoldipine is promising (Sheiban et al., 1997). The nisoldipine was started at the time of reperfusion by primary angioplasty and was combined with an angiotensin-converting enzyme (ACE) inhibitor. Magnesium given at the time of reperfusion but not thereafter should also protect on the basis of animal data (du Toit and Opie, 1992). Despite one large negative megatrial in which intravenous magnesium was given after thrombolysis (ISIS-4, 1995), timing is crucial and further study is now warranted, with magnesium given early and the selection of high-risk patients (Antman, 1995; Antman et al., 1996).

All these clinical observations tie in well with the now established concept that "ischemia does something" that impairs mechanical activity even after the actual ischemic event is over.

OTHER ASPECTS OF REPERFUSION INJURY

Reperfusion Arrhythmias

Experimentally, reperfusion arrhythmias can occur within seconds of the onset of reperfusion. As in the case of stunning, there are two main theories for arrhythmias, namely excess cytosolic calcium and formation of free radicals. During prolonged (30 minutes) or severe hypoxia in the guinea pig papillary muscle, there is a slow steady increase in the diastolic tension, i.e., hypoxic contracture, followed by automaticity upon reoxygenation (Opie, 1989). It is reasonable to suppose that there is a posthypoxic arrhythmogenic increase in calcium (Brooks et al., 1995; Gao et al., 1995; Opie and Coetzee, 1988; Saman et al., 1988).

Direct measurements show large cytosolic calcium oscillations during early reperfusion (Meissner and Morgan, 1995). Restoration of ATP with reperfusion must provide the energy for the excess recycling of calcium. The result is the specific electrophysiologic phenomenon of delayed afterdepolarizations, which probably explain some types of reperfusion arrhythmias (Opie and Coetzee, 1988). Calcium over-cycling repetitively evokes the transient inward current that predisposes to ventricular automaticity (Coetzee and Opie, 1987). Of note, inhibitors of calcium movement in or out of the sarcoplasmic reticulum are able to lessen reperfusion arrhythmias (du Toit and Opie, 1994).

Duration of Ischemia and Arrhythmias. There is a relationship between the incidence of reperfusion arrhythmias and the degree of reversibility of ischemia. No reperfusion arrhythmias arise in dead cells (Corr and Witkowski, 1983; Manning and Hearse, 1984). This postulate is compatible with the idea that energy in the form of ATP is required for the cytosolic recycling of calcium that underlies at least some types of reperfusion arrhythmias. There is a bell-shaped curve of incidence of reperfusion arrhythmias with a peak incidence when the ischemia lasts between 5 and 20 minutes. Thereafter, the incidence decreases (Manning and Hearse, 1984), presumably as the ATP stores run down and calcium ions cannot recycle.

Severity of Ischemia. Relatively little is known about the influence of the severity of ischemic injury on subsequent reperfusion injury. An increased heart rate increases the severity of ischemic injury (Schaper et al., 1987) and increases the incidence of reperfusion arrhythmias (Lederman et al., 1987). Two agents known to reduce heart rate, namely the β-blocker propranolol and the calcium antagonist diltiazem, decrease reperfusion calcium uptake in the case of propranolol (Miyazawa et al., 1986) and reperfusion arrhythmias in the case of diltiazem (Tosaki and Hearse, 1987). Hence, it seems probable that the severity of ischemia is a factor determining the severity of reperfusion arrhythmias, and probably other aspects of reperfusion injury.

Speed of Reperfusion.   Experimentally, sudden rather than gradual reperfusion is associated with a greater degree of reperfusion injury. In patients, reperfusion by thrombolysis is slow over many minutes and not abrupt within seconds, as it is in many animal experiments. This difference may explain why some aspects of reperfusion injury, such as arrhythmias, are less common in humans than in animals. In cases of transient severe coronary spasm, rapid relief of spasm is much faster and may precipitate reperfusion ventricular arrhythmias.

Microvascular Damage and No-Reflow

No-reflow is the phenomenon occurring when removal of coronary occlusion does not lead to restoration of coronary flow (Bernier et al., 1986), or when early complete reperfusiuon is followed by a later close-down (Maes et al., 1995). Clearly, the benefits of reperfusion would be lessened by no-reflow. There are two possible explanations for the no-reflow phenomenon. First, microvascular damage can lead to endothelial cell edema. Second, ischemic contracture of the myocardium can squeeze the coronary arteries and prevent normal flow. Microvascular damage also can decrease formation of vasodilatory substances, such as nitric oxide, from the endothelium and promote formation of vasoconstrictors (see Fig. 9-5). Furthermore, endothelial damage could remove factors inhibiting platelet plugging and neutrophil adherence (Forman et al., 1989). At least some of the microvascular damage is caused by free radicals and is decreased by free radical scavengers (Badylak et al., 1987). A proposed mechanism for the formation of free radicals that damage the endothelium is the reintroduction of neutrophils into the ischemic zone with damage to the endothelium. The end result could be platelet activation, which could explain or contribute to no-reflow (Forde and Fitzgerald, 1997).

Postpump Syndrome, Cytokines, and Neutrophils

Although most patients recover well from cardiopulmonary bypass, in some there is a widespread inflammatory response, thought to be caused by activation of a variety of cells, including monocytes, macrophages, endothelial cells, and T cells. These cells liberate cytokines such as the tumor necrosis factors (TNF) and the interleukins (IL). One of the interleukins, IL-8, is also known as the neutrophil-activating factor, and its messenger RNA is induced in the myocardium during cardiopulmonary bypass (Burns et al., 1995). Neutrophils are attracted to the area of injury, roll on and adhere to the damaged endothelium, and then either return to the blood stream or undergo transendothelial migration, the whole process being known as *neutrophil trafficking*. Neutrophil adhesion is promoted by endothelial surface receptors such as the selectins and intracellular adhesion molecules, which interact with the neutrophil surface. Once inside the vascular interstitial space, the neutrophils are activated and thought to liberate damaging free radicals and leukotrienes. The proposal is that such neutrophil trafficking promotes postsurgery myocardial and whole body damage (Menasché et al., 1995).

Accelerated Cell Death

The prototype experiments on reperfusion damage and cell death were performed by Jennings and co-workers (1960). They found that on reperfusion of a coronary artery, there was a massive increase in the tissue level of calcium, with the appearance of contraction bands and intramitochondrial dense bodies (probably deposits of calcium phosphate). Such changes were much delayed when coronary occlusion was maintained. They proposed that reperfusion led to excess uptake of calcium into the cytosol through a sarcolemma damaged during the ischemic period, with the cytosolic overloading followed by subsequent mitochondrial calcium excess and impaired ability of mitochondrial manufacture of ATP (Jennings and Ganote, 1976). This sequence could explain accelerated reperfusion-related cell necrosis. Their suggestion is that the accelerated demise of cells during reperfusion is limited to those cells so severely damaged by lethal ischemia (see Fig. 18-6) that they would eventually have died in any case had ischemia been continued without reperfusion. According to this concept, reperfusion merely hastens but does not cause cell death.

Reperfusion upregulates the genes p53 and *Bax,* which are tumor suppressors and promoters of apoptosis (Hayashida et al., 1996). Reperfusion has a protective effect in decreasing the extent of ischemic apoptosis, yet provoking a paradoxical acceleration of apoptosis in other cells, which may be those previously destined to die (Fliss and Gattinger, 1996). Yet if ischemic necrosis and apoptosis are two different processes, and if apoptosis is more specifically associated with reperfusion, then it is difficult to avoid the conclusion that reperfusion causes some cells to die that would otherwise have lived.

HIBERNATION AND CHRONIC LEFT VENTRICULAR DYSFUNCTION

Whereas stunning is caused by reperfusion, hibernation is cured by revascularization. Hibernation is a chronic clinical condition in which part of the myocardium does not contract normally (systolic dysfunction) in the presence of severe coronary artery disease, without another obvious cause such as concurrent angina or myocardial infarction, and responding to revascularization by improved mechanical function. The original description of Rahimtoola (1985, 1989) was "a state of persistently impaired myocardial and LV function at rest due to reduced coronary blood flow that can be partially or completely restored to normal if the myocardial oxygen supply/demand relationship is favorably altered, either by improving blood flow and/or by reducing demand." A challenging finding is that the resting blood flow may only be modestly or marginally reduced despite severe coronary artery disease. In any case, the flow reduction is not low enough to damage the myocardium permanently, which would preclude recovery of function after revascularization.

Mechanism of Hibernation

Hibernation poses an interesting challenge to the definition of ischemia already given. On the one hand, blood flow is "too little" for normal contractility, especially during tachycardia (Shen and Vatner, 1995), and it could therefore be said that there is chronic ischemia. On the other hand, the degree of ischemia is mild enough to be "compensated" by the decreased contractility, so that any metabolic impairment is arrested and in fact there is no true ischemia, at least not in a model of acute hibernation described by Heusch and co-workers (Schulz et al., 1993).

The prevailing hypothesis is that there is metabolic downregulation, the major change being inhibited contractile activity (Rahimtoola, 1985), with possibly an additional generalized metabolic hypoactivity as described for brain and liver cells (Hochachka et al., 1996). The latter view suggests that in response to chronic hypoxia, there are not only short-term defense events, but longer term rescue that conserves the limited energy resources. An important alternate proposal explains why myocardial blood flow at rest may be normal, or nearly normal (Fig. 19-6). Severe coronary artery disease is associated with repetitive intermittent and often silent ischemia, giving rise to repetitive episodes of stunning that when summated translate into chronic impairment of LV function (Shen and Vatner, 1995; Vanoverschelde et al., 1993). Alternatively, the myocar-

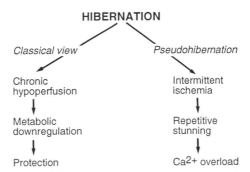

FIG. 19-6. The hibernation controversy. The classical view is that hibernation is associated with chronic hypoperfusion of the hibernating myocardium. A revised view is that intermittent ischemia causes repetitive stunning, which for distinction is here termed "pseudohibernation," but with an appearance similar to that of hibernation.

dial segments with apparently normal coronary flow and reduced contraction could represent remodeled myocardium (Sun et al., 1996).

Unfortunately these controversies cannot be settled by animal models, none of which successfully duplicate the human condition. In any event, whatever the underlying mechanism, after successful coronary artery revascularization, the hibernating segments "wake up" either rapidly (Ferrari et al., 1994) or sometimes only after many months (Rahimtoola, 1989; Vanoverschelde et al., 1993). The long delayed recovery may refer to those hibernating segments that have developed the fetal phenotype as part of the rescue response.

Clinical Significance of Hibernation

If hypocontractile myocardium is still viable and can respond to revascularization, then it is possible to improve LV function in patients with severe coronary disease, thereby easing symptoms and improving prognosis. Hence, the search for viable myocardium undergoing hibernation is now very active (Iskandrian et al., 1996).

Myocardial Viability. Of the various radionucleide methods for assessing viability (Fig. 19-7), positron emission tomography (PET) is often regarded as the metabolic standard for preoperative detection of hibernation (Brunken and Armbrecht, 1990; Uren and Camici, 1992; Vanoverschelde et al., 1993). Viability is indicated by a mismatch pattern whereby the tissue signal of labeled

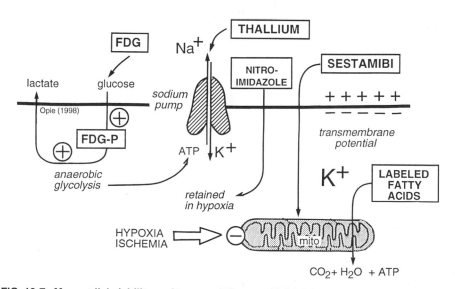

FIG. 19-7. Myocardial viability and tracers. Different radionuclide tracers are able to track different aspects of ischemic metabolism. Thallium here indicates either redistribution or reinjection techniques. FDG, fluorodeoxyglucose; FDG-P, phosphorylated FDG.

deoxyglucose is increased relative to the myocardial blood flow, which is either decreased, low normal, or even normal at rest (see Fig. 11-21). Other methods for detection of viability include a positive inotropic response to dobutamine (Mercier et al., 1982) as shown on the echocardiogram, or a positive redistribution thallium scan (Boden et al., 1996). Thallium is taken up into viable cells by the sodium pump. PET, thallium SPECT (single-photon emission computed tomography), and dobutamine echocardiography when compared give somewhat similar results, with thallium being the least sensitive (Bonow, 1996). In the presence of severe coronary disease, dobutamine, which requires sufficient flow reserve to sustain the β-adrenergic–induced contraction, is less likely to identify viability than is a metabolic indicator such as PET.

Hibernation without Prior Infarction.   Hibernation may be especially common in the early postinfarct phase, with over 40% of patients in one series having a mismatch pattern on PET scanning (Adams et al., 1996). By contrast, and much rarer, hibernation was also found in carefully selected patients without any prior myocardial infarction and with repetitive attacks of angina pectoris (Vanoverschelde et al., 1993). These patients had the major criterion for hibernation in that recovery of poorly functioning segments took place after revascularization. The blood flow in those segments recovering best was only modestly reduced. Yet the surprisingly severe histologic changes found in the hibernating segments raised the possibility of intermittently severe ischemia, compatible with the history of angina pectoris. Intermittent ischemia raises the proposal that repetitive stunning could cause hibernation, as experimentally supported (Shen and Vatner, 1995).

Disuse Atrophy Versus Phenotype Change.   Ventricular unloading can cause shrinkage of myocardial cells, as well as accumulation of collagen and fibroblasts (Kent et al., 1985). Certain changes, such as the loss of myofibrils, are common to the histology of the some hibernating segments (Vanoverschelde et al., 1993), and also to disuse atrophy. A simple hypothesis would therefore be that during sustained hibernation lack of contraction would lead to disuse atrophy. Additionally, in response to an unknown signal, there can be reversion to a fetal "downgraded" phenotype with delayed recovery to the normal pattern (Vanoverschelde et al., 1993). This phenotype has less well differentiated myofibrils with small mitochondria, severely reduced contractile filaments, a reduced content of sarcoplasmic reticulum, and increased glycogen, a combination suggesting adaptation to provide increased energy reserves with decreased mechanical contraction (downgraded myofibrils).

Spectrum of Changes in Hibernation.   It is thus evident that hibernation stretches all the way from one condition in which regional function returns promptly at the operation table upon revascularization (Ferrari et al., 1996), to another condition recognized by a much delayed mechanical recovery and overt histologic changes (Vanoverschelde et al., 1993). Different observers using different techniques are likely to be describing different entities under the same title of hibernation, which in reality is not a uniform condition but rather another spectrum of conditions. Hibernation stretches from acute to chronic hibernation, and from rapid to slow recovery of the contractile elements.

PRECONDITIONING: THE POTENTIAL MODIFIER OF ISCHEMIC STATES

Whereas many repetitive episodes of ischemia should produce cumulative damage, relatively few episodes or even one burst of short-lived severe ischemia followed by complete reperfusion causes preconditioning (Fig. 19-8). When preconditioned, the myocardium is protected against a greater subsequent ischemic insult, with less threat of infarction (Murry et al., 1986; Schott et al., 1990). In addition, there are other surrogates of successful preconditioning such as decreased postischemic stunning (Asimakis et al., 1994) or fewer reperfusion arrhythmias (Lawson and Downey, 1993). Although preconditioning is classically initiated by one or more periods of total ischemia, each followed by reperfusion, nonetheless there are variants. First, ischemic

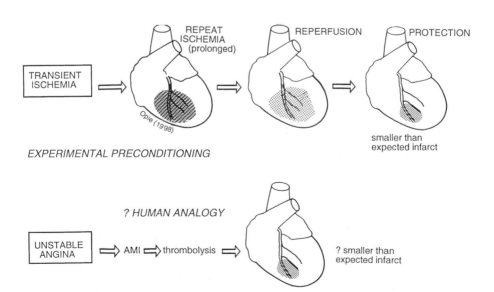

FIG. 19-8. Preconditioning. Top panel shows experimental protocol, bottom panel proposed application in patients. For discussion, see Kloner and Yellon (1994).

preconditioning can be achieved by a partial coronary occlusion (rather than total) and without intermittent reperfusion (Koning et al., 1994), explaining why in the Harris model, when coronary ligation is applied in two stages, there are less fatal arrhythmias than with one single occlusion of equal anatomic size. This finding raises the possibility that myocardial infarction of a "stuttering" pattern of onset may be less severe than expected. Another deviation from the classic pattern of preconditioning is *intraischemic preconditioning,* whereby an initial brief period of no-flow ischemia increases myocardial tolerance to subsequent low-flow ischemia without any intervening reperfusion period (Fig. 19-9) (Ferrari et al., 1996; Schulz et al., 1995). Other variations are that preconditioning can follow transient vigorous β-adrenergic stimulation (Asimakis et al., 1994), or cycles of calcium depletion and repletion (Miyawaki et al., 1996). Thus, preconditioning may be invoked by more stimuli than previously appreciated. Furthermore, whereas the protective effect of preconditioning against subsequent ischemia is generally limited to 2 hours, Yellon's group has described a second window of protection (SWOP) occurring about 24 to 96 hours after the initial preconditioning episode (Baxter et al., 1994).

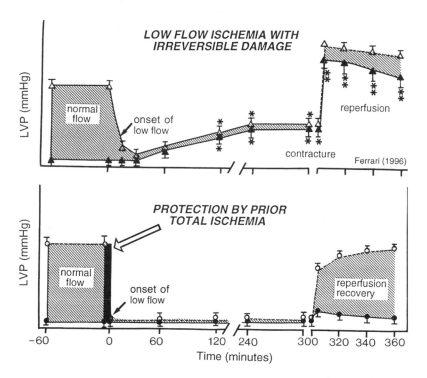

FIG. 19-9. Intraischemic preconditioning. This condition describes "increased tolerance to sustained low-flow ischemia by a brief episode of no-flow ischemia without intermittent reperfusion" (Schulz et al., 1995). This figure is adapted from data of Ferrari et al. (1996).

Mechanism of Preconditioning

The mechanism of the protective effect of preconditioning is still speculative and controversial. A common view is that *adenosine* plays a role in the phenomenon, possibly being linked to activation of protein kinase C (Mitchell et al., 1995; Speechly-Dick et al., 1995; Yao et al., 1994; Ytrehus et al., 1994) and thence to opening of the ATP-sensitive potassium channel (Fig. 19-10). For example, adenosine A_1 receptor stimulation of rat ventricular myocytes activates the δ-protein kinase C isoform (Henry et al., 1996). Alternatively or additionally, there may be an increased activity of the inhibitory G protein, G_i, which links the adenosine receptor to the ATP-senstive potassium channel (Mitchell et al., 1995; Nicroomand et al., 1995; Thornton et al., 1993; Ytrehus et al., 1994). Upregulation of G_i would explain the protective effects of activation of those receptors coupled to it, such as adenosine A_1 and muscarinic M_2 receptors, because of greater inhibition of adenylate cyclase and hence an indirect antiadrenergic effect (Fig. 19-11) (Ashraf et al., 1994; Niroomand et al., 1995; Thornton et al., 1993). In addition, G_i may mediate other potentially protective mechanisms, such as direct inhibition of L-calcium channels and activation of the ATP-sensitive potassium channels (Parratt and Kane, 1994).

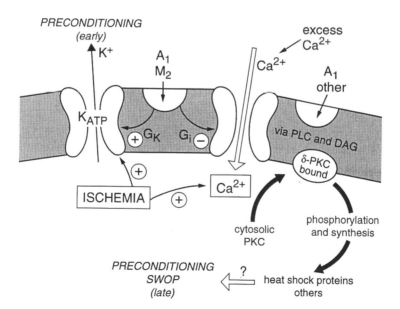

FIG. 19-10. Hypotheses for preconditioning. Adenosine, acting chiefly by A_1 receptors, is thought to play a crucial role and might act in at least four ways: (1) activation of protein kinase C, and particularly the delta-isoform; (2) opening of the ATP-sensitive potassium channel (K_{ATP}), acting via the G protein G_K; (3) inhibition of the L-calcium channel; and (4) increasing the activity of the inhibitory protein G_i (see Fig. 19-11). Note that preconditioning occurs in two phases, early and late (second window of protection, SWOP), the latter possibly involving heat shock proteins. M_2, muscarinic receptor, subtype 2. For ε-isoform of PKC, see Ping et al., *Circ Res* 1997;81:404.

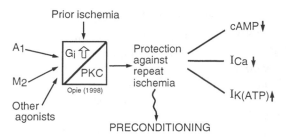

FIG. 19-11. G$_i$ and PKC in preconditioning. Note proposed complementary roles of inhibitory G protein, G$_i$, and protein kinase C (PKC) in mediating effects of preconditioning. The proposal is that prior ischemia (preconditioning episode) upregulates G$_i$ according to Niroomand et al. (1995). G$_i$, by inhibiting formation of cAMP, lessens L-type calcium channel activity and promotes opening of the ATP-dependent K$^+$ channel. Thus, when ischemia is repeated, there is relative protection. A$_1$, subtype 1 of adenosine receptor; M$_2$, subtype 2 of muscarinic receptor; I$_{Ca}$, L-type calcium current; I$_{k(ATP)}$, ATP-dependent potassium current.

Preconditioning in Patients

Preconditioning is therefore an important phenomenon, with probable clinical application because it invokes protection against postischemic and other types of ischemia-related impaired LV dysfunction. Although the clinical evidence for preconditioning is not yet firm, there is increasing evidence that it occurs in humans (Kloner and Yellon, 1994; Pasceri et al., 1996; Speechly-Dick et al., 1995). Patients with effort angina having one attack may be protected from subsequent attacks as in warm-up angina. Those undergoing coronary angioplasty have more severe features of ischemia, such as potassium release and ST-segment elevation on the ECG, when the first is compared with subsequent balloon inflations. Patients with preinfarction angina may experience a less severe infarct than those thought to undergo sudden coronary occlusion without the opportunity for preconditioning (Andreotti et al., 1996; Kloner et al., 1995; Ottani et al., 1995). In contrast, experimental data suggest that patients with multiple short-lived attacks of ischemia might become tolerant to the protection conferred by preconditioning (Cohen et al., 1994).

Thus, not only are there several stimuli to the preconditioned state, but there are also several potential mechanisms, and the consequences are multiple. Hence, the possibility must be considered that preconditioning occurs in any state of repetitive ischemia, as well as in patients.

MIXED ISCHEMIC SYNDROME

"In clinical conditions, ischemia, stunning, hibernation, necrosis and normal myocardium may coexist" (Iskandrian et al., 1996). Furthermore, there may be variations in the myocardial response to ischemia and in the coronary blood supply, as well as the possibility of repetitive ischemic episodes each followed by

TABLE 19-5. *The mixed ischemic syndrome*

(a) *Variations in myocardial response to ischemia*
1. Transient anaerobic metabolism.
2. Anaerobic metabolism plus serious ionic imbalance (Na/Ca/H) with threatened necrosis
3. Tissue necrosis and eventual fibrosis, including inflammatory response and cytokine production
4. Tissue repair including activation of protein synthesis and remodeling/hypertrophy

(b) *Variations in coronary blood supply*
1. Coronary artery disease with one or more of the following:
   (i)   Endothelial damage with impaired production of nitric oxide
   (ii) Increased vascular smooth muscle (vasoconstriction) or if severe and localized, vasospasm
   (iii) Platelet thrombi
   (iv) Plaque rupture
   (v)   Occluding thrombus with or without recanalization
   (vi) Inadequate supply as a result of increased oxygen demand (exercise, emotion, acute hypertension)

(c) *Response to ischemia/reperfusion*
1. Repetitive stunning including maiming
2. Hibernation (may include above)
3. Repetitive preconditioning

reperfusion and stunning, or by preconditioning. The overall clinical picture may therefore comprise one or more of the new ischemic syndromes (stunning, hibernation, and preconditioning) as well as varying degrees of diastolic and or systolic dysfunction (Table 19-5). Several of these entities could overlap in the same patient. To describe this multifarious spectrum of conditions, an appropriate term might be the *mixed postinfarct syndrome* (Opie, 1996).

SUMMARY

1. *Reperfusion injury* refers to a syndrome of related conditions that may follow reperfusion of the ischemic myocardium. For example, thrombolytic reperfusion may bring in its wake arrhythmias, stunning, and no-reflow. Whether reperfusion can actually accelerate cell death remains controversial.

2. *Mechanisms for reperfusion damage* are twofold: cytosolic calcium overload and formation of free radicals. Other important events include endothelial dysfunction, reintroduction of neutrophils into the ischemic area, and microvascular damage.

3. *Stunning* is the delayed recovery of mechanical function after reperfusion. It varies in duration from minutes to hours to days, and can experimentally be averted by a number of interventions, including Na^+/Ca^+ exchange inhibition and calcium antagonists, as well as by a variety of free radical scavengers.

4. *Hibernation* is the state of myocardial dormancy in the presence of severe coronary artery disease that can be revived by revascularization. There is no

good experimental model. Two current hypothesises are a downgrading of myocardial energy requirements and repetitive stunning.

5. *Preconditioning* is the increased myocardial resistance to ischemic reperfusion damage that is evoked by one or more prior episodes of transient ischemia followed by reperfusion. The hypothesis currently favored is that adenosine, released during the period of protective ischemia, activates protein kinase C, which in turn promotes opening of the ATP-sensitive potassium channel, the later being the protective event. Such a sequence remains controversial.

6. *Clinical implications.* The recognition that stunning and especially hibernation can occur in patients with coronary artery disease, and the possibility that preconditioning can also modify the severity of subsequent ischemia, means that the clinical manifestations of ischemia and reperfusion in humans have become very complex. Nonetheless, there is increasing evidence that each of the three new ischemic syndromes, namely stunning, hibernation, and preconditioning, can occur in patients with coronary artery disease. For example, stunning may explain much delayed mechanical recovery after thrombolytic therapy of acute myocardial infarction. Hibernation is now being actively sought in efforts to improve left ventricular function by revascularization.

STUDENT QUESTIONS

1. What are the factors contributing to the large oscillations in internal calcium ion levels found soon after experimental reperfusion?
2. What are the sources and possible dangers of formation of free radicals in the early reperfusion period?
3. What are the naturally occurring defense systems against free radicals?
4. Which nuclear tracers can be used to assess myocardial viability? Which metabolic path is each one testing?
5. What is the proposed role of protein kinase C (PKC) in preconditioning?

CARDIOLOGIST-IN-TRAINING QUESTIONS

1. What are the patterns of recovery of mechanical function in relation to postischemic reperfusion of (a) the hibernating myocardium, (b) the stunned myocardium, and (c) the maimed myocardium?
2. Discuss current hypotheses for stunning. What is thought to be its clinical significance?
3. What is hibernation? Discuss its possible relation to tunning.
4. What is the postpump syndrome? Discuss possible mechanisms.
5. "Postinfarct left ventricular dysfunction has many clinical guises." Do you agree? What mechanism may underlie each clinical condition?

REFERENCES

1. Adams JM, Norton M, Trent RJ, et al. Incidence of hibernating myocardium after acute myocardial infarction treated with thrombolysis. *Heart* 1996;75:442–446.
2. Ambrosio G, Weisfeldt ML, Jacobus WE, Flaherty JT. Evidence for a reversible oxygen radical-mediated component of reperfusion injury: reduction by recombinant human superoxide dismutase administered at the time of reflow. *Circulation* 1987;75:282–291.
3. Andreotti F, Pasceri V, Hackett DR, et al. Preinfarction angina as a predictor of more rapid coronary thrombisis in patients with acute myocardial infarction. *N Engl J Med* 1996;334:7–12.
4. Antman EM. Magnesium in acute MI. Timing is critical. *Circulation* 1995;92:2367–2372.
5. Antman EM, Seelig MS, Fleischmann K, et al. Magnesium in acute myocardial infarction: scientific, statistical and economic rationale for its use. *Cardiovasc Drug Ther* 1996;10:297–301.
6. Ashraf M, Suleiman J, Ahmad M. CA^{2+} preconditioning elicits a unique protection against the Ca^{2+} paradox injury in rat heart. Role of adenosine. *Circ Res* 1994;74:360–367.
7. Asimakis GK, Inners-McBride K, Conti VR, Yang C. Transient beta adrenergic stimulation can precondition the rat heart against posischemic contractile dysfunction. *Cardiovasc Res* 1994;28: 1726–1734.
8. Badylak SF, Simmons A, Turek J, Babbs CF. Protection from reperfusion injury in the isolated rat heart by postischemic deferoxamine and oxypurinol administration. *Cardiovasc Res* 1987;21: 500–506.
9. Baxter GF, Marber MS, Patel VC, Yellon DM. Adenosine receptor involvement in a delayed phase of myocardial protection 24 hours after ischemic preconditioning. *Circulation* 1994;90:2993–3000.
10. Becker LC, Levine JH, DiPaula AF, et al. Reversal of dysfunction in postischemic stunned myocardium by epinephrine and postextrasystolic potentiation. *J Am Coll Cardiol* 1986;7:580–589.
11. Bernier M, Hearse DJ, Manning AS. Reperfusion-induced arrhythmias and oxygen-derived free radicals. Studies with "anti-free radical" interventions and a free radical-generating system in the isolated perfused rat heart. *Circ Res* 1986;58:331–340.
12. Boden W, Messerli F, Hansen JF, Schectman K. Heart rate-lowering calcium channel blockers (diltiazem, verapamil) do not adversely affect long-term cardiac death or non-fatal infarction in post-infarction patients: data pooled from 3 randomized, placebo-controlled clinical trials of 5,677 patients [Abstract]. *J Am Coll Cardiol* 1996;27:319.
13. Boden WE, Brooks WW, Conrad CH, et al. Incomplete, delayed functional recovery late after reperfusion following acute myocardial infarction: "maimed myocardium." *Am Heart J* 1995;130: 922–932.
14. Bolli R. Mechanism of myocardial "stunning." *Ciculation* 1990;82:723–738.
15. Bolli R. Myocardial stunning in man. *Circulation* 1992;86:1671–1691.
16. Bonow RO. Identification of viable myocardium. *Circulation* 1996;94:2674–2680.
17. Bourdillon PD, Lorell BH, Mirsky I, et al. Increased regional myocardial stiffness of the left ventricle during pacing-induced angina in man. *Circulation* 1983;67:316–323.
18. Braunwald E. Stunning of the myocardium: an update. *Cardiovasc Drug Ther* 1991;5:849–851.
19. Braunwald E, Kloner RA. The stunned myocardium: prolonged, postischemic ventricular dysfunction. *Circulation* 1982;66:1146–1149.
20. Brooks WW, Conrad CH, Morgan JP. Reperfusion induced arrhythmias following ischemia in intact rat heart: role of intracellular calcium. *Cardiovasc Res* 1995;29:536–542.
21. Brunken RC, Armbrecht JJ. Detection of hibernating myocardium with positron emission tomography. In: Zipes DP, Rowlands DJ (eds). *Progress in Cardiology.* Philadelphia: Lea & Febriger, 1990;161–179.
22. Burns SA, Newburger JW, Xiao M, et al. Induction of interleukin-8 messenger RNA in heart and skeletal muscle during pediatric cardiopulmonary bypass. *Circulation* 1995;92(suppl II):315–321.
23. Coetzee WA, Opie LH. Effects of components of ischaemia and metabolic inhibition on delayed afterdepolarizations in guinea pig papillary muscle. *Circ Res* 1987;61:157–165.
24. Cohen MV, Yang XM, Downey JM. Conscious rabbits become tolerant to multiple episodes of ischemic preconditioning. *Circ Res* 1994;74:998–1004.
25. Corr PB, Witkowski FX. Potential electrophysiologic mechanisms responsible for dysrhythmias associated with reperfusion of ischemic myocardium. *Circulation* 1983;68(suppl 1):16–24.
26. du Toit E, Opie LH. Role for the Na/H exchanger in reperfusion stunning in isolated perfused rat heart. *J Cardiovasc Pharmacol* 1993;22:877–883.

27. du Toit EF, Opie LH. Modulation of severity of reperfusion stunning in the isolated rat heart by agents altering calcium flux at onset of reperfusion. *Circ Res* 1992;70:960–967.
28. du Toit EF, Opie LH. Inhibitors of Ca^{2+}-ATPase pump of sarcoplasmic reticulum attenuate reperfusion stunning in isolated rat heart. *J Cardiovasc Pharmacol* 1994;24:678–684.
29. Ellis SG, Wynn J, Braunwald E, Henschke CI, et al. Response of reperfusion-salvaged, stunned myocardium to inotropic stimulation. *Am Heart J* 1984;107:13–19.
30. Ferrari R, Bongrazio M, Cargnoni A, et al. Heat shock protein changes in hibernation: a similarity with heart failure. *J Mol Cell Cardiol* 1996;28:2383–2395.
31. Ferrari R, Ceconi C, Curello S, et al. Intracellular effects of myocardial ischemia and reperfusion: role of calcium and oxygen. *Eur Heart J* 1986;7(suppl A):3–12.
32. Ferrari R, La Canna G, Giubbini R, et al. Left ventricular dysfunction due to stunning and hibernation in patients. *Cardiovasc Drug Ther* 1994;8:371–380.
33. Fliss H, Gattinger D. Apoptosis in ischemic and reperfused rat myocardium. *Circ Res* 1996;79: 949–956.
34. Forde RC, Fitzgerald D. Reactive oxygen species and platelet activation in reperfusion injury. *Circulation* 1997;95:787–789.
35. Forman MB, Puett DW, Virmani R. Endothelial and myocardial injury during ischemia and reperfusion: pathogenesis and therapeutic implications. *J Am Cardiol* 1989;13:450–459.
36. Gao WD, Atar D, Backx PH, Marban E. Relationship between intracellular calcium and contractile force in stunned myocardium. Direct evidence for decreased myofilament Ca^{2+} responsiveness and altered diastolic function in intact ventricular muscle. *Circ Res* 1995;76:1036–1048.
37. Hayashida W, Horiuchi M, Zhang L, Dzau VJ. Expression of p53 and Bax genes are induced in the ischemia-reperfused rat ventricle: potential roles in myocardial apoptosis. *Circulation* 1996;94(suppl I):1–225.
38. Hearse DJ, Humphrey SM, Nayler WG. Ultrastructural damage associated with reoxygenation of the anoxic myocardium. *J Mol Cell Cardiol* 1975;7:315–324.
39. Henry P, Demolombe S, Puceat, Escande D. Adenosine A1 stimulation activates delta-protein kinase C in rat ventricular myocytes. *Circ Res* 1996;78:161–165.
40. Heyndrickx GR, Baig H, Nellens P, et al. Depression of regional blood flow and wall thickening after brief coronary occlusions. *Am J Physiol* 1978;234:H653–H659.
41. Heyndrickx GR, Millard RW, McRitchie RJ, et al. Regional myocardial functional and electrophysiological alterations after brief coronary artery occlusion in conscious dogs. *J Clin Invest* 1975;56: 978–985.
42. Hochachka PW, Buck LT, Doll CJ, Land SC. Unifying theory of hypoxia tolerance: molecular/metabolic defense and rescue mechanisms for surviving oxygen lack. *Proc Natl Acad Sci USA* 1996;93: 9493–9498.
43. ISIS-4 Collaborative Group. ISIS-4: A randomised factorial trial assessing early oral captopril, oral mononitrate, and intravenous magnesium sulphate in 58,050 patients with a suspected acute myocardial infarction. *Lancet* 1995;345:669–685.
44. Iskandrian AS, Heo J, Schelbert HR. Myocardial viability: methods of assessment and clinical relevance. *Am Heart J* 1996;132:1226–1235.
45. Ito BR, Tate H, Kobayashi M, Schaper W. Reversibly injured, postischemic canine myocardium retains normal contractile reserve. *Circ Res* 1987;61:834–846.
46. Jennings RB, Ganote CE. Mitochondrial structure and function in acute myocardial ischemic injury. *Circ Res* 1976;38(suppl I):80–91.
47. Jennings RB, Sommers H, Smyth G, et al. Myocardial necrosis induced by temporary occlusion of a coronary artery in the dog. *Arch Pathol* 1960;70:82–92.
48. Kent RL, Uboh CE, Thompson EW, et al. Biochemical and structural correlates in unloaded and reloaded cat myocardium. *J Mol Cell Cardiol* 1985;17:153–165.
49. Kloner RA, Allen J, Cox TA, et al. Stunned left ventricular myocardium after exercise treadmill testing in coronary artery disease. *Am J Cardiol* 1991;68:329–334.
50. Kloner RA, Shook T, Przyklenk K, et al. Previous angina alters in-hospital outcome in TIMI-4. A clinical correlate to preconditioning. *Circulation* 1995;91:37–47.
51. Kloner RA, Yellon DM. Does ischemic preconditioning occur in patients? *J Am Coll Cardiol* 1994;24:1133–1142.
52. Koning MMG, Simonis LAJ, de Zeeuw S, et al. Ischaemic preconditioning by partial occlusion without intermittent reperfusion. *Cardiovasc Res* 1994;28:1146–1151.
53. Lavallee M, Cox D, Patrick TA, Vatner SF. Salvage of myocardial function by coronary artery reperfusion 1, 2 and 3 hours after occlusion in conscious dogs. *Circ Res* 1983;53:235–247.

54. Lawson CS, Downey JM. Preconditioning: state of the art myocardial protection. *Cardiovasc Res* 1993;27:542–550.
55. Lederman SN, Wenger TL, Harrell FE, et al. Effects of different paced heart rates on canine coronary occlusion and reperfusion arrhythmias. *Am J Heart* 1987;113:1365–1369.
56. Maes A, Van de Werf F, Nuyts J, et al. Impaired myocardial tissue perfusion early after successful thrombolysis. Impact on myocardial flow, metabolism and function at late follow-up. *Circulation* 1995;92:2072–2078.
57. Manning AS, Hearse DJ. Reperfusion-induced arrhythmias: mechanisms and prevention. *J Mol Cell Cardiol* 1984;16:497–518.
58. McKenney PA, Apstein CS, Mendes LA, et al. Increased left ventricular diastolic chamber stiffness immediately after coronary artery bypass surgery. *J Am Coll Cardiol* 1994;24:1189–1194.
59. Meerson FZ, Kagan VE, Kozlov Y, et al. The role of lipid peroxidation in pathogenesis of ischemic damage and the antioxidant protection of the heart. *Basic Res Cardiol* 1982;77:465–485.
60. Meissner A, Morgan JP. Contractile dysfunction and abnormal Ca^{2+} modulation during postischemic reperfusion in rat heart. *Am J Physiol* 1995;268:H100–H111.
61. Menasché P, Peynet J, Haeffner-Cavaillon N, et al. Influence of temperature on neutrophil trafficking during clinical cardiopulmonary bypass. *Circulation* 1995;92(suppl II):334–340.
62. Mercier JC, Lando U, Kanmatsuse K, et al. Divergent effects of inotropic stimulation on the ischemic and severely depressed reperfused myocardium. *Circulation* 1982;66:397–400.
63. Mitchell MB, Meng X, Ao L, et al. Preconditioning of isolated rat heart is mediated by protein kinase C. *Circ Res* 1995;76:73–81.
64. Miyawaki H, Zhou X, Ashraf M. Calcium preconditioning elicits strong protection against ischemic injury via protein kinase C signaling pathway. *Circ Res* 1996;79:137–146.
65. Miyazawa K, Fukuyama H, Komatsu E, Yamaguchi I. Effects of propranolol on myocardial damage resulting from coronary artery occlusion followed by reperfusion. *Am Heart J* 1986;111:519–524.
66. Murry CE, Jennings RB, Reimer KA. Preconditioning with ischaemia: a delay of lethal cell injury in ischaemic myocardium. *Circulation* 1986;74:1124–1136.
67. Myers ML, Mathur S, Li GH, Karmazyn M. Sodium hydrogen exchange inhibitors improve postischaemic recovery of function in the perfused rabbit heart. *Cardiovasc Res* 1995;29:209–214.
68. Niroomand F, Weinbrenner C, Weis A, et al. Impaired function of inhibitory G proteins during acute myocardial ischemia of canine hearts and its reversal during reperfusion and a second period of ischemia. Possible implications for the protective mechanism of ischemic preconditioning. *Circ Res* 1995;76:861–870.
69. Opie LH. Reperfusion injury and its pharmacologic modification. *Circulation* 1989;80:1049–1062.
70. Opie LH. Postischemic stunning—the case for calcium as the ultimate culprit. *Cardiovasc Drug Ther* 1991;5:895–900.
71. Opie LH. The multifarious spectrum of ischemic left ventricular dysfunction: relevance of new ischemic syndromes. *J Mol Cell Cardiol* 1996;28:2403–2414.
72. Opie LH, Coetzee WA. Role of calcium ions in reperfusion arrhythmias: relevance to pharmacologic intervention. *Cardiovasc Drug Ther* 1988;2:623–636.
73. Ottani F, Galvani M, Ferrini D, et al. Prodromal angina limits infarct size. A role for ischemic preconditioning. *Circulation* 1995;91:291–297.
74. Parratt JR, Kane KA. KATP channels in ischaemic preconditioning. *Cardiovasc Res* 1994;28:783–787.
75. Pasceri V, Lanza GA, Patti G, et al. Preconditioning by transient myocardial ischemia confers protection against ischemia-induced ventricular arrhythmias in variant angina. *Circulation* 1996;94:1850–1856.
76. Rahimtoola SH. A perspective on the three large multicenter randomized clinical trials of coronary bypass surgery for chronic stable angina. *Circulation* 1985;72(suppl V):123–135.
77. Rahimtoola SH. The hibernating myocardium. *Am Heart J* 1989;117:211–221.
78. Saman S, Coetzee WA, Opie LH. Inhibition by simulated ischemia or hypoxia of delayed afterdepolarizations provoked by cyclic AMP: significance for ischemic and reperfusion arrhythmias. *J Mol Cell Cardiol* 1988;20:91–95.
79. Schaper W, Binz K, Sass S, Winkler B. Influence of collateral blood flow and of variations in MVO2 on tissue-ATP content in ischemic and infarcted myocardium. *J Mol Cell Cardiol* 1987;19:19–37.
80. Schott RJ, Rohmann SS, Braun ER, Schaper W. Ischemic preconditioning reduces infarct size in swine myocardium. *Circ Res* 1990;66:1133–1142.
81. Schulz R, Post H, Sakka S, et al. Intraischemic preconditioning. Increased tolerance to sustained low-flow ischaemia by a brief episode of no-flow ischaemia without intermittent reperfusion. *Circ Res* 1995;76:942–950.

82. Schulz R, Rose J, Martin C, et al. Development of short term myocardial hibernation. Its limitation by the severity of ischemia and inotropic stimulation. *Circulation* 1993;88:684–695.
83. Sheiban I, Tonni S, Chizzoni A, et al. Recovery of left ventricular function following early reperfusion in acute myocardial infarction: a potential role for the calcium antagonist nisoldipine. *Cardiovasc Drug Ther* 1997;11:5–16.
84. Shen YT, Vatner SF. Mechanism of impaired myocardial function during progressive coronary stenosis in conscious pigs. Hibernation versus stunning. *Circ Res* 1995;76:479–488.
85. Speechly-Dick ME, Grover GJ, Yellon DM. Does ischemic preconditioning in the human involve protein kinase C and the ATP dependent K+ channel? Studies of contractile function after simulated ischemia in an atrial in vitro model. *Circ Res* 1995;77:1030–1035.
86. Sun KT, Czernin J, Krivokapich J, et al. Effects of dobutamine stimulation on myocardial blood flow, glucose metabolism and wall motion in normal and dysfunctional myocardium. *Circulation* 1996;94:3146–3154.
87. Thornton JD, Liu GS, Downey JM. Pretreatment with pertussis toxin blocks the protective effects of preconditioning: evidence for a G-protein mechanism. *J Mol Cell Cardiol* 1993;25:311–320.
88. Tosaki A, Hearse DJ. Protective effect of transient calcium reduction against reperfusion-induced arrhythmias in rat hearts. *Am J Physiol* 1987;253:H225–H233.
89. Uren NG, Camici PG. Hibernation and myocardial ischemia: clinical detection by positron emission tomography. *Cardiovasc Drug Ther* 1992;6:273–279.
90. Vanoverschelde J-LJ, Wijns W, Depré C, et al. Mechanisms of chronic regional postischemic dysfunction in humans. New insights from the study of noninfarcted collateral-dependent myocardium. *Circulation* 1993;87:1513–1523.
91. Yao Z, Gross GJ. A comparison of adenosine-induced cardioprotection and ischemic preconditioning in dogs. Efficacy, time course and role of KATP channels. *Circulation* 1994;89:1229–1236.
92. Ytrehus K, Liu Y, Downey JM. Preconditioning protects ischemic rabbit heart by protein kinase C activation. *Am J Physiol* 1994;266:H1145–H1152.

20

Electricity Out of Control: Ventricular Arrhythmias

*"The pain in his arm seizing him, he fell down dead,
without the least motion of any limb"—the mode of
death of the Chancellor of the University of Oxford,
1674.*

R.H. Major, 1945

A useful practical classification of arrhythmias (abnormal heart rhythm, dysrhythmias) is according to their origin, that is, supraventricular or ventricular. Supraventricular arrhythmias may, in turn, be divided into the supraventricular tachycardias or bradyarrhythmias. Ventricular arrhythmias frequently are ischemic in origin and complex in genesis (Fig. 20-1). This chapter concentrates on ventricular tachyarrhythmias; heart block and supraventricular tachycardias are discussed with the conduction system in Chapter 5.

There are three main proposals for the mechanisms underlying the development of ventricular arrhythmias. First, automaticity may develop in otherwise nonautomatic tissue. Second, there may be a re-entry circuit. Third, afterdepolarizations may give rise to triggered activity or atypical ventricular tachycardia.

VENTRICULAR AUTOMATICITY

Automaticity means the development of a new site of depolarization in nonnodal tissue, at the site of an ectopic focus (Greek *ektos,* outside). A single such depolarization can cause an *ectopic beat.* When three or more ventricular ectopic beats occur in rapid succession, a *ventricular tachycardia* results in which there is insufficient time for diastolic filling, so that the cardiac output may decrease with risk of acute myocardial ischemia. By a variety of mechanisms, to be discussed in this chapter, such ischemia predisposes to the development of a totally disorga-

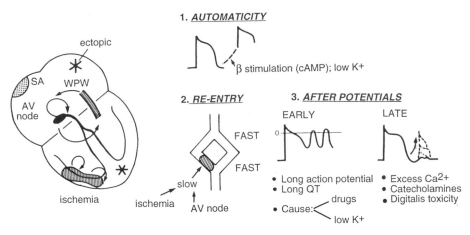

1. _AUTOMATICITY_

ectopic

SA   WPW

AV node

ischemia

β stimulation (cAMP); low K+

2. _RE-ENTRY_

FAST

FAST

slow

ischemia

AV node

3. _AFTER POTENTIALS_

EARLY   LATE

0

• Long action potential
• Long QT
• Cause: — drugs
         — low K+

• Excess Ca2+
• Catecholamines
• Digitalis toxicity

FIG. 20-1. Basic arrhythmogenic mechanisms. Sympathetic stimulation can provoke ectopic beats or, in the presence of re-entry circuits, tachycardia. Supraventricular tachycardias are frequently based on AV nodal re-entry or the existence of a bypass tract. Ventricular tachycardias are often based on the existence of an infarcted or ischemic zone in which the cellular mechanisms may include the development of slow responses or depressed fast channels or lipid-induced changes. Other arrhythmias are the result of increased automaticity, the cellular mechanisms of which include spontaneous depolarization developing in otherwise nonautomatic fibers or the development of afterpotentials. WPW, Wolff-Parkinson-White syndrome with bypass tract.

nized ventricular rhythm called *ventricular fibrillation* (fibrillate, movement of small fibers) in which regular cardiac pumping activity ceases and sudden cardiac death develops unless a strong external electrical current is applied by an external defibrillator. Ventricular automaticity arises especially in Purkinje fibers.

Purkinje fibers, normally quiescent, can develop phase 4 depolarization (as in ischemia) when partially depolarized, so that the threshold for firing is more easily reached. A pacemaker current, I_f, can operate at voltages between -90 and -60 mV (see Fig. 5-4), explaining why partial depolarization caused by ischemia predisposes to automaticity in Purkinje fibers.

Hypokalemia (K+, 2.7 mmol/L) increases phase 4 depolarization, whereas a high normal level (5.4 mmol/L) decreases phase 4 depolarization. If the potassium level is sufficiently high, catecholamine stimulation, which normally also evokes phase 4 depolarization in Purkinje fibers, becomes ineffective. When cyclic adenosine monophosphate (cAMP) is introduced by iontophoresis into spontaneously active cardiac Purkinje fibers, there is a shortened action potential and a steeper rate of phase 4 depolarization, in keeping with catecholamine effects. Catecholamine stimulation and a low external level of potassium should be a potent arrhythmogenic combination. Acute myocardial infarction in humans is characterized by acute liberation of catecholamines, which are known to decrease arterial blood potassium. In addition, some patients with acute infarction will have been given diuretic therapy, a frequent cause of hypokalemia.

Patients with hypokalemia at the time of onset of myocardial infarction have a greater incidence of ventricular arrhythmias, including ventricular fibrillation (Dyckner, 1975).

VENTRICULAR RE-ENTRY CIRCUITS

Ventricular re-entry circuits may develop whenever there is electrical inhomogeneity of the myocardium, which in turn reflects the focal ionic and metabolic abnormalities that cause slow conduction in one limb of a re-entry circuit (Fig. 20-2). Slow conduction is achieved by inhibition of the fast channel with residual slow channel activity, resulting from ischemic or other injury to the conduction tissue. These conditions predispose to the development of re-entry, which when rapid and regular is one cause of ventricular tachycardia (the other being a rapidly firing automatic focus). After myocardial infarction, chronic focal scarring seems to be

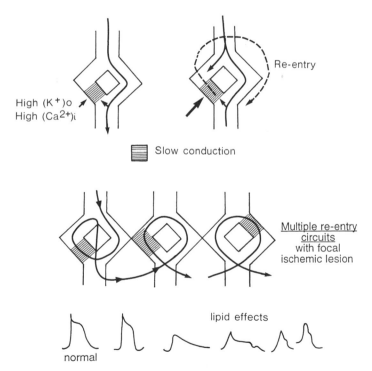

FIG. 20-2. Model for formation of the re-entry circuit. When the conducted impulse reaches a zone of injury, conduction becomes slowed by formation of abnormal action potentials. The slow rate of conduction delays the impulse until the refractory period of the normal impulse has passed, so that re-entry is possible. The bottom panel shows how multiple re-entry circuits could form from multiple ischemic injuries or from the abnormal action potentials (possibly caused by focal glycolytic abnormalities or accumulation of lysophosphoglycerides or a high external K^+, K_o, or high internal Ca^{2+}) so that heterogeneity of function results.

the basis for the re-entry circuits, which cause sustained ventricular tachycardias, again with risk of ventricular fibrillation. In acute ischemic damage, heterogeneous areas of slow conduction can cause *micro-re-entry circuits* that are thought to underlie the development of ventricular fibrillation. The five major theories to explain slow conduction in ischemic tissue are, first, the effect of localized hyperkalemia and partial depolarization. Second, the development of slow responses in completely depolarized tissue may occur when the tissue content of cAMP increases. Third, residual fast channel activity may explain why some apparently slow responses are sensitive to fast channel inhibitors. Fourth, disturbed metabolism of lipids and calcium may directly affect the action potential. Fifth, electrical coupling between cells may be disrupted.

Potassium and Depolarization

In the early 1950s, Harris et al. (1954) found increasing coronary venous potassium values during the onset of arrhythmias after coronary arterial ligation.

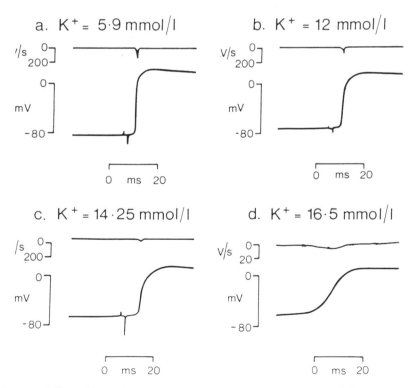

FIG. 20-3. Effect of hyperkalemia on upstroke velocity (dV/dt = V_{max}) of the action potential. There is progressive unmasking of an apparently slow response, which is in reality depressed fast channel activity. Inhibition of the fast response explains the use of a high external potassium in cardioplegia. From Opie et al. (1979).

Since then there has been increasing evidence of links between potassium and arrhythmogenesis. The mechanism whereby potassium loss (see Fig. 17-10) promotes very early arrhythmias after coronary ligation cannot be merely depletion of cell potassium, which requires 2 to 4 hours to become evident. Hyperkalemia, as found in coronary venous blood very early after coronary occlusion, may play a more important role (Fig. 20-3). Theoretical considerations show that when the cell is depolarized to values less negative than −50 mV, the rapid inward current is inactivated and the resting potential approaches the threshold potential for the slow inward current. The intravenous or intra-arterial infusion of potassium salts rapidly produces ectopic activity, possibly by promoting automaticity in Purkinje fibers. Eventually ventricular fibrillation develops, even in otherwise normal hearts.

Calcium and Early Changes in the Action Potential

One of the basic changes in the action potential during early ischemia is the reduction of the resting potential (depolarization), which could be related in part to the early increase in internal calcium found during ischemia, although the evidence is not decisive. Both ischemia and metabolic inhibitors are known to increase internal calcium, depolarize cardiac cells, reduce conduction velocity, and facilitate arrhythmia development. Although potassium loss explains most of ischemic depolarization (see Fig. 17-11), a potassium-independent process also can occur. For example, when the heart rate is increased, depolarization is markedly accelerated, yet very little of this increase is potassium dependent (Blake et al., 1988). The actual mechanism of the potassium-independent depolarization could involve an opening of nonselective calcium-dependent cation channels in the sarcolemma, by the increased cytosolic calcium.

Residual Fast Channel Activity

In some models, apparently slow responses are sensitive to the sodium channel inhibitor tetrodotoxin (Arita et al., 1983), suggesting that the real nature of the action potential depends on residual fast channel activity, as found during progressive hyperkalemia (Fig. 20-3). The practical implication is that antiarrhythmics acting on the fast channel, such as lidocaine, could be effective in suppressing such apparently slow responses.

Shortening and Lengthening of Action Potential Duration

In ischemia, accumulation of lysophosphoglycerides could induce a variety of abnormalities of the action potential, with narrowing in some cells and lengthening in others (Corr et al., 1982; Clarkson and Ten Eick, 1983). These membrane-active agents also may predispose to slow conduction by depressing most of the components of the membrane currents (Cerbai et al., 1997). The action potential duration is shortened by inhibitors of glycolysis, such as iodoacetate, lactate and pyruvate, free fatty acids, and acidosis (Opie et al., 1979). The proposal is that adenosine diphosphate (ATP) made by glycolysis has a special role in maintenance of the action potential duration, as supported by the effects of direct intracellular injection of ATP (Taniguchi et al., 1983). Such metabolic changes can be highly focal. During acute myocardial ischemia, the shortening of the action potential duration can be related to the inhibition of glycolysis in zones with very low blood flow or to an increased cytosolic calcium concentration.

Conversely, the action potential duration is increased in the hypertrophic myocardium (see Fig. 13-9). Variations in the action potential duration between ischemic and nonischemic cells, between sites with different severities of ischemia, and between the shortened action potential of ischemia and the prolonged potential of hypertrophic cells produce the critical differences in the refractory state of the myocardium that explain dispersion of refractoriness and electrical homogeneity.

Cytosolic Calcium and Electrical Alternans

Alterations in cytoplasmic calcium may explain the phenomenon of the alternans pattern in the T wave of the electrocardiogram preceding the onset of ventricular fibrillation in the dog heart. A similar alternation of the action potential duration in the globally ischemic heart is associated with corresponding variations in the amplitude of the intracellular calcium transient (Lee et al., 1988). Local variations of cytosolic calcium can be correlated with the phase relationship of calcium alternans and are thought to be a cause of heterogeneity in the pattern of action potential alternans. Thus, abnormalities of cytosolic calcium can contribute to nonuniformity of the action potential duration across the ventricular surface. This process leads to a dispersion of refractoriness throughout the ventricles, which is an essential precondition for ventricular fibrillation. There is an interesting link between increased acylcarnitine, as found in ischemia, and activation of calcium channels (Huang et al., 1992), which in turn increases the risk of calcium-dependent arrhythmias (Lubbe et al., 1992).

Impaired Intercellular Conduction

Conduction between cells normally proceeds by the gap or nexus junctions (see Fig. 3-9). Two changes found in ischemia, an increased intracellular calcium ion activity and a decreased pH (acidosis), can uncouple intercellular conduction to block conduction and to predispose to arrhythmias (De Mello, 1982). Anatomically, gap junction defects induced by postinfarct remodeling help to define the re-entry paths that underlie some types of ventricular tachycardia (Peters et al., 1997).

AFTERPOTENTIALS

Ventricular myocardium can develop automatic activity in specified experimental conditions that cause *delayed afterdepolarizations* (DADs) or afterpotentials. Normally, ventricular cells have a flat phase 4 with no spontaneous depolarization. Delayed depolarizations are abnormal oscillations found in ventricular or Purkinje cells in certain abnormal circumstances, including digitalis poisoning and microinjection of cAMP in the cell. The factor common to these two stimuli is the increase in cytosolic calcium ion concentration, which induces a transient diastolic inward current (I_{ti}), possibly by promoting sodium–calcium exchange (Fig. 20-4). DAD tends to be a cyclical event with a series of ever smaller waves, which probably reflect calcium ion oscillations in the cytosol because there are accompanying aftercontractions. When reperfusion restores ATP, then the conditions are right for oscillatory movements of calcium ions. Depletion of calcium from the sarcoplasmic reticulum can stop the development of the afterdepolarizations. The current causing the repetitive afterdepolarizations is activated (switched on) by an increased intracellular calcium level. Therefore, the calcium antagonist verapamil and a low external calcium level both inhibit the phenomenon. DADs are thought to underlie the development of ventricular automaticity during digitalis poisoning.

In ventricular muscle, DADs can lead to *triggered automaticity* and hence play a role in converting a focus of automaticity into a sustained ventricular arrhythmia (Fig. 20-4). This sequence seems most likely to occur when there

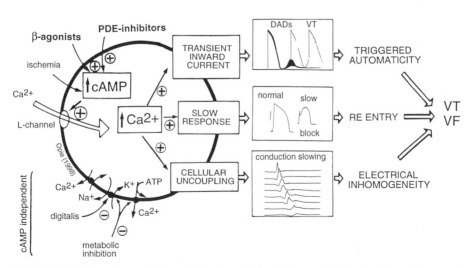

FIG. 20-4. Calcium-dependent arrhythmias. Links between cAMP, cytosolic calcium, and specific calcium-mediated electrophysiologic abnormalities thought to predispose to ventricular tachycardia (VT) and fibrillation (VF). From Lubbe et al. (1992).

is prior inhibition of the sodium pump by digitalis or by a low external potassium concentration. In Purkinje fibers, DADs can develop even at normal external potassium levels and theoretically be a cause of automaticity even in the absence of excess digitalis. Afterdepolarizations are suspected, therefore, of contributing to some of the ventricular arrhythmias of acute myocardial infarction (Opie, 1990) and in the remodeled postinfarct myocardium (Qin et al., 1996).

Early Afterdepolarizations

Besides inducing phase 4 depolarization, hypokalemia can prolong the QT interval by interfering with the repolarizing potassium current with risk of arrhythmia development. Especially dangerous is the combination of diuretic-induced hypokalemia with antiarrhythmic drugs that may also prolong the QT interval, such as quinidine, disopyramide, amiodarone, and sotalol. The type of ventricular arrhythmia resulting is characteristically that with QRS complexes that widen and narrow, called *torsades de pointes* (twisting of the points) or atypical ventricular tachycardia. The danger is ventricular fibrillation. The mechanism is complex and may include (1) differential changes in refractoriness in different parts of the myocardium and (2) development of early afterdepolarizations (EADs) as found in patients when right ventricular action potentials are recorded by suction electrodes. It is very likely that such EADs could contribute triggered activity (Qin et al., 1996). There are a number of differences between EADs and DADs. First, the EADs occur before the end of complete repolarization, whereas the DADs occur well thereafter (Fig. 20-1). Second, the EADs disappear as the heart rate increases, explaining why a bradycardia predisposes to the development of *torsades de pointes* and why tachycardia induced by pacing or isoproterenol is effective in the therapy of that condition. In contrast, tachycardia exaggerates true DADs, perhaps because the rapid repetitive opening of the calcium channel overloads the cell with calcium. A similarity is that both EADs and DADs may develop the same type of triggered activity and ventricular tachycardia in the postinfarct heart (Qin et al., 1996). The cellular mechanisms causing the EADs are not yet confirmed, but may include decreased postinfarct flow of the current I_{to} (Qin et al., 1996).

Inherited Long QT Syndrome

Besides hypokalemia and drug-induced causes of QT prolongation, there are three genetic causes of the long QT syndrome. Either the repolarizing potassium currents must be inhibited or the inward currents prolonged. The abnormal genes that cause these abnormalities have been identified (Fig. 20-5). The gene HERG (human ether-a-go-go related gene) expresses I_{kr} and is defective in one type of

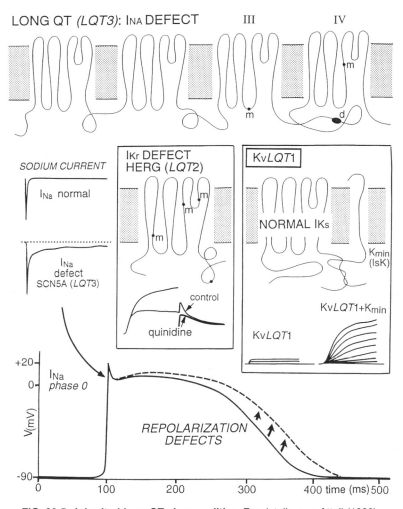

FIG. 20-5. Inherited long QT abnormalities. For details, see Attali (1996).

long QT syndrome (LQT 2). In addition, some drugs such as the class III antiarrhythmic dofetilide (Kiehn et al., 1996) and the antihistaminics may block HERG, thereby producing a similar condition (Roy et al., 1996). Another more recently discovered defect relates to the expression of two structurally different but associated membrane proteins: K_vLQT1 (i.e., the protein that encodes for the potassium channel associated with type 1 long QT syndrome) and K_{min}, also called IsK (Attali, 1996). A third type of long QT (LQT3) can be the result of abnormalities of a sodium channel (SCN5A) that allows increased inward sodium currents.

VENTRICULAR ARRHYTHMIAS IN ACUTE
MYOCARDIAL INFARCTION

In acute myocardial infarction (AMI), ventricular arrhythmias vary from ectopic beats to ventricular tachycardia and fibrillation, indicating an increasing degree of severity because ventricular fibrillation is fatal if untreated. In general, AMI is characterized by an increased sympathetic activity that is proarrhythmic (Fig. 20-6). Four processes currently are held to be basic to the genesis of such cardiac arrhythmias: (1) increased automaticity, (2) slowing of conduction in specific areas of the heart with resultant re-entry and reexcitation, (3) variable shortening or lengthening of the refractory period with an increased dispersion of refractoriness between the ischemic and nonischemic zones, and (4) EADs or DADs (as possible causes of automaticity). Increased dispersion of refractoriness to conduction between the ischemic and the nonischemic zones sets the stage for reentrant arrhythmias. Unidirectional abnormalities of conduction between ischemic and nonischemic zones have been recorded, as have areas of localized fibrillation that are believed to spread from the ischemic to the nonischemic zone.

Localized hyperkalemia and consequent depolarization allow a current of injury to flow from the nonischemic to the ischemic zone, an example of a current of injury (Fig. 20-7). In flowing, the electrons leaving the nonischemic zone will tend to depolarize the nonischemic side of the border zone and, as such, may actually trigger arrhythmias (particularly in Purkinje fibers). Purkinje fibers can

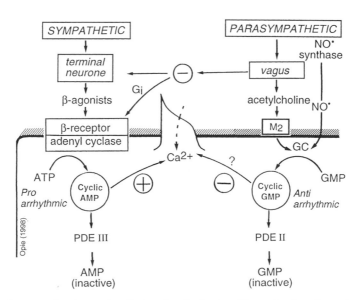

FIG. 20-6. Proposed autonomic effects of arrhythmias. Note role of cyclic nucleotides and calcium.

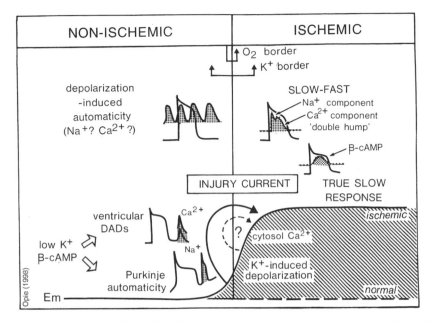

FIG. 20-7. Injury current. Metabolic differences between ischemic and nonischemic tissue that underlie the development of ventricular arrhythmias of early-phase acute myocardial infarction. Points of emphases are the current of injury between ischemic and nonischemic zones, the development of Purkinje fiber automaticity, especially when arterial potassium is low and there is α-adrenergic stimulation (α-cAMP), and DADs, which can give rise to triggered ventricular automaticity. Note also the formation of abnormal action potentials in the ischemic zone that predispose to abnormalities of impulse conduction and hence to re-entry (see Fig. 20-2). Slow-fast action potentials have the fast sodium component inhibited by ischemic depolarization, which tends to close the sodium channel and allows the calcium channel to become more dominant, giving the action potential a double-hump appearance. The true slow response is also found in totally depolarized fibers stimulated by cAMP. Such action potentials also predispose to conduction abnormalities. Em, resting membrane potential.

be the site of origin both of slowly conducted normal impulses and of ectopic foci.

The actual initiating ectopic beat may arise in the nonischemic zone. Purkinje fibers of the infarcted zone may be another source of arrhythmias. Impulses originating in surviving Purkinje fibers have a reduced diastolic potential, a decreased action potential amplitude, and a decreased upstroke velocity (Friedman et al., 1973) and resemble the slow response. The action potential duration can be extraordinarily prolonged. The proposed explanation is that the density of the repolarizing current I_{to} is decreased (Qin et al., 1996). Therefore, EADs are more likely to develop.

Apart from the differential rate of involvement of epicardium and endocardium in some models and the superior survival of Purkinje fibers, the persistence of a variable collateral circulation introduces further metabolic and histologic heterogeneity. Complex and multiple metabolic lesions induce numerous and varying changes in the action potential pattern (Fig. 20-7). Changes in receptor density (such as increased numbers of β-adrenergic receptors), hypokalemia, and other general metabolic disturbances all may play a role. There probably is no unique causal event to link metabolic changes and ischemic arrhythmias. Rather, a variety of factors, each arrhythmogenic in certain specific experimental conditions, could be contributing to the very complex situation in patients with acute myocardial infarction. Such multiple mechanisms may explain the difficulties frequently encountered in treating the ventricular arrhythmias of acute infarction.

REPERFUSION ARRHYTHMIAS

These ventricular arrhythmias, occurring predictably and very soon after the start of experimental reperfusion, are specific to the reperfusion process and a manifestation of reperfusion injury (Opie, 1989). In patients undergoing reperfusion by thrombolytic therapy, reperfusion arrhythmias are much less common for complex reasons, probably including a much slower rate of reperfusion. The two main theories for the development of these arrhythmias are excess intracellular calcium cycling and formation of free radicals.

Calcium Transients and Reperfusion Arrhythmias. New techniques show excess cytosolic calcium levels during reperfusion (Kusuoka et al., 1990), supporting the proposal that excess calcium levels with recycling underlie these arrhythmias (Fig. 20-8).

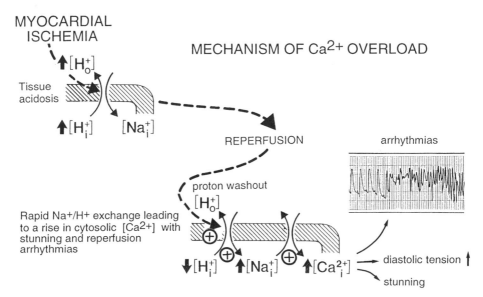

FIG. 20-8. Reperfusion arrhythmias. Rapid Na^+/H^+ exchange leading to an increase in cytosolic (Ca^{2+}) with reperfusion arrhythmias.

Free Radicals and Reperfusion Arrhythmias.   Hearse (1991) has proposed tight links between formation of free radicals and reperfusion ventricular fibrillation. One proposed mcehanism is that free radicals in sufficiently high concentrations can damage the sarcoplasmic reticulum (Xu et al., 1997) to cause calcium overload and promote calcium-dependent arrhythmias (Fig. 20-4).

ANTIARRHYTHMIC DRUGS

Antiarrhythmic agents, currently divided into four classes (Table 20-1), should be active on two of the major factors provoking arrhythmias: automaticity and re-entry circuits. The development of ectopic beats depends on opening of the fast channel even if it does not open as rapidly as normal. Therefore, it may be anticipated that the sodium channel inhibitors (class I, Fig. 20-9) are potentially antiarrhythmic agents. A critical feature is that these agents act preferentially on partially inactivated sodium channels so that they inhibit ectopic beats arising in the relative refractory or vulnerable period and in partially depolarized (ischemic) tissue. Thus, class I antiarrhythmics preferentially inhibit abnormal depolarizations. As a class, these drugs exert use-dependent block, so that their effect is greater at high heart rates (Fei et al., 1997). But it must not be supposed that class 1 drug action is simple or well understood. For example, the drug lidocaine acts in part by termination of re-entry circuits, a property linked to the rapid rate of recovery from use-dependent block (Fei et al., 1997), and in part by block of the ATP-dependent potassium channel K_{ATP} so that ischemic potassium loss and regional inhomogeneity are lessened (Olschewski et al., 1996). Lidocaine also inhibits DADs, probably by a reduction of internal calcium as the internal sodium decreases with channel blockade (Eisner et al., 1983).

TABLE 20-1. *Classification of antiarrhythmic agents*

Class	Drugs
1. *Sodium channel blockers*	Quinidine and quinidine-like agents (major effect, inhibition of fast Na^+ channel; action potential duration lengthened)
	Lidocaine and lidocaine-like agents (major effect: fast channel inhibition, also action potential duration shortening)
	Sodium channel blocking agents with powerful inhibitory effects on the conduction system: encainide, flecainide, and others
2. *Beta-blocking agents (cAMP inhibitors)*	Propranolol and all other β-blockers
3. *Potassium channel inhibitors* (repolarizing K^+ current); agents widening action potential duration as their major effect	Amiodarone and others
4. *Calcium channel antagonist agents* active on the AV node	Verapamil and diltiazem; adenosine and other potassium channel openers (acting indirectly to inhibit calcium channel)

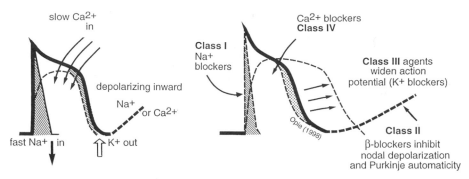

FIG. 20-9. The classic four types of antiarrhythmic agents. Class I agents decrease phase 0 of the rapid depolarization of the action potential (rapid sodium channel). Class II agents, β-blocking drugs, have complex actions including inhibition of spontaneous depolarization (phase 4) and indirect closure of calcium channels, which are less likely to be in the open state when not phosphorylated by cAMP. Class III agents block the outward potassium channel to prolong the action potential duration and hence refractoriness. Class IV agents, verapamil and diltiazem and the indirect calcium antagonist adenosine, all inhibit the inward calcium channel, which is most prominent in nodal tissue, particularly the AV node. Most antiarrhythmic drugs have more than one action.

β-adrenergic blocking agents constitute class II antiarrhythmic agents. β-adrenergic stimulation enhances automaticity by several mechanisms. First, phase 4 depolarization in Purkinje fibers is stimulated. Second, DADs are provoked. Third, the slow response may develop in completely depolarized cells.

Drugs prolonging the duration of the refractory period (class III agents) may slow or stop conduction through one limb of the circuit besides lessening ectopic formation. These agents generally inhibit the rapid component of the delayed rectifier repolarizing current (I_{Kr}). Not only do they prolong the action potential duration, but they all have as a potential side-effect *torsades de pointes* (Roden, 1996).

Class IV agents inhibit the calcium channel of the atrioventricular node, or part of it, to stop supraventricular re-entry arrhythmias (Fig. 20-1).

Refractory Period

For an impulse to fire requires depolarization; therefore, throughout the period of depolarization associated with phases 0, 1, and 2 of the action potential, no further depolarization is possible, and the cardiac cell is resistant or in the refractory period. As repolarization occurs, so does the capacity for depolarization come back, and phase 3 of the cardiac action potential therefore reflects the *relative refractory period* during which sensitivity to a depolarizing stimulus is returning. When the highly focal and variable metabolic abnormalities occurring in ischemia are associated with variable action potential patterns

(Fig. 20-7), the refractory state is correspondingly highly variable, so that a state of *dispersion of refractoriness* exists, predisposing to electrophysiologic heterogeneity (Greek *hetero,* different). When there is marked heterogeneity of this variety, an ectopic depolarization is much more likely to develop into a re-entry circuit (Fig. 20-2) with risk of ventricular tachycardia.

Antiarrhythmic agents of the class III variety owe their antiarrhythmic mechanism to prolongation of the action potential duration and, hence, an increased refractory period of the myocardium. Thus, it is more difficult for ectopic foci to arise. In addition, class III agents, such as amiodarone, seem to make the refractory period throughout the myocardium more uniform, thereby lessening any tendency to dispersion of refractoriness.

Proarrhythmic Effect of Antiarrhythmic Agents

Postinfarct patients have a risk of sudden death, and the mechanism is thought to be at least in part the development of ventricular tachycardia or fibrillation. A simple hypothesis is that postinfarct ventricular arrhythmias predispose to potentially fatal arrhythmias. Therefore, it has seemed logical to test the effect of ventricular antiarrhythmics on postinfarct arrhythmias. The first such study was with mexiletine, in which a variety of ventricular arrhythmias were treated by mexiletine with suppressive effects in the postinfarct period. Nonetheless, the overall mortality in the mexiletine group tended to be higher, and although this was not statistically significant, it was a warning. Definite confirmation of the potential harm of at least two antiarrhythmic agents, flecainide and encainide, came with the CAST study (1989). In that study, patients required only a low incidence of ventricular premature systoles, more than six per hour, to enter. The agents encainide and flecainide both increased the risk of death or nonfatal cardiac arrest by 3.6 times. Total mortality increased by 2.6 times in the drug-treated group. These agents belong to a subdivision of class I, class IC, with a powerful inhibitory effect on the conduction system and differential electrophysiologic changes on the conduction system and nonconducting ventricular muscle, so that these agents may well predispose to electrical heterogeneity and to re-entry arrhythmias (Fig. 20-7).

In addition, class III agents and IA agents (the latter are quinidine-like) prolong the action potential duration, may predispose to EADs, triggered ventricular activity and the ventricular arrhythmia called *torsades de pointes.* In the SWORD study, d-sotalol, a pure class III agent, increased mortality in survivors of myocardial infarction, probably due to provocation of *torsades de pointes* (Waldo et al., 1996).

Although there are many possible explanations for these negative or harmful studies, the point has been clearly made that prophylactic postinfarct antiarrhythmic therapy cannot be justified, with the exception of the proven beneficial effects of β-blockade, which decreases postinfarct mortality.

ARRHYTHMIAS IN HEART FAILURE

Congestive heart failure is a serious condition, still often fatal, and lethal arrhythmias are thought to be a common mode of exit. There are many mechanisms that act to promote arrhythmias in heart failure (Fig. 20-10). For example, diuretic drugs may cause hypokalemia as a side effect, thereby predisposing afterpotentials. Increased circulating concentrations of catecholamines and angiotensin II tend to increase cell calcium. The dilated left ventricle may activate stretch receptors that, in turn, directly or indirectly increase cell calcium (see Fig. 13-5). Failing myocytes may have abnormal electrophysiologic properties, such as the hyperpolarizing activated current, I_f, or prolonged action potentials resulting from prior hypertrophy. It is increasingly evident that agents that are positive inotropes and act by increasing cell calcium are potentially arrhythmogenic.

Proarrhythmic Risks of Positive Inotropic Agents. Digitalis agents, besides being positively inotropic by inhibition of the sodium–potassium pump, are potentially arrhythmogenic at toxic blood levels. DADs, resulting from cytoso-

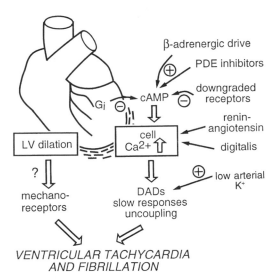

FIG. 20-10. Arrhythmias of heart failure. Proposed proarrhythmic mechanisms in left ventricular (LV) failure and arrhythmias, most of which are thought to act by means of an increase in cellular calcium. Impaired function of the sarcoplasmic reticulum may account for the prolonged calcium transients. In left ventricular failure, formation of cAMP is impaired and myocardial function can be improved by the combined administration of both phosphodiesterase (PDE) inhibitors and β-stimulation, but with risks of ventricular arrhythmias. G_i, inhibitory G protein.

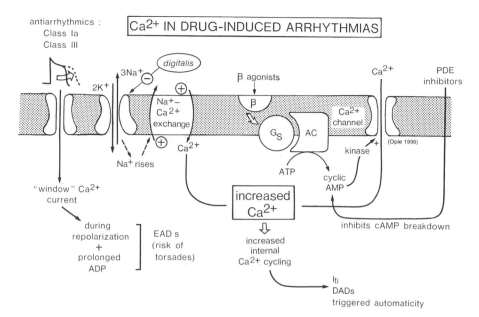

FIG. 20-11. Drug-induced abnormalities of calcium ions. On the left is the proposed mechanism whereby agents prolonging the action potential duration (APD) enable the window calcium current to flow, with development of EADs and risk of *torsades de pointes*. On the right are the effects of agents that increase cytosolic Ca^{2+}, with risk of excess internal recycling of Ca^{2+} in and out of the sarcoplasmic reticulum and formation of DADs. PDE, phosphodiesterase.

lic calcium overload and excess calcium recycling, are thought to underlie the development of ventricular automaticity during digitalis poisoning.

β-agonists and phosphodiesterase inhibitors produce a positive inotropic effect by elevating cellular cAMP and hence the cytosolic calcium level (Fig. 20-11). Because excess cytosolic calcium is potentially arrhythmogenic (Fig. 20-4), such positive inotropes have an implicit risk of arrhythmia development. The risk is increased when there is hypokalemia, frequently found in patients with severe heart failure treated by excess diuretics.

SUMMARY

1. *Mechanisms for ventricular arrhythmias.* The major three are (1) the development of automaticity, (2) re-entry circuits, and (3) abnormalities of repolarization, such as early and late afterdepolarizations. Automaticity in Purkinje fibers is particularly predisposed to by hypokalemia or by catecholamine stimulation. Ventricular re-entry circuits presuppose electrical heterogeneity, such as localized depolarization. Focal changes in extracel-

lular potassium and intracellular calcium could contribute significantly. For example, differing intracellular calcium concentrations in ischemic tissue are thought to predispose to electrical alternans, which is a risk factor for ventricular fibrillation.

2. *Afterdepolarizations.* Delayed afterdepolarizations (DADs) particularly occur in conditions of cytosolic calcium overload, such as early reperfusion or digitalis intoxication or excess therapy with some inotropic agents. Early afterdepolarizations (EADs) are associated with prolongation of the QT interval and with certain antiarrhythmic drugs. They predispose to a potentially lethal arrhythmia called *torsades de pointes.*

3. *Long QT syndrome.* The genes responsible for the abnormalities of the repolarizing potassium currents and of the inward sodium current have been identified.

4. *Ventricular arrhythmias of acute myocardial infarction.* The initiating ectopic beat, which may trigger micro and macro re-entry circuits, is thought to be in the nonischemic zone. The current flowing from the nonischemic to the ischemic zone is the current of injury. Reperfusion arrhythmias basically have two origins: cytosolic calcium overload with DADs and formation of free radicals.

5. *Antiarrhythmic drugs* may promote arrhythmias (proarrhythmic effect) and therefore should be used with care and only for specific actions.

STUDENT QUESTIONS

1. Hypokalemia predisposes to arrhythmias, yet regional loss of potassium with local hyperkalemia is arrhythmogenic. Explain this apparent contradiction.
2. Describe how abnormalities of internal calcium could be arrhythmogenic in ischemic and in reperfusion arrhythmias.
3. What are the differences between early and delayed afterdepolarizations?

CARDIOLOGIST-IN-TRAINING QUESTIONS

1. What is a re-entry circuit? When might it be arrhythmogenic?
2. What is HERG? Describe the abnormalities of the long QT syndrome.
3. What is the cellular and electrophysiologic origin of the current of injury?
4. Why are patients with congestive heart failure prone to ventricular arrhythmias?
5. How can drugs cause arrhythmias?

REFERENCES

1. Arita M, Kiyosue T, Aomine M, Imanishi S. Nature of "residual fast channel"–dependent action

potentials and slow conduction in guinea pig ventricular muscle and its modification by isoproterenol. *Am J Cardiol* 1983;51:1433–1440.

2. Attali B. A new wave for heart rhythms. *Nature* 1996;384:24–25.
3. Blake K, Clusin WT, Franz MR, Smith NA. Mechanism of depolarization in the ischemic dog heart: discrepancy between T-Q potentials and potassium accumulation. *J Physiol* 1988;397:307–330.
4. Cardiac Arrhythmia Suppression Trial (CAST). Preliminary report: effect of encainide and flecainide on mortality in a randomized trial of arrhythmia suppression after myocardial infarction. *N Engl J Med* 1989;321:406–412.
5. Cerbai E, Pino R, Porciatti F, et al. Characterization of the hyperpolarization-activated current, I_f, in ventricular myocytes from human failing heart. *Circulation* 1997;95:568–571.
6. Clarkson CW, Ten Eick RE. On the mechanism of lysophosphatidylcholine-induced depolarization of cat ventricular myocardium. *Circ Res* 1983;52:543–556.
7. Corr PB, Gross RW, Sobel BE. Arrhythmogenic amphiphilic lipids and the myocardial cell membrane [Editorial]. *J Mol Cell Cardiol* 1982;14:619–626.
8. De Mello WC. Intercellular communication in cardiac muscle. *Circ Res* 1982;51:1–9.
9. Dyckner T, Helmers C, Lundman T, et al. Initial serum potassium level in relation to early complications and prognosis in patients with acute myocardial infarction. *Acta Med Scand* 1975;197:207–210.
10. Eisner DA, Lederer WJ, Sheu S. The role of intracellular sodium activity in the antiarrhythmic action of local anaesthetics in sheep Purkinje fibres. *J Physiol Lond* 1983;340:239–257.
11. Fei H, Yazmajian D, Hanna MS, Frame LH. Termination of reentry by lidocaine in the tricuspid ring in vitro. Role of cycle-length oscillation, fast use-dependent kinetics, and fixed block. *Circ Res* 1997;80:242–252.
12. Friedman I, Moravec J, Reichart E, Hatt PY. Subacute myocardial hypoxia in the rat. An electron microscopic study of the left ventricular myocardium. *J Mol Cell Cardiol* 1973;5:125–132.
13. Harris AS, Bisteni A, Russell RA, Brigham JC, Firestone JE. Excitatory factors in ventricular tachycardia resulting from myocardial ischemia: potassium a major excitant. *Science* 1954;119:200–203.
14. Hearse DJ. Reperfusion-induced injury: a possible role for oxidant stress and its manipulation. *Cardiovasc Drugs Ther* 1991;5:225–236.
15. Huang J-C, Xian H, Bacaner M. Long-chain fatty acids activate calcium channels in ventricular myocytes. *Proc Natl Acad Sci USA* 1992;89:6452–6456.
16. Kiehn J, Lacerda AE, Wible B, Brown AM. Molecular physiology and pharmacology of HERG. Single-channel currents and block by dofetilide. *Circulation* 1996;94:2572–2579.
17. Kusuoka H, Koretsune Y, Chacko VP, et al. Excitation-contraction coupling in postischemic myocardium. Does failure of activator Ca transients underlie stunning? *Circ Res* 1990;66:1268–1276.
18. Lee H-C, Mohabir R, Smith N, et al. Effect of ischemia on calcium-dependent fluorescence transients in rabbit hearts containing indo 1. Correlation with monophasic action potentials and contraction. *Circulation* 1988;78:1047–1059.
19. Lubbe WH, Podzuweit T, Opie LH. Potential arrhythmogenic role of cyclic adenosine monophosphate (AMP) and cytosolic calcium overload: implications for prophylactic effects of beta-blockers in myocardial infarction and proarrhythmic effects of phospodiesterase inhibitors. *J Am Coll Cardiol* 1992;19:1622–1633.
20. Major RH. In: *Classic Descriptions of Disease*. Springfield, IL: Charles C Thomas, 1945.
21. Olschewski A, Brau ME, Olschewski H, Hempelmann G. ATP-dependent potassium channel in rat cardiomyocytes is blocked by lidocaine. Possible impact on the antiarrhythmic action of lidocaine. *Circulation* 1996;93:656–659.
22. Opie LH. Reperfusion injury and its pharmacologic modification. *Circulation* 1989;80:1049–1062.
23. Opie LH. Cellular mechanism for ischemic ventricular arrhythmias. *Ann Rev Med* 1990;41:231–238.
24. Opie LH, Nathan D, Lubbe WF. Biochemical aspects of arrhythmogenesis and ventricular fibrillation. *Am J Cardiol* 1979;43:131–148.
25. Peters NS, Coromilas J, Severs NM, Wit AL. Disturbed connexin-43 gap junction distribution correlates with the location of reentrant circuits in the epicardial border zone of healing canine infarcts that cause ventricular tachycardia. *Circulation* 1997;95:988–996.
26. Qin D, Zhang Z-H, Caref EB, et al. Cellular and ionic basis of arrhythmias in postinfarction remodeled ventricular myocardium. *Circ Res* 1996;79:461–473.
27. Roden DM. Ibutilide and the treatment of atrial arrhythmias. A new drug—almost unheralded—is now available to US physicians. *Circulation* 1996;94:1499–1502.
28. Roy M-L, Dumaine R, Brown AM. HERG, a primary human ventricular target of nonsedating antihistamine terfenadine. *Circulation* 1996;94:817–823.

29. Russell DC. Early ventricular arrhythmias: relationship of electrophysiology to blood flow and metabolism. In: Parratt JR (ed). *Early Arrhythmias Resulting from Myocardial Ischemia.* London: Macmillan, 1982;37–56.
30. Taniguchi J, Noma A, Irisawa H. Modification of the cardiac action potential by intracellular injection of adenosine triphosphate and related substances in guinea pigs single ventricular cells. *Circ Res* 1983;53:131–139.
31. Waldo AL, Camm AJ, deRuyter H, for the SWORD Investigators. Effect of *d*-sotalol on mortality in patients with left ventricular dysfunction after recent and remote myocardial infarction. *Lancet* 1996;348:7–12.
32. Xu KY, Zweier JL, Becker LC. Hydroxyl radical inhibits sarcoplasmic reticulum Ca^{2+}-ATPase function by direct attack on the ATP binding site. *Circ Res* 1997;80:76–81.

Glossary

α Alpha-adrenergic

ACE inhibitor   Angiotensin-converting enzyme inhibitor

ACh   Acetylcholine

ADP   Adenosine diphosphate

AMI   Acute myocardial infarction

AMP   Adenosine monophosphate

AII or Angio II   Angiotensin II

ANP   Atrial natriuretic peptide (also called atrial natriuretic factor, ANF)

ATP   Adenosine triphosphate

β Beta-adrenergic

BP   Blood pressure

Ca^{2+} Calcium ions

cAMP   Cyclic adenosine monophosphate

cGMP   Cyclic guanosine monophosphate

CHF   Congestive heart failure

CO   Cardiac output

CP   Creatine phosphate = PCr = phosphocreatine

Echo   Echocardiogram

ECG   Electrocardiogram (also abbreviated as EKG)

EDRF   Endothelium-derived relaxation factor

E or Epi   Epinephrine, also called adrenaline

GC   Guanylate cylcase

G_i Inhibitory G-protein

G_s Stimulatory G-protein

I   Current

I_{Ca-L} Calcium current, long lasting

I_{Ca-T} Calcium current, transient

I_K Potassium current, voltage-operated (also called delayed rectifier, including K_r and K_s)

I_{K1} Inward rectifier potassium current (also called K_{ir})

I_{KATP} ATP-sensitive potassium current

I_{Na} Sodium current

IP$_3$ Inositol trisphosphate

LV Left ventricle

LVH Left ventricular hypertrophy

MAPK Mitogen activated protein kinase, also called ERK

NAD or NAD$^+$ Nicotinamide adenine dinucleotide, which forms a redox couple, together with NADH$_2$ (or NADH + H$^+$)

NADH$_2$ or NADH Reduced nicotinamide adenine dinucleotide

NE Norepinephrine, also called noradrenaline

NO Nitric oxide

PKC Protein kinase C

PLC Phospholipase C

PV Pressure-volume

PVR Peripheral vascular resistance, also called systemic vascular resistance

SR Sarcoplasmic reticulum

SV Stroke volume

SVR Systemic vascular resistance, also called peripheral vascular resistance

μm Micrometers, also called microns

Subject Index

A

A band (anisotropic band), 47
ACE. *See* Angiotensin-converting enzyme
ACE inhibitors. *See* Angiotensin-converting enzyme inhibitors
^{11}C-Acetate, 335
Acetylcholine
  functions, 40
  release, 28
  vasodilation, 278–279
Acetylcholine-regulated potassium channel, 121–122, 122*f*
Acidosis, ischemic, 524–525
Actin
  α-actin, 59*t*, 210*t*
  β-actin, 210*t*
  characteristics, 210*t*
  filaments, 45, 47, 46*f*, 47*f*
  interaction with myosin, 151, 223, 238*f*, 349
  mechanical overload and, 222*t*
  microanatomy, 211
α-Actinin, 58
Action potential
  changes
    in hypertrophy, 408–409, 408*f*
    in ischemia, 529, 531*f*
  definition of, 51
  duration, ventricular re-entry circuits and, 593–594
  ionic conductances during, 85*f*
  patterns, from SA node to ventricle, 124–125, 124*f*
  phases, 71, 73*f*
  plateau, 51
  Purkinje fiber, 102, 103*f*
  sodium-calcium exchanger and, 104, 105*f*
  vascular smooth muscle, 65
  ventricular, 74*f*, 100–102
    computed currents, 101*f*
    epicardial *vs.* endocardial, 100, 102*f*
    phase 0, 100

    phase 1, 100
    phase 2, 100
    phase 3, 99*f*, 100,
    phase 4, 100–101
    ventricular re-entry circuits and, 593
Activation gate (m gate), 82
Activation threshold, 118
Acute myocardial infarction. *See* Myocardial infarction
Adenosine
  formation, 327*t,* 337
  functions, 324–325
  inhibition, of atrioventricular node, 128–129, 129*f*
  for ischemic injury, 333
  myocardial cAMP levels and, 189*t*
  neuroregulation and, 31–32
  potassium current, adenosine sensitive, 97, 98
  in preconditioning, 581
  regulation, of coronary vascular tone, 272–275, 273*f,* 274*f*
  signaling, 325, 325*f*
  sinus bradycardia and, 138*t*
  stimulation, of cAMP formation, 190, 190*f*
  vasodilatory activity, 26, 267, 273–274, 274*f*
Adenosine deaminase, 273–274, 274*f*
Adenosine diphosphate (ADP)
  breakdown, 324
  in heart, 324
  phosphorylation, 315
Adenosine monophosphate (AMP), 273
Adenosine triphosphate (ATP)
  breakdown, 311–312
    in ischemia, 325–327, 327*t*
    physiologic, 323–324, 323*f*
  compartmentation, 322–323, 321*f*
  conversion, 25
  energy transfer, 320
  in exercise, 464
  free energy of hydrolysis, 327
  in irreversible ischemic damage, 550, 551*f*

definition of, 563
experimental conditions, 565–566
ischemia duration and, 566
mechanism of
 antioxidant defense against, 570–571,
  570*t*, 571*f*
 cystolic calcium and, 566*f*, 567–568, 567*f*
 free radicals and, 568–570,
  569*f*, 569*t*, 570*t*
 time frame, 565, 565*f*
Subsarcolemmal cisternae (junctional
 components), 53
Suction, ventricular diastolic, 346
Sudden cardiac death,
 psychological stress and, 469
Sulfonylureas, inhibition of ATP-sensitive
 potassium channels, 96
Superior vena cava, 9
Swan-Ganz catheterization, 454
Sympathetic nervous system
 functions, 17, 18*f*
 interaction with parasympathetic system,
  199, 200*f*
 stimulation
  effects on sinus node, 23, 25, 25*f*
  in heart failure, 495
  mechanisms of, 17, 19*f*
  rapid, effects of, 23, 24*f*
  terminal nerves, norepinephrine release from,
   27–28, 28*f*
Synaptic gap or junction, 17
Syncytium, 57
Syndrome X (metabolic cardiovascular
 syndrome), 440–441, 440*f*
Systemic vascular resistance. *See* Peripheral
 vascular resistance
Systole
 coronary blood flow during, 279, 280*f*
 definition of, 346
 failure, in supply ischemia, 527
 mitral valve in, 7, 7*f*
 physiologic *vs.* cardiologic, 346–347, 347*t*
 physiology, 343, 345
 ventricular interaction in, 383
 wall stress in, 437

T

T-type calcium channels, 89*f*, 90*t*
Tachycardia
 atypical ventricular, 596
 sinus, 137, 138
 ventricular, 589
Talin, 59*t*

Tau, 379
Taurine, 335
Tension, 362. *See also* Wall stress
Terminal cisternae, functions, 48*t*
Terminal varicosities, norepinephrine release
 from, 27–28, 28*f*
Tetrodotoxin (TTX), 85
TGF-β, 404
Thallium 201, 290
Thapsigargin, effect on sarcoplasmic reticulum,
 158–159, 159*t*
Thermodilution technique, for
 cardiac output measurement, 454
Third messengers, 186, 188, 188*f*
Threshold of activation, 83, 83*t*
Thrombolytic agents, 563, 572
Thrombosis, endothelial damage and,
 259–260, 260*f*
Thromboxane A₂, 249, 251*f*, 288
Thyroid hormones, stimulation of cAMP
 formation, 190
Thyrotoxic hypertrophy, 409–410
Thyrotoxicosis, 221
Time-tension index, 457*t*
Titin
 characteristics, 210*t*
 function, 45
 microanatomy, 213
Tolerance, 183
Torsades de pointes, 596, 602, 603, 605*f*
Transplantation, cardiac, 204
Transcription, 395, 395*f*
Transduction, 396
Transfer RNA, 55
Transforming growth factor-β (TGF-β), 404
Transgenic models, of heart failure, 488
Transient inward current, 104
Transitional cells, 117
Translocase, 318
Transverse tubular system, 51–53, 52*f*
Trauma, hemostatic response to, 259–260, 260*f*
Treppe phenomenon (Bowditch staircase
 effect), 356, 356*f*, 358, 384, 452
Triads, 53
Tricuspid valve, 9
Triglycerides, 297
Tropomodulin, 211
Tropomyosin, 210*t*, 211, 215, 216
Troponin-C
 calcium affinity, 216*f*, 219
 calcium binding sites, 217
 calcium interaction, 151
 characteristics, 210*t*